Physical Rehabilitation of the Injured Athlete

Second Edition

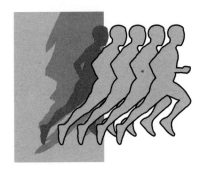

James R. Andrews, M.D.
Clinical Professor of Orthopaedics
  and Sports Medicine
University of Virginia School of
  Medicine
Charlottesville, Virginia
Chairman, American Sports
  Medicine Institute
Birmingham, Alabama

Gary L. Harrelson, Ed.D., A.T.,C.
Adjunct Assistant Professor
Athletic Training Education Program
The University of Alabama
Manager, Educational Services and
  Technology
DCH Regional Medical Center
Tuscaloosa, Alabama

Kevin E. Wilk, P.T.
Adjunct Assistant Professor
Programs in Physical Therapy
Marquette University
Milwaukee, Wisconsin
National Director, Research and
  Clinical Education
HealthSouth Rehabilitation
  Corporation
Associate Clinical Director
HealthSouth Sports Medicine and
  Rehabilitation Center
Director of Rehabilitative Research
American Sports Medicine Institute
Birmingham, Alabama

W.B. SAUNDERS COMPANY
An Imprint of Elsevier Science
Philadelphia   London   New York   St. Louis   Sydney   Toronto

W.B. SAUNDERS COMPANY
An Imprint of Elsevier Science

The Curtis Center
Independence Square West
Philadelphia, Pennsylvania 19106

Library of Congress Cataloging-in-Publication Data

Physical rehabilitation of the injured athlete / [edited by] James R. Andrews,
Gary L. Harrelson, Kevin E. Wilk.—2nd ed.

p.   cm.

Includes bibliographical references and index.

ISBN 0–7216–6549–7

1. Sports injuries—Treatment.   2. Sports physical therapy.   I. Andrews,
   James R. (James Rheuben).   II. Harrelson, Gary L.   III. Wilk, Kevin E.
   [DNLM: 1. Athletic Injuries—rehabilitation.   2. Physical Therapy.
   QT 261 P578 1998]

RD97.P49 1998   617.1′027—dc21

DNLM/DLC   97-9769

PHYSICAL REHABILITATION OF THE INJURED ATHLETE   ISBN 0–7216–6549–7

Printed in the United States of America.

Last digit is the print number: 9   8   7   6   5

To my wife Lisa for her unyielding love, understanding, and support as I chase my vision; to my mother, who has always encouraged me to pursue my vision; and in memory of my father, who showed me how to live a vision.

GLH

To my wife Debbie and children Justin, Summer, and Brittany, whose love, patience, and understanding have allowed me to achieve so much.

KEW

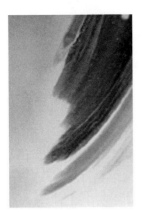

Contributors

Christopher Arrigo, M.S., P.T., A.T.,C.
Administrator
HealthSouth Rehabilitation Center
Arlington, Texas
Shoulder Rehabilitation

Terri Chmielewski, M.A., P.T.
Coordinator Clinical Services
HealthSouth Sports Medicine and
    Rehabilitation Center
Birmingham, Alabama
Shoulder Rehabilitation

Ron Courson, A.T.,C., P.T.
Director of Sports Medicine
University of Georgia
Athens, Georgia
*Role of Evaluation in the Rehabilitation
    Program*

**George J. Davies, M.Ed. P.T., S.C.S.,
A.T.,C., C.S.C.S.**
Professor of Physical Therapy
University of Wisconsin–LaCrosse
Director
Clinical and Research Services
Gundersen Lutheran Sports
    Medicine
LaCrosse, Wisconsin
President—Sports Physical Therapy
    Section
American Physical Therapy
    Association
*Application of Isokinetics in Testing and
    Rehabilitation*

**Todd S. Ellenbacker, M.S., P.T.,
S.C.S., C.S.C.S.**
Clinic Director

Physiotherapy Associates—
    Scottsdale Sports Clinic
Scottsdale, Arizona
*Application of Isokinetics in Testing and
    Rehabilitation*

Cheryl S. Fuller, M.S., A.T.,C.
Aquatics Director
University of Alabama Hospital
Spain Rehabilitation Center
Birmingham, Alabama
Aquatic Rehabilitation

James B. Gallaspy, M.Ed., A.T.,C.
Associate Professor
Coordinator of Athletic Training
    Education
University of Southern Mississippi
Hattiesburg, Mississippi
*Hamstring, Quadriceps, and Groin
    Rehabilitation*

Joe Gieck, Ed.D., A.T.,C., P.T.
Professor, Curry School of
    Education
Professor of Clinical Orthopaedics
University of Virginia
Charlottesville, Virginia
Rehabilitation of Wrist and Hand Injuries

Gary L. Harrelson, Ed.D., A.T.,C.
Adjunct Assistant Professor
Athletic Training Education
    Program
The University of Alabama
Manager, Educational Services and
    Technology
DCH Regional Medical Center
Tuscaloosa, Alabama
Physiologic Factors of Rehabilitation;

Measurement in Rehabilitation; Use of Modalities in Rehabilitation; Range of Motion and Flexibility; Introduction to Rehabilitation; Shoulder Rehabilitation; Elbow Rehabilitation; Knee and Leg Rehabilitation Exercises; Interval Rehabilitation Programs

Tim Holbrook, P.T., Cert. MDT
Manager, Outpatient Rehabilitation
Northport Hospital DCH Sports and Medicine Building
Northport, Alabama
Low Back Rehabilitation

Deidre Leaver-Dunn, M.Ed., A.T.,C.
Instructor
The University of Alabama
Research Assistant and Certified Athletic Trainer
DCH SportsMedicine
Tuscaloosa, Alabama
Use of Modalities in Rehabilitation; Range of Motion and Flexibility; Introduction to Rehabilitation; Elbow Rehabilitation

Edward P. Mulligan, M.S., P.T., S.C.S., A.T.,C.
Adjunct Faculty
Texas Women's University
Dallas, Texas
National Director of Clinical Education
HealthSouth Rehabilitation Corporation
Grapevine, Texas
Lower Leg, Ankles, and Foot Rehabilitation

Dale G. Pease, Ph.D.
Associate Professor
Department of Health and Human Performance
University of Houston
Houston, Texas
Psychologic Factors of Rehabilitation

Sejal Shah, O.T.R./L.
Staff Occupational Therapist

The Human Performance and Rehabilitation Center
Columbus, Georgia
Rehabilitation of Wrist and Hand Injuries

Tim L. Uhl, M.S., P.T., A.T.,C.
Graduate Assistant Athletic Trainer
University of Virginia
Charlottesville, Virginia
Rehabilitation of Wrist and Hand Injuries

A. Nelson Ware, A.T.,C., P.T.
Assistant Director of Physical Therapy
University of Mississippi Medical Center
Jackson, Mississippi
Knee Rehabilitation

Mark D. Weber, M.S., A.T.,C., P.T., S.C.S.
Assistant Professor of Physical Therapy
University of Mississippi Medical Center
Jackson, Mississippi
Use of Modalities in Rehabilitation; Knee Rehabilitation

Kevin E. Wilk, P.T.
Adjunct Assistant Professor
Programs in Physical Therapy
Marquette University
Milwaukee, Wisconsin
National Director, Research and Clinical Education
HealthSouth Rehabilitation Corporation
Associate Clinical Director
HealthSouth Sports Medicine and Rehabilitation Center
Director of Rehabilitative Research
American Sports Medicine Institute
Birmingham, Alabama
Shoulder Rehabilitation; Upper Extremity Plyometrics; Throwers' Ten Exercise Program; Interval Rehabilitation Programs

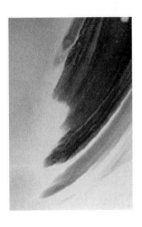

Preface

Therapeutic rehabilitation has long been a product of philosophies based on tradition handed down through the years from clinician to clinician. These concepts have usually been based on the premise, "Well, it has always worked for me," with the subsequent blending of these philosophies and/or exercises into therapeutic rehabilitation programs without an underlying scientific rationale for their implementation. Many early rehabilitation concepts and exercises were extrapolated from scientific models using biomechanical principles without empiric research data to support the theories. Over the past decade, rehabilitation research, specifically orthopedic sports medicine, has begun to "catch up" to the ever-expanding profession of orthopedic surgery. And we are forever indebted to the reseachers who have contributed to the scientific base for rehabilitation. Since the first edition of this book, a plethora of research on rehabilitation has been published.

The material within this book is based on a thorough review of the scientific literature. A scientific premise for rehabilitation and the vital importance of early motion are addressed. Stress is placed on the treatment of the entire kinetic chain, rather than on the isolation of the injured joint or structure. Emphasis is placed on the use of all types of exercises (open- and closed-chain) across a functional progression. The clinician should take into account the biomechanical demands of the athlete's sport and structure the rehabilitation program accordingly. Protocols are used throughout the book as guidelines for rehabilitation and are by no means "the only way to do it." Rather, advancement through a rehabilitation program should be based on the known healing-restraint time of injured structures, the athlete's pain tolerance level, the amount of joint effusion, and achievement of specific criteria. Surgeons vary their surgical techniques for specific lesions, and this must be considered when developing a rehabilitation regimen. Rehabilitation can by no means be "cookbooked," with one program developed for every injury and applied to all athletes, because individuals heal at varying rates and tolerate pain differently. Each athlete brings a unique set of personal qualities that must be addressed by the clinician to facilitate the athlete's rehabilitation. More than anything else, this book attempts to bring together an abundance of rehabilitation research upon which to base the advancement of an injured athlete through a rehabilitation protocol and implementation of specific exercises.

Readers will find the second edition of *Physical Rehabilitation of the Injured Athlete* to be expanded with the addition of chapters on isokinetics, wrist and rehabilitation, and low back rehabilitation, as well as expansion and updating of the chapters from the first edition. Additionally, all the protocols were updated and new ones added where appropriate. As in the first edition, areas of vital importance in implementing a rehabilitation regimen are examined, including the psychologic aspect of the injured athlete, goniometry, joint mobilization, evaluation of the injured athlete and how it relates to program implementation, types of exercise, the kinetic chain, components of rehabilitation, and aquatic therapy. Exercises have been expanded to help the clinician in the implementation of a rehabilitation program, with discussion of contraindications for exercises for specific problems.

It is our hope that *Physical Rehabilitation of the Injured Athlete* will serve as a clinician's reference source to enhance health care of athletes and will provide students with the basic knowledge for the development and implementation of rehabilitation programs for the injured athlete.

JAMES R. ANDREWS
GARY L. HARRELSON
KEVIN E. WILK

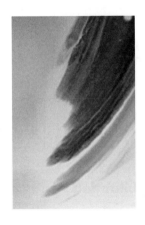

Table of Contents

Chapter 1
Psychologic Factors of Rehabilitation 1
Dale G. Pease, Ph.D.

Chapter 2
Physiologic Factors of Rehabilitation 13
Gary L. Harrelson, Ed.D., A.T.,C.

Chapter 3
Role of Evaluation in the Rehabilitation Program ... 38
Ron Courson, A.T.,C., P.T.

Chapter 4
Measurement in Rehabilitation 55
Gary L. Harrelson, Ed.D., A.T.,C.

Chapter 5
Use of Modalities in Rehabilitation 82
Gary L. Harrelson, Ed.D., A.T.,C.,
Mark D. Weber, M.S., A.T.,C., P.T., S.C.S.,
and Deidre Leaver-Dunn, M.Ed., A.T.,C.

Chapter 6
Range of Motion and Flexibility 146
Gary L. Harrelson, Ed.D., A.T.,C., and
Deidre Leaver-Dunn, M.Ed., A.T.,C.

Chapter 7
Introduction to Rehabilitation 175
Gary L. Harrelson, Ed.D., A.T.,C., and
Deidre Leaver-Dunn, M.Ed., A.T.,C.

Chapter 8
Application of Isokinetics in Testing and Rehabilitation 219
George J. Davies, M.Ed., P.T., S.C.S,
A.T.,C., C.S.C.S., and
Todd S. Ellenbecker, M.S., P.T., S.C.S,
C.S.C.S.

Chapter 9
Lower Leg, Ankle, and Foot Rehabilitation 261
Edward P. Mulligan, M.S., P.T., S.C.S.,
A.T.,C.

Chapter 10
Knee Rehabilitation 330
Mark D. Weber, M.S., A.T.,C., P.T., S.C.S.,
and A. Nelson Ware, A.T.,C., P.T.

Chapter 11
Hamstring, Quadriceps, and Groin Rehabilitation . 405
James B. Gallaspy, M.Ed., A.T.,C.

Chapter 12
Low Back Rehabilitation .. 426
Tim Holbrook, P.T., Cert. MDT

Chapter 13
Shoulder Rehabilitation ... 478
Kevin E. Wilk, P.T.,
Gary L. Harrelson, Ed.D., A.T.,C.,
Christopher Arrigo, M.S., P.T., A.T.,C.,
and Terri Chmielewski, M.A., P.T.

Chapter 14
Elbow Rehabilitation 554
Gary L. Harrelson, Ed.D., A.T.,C., and
Deidre Leaver-Dunn, M.Ed., A.T.,C.

ix

Chapter 15
**Rehabilitation of Wrist
and Hand Injuries** 589
Tim L. Uhl, M.S., P.T., A.T.,C.,
Sejal Shah, O.T.R./L., and
Joe Gieck, Ed.D., A.T.,C., P.T.

Chapter 16
Aquatic Rehabilitation 615
Cheryl S. Fuller, M.S., A.T.,C.

Appendix A
**Upper Extremity
Plyometrics** 632
Kevin E. Wilk, P.T.

Appendix B
**Knee and Leg
Rehabilitation Exercises** ... 636
Gary L. Harrelson, Ed.D., A.T.,C.

Appendix C
**Throwers' Ten Exercise
Program** 663
Kevin E. Wilk, P.T.

Appendix D
**Interval Rehabilitation
Programs** 670
Gary L. Harrelson, Ed.D., A.T.,C.,
and Kevin E. Wilk, P.T.

Index 679

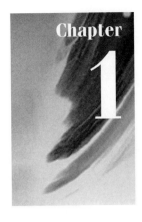

Chapter 1

Psychologic Factors of Rehabilitation

Dale G. Pease, Ph.D.

Although coaches, athletes, and spectators involved in sports have recognized that physical injury is an inherent risk factor of participation, the psychologic aspects of participation and injury have often been overlooked. Until recently, many individuals in sports treated the body and mind as a dichotomous unit, an approach that resulted in the development of training programs that focused on the body and, in some cases, that treated the mind with scorn. Following the lead of those in other fields of medicine, practitioners of sports medicine are now moving toward a more holistic approach, recognizing that the psychologic state of the athlete is as important as, and sometimes more important than, the athlete's physical state (Fig. 1–1).

With the growth and recognized importance of the field of sports psychology, there has been increasing interest in the relationship between psychologic factors and the occurrence and treatment of sports injuries. The intent in this chapter is to help the clinician understand this relationship, especially in regard to the following: (1) potential risk factors, (2) responses to injury, (3) influence on the recovery period, and (4) "slumps" resulting from injury.

PSYCHOLOGIC RISK FACTORS

Are there psychologic factors that could help identify athletes who are more injury prone than others? Early attempts to investigate this question used the "trait" approach, in which specific and enduring personality dispositions were identified in athletes with a history of injury. The personality studies included traits such as introversion or extroversion,* locus of control,† self-concept, anxiety, aggressiveness, and dominance, which could be identified with written tests. For example, it was believed that an athlete with a strong anxiety trait would have greater body tension and would be less able to focus effectively on critical information involving performance and would therefore be more susceptible to injury.

A second example involves athletes with an external locus of control, who perceive themselves as having less control over the events around them and thus have a greater potential for injury. By identifying certain psychologic traits

---

*Introverts tend to withdraw into themselves (introversion), whereas extroverts extend or seek out external stimulation (extroversion).

†Locus of control is the responsibility people feel for their behavior by referring to internal causes, such as those attributed to their own actions, or to external causes, in which they have little control over the events in their lives.

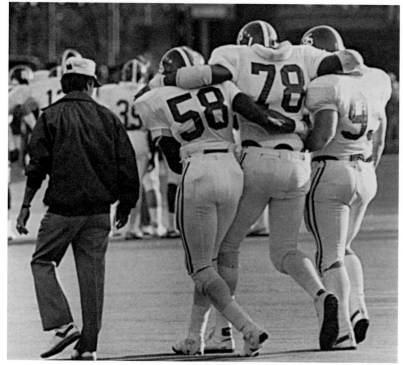

Figure 1–1. Risk factors have been recognized as inherent with sport participation. Until recently, the athlete's body and mind were treated as a single unit, with the latter receiving little or no attention. (From Philpot, D. [1986]: Evaluation of the injured ankle. Sports Med. Update, 1:5.)

as factors contributing to potential injury, an athlete with such traits might be advised to select sports with a low injury risk factor or to take special precautions if participating in a sport with a high injury risk factor.

Research using the trait approach has shown limited significant findings involving the relationship of psychologic traits and the occurrence of athletic injuries. It was found that football players who were more "tender-minded" and reserved were more susceptible to injury.[10, 11] Contrary to this finding, a recent study of female volleyball players found that players who were more tough-minded (e.g., assertive, independent) experienced higher injury rates than did athletes who were more tender-minded.[23] This study supported a previous study that reported that female basketball players with a higher incidence of injury scored more positively on self-concept and identity and on physical and personal self-factors than did noninjured female players.[24] It was suggested that these injured volleyball and basketball players were more likely to take risks because of greater self-confidence, and consequently they increased their potential for injury. Thus, although some studies have provided limited support for the notion that there is a direct relationship between some personality traits and the occurrence of injury, most researchers believe that other interacting factors need to be investigated.

As a result of findings from these trait studies, research focus has shifted to exploring the relationship of stress to injury. The concept that stressful life events may be related to the occurrence of athletic injuries was initially based on reports in the general medical literature. Studies have shown a positive correlation between stressful life events, especially those associated with high negative stress levels, and the occurrence of injury and disease. Using these reports, Anderson and Williams[1] developed a theoretic model showing factors that could contribute to the stress–injury relationship in the sports setting (Fig. 1–2).

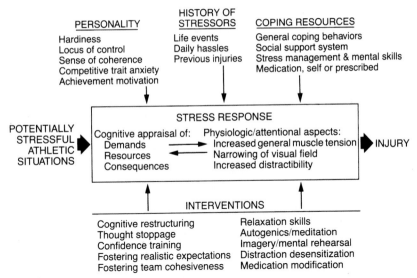

Figure 1–2. A model of stress and athletic injury. (From "A Model of Stress and Athletic Injury: Prediction and Prevention" by M.B. Andersen and J.M. Williams, 1988, *Journal of Sport and Exercise Psychology, 10,* p. 297. Copyright 1988 by Human Kinetics Publishers, Inc. Reprinted by permission.)

Although this model includes the personality traits previously discussed, it uses these traits as contributors to an individual's history of stress events or as factors that have a direct impact on the stress response. Their model also includes the coping resources and interventions that can serve as modifiers of a potential stress response. The model should be reviewed to understand the factors contributing to the stress response and the proposed relationship among the factors. It is also referred to later in this chapter.

Several studies have investigated the relationship of life stress to sports injuries. Bramwell and associates[3] studied the life changes of 79 varsity collegiate football players for 1- and 2-year periods prior to their playing season and found that a greater percentage of injuries occur in those in the group with many changes in their lives resulting in greater stress. In their study of two college football teams, Passer and Seese[16] found a significant relationship between negative life stress and injury on one team but not on the other. A study of elite female gymnasts revealed that stressful life events are related significantly to both the number and the severity of injuries.[12] In this study, factors such as anxiety, locus of control, and self-concept were not significant predictors of injury. Although several studies have noted a relationship between high life stress (especially negative stress) and injuries, a study involving male and female intercollegiate volleyball players showed no relationship between life stress and injury.[22] The type of sport and the predominate types of injuries found in a sport may be important variables in the stress–injury relationship, but at present no published reports have addressed this hypothesis.

In the studies mentioned in the preceding paragraph, the primary focus was on negative life events. However, positive life events can also create stress that has been related to athletic injury.[9] Events such as being named a team leader, which increases the team responsibility role, being named to a preseason all-star team, or receiving a performance award may increase the performance expectations of the athlete, resulting in increased levels of stress and making the athlete more prone to injury.

To explore the stress–injury relationship further, the physiologic and psychologic changes in response to stress must be understood, as shown in a model by Nideffer[15] (Fig. 1–3). With regard to physiologic changes, there is increasing

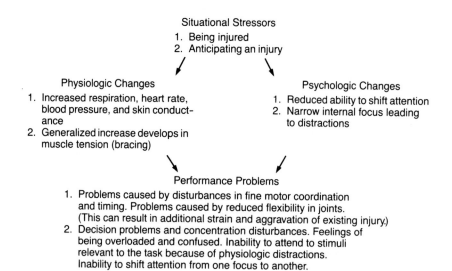

Figure 1–3. Physical and psychologic changes accompany increases in pressure as a result of injury or the fear of injury. Problems in performance resulting from stress and reduced physiologic and psychologic flexibility can become chronic. Disturbances in physical flexibility affect concentration, and as the athlete becomes upset at his or her own failure (frustration or anxiety increases), the attentional and physiologic disturbances become stronger and more intractable. (Modified from Nideffer, R.M. [1983]: The injured athlete: Psychological factors in treatment. Orthop. Clin. North Am., 14:373–385.)

concern about the muscle tension produced as a result of the stress response. Increased tension in the antagonistic and agonistic muscle groups results in a reduction of flexibility and a loss of motor coordination. Another significant factor related to increased muscular tension is a slowed reaction time, which reduces the athlete's ability to respond to environmental events. Therefore, the maintenance of appropriate muscle tension to achieve a desired result appears to be essential in the prevention of injuries.

It is seen from the Nideffer model (see Fig. 1–3) that an important psychologic variable is the ability of the athlete to select and process information, because stress has been shown to narrow or switch the attentional focus. For example, a player under heavy stress in football might not process information in the peripheral areas of the visual field, resulting in a lack of response to oncoming physical contact (e.g., there is a greater potential for a blind-side hit). Another important aspect of attentional focus involves the athlete's thoughts at the time of injury. From the Nideffer model, it is proposed that an athlete under stress, especially negative stress, may be thinking about the events causing the stress and not thinking about what is currently happening in the environment. Therefore, the athlete does not process relevant information that could result in a protective response. For example, a linebacker in football who has just learned of the divorce plans of his parents may be thinking of what his future holds (internal focus) and not attending well to information involving what is happening on the field (external focus). Hence, there would be a greater potential for injury for this athlete.

A discussion of the importance of attentional focus in athletic injuries must address the interest in recent studies on the psychologic phenomenon of mood congruence. It has been shown that we attend, encode, and retrieve information that is congruent with our mood state.[2] For example, if the mood state of the athlete described above is depression, resulting from knowledge of the parents' divorce, the information he attends to probably contains affect-congruent information. In this case, it is negative information from the environment (external focus) and negative thoughts (internal focus) that are affecting his thought process. If the mood state is anger as a result of the divorce plans, a high level of activation would be expected, which also disrupts the attentional ability and the processing of relevant information. With the occurrence of either emotion, depression or anger, the ability to control attention and process correct information is inhibited, thus increasing the potential for injury. The ability to control attention and block out irrelevant information depends greatly on the individual, with a wide variation among athletes.

For the athlete returning to competition after recovery from injury, attentional focus and muscular tension can be problematic. Fear or worry about a second injury can place an athlete into an internal mode of thought processing, causing increased muscular tension. There has been interest in the role of psychologic hardiness as it relates to return from injury. Hardiness can be defined as a combination of commitment, control, and the ability to meet challenge on the part of an individual, and it seems to be a moderating factor in the stress–illness relationship.[13] It is believed that athletes who exhibit this trait to a greater degree are better able to control the attentional processing of information and hence are able to reduce the potential for occurrence of a second injury. At present, however, not enough studies have been done on hardiness and its relationship to injury to warrant definite conclusions' being reached.

Fatigue, the final factor to be discussed here, has been recognized to be a contributor to injury, usually only as a physical factor. However, mental fatigue may be more important. Maintaining a high level of concentration (attention) requires a large amount of energy, and in combination with a demanding training program, attention is reduced as both physical and mental fatigue sets in. Reduced attention results in slowed response times, and this, together with the loss of neuromuscular coordination, increases the potential for injury.

In moving beyond the general physical effects of stress, as discussed above, recent research has shown the importance of the social support systems available to the athlete in coping with the stress response. Petrie[17] reported that female collegiate gymnasts with less social support were most vulnerable to the effects of life stress that was positively correlated to the incidents of injury. In a second study with collegiate football players, Petrie[18, 19] reported a significant relationship for the starting players on the teams involved. The number of severe injuries, days missed due to injury, and games missed were related to negative life stress with social support serving as a moderating variable. In other words, if an athlete had a strong social support system, the life stressors encountered would not have resulted in as high an injury potential. This relationship of social support to stress and injury did not exist for the nonstarting players. It is also important to note that Petrie reports that players with high social support and low life stress were more likely to experience injury than were those reporting low levels of support with low life stress. One explanation is that in situations of low stress and high support, athletes may have a greater sense of confidence and security and therefore exhibit greater risk-taking behaviors that would increase the potential for injury. From the current research it appears that social support is an important moderating variable, in either high or low life-stress situations, of the potential for injury in sports situations.

Thus, although there are only a few studies pertaining to psychologic risk factors and injury, current evidence supports the importance of the stress response (as presented in the Anderson and Williams model; see Fig. 1–2).

OCCURRENCE OF INJURY

When an athlete is injured, the primary focus of trainers, coaches, teammates, doctors, parents, and even spectators is generally on tangible evidence of the injury. "How severe is the injury?" "Will surgery be required?" These questions are followed by others. "How long will the athlete be out of competition?" "Who will replace this athlete in the lineup?" And, if the athlete is a critical player (e.g., a quarterback or a pitcher), many of the significant people working with this athlete might think of the season "going down the drain."

Initial treatments, such as cryotherapy and immobilization, are usually provided quickly; these are followed by a rehabilitation program that includes a regimen for regaining strength and flexibility. Although the physical needs of an injured athlete are taken care of, other major needs that may create more pain than the physical aspect of the injury are often overlooked. If an athlete is injured, the thoughts and feelings of the athlete are often disregarded or given a low priority. These thoughts and feelings, reflecting on past experiences involving injury to self or to others and on how this injury may change the future, can produce psychologic pain that is greater and that lasts longer than the physical pain. Well-intended comments to an injured athlete (e.g., "You will be okay" or "Just hang in there") are often heard, but these do not really address the psychologic problems the athlete is experiencing.

As the initial physical pain of the injury subsides, the athlete encounters an array of psychologic reactions. Emotional responses, such as "Why me?", "Why now?", and "This can't be happening," take over the thoughts of the athlete. Other emotions, such as anger, depression, anxiety, and panic are common responses.

Sometimes these emotions cannot be expressed overtly by the athlete, because this type of behavior is unacceptable in the macho world of athletics. When an athletic career is interrupted or perhaps terminated as a result of an injury, the years of expectations and hard work seem wasted, and a strong emotional response, overt or hidden, must be expected.

Although an injury can be psychologically devastating to many athletes, some athletes view the injury with relief. For some athletes, the injury provides them with attention and support from others that they may not have received before the injury. For others, the injury relieves the pressure to perform, and the respite from training and competition may be welcomed. This gives the athlete a chance to enjoy other aspects of life and provides time for re-evaluating the commitment to the sport. The idea that an athlete may obtain satisfaction from an injury, however, is often difficult for a trainer, especially a coach, to understand. With the emphasis on sports in today's society, which produces enormous pressure on the athlete to perform and be successful, there is increasing evidence that more athletes are using injury as a means of coping through escape from the pressures of performing.

As stated previously, various psychologic responses can be observed immediately after injury, and these can continue long after recovery. The nature and intensity of these responses depend on several factors, such as the type of injury, its importance to performing the skills essential to the sport, the time of injury with regard to the season and major competitive events, and the importance of participation to the athlete. The major variable related to these factors seems to be the athlete's perception of the injury and its effect on the future. Although the injury might seem minor to the trainer or the physician, the athlete might believe that it is more severe and therefore could exhibit emotional responses that seem unwarranted to others. Of significance here is acceptance by the athlete of the trainer's or physician's appraisal of the injury. If the athlete lacks confidence in the ability of medical personnel to appraise and treat the injury properly, the athlete can reject and ignore the medical advice, which would result in a stronger negative emotional response.

Lynch[14] has reported that severely injured athletes go through emotional stages of denial, anger, bargaining, depression, and acceptance. This suggested orderly process for emotional behavior following injury, often referred to as a stage model, has not been supported in a recent review of athletic injury research.[4] It was found that the emotional reaction to injury varies among individuals, depending on the stress resulting from the athlete's appraisal of the injury. Personal factors (e.g., motivation, coping skills, self-esteem, or personality) and situational factors (e.g., injury severity, timing, impact on daily life, or social pressures) cause athletes to alternate among emotional states and to reflect feelings of fear, panic, and even learned helplessness.

What about gender differences? Do male and female athletes respond differently to injury? Most athletic injury studies have not included a gender comparison in studying the emotional responses of injured athletes. A study by Quackenbush and Crossman[20] is one of the few studies comparing gender behaviors. After studying recovering athletes at three sports medicine clinics, they reported significant emotional differences between male and female athletes. The women were found to express more emotional responses, both positive and negative, than did the men. Immediately after injury, the male and female athletes were equally frustrated, angry, and discouraged; however, the men were more irritable, whereas the women were more cooperative, optimistic, and hopeful. During the recovery period, women showed more positive signs toward returning to practice. These researchers concluded that socialization differences impact the expression of psychologic feelings and thoughts, suggesting that the gender of the injured athlete must be a consideration in the psychologic rehabilitation process.

These psychologic responses, coupled with the physical pain from the injury, result in a threat to self-esteem and in feelings of incompetence and may have a major influence on the recovery period. This seems to be especially true if the athlete has no strong social support system. During recovery, stress from the injury can be a major problem; however, it is the perceived stress experienced by the athlete that is important. For example, the coach may plan for the injured athlete to return to his or her starting position after recovery and may discuss these plans with the athlete. If the athlete perceives his or her starting role to be in jeopardy, however, there can be additional stress on the athlete that others may not observe or understand. This stress, from whatever source, causes increased muscle tension and can reduce the ability of the circulatory system to supply blood to the injured area. This stress can also reduce the ability of the athlete to perform the simple physical movement patterns necessary for rehabilitation.

Of prime importance in providing medical services to an athlete during recovery is the availability of a strong social support system. Extensive medical research has shown the value of support systems as buffers or moderators of the negative stress resulting from disease or injury. Results of studies involving sports settings have also suggested a positive correlation between desired behavior on the part of the athlete during the recovery period and the support provided by significant others.[6, 7] Weiss and Troxell[21] have presented a strong case for the role of the athletic trainer in the support system. The presence and positive support of others who understand the needs of the athlete and why certain behaviors are occurring are valuable in helping the athlete cope with various problems during the recovery period. This understanding is especially necessary because the injured athlete might be depressed and, as a result, could reject the efforts of people close to him or her. Within a short period, however, this athlete may be seeking assurance and reinforcement from these same individuals.

Those in the support system, which must include the athletic trainer, the physical therapist, and the physician, therefore play an extremely important role in understanding and guiding the athlete through these emotional times during recovery.

ADHERENCE AND RECOVERY PROBLEMS

During the recovery period, a disturbing behavior on the part of the athlete sometimes emerges. The athlete misses assigned therapy sessions or, when attending the session, does not put forth the necessary effort for effective rehabilitation. This becomes extremely disturbing to coaches, trainers, teammates, and others who are influenced by this lack of adherence and commitment on the part of this athlete. Some athletes may regard the occurrence of an injury as a positive event, in that it may relieve them of the pressures of competition, gain them attention, or allow them time to re-evaluate the importance of participation in sports.

Why don't athletes adhere to rehabilitation programs? The study by Duda and colleagues[6] is one of the few that have investigated why athletes do not adhere to rehabilitation programs. Their study involved 40 intercollegiate athletes who had sustained a sports injury of at least second-degree severity that resulted in scheduled rehabilitation sessions for 3 weeks or more. They measured the attendance and the completion of the exercise protocol and observed the exercise intensity of the injured athletes. The study shows that perceived value of the treatment, social support, degree of self-motivation, and task involvement in sports are significant predictors of adherence behaviors.

How do these factors relate to the participation of a sports medicine team in treatment of an injury? Educating the athlete about the nature and value of the treatment is a responsibility of the trainer and the physician, with the aid of the coach and the parents. Often, treatments and drug therapy are prescribed without the patient's being provided information about how these influence the rehabilitation process.

This problem arises because it is often assumed that the athlete already knows why a treatment is prescribed or because, when large numbers of players are involved, such as on a football team, there is not enough time to provide individual attention. The educational process is part of the responsibility of those who provide social support in the recovery period. Two factors—self-motivation and task involvement—are sometimes the most misunderstood variables when one is working with athletes, because most people assume that highly successful athletes have high levels of self-motivation and a high degree of involvement and commitment to their sport. This assumption, however, is not true. For example, some athletes with great natural abilities have low need achievement levels and a limited commitment to the sport for which they are recognized. Such athletes usually lack self-directed goals that can help provide the intrinsic drive necessary to gain maximum value from their natural abilities. Therefore, when this type of athlete is injured, the lack of internal drive and goals results in problems with regard to adherence to a prescribed rehabilitation program, which takes time and effort to complete. Also, the lack of adherence could be the result of the athlete's not viewing the reward system (extrinsic motivation) as providing the necessary returns for overcoming that lack of internal motivation to complete the rehabilitation program successfully.

These adherence variables are consistent with those found in the medical literature.[5] Sports adherence studies are limited, and the influence of several variables needs to be clarified to understand this problem. These include the type of sport, the gender of the athlete, the time during the season when the injury occurs, and the perceived cause of the injury. Injury is an inherent variable in sports participation, so factors that influence the adherence to rehabilitation programs are important for the effective functioning of a sports medicine team.

A behavior observed by coaches and trainers on return of an athlete to competition after an injury is that the athlete does not have the same intensity and dedication to the sport as had been observed before the injury. This loss of focus and intensity can contribute to adherence problems but becomes more serious after the return to practice and competition.

It is generally believed that the athlete has a fear of being reinjured, and to some extent this is true. It may also be the case, however, that the athlete has had time to reflect on the role of sports in his or her life, has questioned its importance and rewards, and as a result, has established new priorities. One athlete, currently in her middle teens, after having to take time off from swimming because of a car accident injury, reported that "I never thought there were so many other fun things to do." This swimmer had been attending twice-a-day workouts for the past 10 years of her life, and everything she did was related to swimming. The "time out" gave her a chance to participate in other activities and changed her thinking about the importance of sports in her life.

Trainers, coaches, and significant others play important roles in the recovery period. Their understanding of the problems that an athlete can encounter during this period is critical to satisfactory recovery. They can provide the motivation for the athlete to adhere to rehabilitation programs and to return to practice and competition with a positive mental attitude (Fig. 1–4).

SLUMPS AND INJURIES

Most athletes at some time experience declines in performance, commonly referred to as "slumps." These can result from physical, technical, or psychologic problems or from some combination of these. The prescription for a slump can range from "work harder and work your way through it" to a "time out" during which the athlete has a period of total rest from the sport. How do athletic injuries and psychologic variables further relate to slumps?

The most frequent cause of a slump is probably the physical component. Fatigue caused by overtraining and injury, especially nagging minor injuries that receive little attention, creates problems in executing the skill and results in a lower performance level. As the athlete senses the declining physical performance, psychologic factors lead to anxiety, loss of concentration, and confidence, which become a major source of future problems.

The increased anxiety results in greater muscle tension, which interferes with coordination in the muscular system and results in a lower performance level and in an increased risk of further injury. Because a slump can be extremely draining, it adds to the general fatigue problem, and the athlete's ability to concentrate on important information can be hindered still more.

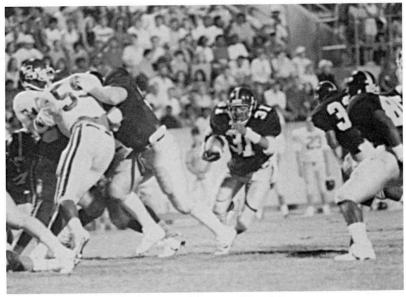

Figure 1–4. The return of an athlete to his or her sport involves not only the physical rehabilitation program but also the athlete's mental health. Of the support personnel available, the athletic trainer can be the best qualified to address these concerns.

Sometimes slumps are the result of problems that are not directly related to sports participation. Marital or financial problems or family illness could be the cause of a slump. Again, the problem of lack or loss of concentration increases the potential for injury to occur. In some cases the athlete may use the injury as a means of explaining the slump and of escaping the pressure of performance and the need to explain the real problem to others.

It is therefore important that the members of the sports medicine team do not write off a slump as only a psychologic problem related to athletic performance. Often the antecedents to the observed psychologic responses, such as injury, fatigue, or outside influences, are the true source of the slump.

COPING STRATEGIES

The Anderson and Williams model (see Fig. 1–2) has two parts that show the importance of coping strategies. The first part is listed under coping resources, which shows the importance of social support systems, stress management and mental skills, and general coping behaviors in mediating the life stress factors and in interacting directly with the stress response. The second aspect of the model deals with the interventions that can be used in response to stress. Although this model was designed to explain the psychologic phenomena that are antecedents of an injury, the model can also be useful for understanding the psychologic components of postinjury responses. Therefore, it is important for the athlete to have coping strategies available both before and after injury.

Space limitations prevent a detailed discussion of the many coping resources and interventions available, but one example is that of relaxation techniques. Because many athletes and coaches are concerned about stress management, it can be important for an athlete to know some basic relaxation techniques. Athletes who have knowledge of such skills as breathing techniques, ways of detecting and reducing muscular tension, and use of imagery can help prevent or reduce the severity of injury. For example, Green[8] has shown how athletes trained in the use of imagery can potentially reduce stress that may lead to injury and how imagery can be used during the rehabilitation process. If injury does occur, the knowledge and the ability to use psychologic techniques can be very valuable during the recovery period.

Only recently have coaches shown an interest in having their athletes taught psychologic skills such as relaxation and imagery. Sometimes the coach has had the proper training for teaching such skills, but often the acquisition of these techniques is left to the athlete or some other interested person. Many teams do not have access to a sports psychologist or cannot afford to have one on staff. In such cases it is believed that the athletic trainer, who has the best general relationship with the athletes, can implement and carry out psychologic development programs most effectively.

SUGGESTIONS

The suggestions for members of a sports medicine team to handle some of the problems discussed in this chapter include the following:

1. We must educate the athlete about the importance of the mind-body connection as part of the daily training program. This is based on the assumption that athletes who have developed cognitive strategies (e.g., relaxation, imagery, concentration) along with their physical skills have a better chance of

preventing injury and are better equipped to cope with an injury if one does occur.

2. We must establish communication and support structures. In many sports, communication between the coach and the athlete is limited and, at best, superficial. Some athletes do not feel confident about talking with the coach about their thoughts and feelings. It is with respect to this that the trainer and other members of the sports medicine team can be extremely important in providing a means for athletes to express their thoughts and feelings.

3. We must ensure that the athletic trainer has knowledge and training about the psychologic aspects of sports participation. The trainer already has major responsibilities for the prevention and care of the physical aspect of injuries and thus may be the best person to be involved in a psychologic training program if other resources are not available. The relationship of the athletic trainer to the athlete may be more flexible, open, and less threatening, and the athlete may feel more comfortable in discussing his or her mental needs with the trainer.

References

1. Anderson, M.B., and Williams, J.M. (1988): A model of stress and athletic injury: Prediction and prevention. J. Sport Exerc. Psychol., 10:294–306.
2. Blaney, P.H. (1986): Affect and memory: A review. Psychol. Bull., 99:229–246.
3. Bramwell, S.T., Masuda, M., Wagner, N.N., and Holmes, T.H. (1975): Psychosocial factors in athletic injuries: Development and application of the social and athletic readjustment rating scale. J. Human Stress, 1:6–20.
4. Brewer, B.W. (1994): Review and critique of models of psychological adjustment to athletic injury. J. Appl. Sport Psychol., 6:87–100.
5. Dishman, R.K. (1986): Exercise compliance: A new view for public health. Physician Sportsmed., 14:127–145.
6. Duda, J.L., Smart, A.E., and Tappe, M.K. (1989): Predictors of adherence in the rehabilitation of athletic injuries: An application of personal investment theory. J. Sport Exerc. Psychol., 11:367–381.
7. Fisher, A.C., Domm, M.A., and Wuest, D.A. (1988): Adherence to sports-injury rehabilitation programs. Physician Sportsmed., 16:47–52.
8. Green, L.B. (1992): The use of imagery in the rehabilitation of injured athletes. Sport Psychologist, 6:416–428.
9. Hanson, S.J., McCullagh, P., and Tonymon, P. (1992): The relationship of personality characteristics, life stress, and coping resources to athletic injury. J. Sport Exerc. Psychol., 14:262–272.
10. Irwin, R.F. (1975): Relationship between personality and the incidence of injuries to high school football participants. Dissertation Abstr. Int., 36:4328A.
11. Jackson, D.W., Jarrett, H., Bailey, D., et al. (1978): Injury prediction in the young athlete: A preliminary report. Am. J. Sports Med., 6:6–14.
12. Kerr, G., and Minden, H. (1988): Psychological factors related to the occurrence of athletic injuries. J. Sport Exerc. Psychol., 109:167–173.
13. Kobasa, S.C., Maddi, S.R., and Puccetti, M.C. (1982): Personality and exercise as buffers in the stress-illness relationship. J. Behav. Med., 5:391–404.
14. Lynch, C.P. (1988): Athletic injuries and the practicing sport psychologists: Practical guidelines for assisting athletes. Sport Psychologist, 2:161–167.
15. Nideffer, R.M. (1983): The injured athlete: Psychological factors in treatment. Orthop. Clin. North Am., 14:373–385.
16. Passer, M.W., and Seese, M.D. (1983): Life stress and athletic injury: Examination of positive versus negative events and three moderator variables. J. Human Stress, 9:11–16.
17. Petrie, T.A. (1992): Psychosocial antecedents of athletic injury: The effects of life stress and social support on women collegiate gymnasts. Behav. Med., 18:127–138.
18. Petrie, T.A. (1993): The moderating effects of social support and playing status on the life stress-injury relationship. J. Appl. Sport Psychol., 5:1–16.

19. Petrie, T.A. (1993): Coping skills, competitive trait anxiety, and playing status: Moderating effects on the life stress-injury relationship. J. Sport Exerc. Psychol., 15:261–274.
20. Quackenbush, N. and Crossman, J. (1994): A study of emotional responses. J. Sport Behav., 17:178–187.
21. Weiss, M.R., and Troxell, R.K. (1986): Psychology of the injured athlete. Athl. Train., 21:104–110.
22. Williams, J.M., Tonymon, P., and Wadsworth, W.A. (1986): Relationship of stress to injury in intercollegiate volleyball. J. Human Stress, 12:38–43.
23. Wittig, A.F., and Schurr, K.T. (1994): Psychological characteristics of women volleyball players: Relationships with injuries, rehabilitation, and team success. Pers. Soc. Psychol. Bull., 20:322–330.
24. Young, M.L., and Cohen, D.A. (1981): Self-concept and injuries among high school basketball players. J. Sports Med., 21:55–61.

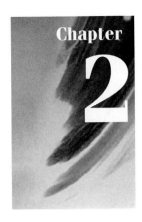

Physiologic Factors of Rehabilitation

Gary L. Harrelson, Ed.D., A.T.,C.

The effects of immobilization on bone and connective tissue have been widely reported in the literature. The use of early range-of-motion exercises to prevent the deleterious effects of immobilization has become accepted practice in the orthopedic community. The proper use of exercise can speed up the healing process, whereas the lack of exercise during the early stages of rehabilitation can result in permanent disability. Caution must be observed, however, because exercise that is too vigorous can also result in permanent damage. Immobilization initially results in loss of tissue substrate, with a subsequent loss of basic tissue components. The reversibility of these changes appears to be dependent on the length of immobilization.

To understand the body's response to immobilization and remobilization, its normal reaction to injury must be addressed. The enzymes released when trauma occurs to a joint can cause cartilage degradation, chronic joint synovitis, and stretching of the joint capsule as a result of increased effusion.

REACTION TO INJURY

Inflammation is the body's response to injury, and optimally, it results in healing of injury and replacement of damaged and destroyed tissue, with an associated restoration of function.[38] Continued injury or microtrauma to an area, however, can cause a chronic inflammatory response that results in adverse effects to the joint and its surrounding structures. The inflammatory response is the same, regardless of the location and nature of the injurious agent, and consists of chemical, metabolic, permeability, and vascular changes, followed by some form of repair.[57]

Figure 2–1 illustrates the primary and secondary injuries affiliated with trauma and the associated inflammation and repair processes. Primary injury is the result of trauma that directly injures the cells themselves. Secondary injury (sometimes referred to as secondary hypoxia) is precipitated by the body's response to trauma. This response includes decreased blood flow to the traumatized region as a result of vasoconstriction, which decreases the amount of oxygen to the injured area. Thus, additional cells die because of secondary hypoxia; these dead cells organize and ultimately form a hematoma.

Cell degeneration or cell death perpetuates the release of potent substances that can induce vascular changes. The most common of these substances is histamine, which increases capillary permeability and allows the escape of fluid and blood cells into the interstitial spaces. In the noninjured state, plasma and blood proteins escape from capillaries by osmosis and diffusion into the intersti-

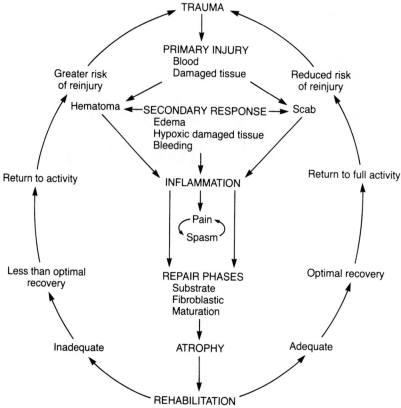

Figure 2–1. Cycle of athletic injury. (Reproduced by permission from Booher, James M., and Thibodeau, Gary A.: Athletic Injury Assessment. St. Louis, 1989, Times Mirror/ Mosby College Publishing.)

tial spaces but are reabsorbed. This homeostasis is maintained by colloids present within the blood system. However, trauma leads to increased capillary permeability as a result of the release of cell enzymes, allowing blood plasma and proteins to escape into surrounding tissues. Concurrently, the concentration of colloids greatly increases in the surrounding tissues, thus reversing the colloidal effect. Rather than the colloids' pulling fluid back into the capillaries, the presence of the colloids outside the vessels causes additional fluid to be pulled into the interstitial tissues, resulting in swelling and edema.

The body's reaction postinjury is mobilization and transport of the defense components of the blood to the injured area. Initially, blood flow is reduced, allowing white blood cells to migrate to the margins of the blood vessels. These cells adhere to the vessel walls and eventually travel into the interstitial tissues. Once in the surrounding tissues, the white cells remove irritating material by the process of phagocytosis. Neutrophils are the first white blood cells to arrive, and they normally destroy bacteria. However, because bacteria are not usually associated with athletic injuries, these neutrophils die.[57] Then, macrophages appear and phagocytize the dead neutrophils, cellular debris, fibrin, red cells, and other debris that may impede the repair process.[57] Unfortunately, the destruction of the neutrophils results in the release of active proteolytic enzymes (i.e., enzymes that hasten the hydrolysis of proteins into simpler substances), which can attack joint tissues, into the surrounding inflammatory fluid.[45] Although this is the natural response of ridding the body of toxic or foreign materials, prolongation of this process can damage surrounding joint structures.

Once the inflammatory debris has been removed, repair can begin. Cleanup by the macrophages and repair often occur simultaneously. However, for repair to occur, enough of the hematoma must be removed to permit ingrowth of new tissue. Thus, the size of the hematoma or the amount of the exudate is directly related to the total healing time. If the size of the hematoma can be minimized, healing can begin earlier and total healing time is reduced.[57]

Response of Joint Structures to Injury

As a result of the inflammatory process, each joint component responds differently to injury (Fig. 2–2). The reaction of the synovial membrane to injury involves the proliferation of surface cells, an increase in vascularity, and a gradual fibrosis of the subsynovial tissue. Posttraumatic synovitis is not uncommon after most injuries. Continued mechanical irritation can produce chronic synovitis, which results in the reversal of normal synovial cell ratios.[45, 92] Changes in synovial fluid occur as a result of alterations in the synovial membrane. Cells are destroyed as a consequence of the synovitis; the white blood cells ingest lysosomes and proteolytic enzymes. This ingestion and the subsequent death of white blood cells in the transudate result in the further release of proteolytic enzymes. The overall consequence is the spawning of a vicious inflammatory cycle, which can keep reactive synovitis active for some time, even without further trauma (Fig. 2–3).[10] As chronic posttraumatic effusions occur, changes of the synovial membrane can continue, with progressing sclerotic alterations as a sequel.[105] If conservative treatment consisting of anti-inflammatory medications,

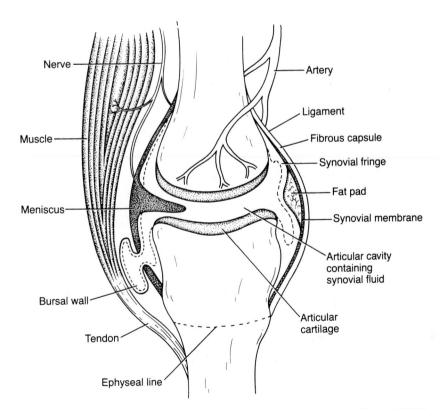

Figure 2–2. Synovial joint structures. (From Wright, V., Dowson, D., and Kerry, J. [1973]: The structure of joints. Int. Rev. Connect. Tissue Res., 6:105–125.)

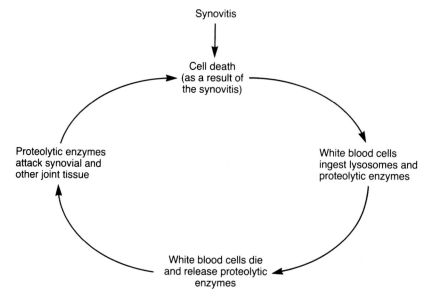

Figure 2–3. Continued mechanical irritation of a joint can result in chronic synovitis that is perpetuated by a vicious inflammatory cycle. This keeps the reactive synovitis alive even without further trauma.

rest, aspiration, and cold applications does not relieve the symptoms, a synovectomy may be necessary.

Meniscus lesions within the knee are invariably accompanied by increased synovial effusion. Once the problem is corrected, the synovial irritation usually subsides. If, however, the problem is left uncorrected, tissues not injured by the original trauma can be damaged from the prolonged inflammation, resulting in progressive degradation of the synovial membrane.

Fortunately, once the inflammation begins to abate, synovial tissue can regenerate remarkably well, an ability that possibly stems from its excellent blood supply and origin. Synovium regenerates completely within several months into tissue that is indistinguishable from the normal tissue.[45]

Acute and chronic synovitis directly affect the amount and content of synovial fluid produced. Synovitis can result in an increased protein level within the synovial fluid. In addition, chronic synovitis can cause a decrease in synovial fluid viscosity and a decrease in the concentration of hyaluronic acid.[17] The concentration of hyaluronic acid is directly related to synovial fluid viscosity. Minor joint trauma results in no change in either the concentration or the molecular weight of the hyaluronic acid.[17] As trauma severity increases, however, the hyaluronic acid concentration decreases to levels below normal, and when the inflammatory process becomes sufficiently disruptive, joint lining cells fail not only to maintain hyaluronic acid concentration but also to maintain normal polymer weight.[17]

A hemarthrosis can result in the synovial fluid's having a lower sugar concentration; blood clots can be detected in the synovial fluid; and fibrinogen, which normally is not found in synovial fluid, can be detected as a result of bleeding into the joint. Because blood is quickly absorbed by phagocytic cells in the synovial membrane, it may not be evident in the synovial fluid until several days posthemarthrosis.[45]

The effect of a hemarthrosis on the synovial lining is synovium proliferation and an increased rate of blood absorption with each repeated hemarthrosis. The stimulus for the production of this proliferative synovitis appears to be the iron released from the red blood cells.[45]

The absorption rate of solutions from the joint space is inversely proportional to the size of the solutes; the larger the molecules, the slower the clearance. Clinically, absorption from a joint is increased by active or passive range of motion, massage, intra-articular hydrocortisone, or acute inflammation, whereas the effect of external compression is variable.[112]

The reaction of the joint capsule to injury is similar to that of the synovial membrane. If the inflammatory process continues, the joint capsule eventually becomes a more fibrous tissue, and effusion into the joint cavity can lead to stretching of the capsule and its associated ligaments. The higher the hydrostatic pressure and volume of effusion, the faster the fluid reaccumulates after aspiration.[45, 46] Conversely, a significant rise in intra-articular hydrostatic pressure contributes to joint damage by stretching the capsule and associated ligaments.

The load-carrying surfaces of the synovial joint are covered with a thin layer of specialized connective tissue, referred to as articular cartilage. The response of the articular cartilage to trauma is not unlike that of the other structures within the joint. The mechanical properties of articular cartilage are readily affected by enzymatic degradation of cartilage components. This can occur after acute inflammation, synovectomy, immobilization, or other seemingly minor insults.[104] When articular cartilage loses its content of proteoglycan (a protein aggregate that helps establish the resiliency and resistance to deformation of articular cartilage), the physical properties of the cartilage are changed; this renders the collagen fibers susceptible to mechanical damage.[104] As a result of this enzymatic degradation, articular cartilage can erode and leave denuded bone, resulting in early, irreversible osteoarthritis or degenerative joint disease (Fig. 2–4).

The reduction of posttraumatic joint effusion is paramount in the early rehabilitation process and is important in the restoration of joint kinematics. Prolonged effusion, if left unchecked, can result in reactive synovitis, damage of the joint capsule, and degradation of articular cartilage. The early use of mobilization techniques such as continuous passive motion and of modalities such as cryotherapy and vasopneumatic compression can aid in reducing joint effusion.

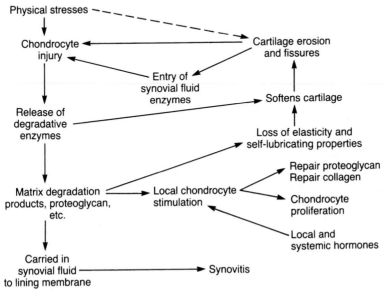

Figure 2–4. Postulated final pathway of cartilage degeneration. (Reproduced by permission from Howell, David S.: Osteoarthritis—etiology and pathogenesis. *In*: American Academy of Orthopaedic Surgeons: Symposium on osteoarthritis, St. Louis, 1976, The C.V. Mosby Co.)

EFFECTS OF IMMOBILIZATION
Muscle

One of the first and most obvious changes that occur as a result of immobilization is loss of muscle strength. This correlates with a reduction in muscle size and a decrease in tension per unit of muscle cross-sectional area.[7, 71, 72] MacDougall and colleagues[72] have reported that 6 weeks of elbow cast immobilization results in a greater than 40% decrease in muscle strength. In addition, this strength deficit is correlated with a loss of fiber cross-sectional area and, therefore, with a decrease in muscle mass. Animal studies have confirmed general correlations among loss of muscle strength and volume and maintenance of specific strength; loss of muscle strength and volume can be measured as functional muscle strength for cross-sectional area in a muscle.[7] The rate of loss appears to be most rapid during the initial days of immobilization. Lindboe and Platou[67] have reported that in humans, muscle fiber size is reduced by 14% to 17% after 72 hours of immobilization. After 5 to 7 days of immobilization, the absolute loss in muscle mass appears to slow considerably.[7]

Both fast-twitch (type I) and slow-twitch (type II) muscle fibers atrophy. Studies suggest that there is no selective loss of muscle mass in slow-twitch fibers compared with fast-twitch fibers, and it is still unclear whether there is differential atrophy between fast-twitch and slow-twitch fibers or whether one fiber type is involved more than the other.[20, 36, 72] However, it is generally accepted that with immobilization there is a greater degeneration of slow-twitch fibers compared with fast-twitch fibers.[9, 41, 42, 73, 110]

In addition to causing changes in muscle size and volume, immobilization also results in histochemical changes. These include a reduction in the levels of adenosine triphosphate (ATP), adenosine diphosphate (ADP), creatine, creatine phosphate (CP), and glycogen and a greater increase in lactate concentration with work. Furthermore, the rate of protein synthesis decreases within 6 hours of immobilization.[7, 9, 72, 73, 117]

Immobilization also causes an increase in muscle fatigability as a result of decreased oxidative capacity. Reductions occur in maximum oxygen consumption, glycogen levels, and high-energy phosphate levels.[7, 8, 18, 72, 76] Rifenberick and Max[90] have reported fewer mitochondria in atrophic muscle and a significant decrease in mitochondrial activity by day 7 postimmobilization, causing a reduction in cell respiration and contributing to decreased muscle endurance. The following is a summary of the effects of immobilization on muscle:

1. Decrease in muscle fiber size
2. Decrease in size and number of mitochondria
3. Decrease in total muscle weight
4. Increase in muscle contraction time
5. Decrease in muscle tension produced
6. Decrease in resting levels of glycogen and ATP
7. More rapid decrease in ATP level with exercise
8. Increase in lactate concentration with exercise
9. Decrease in protein synthesis

It appears that there is selective muscle atrophy with immobilization. For example, immobilization of the thigh is often associated with selective atrophy of the quadriceps femoris muscle.[50] It was traditionally believed that the vastus medialis muscle atrophies more than the other quadriceps muscles. However, of the studies available, none supports this theory, and the results of these studies are more suggestive of a uniform atrophy.[66, 137] Clinically, it is observable that quadriceps atrophy is greater than that of the hamstrings. This observation is supported by muscle biopsy, which shows that the loss in muscular bulk is virtually confined to the quadriceps muscle. This has been further supported by computed tomography (CT) studies.[50, 69, 98]

Also, investigators using CT and ultrasonography to measure quadriceps atrophy have reported that thigh circumference measurements, even if supplemented by caliper measurements of subcutaneous fat, underestimate the amount of quadriceps atrophy.[110, 138] Although the knee is the area traditionally noted for selective atrophy, this phenomenon can also be observed in the triceps brachii of an immobilized elbow.[71]

Reflex inhibition can also lead to selective atrophy, particularly in the quadriceps. This type of muscle atrophy is called "arthrogenous muscle wasting," which refers to muscular weakness resulting from injury or from an inflamed joint (Fig. 2–5). This is commonly observed in the quadriceps muscle, and athletes describe it as an inability to contract the quadriceps muscle or as a lack of control over that muscle ("quad shutdown"). This condition was originally ascribed to pain[27] but can have various underlying causes, the least common of which is pain. Most researchers have postulated that this is a reflex phenomenon having several causes, with no single factor being responsible.

The level of quadriceps activation can be determined through electromyography (EMG). The degree of unilateral quadriceps inhibition can be judged by the difference in maximum voluntary activation (MVA) between the two limbs. Research has shown[110] that quadriceps recruitment (quadriceps setting) is severely inhibited after an arthrotomy (with or without a meniscectomy). Maximum voluntary contraction is reduced by 70% to 90% for 3 to 4 days and is usually still about 40% lower than its preoperative level 2 weeks after surgery. Quadriceps inhibition 24 hours after arthroscopy (with or without a meniscectomy), however, is only about one half of that measured after an arthrotomy (with or without a meniscectomy).[102, 110]

It has been postulated that the greater magnitude of quadriceps shutdown after an arthrotomy is a result of the small amount of capsular damage from an arthroscopy versus the "taking down" of the capsule, as in an arthrotomy.[110] The tension in the arthrotomy suture line can evoke afferent impulses from the same receptors that are activated by an increase in intra-articular pressure resulting from an effusion.[129]

Pain has traditionally been regarded as the general cause of reflex inhibition. The perception of fear of pain can greatly affect muscular strength. Athletes who fear that muscle contraction will result in pain may be very apprehensive about contracting those particular muscles, but severe inhibition of muscle strength is seen even after pain subsides.[99] Stokes and Young[110] have noted that postmeniscectomy pain during contraction can be severe during the first 24 hours but, unlike the pain of inhibition, it is usually only mild for the next 3 to 4 days.[101] Ten to 15 days postoperatively, pain is mild or absent, but the athlete may

Figure 2–5. "Vicious cycles" of arthrogenous muscle weakness. (From Stokes, M., and Young A. [1984]: The contribution of reflex inhibition to arthrogenous muscle weakness. Clin. Sci., 67:7.)

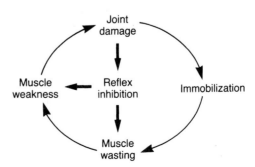

still have quadriceps shutdown. In addition, injection of the meniscal bed and surrounding tissues with an anesthetic temporarily blocks most of the pain, but no change can be detected in quadriceps inhibition.[139]

Tourniquet ischemia has also been thought to contribute to quadriceps shutdown. However, a study involving tourniquet application on normal subjects revealed that quadriceps MVA is unaltered after voluntary ischemia.[109]

Research has shown that a knee distended with plasma can lead to quadriceps shutdown and subsequent quadriceps weakening in normal individuals, even in the absence of pain.[19, 52, 56] Stimuli from a distended knee joint might reflexively inhibit development of muscle strength by a central nervous system pathway.[19] Aspiration of the effusion may decrease the severity of inhibition but rarely abolishes it.[110] Young and associates[138] and others[56] have reported that injection of small volumes of fluid (20 to 30 ml) into normal knees results in a 60% quadriceps inhibition, with the inhibition increasing as infusion increases.

Joint angle has also been shown to have an effect not only on quadriceps inhibition but also on selective atrophy of muscles with regard to the angle of immobilization. Stratford[111] has reported that effusion inhibits quadriceps contraction less when the knee is in 30° of flexion than when it is fully extended. Similar results are found even after arthrotomy with meniscectomy, in that isometric quadriceps contraction is inhibited less in flexion than in extension.[58, 99, 110] It has been postulated that this is because intra-articular pressure is less when the knee is in 30° of flexion versus being in extension.[30, 52, 64, 65, 99]

The length at which the muscle is immobilized also affects selective atrophy. Tardieu and colleagues[114] have suggested that muscle fibers under stretch lengthen by adding sarcomeres in series, whereas those immobilized in a shortened position lose sarcomeres. Thus, when a muscle is immobilized in a lengthened position, the length of the muscle fibers increases to accommodate the muscle's new length, along with occurrence of other connective tissue changes. A similar adjustment occurs with muscle that is immobilized in a shortened position. In this case, the length of the fibers decreases, and the number of sarcomeres is reduced to achieve the physiologic change.[128] Immobilization of a muscle in a shortened position leads to increased connective tissue and reduced muscle extensibility.[114] Garrett[36] has pointed out that muscle immobilization in a lengthened position maintains muscle weight and fiber cross-sectional area better than does immobilization in a shortened position, which may explain selective atrophy of the quadriceps. Because the knee is usually immobilized in an extended or slightly flexed position, the hamstrings are placed in a lengthened position and the quadriceps are in a shortened position.

Although effusion and periarticular damage are plausible reasons for quadriceps inhibition, it appears that inhibition may also be a multifocal phenomenon, with an additional neurophysiologic basis involving the H reflex. The H reflex is a monosynaptic reflex that produces a small muscle contraction in response to low-intensity stimulation of mixed nerves. Infusion of sterile saline solution into the normal knee inhibits the quadriceps H reflex at rest,[49, 106] with the inhibition being more severe during submaximal voluntary contraction.[52]

The measured muscular strength output during a large portion of the rehabilitation period after injury is less a function of innate muscle strength than of the amount of voluntary effort. Various factors appear to affect muscle inhibition in producing a maximal voluntary effort.[36]

Periarticular Connective Tissue

Periarticular connective tissue consists of ligaments, tendons, synovial membrane, fascia, and joint capsule. As a result of immobilization, biochemical and histologic changes occur in periarticular tissue around synovial joints, resulting in arthrofibrosis.

Arthrofibrosis has been referred to as ankylosis, joint stiffness, or a joint contracture.[48] It is a term that describes the pathologic formation of scar tissue around a joint following a surgical procedure or traumatic injury.[86, 107] The characteristic feature is the formation of scar tissue within the joint capsule, the synovium, or the intra-articular spaces.[51]

The two main components of fibrous connective tissue are the cells and an extracellular matrix. The matrix consists primarily of collagen and elastin fibers and a nonfibrous ground substance. Fibrocytes, located between the collagen fibers in fibrous connective tissue, are the main collagen-producing cells. As collagen fibers mature, intra- and intermolecular bonds or cross-links are formed, and these increase in number, thereby providing tensile strength to the fibers.[33, 34, 87] On the basis of the arrangement of its collagen fibers, connective tissue is commonly classified into two types: irregular and regular.[43] The irregular type of connective tissue is characterized by fibers running in different directions in the same plane.[22] This is of functional value for capsules, aponeuroses, and sheaths, which are physiologically stressed in many directions.[22, 43] Conversely, in the regularly arranged tissues, collagen fibers run more or less in the same plane and in the same linear direction.[22] This arrangement affords great tensile strength to ligaments and tendons, which physiologically receive primarily unidirectional stress.[22]

The extracellular matrix is often referred to as ground substance and is composed of glycosaminoglycans (GAGs) and water. To understand the changes that occur with immobilization it is important to be familiar with GAGs and their effect on connective tissue extensibility.[22] Four major GAGs are found in connective tissue: hyaluronic acid, chondroitin-4-sulfate, chondroitin-6-sulfate, and dermatan sulfate. Generally, GAGs are bound to a protein and are collectively referred to as proteoglycans. In connective tissue, proteoglycans combine with water to form a proteoglycan aggregate.

Water constitutes 60% to 70% of the total connective tissue content. GAGs have enormous water-binding capacity and are responsible for this large water content. Together, GAGs and water form a semifluid viscous gel in which collagen and fibrocytes are embedded. Hyaluronic acid with water is thought to serve as a lubricant between the collagen fibers.[4, 43, 113] This lubricant maintains a distance between the fibers, thereby permitting free gliding of the fibers past each other and perhaps preventing excessive cross-linking. Such free gliding is essential for normal connective tissue mobility.[4]

The sliding of collagen fibers across each other, the collagen weave pattern, and the cross-links all can be illustrated by the Chinese finger-trap analogy.[22] When tension is applied to the Chinese finger trap, the trap lengthens to a certain point, as the straw-weave patterns of the trap move across one another (Fig. 2–6). If tension continues to increase once the end point of the trap is reached, the straw fibers will begin to fail. This illustration is not unlike how body connective tissue functions.

Arthrofibrosis is induced primarily by immobilization, which results in a significant reduction in GAG content with subsequent water loss, contributing to abnormal cross-link formation and joint restriction. In addition, within the joint space and recesses, there is excessive connective tissue deposition in the form of fatty fibers, which later mature to form scar tissue that adheres to intra-articular surfaces and restricts motion further.[22]

The most significant reduction of GAG content occurs within the matrix. Akeson and associates[1-4] have reported a 40% decrease in hyaluronic acid and 30% decreases in chondroitin-4-sulfate and chondroitin-6-sulfate; collagen mass decreases by about 10%, and collagen turnover increases, with accelerated degradation and synthesis.[2]

The effects of immobilization on connective tissue can be summarized as follows:

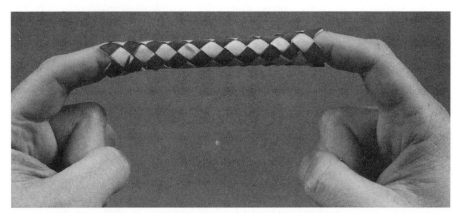

Figure 2–6. Chinese finger trap. The trap can be used to illustrate the sliding of collagen fibers over each other in normal connective tissue.

1. Reduction in water and GAG content, which decreases the extracellular matrix
2. Reduction in extracellular matrix, which is associated with decrease in lubrication between fiber cross-links
3. Reduction in collagen mass
4. Increase in rate of collagen turnover, degradation, and synthesis
5. Increase in abnormal collagen fiber cross-links

The pathophysiology of arthrofibrosis appears to be the reduction in the semifluid gel as a result of loss of GAG and water, causing a decrease in the critical fiber distance between collagen fibers.[22] Friction is created between fibers, thus reducing collagen extensibility. Furthermore, with joint immobilization, the lack of movement perpetuates a random orientation of newly synthesized collagen fibrils, facilitating the development of irregular cross-links in strategic regions of the collagen weave pattern (Fig. 2–7).

Currently, arthrofibrosis most commonly affects the knee joint, particularly as a complication after anterior cruciate ligament (ACL) reconstructive surgery, in which the operative knee develops a thicker joint capsule and a secondary flexion contracture. Arthrofibrosis of the knee joint is characterized by a lack of flexion as well as of extension (the most commonly involved motion is extension). Prolonged joint immobilization is the most recognized risk factor for the development of arthrofibrosis. Microscopic examination of a knee with

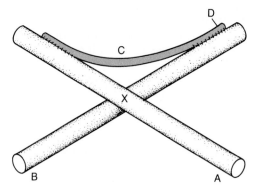

Figure 2–7. Idealized model of the interaction of collagen cross-links at the molecular level. A, B, pre-existing fibers; C, newly synthesized fibril; D, cross-links created as the fibril becomes incorporated into the fiber; X, point at which adjacent fibers are normally freely movable past each other. (Reprinted from Biorheology, 17, W.H. Akeson, D. Armiel, and S. Woo, Immobility effects of synovial joints: The pathomechanics of joint contracture, 95, 1980, with permission from Elsevier Science Ltd, The Boulevard, Langford Lane, Kidlington 0X5 1GB, UK.)

arthrofibrosis shows a proliferation of fibroblasts and an associated accumulation of extracellular matrix. The principal component of the matrix is type I collagen that is specifically found as an unorganized network of fibers.[5] Although these findings are well-recognized, the etiology underlying the formation of the exuberant scar tissue is less clear.

With a lack of experimental studies and suitable animal models, the pathophysiology of arthrofibrosis remains poorly understood. However, several theories have been proposed to explain and prevent this condition. Shelbourne et al[100] have recommended delaying reconstructive surgery on acutely injured ACLs until the knee joint recovers from the initial trauma. The authors have suggested delaying surgery by at least 3 weeks from the time of the acute ACL injury, thus enabling the knee-joint swelling and inflammation to diminish, pain to subside, and motion to improve. Although these guidelines appear clinically relevant, other theories exist.

Other researchers suggest that arthrofibrosis is more a variation of a normal healing response than an entirely abnormal reaction to surgery or injury. Wound healing within the joint capsule normally follows a well-characterized cascade of cellular and molecular events (discussed previously). In this cascade, each cellular phase and subsequent matrix synthesis phases have a well-regulated onset and conclusion. Once scar tissue has formed within the wound, a complete and highly regulated remodeling process replaces that scar tissue with more differentiated and specialized capsular tissue. This step is essential in the wound healing process because the demands on the knee require joint capsular tissue that has specific biomechanical properties such as strength and elasticity. Arthrofibrosis is the result of a breakdown at any step of the complex repair process.

Fibrosis results from increased numbers of collagen-synthesizing cells (from proliferation and from recruitment), increased synthesis by existing cells, or deficient collagen degradation with continued collagen synthesis.[125] Injury-induced inflammation precedes the repair process; therefore, precise regulation and control of the inflammatory response will have a direct impact on the timing and amount of fibrosis during healing. Growth factors present within the injury hematoma, such as transforming growth factor-β, have been shown to directly stimulate fibrosis in a dose-dependent fashion.[53] Inhibition of these factors may ultimately reduce the occurrence or severity of arthrofibrosis, independent of joint immobilization. Another possibility for the prevention of arthrofibrosis focuses on the accumulation of interstitial collagens. In fibrosis, the pathologic accumulation of collagen may reflect alteration not only in matrix synthesis but also in matrix degradation. Enzyme-enhanced degradation of collagen may be beneficial in fibrotic tissue, but further understanding of this process is required before specific regulation of enzymatic matrix degradation can be attempted. A fine balance between matrix synthesis and degradation must be maintained to achieve a strong repair without excessive matrix production and its associated arthrofibrosis.

Early recognition of arthrofibrosis is important, and its prevention is paramount. Arthrofibrosis can be divided into three phases (Table 2–1). Decreasing joint effusion, early muscle turn-on, and pain modulation are key components affecting the arthrofibrotic loop (Fig. 2–8). Arthrofibrotic lesions can usually be prevented by the following[74]: (1) early turn-on of muscle; (2) control of hemarthrosis; (3) control of pain; (4) control of postsurgical scarring; and (5) preoperative education of patients to increase rehabilitation compliance.

Movement is essential in the prevention of contractures and the formation of adhesions within joints. Physical forces and motion modulate the synthesis of proteoglycans and collagen in normal joints. Stress and motion also influence the deposition of newly synthesized collagen fibers, allowing for proper orientation of collagen to resist tensile stress. Motion appears to inhibit periarticular tissue contractures by the following mechanisms[133]:

Table 2-1. Stages of Arthrofibrosis

STAGE	PHASE	COMMENTS
I	Acute (first 3 weeks)	*Goal:* Prevention of complications 1. Early identification of a problem that could lead to complications 2. Early muscle turn-on to avoid "shutdown" 3. Reduction of hemarthrosis
II	Subacute (weeks 3 to 8)	1. Constant evaluation necessary because 10% of patients may enter the fibrosis stage as early as 10 days postoperatively 2. Rehabilitation geared toward controlling stress on contracted tissues; includes joint mobilization techniques, low-force overpressure, isometrics in the shortened position, and a home program for motion restoration 6–8 times daily 3. Neurophysiologic response of the muscle increased through electrical muscle stimulation and proprioception techniques
III	Chronic (more than 10 weeks)	The patient, through a conservative program or lack of compliance, enters a dangerous period, during which reversal may not occur in 10% of patients *Goal:* Reversal of loss of motion and scar tissue buildup 1. Characterized by ingrowth of tissue into the joint and tightness of periarticular structures 2. Treatment consists of careful manipulation or surgical lysis, followed by NSAIDs and careful implementation of a rehabilitation program

Data from Mangine, R. (1990): The complicated knee: A loss of motion. *In*: 1990 Advances on the Knee and Shoulder. Cincinnati, Cincinnati Sports Medicine and Deaconess Hospital, Symposium held April 2–4, 1990. NSAIDs, Nonsteroidal anti-inflammatory drugs.

1. Stimulation of proteoglycan synthesis, thereby lubricating and maintaining a critical distance between existing fibers
2. Ordering (rather than randomizing) the disposition of new collagen fibers to resist tensile stress
3. Preventing formation of anomalous cross-links in the matrix by preventing a stationary fiber-fiber attitude at intercept points

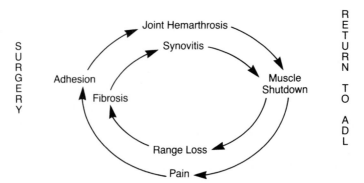

Figure 2-8. Arthrofibrotic loop. *Outer loop*, Acute phase. *Inner loop*, Subacute phase. (From Mangine, R. [1990]: The complicated knee: A loss of motion. *In*: 1990 Advances on the Knee and Shoulder. Cincinnati, Cincinnati Sports Medicine and Deaconess Hospital. Symposium held April 2–4, 1990.)

The matrix changes associated with immobilization (noted above) are relatively uniform in ligaments, capsules, tendons, and fasciae. These changes involve extracellular water loss and GAG depletion, along with collagen cross-link changes.

Articular Cartilage

Articular cartilage is a thin covering on the ends of bones that creates the moving surfaces of synovial joints.[127] It varies from 1 to 7 mm in thickness, with the cartilage covering larger, weight-bearing joints (e.g., hip and knee joints) being thicker than that covering smaller, non–weight-bearing joints.[127, 134] Articular cartilage consists of fibers, ground substance, and cells. The fibers are composed of collagen and make up 57% to 75% of the dry weight of the cartilage.[120] The ground substance is similar to that of periarticular tissue and consists of water (70% to 80%) and proteoglycans (15% to 30%).[24, 120, 126] The quantity of proteoglycans in articular cartilage depends on joint location, with weight-bearing joints having a higher proteoglycan content than non–weight-bearing joints.[119] Both collagen and proteoglycans are produced by chondrocytes.

Articular cartilage is avascular, and its nutritional requirements are met through diffusion and osmosis. Diffusion occurs through a hydraulic pressure gradient. Low hydraulic pressure has no effect, whereas constant pressure interferes with nutrition.[127] High intermittent pressure loading does not contribute much to the diffusion rate.[75] Joint motion, however, increases the diffusion rate to three to four times the static level,[75] but joint motion in the absence of loading fails to maintain the nutrition of articular cartilage.[85]

The various effects of immobilization appear to depend on the length of immobilization, the position of immobilization, and joint loading. Cartilage degradation has been reported in rabbits as early as 1 week after immobilization,[16, 56] with a gradual progression of the degenerative process as immobilization continues.[170] Prolonged knee-joint immobilization in forced full extension results in full-thickness loss of articular cartilage and infiltration of intra-articular adhesions.[95] Even periodic short-term immobilization results in cumulative, harmful effects to joints.[122] Periodic immobilization longer than 30 days can lead to progressive osteoarthritis.[123]

The effects of immobilization on articular cartilage can be separated into contact and noncontact effects. In contact areas, the seriousness of the changes depends mainly on the degree of compression; in noncontact areas, it depends on the ingrowth of connective tissue on the articular surface.[55] Compression of articular cartilage decreases the synovial fluid diffusion rate and leads to pressure necrosis and chondrocyte death as a result of constant joint compression.[88, 121] Whether the lesions are reversible depends directly on the duration of continuous compression.[95] Also, loss of contact between opposed articular surfaces in weight-bearing and non–weight-bearing joints appears to lead to degenerative changes, suggesting a functional relationship between joint motion and normal articular cartilage surface contact.[42, 121]

The effects of immobilization on articular cartilage can be summarized as follows:

1. Decrease in proteoglycan synthesis
2. Softening of articular cartilage
3. Decrease in articular cartilage thickness
4. Adherence of fibrofatty connective tissue to cartilage surfaces
5. Pressure necrosis at points of cartilage-cartilage contact
6. Death of chondrocytes

Intermittent joint loading appears to have a critical role in maintaining healthy articular cartilage. The formation and circulation of synovial and interstitial fluids are stimulated with intermittent joint loading and retarded in its absence. Because synovial fluid is important in cartilage nourishment and lubrication, intermittent pressure can facilitate chondrocyte nourishment and is important for cell function.[11, 23, 25] Conversely, joint immobilization in which the joint is constantly loaded or unloaded can compromise the metabolic exchange necessary for proper structure and function, eventually leading to cartilage degradation and eburnation.[28, 61, 102, 117] Immobilization of knees in extension leads to irreversible and progressive osteoarthritis. The compression between articular surfaces increases in the immobilized knee and, after 4 weeks of immobilization, reaches a level that is three times greater than the initial level.[122] Further evidence in support of the concept of intermittent joint compression is that joint motion without loading during the immobilization period does not prevent deterioration of the articular cartilage.[42]

As a result of immobilization, articular cartilage undergoes structural, biochemical, and physiologic changes at the cellular and ultrastructural levels.[127] Consistently reported changes include the following: fibrillation, fraying, cyst formation, and loss of staining characteristics of the extracellular ground substance; varying degrees of chondrocyte degeneration, causing cell death and necrosis; cartilage proliferation at joint edges; atrophy in weight-bearing areas and regional bony eburnation; sclerosis; and cartilage resorption after 2 weeks of immobilization. These changes are generally irreversible, but the length of immobilization is important in determining whether the articular changes are irreversible.

Ligaments

Ligaments, like other connective tissue, undergo the same changes in structure as do other elements in periarticular tissue. However, because of the function of ligaments and because of the bone-ligament interface, additional factors must be considered to understand the response of ligaments to immobilization.

Like bone, a ligament appears to remodel in response to the mechanical demands placed on it. Stress results in a stiffer, stronger ligament, whereas inactivity yields a weaker, more compliant structure.[15] These changes in properties appear to be caused more by an alteration in the mechanical properties of ligaments and by subperiosteal resorption at the bone-ligament junction than by actual ligament atrophy.[63, 82] The alterations lead to a decrease in the tensile strength of the ligament and thus reduce the ability of ligaments to provide joint stability. Ligaments respond to immobilization by undergoing various alterations.[2, 6, 35, 81, 131]

1. Significant decrease in linear stress, maximum stress, and stiffness
2. Decrease in cross-sectional area of the ligament fibril, resulting in reduction of fibril size and density
3. Decrease in synthesis and degradation of collagen
4. Haphazard arrangement of new collagen fibers
5. Reduction in load and in energy-absorbing capabilities of the bone-ligament complex
6. Decrease in GAG level
7. Increase in osteoclastic activity at the bone-ligament junction, causing an increase in bone resorption in that area

Chemical changes in the medial collateral ligament (MCL) of the knee can be detected as early as 2 weeks after immobilization. By 9 weeks there is significant collagen degradation, with an additional decline in mechanical properties at 12 weeks postimmobilization.[35, 131, 132] This results in a decrease of tensile properties, with a decreased time to failure. In primates, immobilization of the lower limbs led to a 40% decrease in maximum load to failure and to a significant decrease in energy absorbed before failure in their ACLs.[81] Most of these failures occurred at the bone-ligament junction.[81, 116] Furthermore, 5 months of postimmobilization reconditioning proved ineffective in restoring the ligament complex to its original state.[81, 87] However, at 12 months, the strength and stiffness characteristics of the ligament were equal to those in the original state; but increased strength at the insertion site may be restored more slowly.[81, 87]

High-frequency, low-duration endurance exercises have been shown to have a positive influence on the mechanical properties of ligaments.[15] Such exercises may even lead to ligament hypertrophy as a result of increased collagen production and hypertrophy of the fiber bundle.[1] It appears, however, that an isometric exercise program during immobilization cannot stimulate or substitute for the normal physiologic loading of weight bearing and, therefore, cannot prevent ligaments from decreasing in strength.[10]

Bone

The effects of immobilization on bone are similar to those on other connective tissues. A consistent finding in response to diminished weight bearing and muscle contraction is bone loss. Bone changes can be detected as early as 2 weeks after immobilization.[44, 79, 119] Although the pathogenesis of immobilization osteoporosis is unclear, animal studies have shown decreased bone formation and increased bone resorption.[14, 32, 37, 60] Similar findings were noted in patients for whom total bed rest was prescribed.[21]

Bone hardness decreases steadily with the duration of immobilization, dropping to 55% to 60% of normal by 12 weeks.[108] There is also a decline in elastic resistance—the bone becomes more brittle and thus more susceptible to fracture.

It appears that mechanical strain influences osteoblastic and osteoclastic activity on the bone surface.[26] Bone loss from disuse atrophy occurs at a rate 5 to 20 times greater than that resulting from metabolic disorders affecting bone.[77] The primary cause of this immobilization osteoporosis appears to be the mechanical unloading, which may be responsible for the inhibition of bone formation during immobilization.[135] Therefore, non–weight-bearing immobilization of an extremity should be limited to as short a period as possible.

CONTINUOUS PASSIVE MOTION

Salter,[94] in 1970, originated the biologic concept of continuous passive motion (CPM) of synovial joints to stimulate healing, regenerate articular tissue, and avoid the harmful effects of immobilization.[68] In 1978, Salter and Saringer (an engineer) collaborated to develop the first CPM device for humans (Fig. 2–9).[94] A CPM machine is an electrical, motor-driven device that helps support the injured limb. It is used to move a joint at variable rates through progressively increasing ranges of motion; no muscular exertion is required of the patient.

Salter and colleagues[94, 95] provided the first histologic evidence in support of CPM. They reported[94, 97] that CPM significantly stimulates healing of articular tissues, including cartilage, tendons, and ligaments; it prevents adhesions and joint stiffness; it does not interfere with healing of incisions over the moving joint; and it influences the regeneration of articular cartilage through neochondrogenesis.

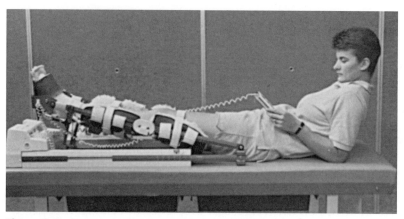

Figure 2–9. Continuous passive motion device for the knee.

When compared to immobilization of tendons, CPM has proved effective in increasing linear and maximum stress, linear load, and ultimate strength for tendons.[68] Salter and Minster[96] have also reported preliminary results of semi-tendinous tenodesis for MCL reconstruction in experimental animals, in which increased strength was reported after CPM. The application of early tensile forces appears to facilitate the proper alignment of collagen fibers during the initial healing process. Also, decreases in medication requests and decreases in wound edema and effusion in operative knees were reported in patients undergoing CPM.[87, 84] The greatest benefit of CPM appears to be the prevention of articular cartilage degradation. Salter[94] has reported that there appears to be more rapid and complete healing in cartilage defects in rabbits when CPM is used.

There has been some concern about the early use of CPM after autogenous patellar tendon reconstruction of the ACL with respect to potentially detrimental damage to the graft. The literature does support the early use of CPM in this patient population; CPM resulted in greater knee range of motion, less swelling and effusion, use of less pain medication, and no change in joint stability when comparisons were made to subjects who did not use CPM.[83, 136] More recently, the use of CPM and its effect on outcomes after ACL surgery have been assessed. There has been concern that the use of immediate passive motion after ACL surgery may stretch or rupture the graft.[12] However, other studies support the early use of passive motion and report the following benefits[78, 83, 136]:

- No deleterious effects on the stability of the ligament
- Decrease in joint swelling and effusion
- Decrease in pain medication taken
- Increase in knee range of motion sooner

More recently, Rosen and colleagues[91] found no significant differences between those patients who began early motion and those patients who began early active motion with no CPM. They did not find an improvement in the results after the routine use of postoperative CPM when compared to results obtained after initiation of early mobilization and supervised rehabilitation within the first month of rehabilitation.

CPM units are considered an acceptable practice after most orthopedic surgeries. Although initially designed for the lower extremities, CPM units are now available for the upper extremities as well. CPM has helped stem the deleterious effects of immobilization by allowing early motion, even in a protected range of motion. Some indications for the use of CPM include ligament reconstruction or repair, total joint replacement, joint contracture release, tendon repair, open reduction of fractures, and articular cartilage defects.

EFFECTS OF REMOBILIZATION

Physical forces provide important stimuli to tissues for the development and maintenance of homeostasis.[130] The lack of or denial of mobilization results in deleterious effects on bone, muscle, connective tissue, and articular cartilage. The advent of CPM in the late 1970s and early 1980s provided an impetus for initiating early motion to repair tissues and for using early electrical stimulation of muscle to decrease atrophy and promote early muscle re-education. In addition, the emergence of hinged braces, which allow for early protected motion, has helped foster early mobilization.

Early motion and loading and unloading of joints through partial weight bearing promote the diffusion of synovial fluid to nourish articular cartilage, meniscus, and ligaments. Moreover, research has shown that motion enhances this transsynovial nutrient flow.[65, 75, 89] Regardless of the cell-stimulating mechanism, it is clear that the fibroblasts and chondrocytes respond to physical forces by increasing their rate of synthesis, and extracellular degradation of matrix components is similarly controlled.[2]

Immobilization through casting techniques is still used, however, in the treatment of many ligamentous reconstructions and fractures. It is not known whether the deleterious effects of prolonged immobilization can be reversed with remobilization techniques. These structural changes generally appear to depend on the duration and angle of immobilization and on the weight-bearing status.

Muscle

Muscle responds to remobilization more readily than do other connective tissue structures. Muscle regeneration begins within 3 to 5 days after initiation of a reconditioning program.[18, 141] By 6 weeks postimmobilization, it appears that both fast-twitch and slow-twitch muscle fibers can recover completely.[129] Protein synthesis is rapidly increased in response to major changes in muscle contractile activity.[118] Booth and Seider[9] have reported that in rats, after 90 days of immobilization, ATP, glycogen, and protein concentrations return to control levels by recovery day 60. Soleus muscle wasting and protein content return to control levels by day 14. Maximum isometric tension does not return to normal, however, until day 120. Thus, the biochemical and physiologic changes that occur after skeletal muscle immobilization do return to normal, but at differing times following termination of immobilization.

It has been theorized that electrical muscle stimulation (EMS) can provide enough muscle activity to deter atrophy and the deleterious effects of immobilization on muscle. Most studies on the effects of EMS have been on normal muscle, and investigations concerning effects on diseased, traumatized, or immobilized muscle have not been as well reported. Initial investigations yielded promising results, but more recent studies have been less encouraging. Sisk and colleagues[103] have reported that EMS in conjunction with exercise after ACL reconstruction has no significant benefit compared to 9 weeks of exercise alone. Also, EMS to the quadriceps muscle appears not to be significant enough to alter quadriceps atrophy[39-41, 80] or to affect the muscle enzyme changes that result from immobilization.[40, 41]

Although research has shown that EMS does not significantly change the process of muscle atrophy, it has been postulated that using EMS may be better than not exercising at all.[59, 80] EMS can be most helpful in re-educating muscle, abating pain and spasm, and decreasing effusion through the pumping action of the muscle as it contracts.

Unfortunately, it appears that neither EMS nor isometric exercise is of enough help to prevent disuse atrophy.[39–41] Although the use of EMS and of braces that allow for early limited range of motion can decrease atrophy to some extent, they do not adequately replace the amount and type of contractile activity.[7] It appears that the only way to prevent muscle atrophy in immobilized limbs is to replace the muscle usage lost through limb immobilization with muscle contractions of equivalent quantity and quality.

Articular Cartilage

The effects of remobilization on articular cartilage seem to be time-dependent. Many studies have examined the effects on articular cartilage of remobilization after a period of immobilization. Evans and coworkers[29] have reported alterations in cartilage such as matrix fibrillation, cleft formation, and ulceration that are not reversible in rats after immobilization for up to 90 days. They noted, however, that soft tissue changes are reversible if the period of immobilization does not exceed 30 days. Finsterbush and Friedman[31] also noted similar irreversible damage in remobilization experiments. Articular cartilage generally responds favorably to mechanical stimuli, with structural modifications noted after exercise.[47, 93] Furthermore, studies showed that exercising on a treadmill for 1 to 6 hours daily did not contribute to an increased occurrence of joint degeneration in mice.[62] This observation has been further supported by Jurvelin and colleagues,[54] whose animal studies revealed remarkable changes in articular cartilage within the first week of immobilization; running exercises up to 8 weeks, however, elicited only transitory to minor alterations in articular surface.

It has been speculated that the limitation of joint movement, whether there is contact or loss of contact between joint surfaces, produces changes by interfering with cartilage nutrition, which relies on loading and unloading of a joint for nourishment and diffusion. This is supported by research showing that articular cartilage changes still occur, even in mobilized joints, if weight bearing is not allowed.[42]

Bone

Immobilization results in disuse osteoporosis, which may not be reversible on remobilization of the limb. The reversibility is related to the severity of changes and to the length of immobilization. Permanent osseous changes appear to occur with an immobilization period exceeding 12 weeks.[140] Even though bone lost in the first 12 weeks is regained, the period of recovery is at least as long as and may be many times longer than the immobilization period.[13] The most effective means of modifying osteoporosis caused by reduced skeletal loads appears to be through exercise. Isotonic and isometric exercises decreased bone loss in subjects who were exposed to prolonged periods of weightlessness and bed rest.[70, 124] Activity increases bone formation in these situations and can hasten recovery after return to a normal loading environment. If an appropriate environment can be maintained during immobilization of a limb, the deleterious effects of disuse on bone can be partially prevented, and rehabilitation can be accelerated.[13]

Ligaments

Remobilization after immobilization of ligaments occurs in an asynchronous fashion. It appears that the bone-ligament junction recovers at a much slower rate than do the mechanical or midsubstance properties of the ligament.[131, 132] Cabaud and colleagues[15] have reported that ligament strength and stiffness in rat ACLs can increase with endurance-type exercises. Others have noted similar results.[54, 55] Moreover, not only does the injured ligament result in weaker mechanical properties at midsubstance and at the bone-ligament complex, but nontraumatized ligaments become weaker as a result of immobilization. These weakened mechanical ligament properties must be considered when a rehabilitation program is being planned.

Recovery from immobilization depends on the duration of immobilization. Woo and associates[131] have noted that 1 year of remobilization is required before the architectural components of the MCL-tibia junction return to normal after 12 weeks of immobilization. Noyes[81] has reported that in primates, after 5 months of remobilization following total body immobilization, there is only partial recovery in ligament strength, although ligament stiffness and compliance parameters return to control values. It was reported that 12 months are required for complete recovery of ligament strength parameters.[81] Tipton and coworkers[115] have observed a recovery of 50% of normal strength in a healing ligament by 6 months, of 80% after 1 year, and of 100% after 1 to 3 years, depending on the type of stresses placed on the ligament and on the prevention of repeated injury.

It appears that properties of ligaments return to normal with remobilization, but this depends on the duration of the immobilization, with the bone-ligament junction taking longer to return to normal after immobilization.

Connective Tissue

Few studies have documented the effects of remobilization after immobilization on formation of cross-links.[22] Movement maintains lubrication and critical fiber distance within the matrix and ensures an orderly deposition of collagen fibrils, thereby preventing abnormal cross-link formation.[22] Often, for range of motion to be restored, forceful manipulation that breaks the intracapsular fibrofatty adhesions may have to be performed.[22] Although range of motion is restored, it has been speculated that there is peeling of the fibrofatty tissue from the bone ends, with ragged edges of adhesions remaining in the joint.[25, 29] There is also increased joint inflammation from the manipulation, enhancing the potential for chronic synovitis.

SUMMARY

Motion problems should be detected early, joint end-feel should be assessed by palpation, and the reason for the motion problem should be determined. If manipulation is the treatment of choice, it should be performed early in the recovery process to decrease the amount of joint damage resulting from a manipulation and to prevent the connective tissue changes from becoming morphologic changes.

The deleterious effects of immobilization on bone and connective tissue have been widely reported. The efficacy of early, controlled mobilization to allow orderly organization of collagen along lines of stress and to promote healthy joint arthrokinematics is supported by many studies. Acute injury that is not treated adequately by early concentration on decreasing joint effusion and pain and restoration of normal joint arthrokinematics can result in a vicious inflammatory cycle; this perpetuates the degradation of articular cartilage by the enzymes released after cell death. This articular cartilage damage is a secondary injury induced by inadequate attention to decreasing the severity of the early inflammatory process.

The harmful effects of immobilization on muscle are the most obvious changes.

Muscle atrophy can be detected as early as 24 hours after immobilization. Muscle responds to immobilization by decreases in muscle fiber size, total muscle weight, mitochondria size and number, muscle tension produced, resting levels of glycogen and ATP, and protein synthesis. With exercise, there is an increase in the muscle contraction time and in the lactate level.

Muscle shutdown is a phenomenon generally seen after immobilization, but it can also be readily detected after most surgeries. It is observed in the quadriceps muscle after knee surgery. Although many reasons for muscle shutdown have been postulated, it appears to be affected by one or more of the following factors: joint effusion, angle of joint immobilization, periarticular tissue damage from surgery or trauma, and the H reflex.

Immobilization leads to biochemical and histochemical changes in the periarticular tissue, ultimately contributing to arthrofibrosis. Immobilization-induced arthrofibrosis has been widely documented, although the exact mechanism is still speculative. Connective tissue usually responds to immobilization by a reduction in water and glycosaminoglycan content; a decrease in the extracellular matrix, which leads to a reduction in the lubrication between fiber cross-links; a decrease in collagen mass; an increase in collagen turnover, degradation, and synthesis rates; and an increase in abnormal collagen fiber cross-links.

Ligaments are similarly affected by immobilization. It appears that the bone-ligament junction undergoes an increase in osteoclastic activity, resulting in a weaker bone-ligament junction. There is also ligament atrophy, with a corresponding decrease in linear stress, maximum stress, and stiffness.

The greatest insult from immobilization appears to be on the articular cartilage. The intermittent loading and unloading of synovial joints promotes the metabolic exchange necessary for the proper structure and function of articular cartilage. Joint immobilization, in which articular cartilage is in constant contact with opposing bone ends, can cause pressure necrosis. Conversely, noncontact between joint surfaces can promote ingrowth of connective tissue into the joint. Diminished weight bearing and loading and unloading of an extremity also cause an increase in bone resorption in that area.

CPM devices allow for early joint motion, with no detrimental side effects. CPM has a significantly stimulating effect on healing articular tissues, including cartilage, tendons, and ligaments, and also prevents joint adhesions and stiffness. Patients using CPM devices have shown a decrease in joint hemarthrosis and in requests for pain medication.

Tissues appear to recover at different rates with remobilization after immobilization, with muscle recovering the fastest. Although few studies on the effects of remobilization on immobilized connective tissue have been reported, it has been proved that early mobilization maintains lubrication and a critical fiber distance among collagen fibrils in the matrix, thus preventing abnormal cross-link formation. After immobilization, articular cartilage and bone respond the least favorably to remobilization. Changes in articular cartilage depend on the length and angle of immobilization. Prolonged immobilization can result in irreversible changes in articular cartilage .

Early protected motion and weight bearing, as healing restraints allow, are therefore advocated to avoid the deleterious effects of immobilization and to deter the secondary problems perpetuated by immobilization.

References

1. Akeson, W.H., Woo, S.L.-Y., Amiel, D., et al. (1984): The chemical basis of tissue repair. *In:* Hunter, L.Y., and Funk, F.J. (eds.): Rehabilitation of the Injured Knee. St. Louis, C.V. Mosby, pp. 93–148.
2. Akeson, W.H., Amiel, D., Abel, M.F., et al. (1987): Effects of immobilization on joints. Clin. Orthop., 219:28–37.
3. Akeson, W.H., Amiel, D., and LaViolette, D. (1967): The connective tissue response to immobil-

ity: A study of the chondroitin-4- and 6-sulfate and dermatan sulfate changes in periarticular connective tissue of control and immobilized knee of dogs. Clin. Orthop., 51:183–197.

4. Akeson, W.H., Amiel, D., and Woo, S. (1980): Immobility effects of synovial joints: The pathomechanics of joint contracture. Biorheology, 17:95–110.

5. Akeson, W.H., Woo, SL-Y, Amiel, D., et al. (1973): The connective tissue response to immobility: Biochemical changes in periarticular connective tissue of the immobilized rabbit knee. Clin. Orthop., 356-362.

6. Binkley, J.M., and Peat, M. (1986): The effects of immobilization on the ultrastructure and mechanical properties of the medial collateral ligament of rats. Clin. Orthop. Rel. Res., 203:301–308.

7. Booth, F.W. (1987): Physiologic and biochemical effects of immobilization on muscle. Clin. Orthop. Rel. Res., 219:15–20.

8. Booth, F.W., and Kelso, J.R. (1973): Effect of hindlimb immobilization on contractile and histochemical properties of skeletal muscle. Pflugers Arch., 342:231–238.

9. Booth, F.W., and Seider, M.J. (1979): Recovery of skeletal muscle after 3 months of hindlimb immobilization in rats. J. Appl. Physiol., 47:435–439.

10. Bozdech, Z. (1976): Posttraumatic synovitis. Acta Chir. Orthop. Traumatol. Cech., 43:244–247.

11. Broom, N.D., and Myers, D.B. (1980): A study of the structural response of wet hyaline cartilage to various loading situations. Connect. Tissue Res., 7:227–237.

12. Burks, R., Daniel, D., and Losse, G. (1984). The effect of continuous passive motion on anterior cruciate ligament reconstruction stability. Am. J. Sports Med., 12:323–327.

13. Burr, D.B., Frederickson, R.G., Pavlinch, C., et al. (1984): Intracast muscle stimulation prevents bone and cartilage deterioration in cast-immobilized rabbits. Clin. Orthop. Rel. Res., 189:264–278.

14. Burdeaux, B.D., and Hutchinson, W.J. (1953): Etiology of traumatic osteoporosis. J. Bone Joint Surg. [Am.], 35:479–488.

15. Cabaud, H.E., Chatty, A., and Gildengorin, V. (1980): Exercise effects on the strength of the rat anterior cruciate ligament. Am. J. Sports Med., 8:79–86.

16. Candolin, T., and Videman, T. (1980): Surface changes in the articular cartilage of rabbit knee during immobilization. A scanning electron microscopic study of experimental osteoarthritis. Acta Pathol. Microbiol. Immunol. Scand., 88:291–296.

17. Castor, C.W., Prince, R.K., and Hazelton, M.J. (1966): Hyaluronic acid in human synovial effusions: A sensitive indicator of altered connective tissue cell function during inflammation. Arthritis Rheum., 9:783–794.

18. Cooper, R.R. (1972): Alternatives during immobilization and regeneration of skeletal muscle in cats. J. Bone Joint Surg. [Am.], 54:919–953.

19. DeAndrade, J.R., Grant, C., and Dixon, A. (1965): Joint distension and reflex inhibition in the knee. J. Bone Joint Surg. [Am.], 47:313–322.

20. Dickinson, A., and Bennett, K.M. (1985): Therapeutic exercise. Clin. Sports Med., 4:417–429.

21. Donaldson, C.L., Hulley, S.B., Vogel, J.M., et al. (1970): Effect of prolonged bed rest on bone mineral. Metabolism, 19:1071–1084.

22. Donatelli, R., and Owens-Burkhart, A. (1981): Effects of immobilization on the extensibility of periarticular connective tissue. J. Orthop. Sports Phys. Ther., 3: 67–72.

23. Ekholm, R. (1955): Nutrition of articular cartilage: A radioautographic study. Acta Anat., 24:329–338.

24. Elliot R.J., and Gardner, D.L. (1979): Changes with age of the glycosaminoglycans of human cartilage. Ann. Rheum. Dis., 38:371–377.

25. Enneking, W.F., and Horowitz, M. (1972): The intra-articular effects of immobilization on the human knee. J. Bone Joint Surg. [Am.], 54:973–985.

26. Epker, B.N., and Frost, H.M. (1965): Correlation of bone resorption and formation behavior of loaded bone. J. Dent. Res., 44:33–41.

27. Eriksson, E. (1981): Rehabilitation of muscle function after sports injury—major problem in sports medicine. Int. J. Sports Med., 2:1–6.

28. Eronen. I., Videman, T., Friman, C., and Michelesson, J.E. (1978): Glycosaminoglycan metabolism in experimental osteoarthritis caused by immobilization. Acta Orthop. Scand., 49:329–334.

29. Evans, E.B., Egger, G.W.N., Butler, M., and Blumel, J. (1960): Experimental immobilization and remobilization of rat knee joints. J. Bone Joint Surg. [Am.], 42:737–758.

30. Eyring, E.J., and Murray, W.R. (1964): The effect of joint position on the pressure of intra-articular effusion. J. Bone Joint Surg. [Am.], 46:1235–1241.

31. Finsterbush, A., and Friedman, B. (1975): Reversibility of joint changes produced by immobilization in rabbits. Clin. Orthop., 111:290–298.

32. Fleisch, H., Russell, R.G., Simpson, B., and Muhlbauer, R.C. (1969): Prevention by a diphosphonate of immobilization osteoporosis in rats. Nature, 223:211:212.

33. Freeman, M.A.R. (1979): Adult Articular Cartilage, 2nd ed. Tunbridge Wells, U.K., Pitman Medical, pp. 183–196.

34. Fujimoto, D., Moriquichi, T., Ishida, T., and Hayashi, H. (1978): The structure of pyridinoline, a collagen cross link. Biochem. Biophys. Res. Commun., 84:52–57.

35. Gamble, J.G., Edwards, C.C., and Max, S.R. (1984): Enzymatic adaptation in ligaments during immobilization. Am. J. Sports Med., 12:221–228.

36. Garrett, G.E. (1989): Effects of injury on muscle and the patellofemoral joint. In: 1989 Advances

on the Knee and Shoulder. Cincinnati, Cincinnati Sports Medicine and Deaconess Hospital, Symposium held March 6–8, 1989.

37. Geiser, M., and Trueta, J. (1985): Muscle action, bone rarefaction, and bone formation. J. Bone Joint Surg. [Br.], 40:282–311.

38. Golden, A. (1980): Reaction to injury in the musculoskeletal system. *In:* Rosse, C., and Clawson, D.K. (eds.): The Musculoskeletal System in Health and Disease. New York, Harper & Row, pp. 89–93.

39. Halkjaer-Kristensen, J., and Ingemann-Hansen, T. (1985): Wasting of the human quadriceps muscle after knee ligament injuries. I. Anthropometrical consequences. Scand. J. Med. (Suppl.), 13:5–11.

40. Halkjaer-Kristensen, J., and Ingemann-Hansen, T. (1985): Wasting of the human quadriceps muscle after knee ligament injuries. II. Muscle fibre morphology. Scand. J. Med. (Suppl.), 13:12–20.

41. Halkjaer-Kristensen, J., and Ingemann-Hansen, T. (1985): Wasting of the human quadriceps muscle after knee ligament injuries. III. Oxidative and glycolytic enzyme activities. Scand. J. Med. (Suppl.), 13:21–28.

42. Hall, M.C. (1963): Cartilage changes after experimental relief of contact in the knee of the mature rat. J. Bone Joint Surg. [Am.], 45:36–44.

43. Ham, A.C., and Cormack, D. (1979): Histology, 8th ed. Philadelphia, J.B. Lippincott.

44. Hardt, A.B. (1972): Early metabolic responses of bone to immobilization. J. Bone Joint Surg. [Am.], 54:119–124.

45. Hettinga, D.L. (1979): I. Normal joint structures and their reaction to injury. J. Orthop. Sports Phys. Ther., 1:16–22.

46. Hettinga, D.L. (1979): II. Normal joint structures and their reaction to injury. J. Orthop. Sports Phys. Ther., 1:83–88.

47. Holmdahl, D.E., and Ingelmark, B.E. (1948): Des Gelenkknorpels unter verschiedenen funktionellen Verhältnissen. Acta Anat. (Basel), 7:309–375.

48. Hughston, J.C. (1985). Complications of anterior cruciate ligament surgery. Orthop. Clin. North Am., 16: 237–240.

49. Iles, J.F., Stokes, M., and Young, A. (1985): Reflex actions of knee joint receptors on quadriceps in man. J. Physiol., 360:48P.

50. Ingemann-Hansen, T., and Halkjaer-Kristensen, J. (1980): Computerized tomographic determination of human thigh components. The effects of immobilization in plaster and subsequent physical training. Scand. J. Rehabil. Med., 12:27–31.

51. Jackson, D.W., and Shafer, R.K. (1987): Cyclops syndrome: loss of extension following intra-articular anterior cruciate ligament reconstruction. Arthroscopy, 6:171–178.

52. Jayson, M.I.V., and Dixon, A. (1970): Intra-articular pressure in rheumatoid arthritis of the knee. III. Pressure changes during joint use. Ann. Rheum. Dis., 29:401–408.

53. Joyce, M.E., Aoki, M., Lou, J., and Manske, P.R. (1994). Molecular mechanism of adhesion formation during flexor tendon healing (Absract). American Society of Surgery of the Hand, Cincinnati, OH., Oct. 1994.

54. Jurvelin, J., Helminen, H.J., Laurisalo, S., et al. (1985): Influences of joint immobilization and running exercise on articular cartilage surfaces of young rabbits. Acta Anat., 122:62–68.

55. Jurvelin, J., Kiviranta, I., Tammi, M., and Helminen, J.H. (1986): Softening of canine articular cartilage after immobilization of the knee joint. Clin. Orthop. Rel. Res., 207:246–252.

56. Kennedy, J.C., Alexander, I.J., and Hayes, K.C. (1982): Nerve supply of the human knee and its functional importance. Am. J. Sports Med., 10:329–335.

57. Knight, K. (1976): The effects of hypothermia on inflammation and swelling. Athl. Train., 11:7–10.

58. Krebs, D.E., Staples, W.H., Cuttita, D., and Zickel, R.E. (1983): Knee joint angle: Its relationship to quadriceps femoris activity in normal and post-arthrotomy limbs. Arch. Phys. Med. Rehabil., 64:441–447.

59. Kubiak, R.J., Whitman, K.M., and Johnston, R.M. (1987): Changes in quadriceps femoris muscle strength during isometric exercise versus electrical stimulation. J. Orthop. Sports Phys. Ther., 8:537–541.

60. Landry, M., and Fleisch, H. (1964): The influence of immobilization on bone formation as evaluated by osseous incorporation of tetracyclines. J. Bone Joint Surg. [Br.], 46:764–771.

61. Langenskiold, A., Michelsson, J.E., and Videman, T. (1979): Osteoarthritis of the knee in the rabbit produced by immobilization. Attempts to achieve a reproducible model for studies on pathogenesis and therapy. Acta Orthop. Scand., 50:1–14.

62. Lanier, R.R. (1946): The effects of exercise on the knee joints of inbred mice. Anat. Rec., 94:311–319.

63. Laros, G.S., Tipton, C.M., and Cooper, R.R. (1971): Influence of physical activity on ligament insertions in the knees of dogs. J. Bone Joint Surg. [Am.], 53:275–286.

64. Levick, R.J. (1983): Joint pressure-volume studies: Their importance, design and interpretation. J. Rheumatol., 10:353–357.

65. Levick, R.J. (1983): Synovial fluid dynamics: The regulation of volume and pressure. *In:* Holborrow, E.J., and Maroudas, A. (eds.): Studies in Joint Disease. London, Pitman Medical, pp. 153–240.

66. Lieb, F.J., and Perry, J. (1968): Quadriceps function: An anatomical and mechanical study using amputated limbs. J. Bone Joint Surg. [Am.], 50:1535–1548.
67. Lindboe, C.F., and Platou, C.S. (1984): Effects of immobilization of short duration on muscle fibre size. Clin. Physiol., 4:183–188.
68. Loitz, B.J., Zernicke, R.F., Vailas, A.C., et al. (1989): Effects of short-term immobilization versus continuous passive motion on the biomechanical and biochemical properties of the rabbit tendon. Clin. Orthop., 244:265–271.
69. LoPresti, C., Kirkendall, D., Street, G., et al. (1984): Degree of quadriceps atrophy on a 1-year postanterior cruciate repair. Med. Sci. Sports Exerc., 16:204.
70. Lynch, T.N., Jensen, R.L., Stevens, D.M., et al. (1967): Metabolic effects of prolonged bed rest: Their modification by simulated altitude. Aerospace Med., 38:10–20.
71. MacDougall, J.D., Elder, G.C.B., Sale, D.G., et al. (1980): Effects of strength training and immobilization on human muscle fibers. Eur. J. Appl. Physiol., 43:25–34.
72. MacDougall, J.D., Ward, G.R., Sale, D.G., and Sutton, J.R. (1977): Biochemical adaptation of human skeletal muscle to heavy resistance training and immobilization. J. Appl. Physiol., 43:700–703.
73. Maier, A., Crockett, J.L., Simpson, D.R., et al. (1976): Properties of immobilized guinea pig hindlimb muscles. Am. J. Physiol., 231:1520–1526.
74. Mangine, R.E. (1990): The complicated knee: A loss of motion. In: 1990 Advances on the Knee and Shoulder. Cincinnati, Cincinnati Sports Medicine and Deaconess Hospital. Symposium held April 2–4, 1990.
75. Maroudes, A., Bullough, P., Swanson, S., and Freeman, M. (1968): The permeability of articular cartilage. J. Bone Joint Surg. [Br.], 50:166–177.
76. Max, S.R. (1972): Disuse atrophy of skeletal muscle: Loss of functional activity of mitochondria. Biochem. Biophys. Res. Commun., 46:1394–1398.
77. Mazess, R.B., and Whedon, G.D. (1983): Immobilization and bone. Calcif. Tissue Int., 35:265–267.
78. McCarthy, M.R., Buxton, B.P., and Yates, C.K. (1993): Effects of continuous passive motion on anterior laxity following ACL reconstruction with autogenous patellar tendon grafts. J. Sports Rehab., 2:171–178.
79. Minaire, P., Meunier, P., Edouard, C., et al. (1974): Quantitative histological data on disuse osteoporosis. Calcif. Tissue Res., 17:57–65.
80. Morrissey, M.C., Brewster, C.E., Shields, C.L., and Brown, M. (1985): The effects of electrical stimulation on the quadriceps during postoperative knee immobilization. Am. J. Sports Med., 13:40–45.
81. Noyes, F.R. (1977): Functional properties of knee ligaments and alterations induced by immobilization. Clin. Orthop. Rel. Res., 123:210–242.
82. Noyes, F.R., Mangine, R.E., and Barber, S. (1974): Biomechanics of ligament failure. II. An analysis of immobilization, exercise, and reconditioning effects in primates. J. Bone Joint Surg. [Am.], 56:1406–1418.
83. Noyes, F.R., Mangine, R.E., and Barber, S. (1987): Early knee motion after open and arthroscopic anterior cruciate ligament reconstruction. Am. J. Sports Med., 15:149–160.
84. O'Driscoll, S.W., Kumar, A., and Salter, R.B. (1983): The effect of continuous passive motion on the clearance of a hemarthrosis from a synovial joint: An experimental investigation in the rabbit. Clin. Orthop., 176:305–311.
85. Palmoski, M.J., Colyer, R.A., and Brandt, K.D. (1980): Joint motion in the absence of normal loading does not maintain articular cartilage. Arthritis Rheum., 23:325–334.
86. Paulos, L., Rosenberg, T., Drawbert, J., et al. (1987). Infrapatellar contracture syndrome: An unrecognized cause of knee stiffness with patella entrapment and patella infera. Am. J. Sports Med., 15:331–342.
87. Peacock, E.E., Jr. (1981): Wound Repair, 3rd ed. Philadelphia, W.B. Saunders.
88. Radin, E.L., Paul, I.L., and Pollock, D. (1970): Animal joint behavior under excessive loading. Nature, 266:554–555.
89. Renzoni, S.A., Amiel, D., Harwood, F.L., and Akeson, W.H. (1984): Synovial nutrition of knee ligaments. Trans. Orthop. Res. Soc., 9:277–283.
90. Rifenberick, D.H., and Max, S.R. (1974): Substrate utilization by disused rat skeletal muscles. Am. J. Physiol., 226:295–297.
91. Rosen, M.A., Jackson, D.W., and Atwell, E.A. (1992): The efficacy of continuous passive motion in the rehabilitation of anterior cruciate ligament reconstructions. Am. J. Sports Med., 20:122–127.
92. Roy, S., Ghadially, F.N., and Crane, W.A.J. (1966): Synovial membrane and traumatic effusion: Ultrastructure and autoradiography with tritiated leucine. Ann. Rheumatol. Dis., 25:259–271.
93. Saaf, J. (1950): Effect of exercise on adult cartilage. Acta Orthop. Scand. Suppl., 7:1–83.
94. Salter, R.B. (1989): The biologic concept of continuous passive motion of synovial joints. Clin. Orthop., 242:12–25.
95. Salter, R.B., and Field, P. (1960): The effects of continuous compression on living articular cartilage. J. Bone Joint Surg. [Am.], 42:31–49.
96. Salter, R.B., and Minster, R.R. (1982): The effect of continuous passive motion on a semitendinous tenodesis in the rabbit knee (abstr.). Orthop. Trans., 6:292.
97. Salter, R.B., Simmonds, D.F., Malcolm, B.W., et al. (1975): The effect of continuous passive

motion on the healing of articular cartilage defects: An experimental investigation in rabbits (abstr.). J. Bone Joint Surg. [Am.], 57:570.

98. Sargeant, A.J., Davies, C.T.M., Edwards, R.H.T., et al. (1976): Functional and structural changes after disuse of human muscle. Clin. Sci., 52:337–342.

99. Shakespeare, D.T., Stokes, M., Sherman, K.P., and Young, A. (1983): The effect of knee flexion on quadriceps inhibition after meniscectomy. Clin. Sci., 65:64P–65P.

100. Shelborne, K.D., Wilchkens, J.H., Mollabashy, A., and DeCarlo, M. (1991). Arthrofibrosis in acute anterior cruciate ligament reconstruction: The effect of timing on reconstruction and rehabilitation. Am. J. Sports Med., 19:332–336.

101. Sherman, K.P., Shakespeare, D.T., Stokes, M., and Young, A. (1983): Inhibition of voluntary quadriceps activity after meniscectomy. Clin. Sci., 64:70P.

102. Sherman, K.P., Young, A., Stokes, M., and Shakespeare, D.T. (1984): Joint injury and muscle weakness. Lancet, 2:646–651.

103. Sisk, D.T., Stralka, S.W., Deering, M.B., and Griffin, J.W. (1987): Effect of electrical stimulation on quadriceps strength after reconstructive surgery of the anterior cruciate ligament. Am. J. Sports Med., 15:215–220.

104. Sledge, C.B. (1975): Structure, development, and function of joints. Orthop. Clin. North Am., 6:619–628.

105. Soren, A., Rosenbauer, K.A., Klein, W., and Huth, F. (1973): Morphological examinations of so-called posttraumatic synovitis. Beitr. Pathol., 1950:11–30.

106. Spencer, J.D., Hayes, K.C., and Alexander, I.J. (1984): Knee joint effusion and quadriceps reflex inhibition in man. Arch. Phys. Med. Rehabil., 65:171–177.

107. Sprangue, N.F., O'Conner, R.L., and Fox, J.M. (1982). Arthroscopic treatment of postoperative knee fibroarthrosis. Clin. Orthop., 166:165–172.

108. Steinberg, F.U. (1980): The Immobilized Patient: Functional Pathology and Management. New York, Plenum Press.

109. Stokes, M., Mill, K., Shakespeare, D., et al. (1984): Post-operative inhibition: Voluntary ischemia does not alter quadriceps function in normal subjects. In: Wittle, M.W., and Harris, J.D. (eds.): Biomechanical Measurement in Orthopaedic Practice. New York, Oxford University Press, pp. 188–193.

110. Stokes, M., and Young, A. (1984): The contribution of reflex inhibition to arthrogenous muscle weakness. Clin. Sci., 67:7–14.

111. Stratford, P. (1981): Electromyography of the quadriceps femoris muscles in subjects with normal knees and acutely effused knees. Phys. Ther., 62:279–289.

112. Stravino, V.D. (1972): The synovial system. Am. J. Phys. Med., 51:312–320.

113. Swann, D., Radin, E., and Nazimiec, M. (1976): Role of hyaluronic acid on joint lubrication. Ann. Rheum. Dis., 33:318–326.

114. Tardieu, C., Tabary, J.C., Tabary, C., and Tardieu, G. (1982): Adaptation of connective tissue length to immobilization in the lengthened and shortened positions in cat soleus muscle. J. Physiol., 78:214–217.

115. Tipton, C.M., James, S.L., Mergner, W., et al. (1970): Influence of exercise on strength of medial collateral knee ligament of dogs. Am. J. Physiol., 218:894–902.

116. Tipton, C.M., Marrhes, R.D., Maynard, J.A., and Carey, R.A. (1975): The influence of physical activity on ligaments and tendons. Med. Sci. Sports, 7:165–175.

117. Trias, A. (1961): Effects of persistent pressure on articular cartilage. J. Bone Joint Surg. [Am.], 43:376–386.

118. Tucker, K.R., Sider, M.J., and Booth, F.W. (1981): Protein synthesis rates in atrophied gastrocnemius muscles after limb immobilization. J. Appl. Physiol., 51:73–77.

119. Uhthoff, H.K., and Jaworski, Z.F.G. (1978): Bone loss in response to long-term immobilization. J. Bone Joint Surg. [Br.], 60:420–429.

120. Venn, M.F. (1979): Chemical composition of human femoral head cartilage: Influence of topographical position and fibrillation. Ann. Rheum. Dis., 38:57–62.

121. Videman, T. (1981): Changes of compression and distances between tibial and femoral condyles during immobilization of rabbit knee. Arch. Orthop. Trauma Surg., 98:289–294.

122. Videman, T. (1982): Experimental osteoarthritis in the rabbit. Comparison of different periods of repeated immobilization. Acta Orthop. Scand., 53:339–347.

123. Videman, T. (1987): Connective tissue and immobilization. Clin. Orthop. Rel. Res., 221:26–32.

124. Vogt, F.B., Mack, P.B., Beasley, W.G., et al. (1965). The effect of bed rest on various parameters of physiological function. Part XII. The effect of bed rest on bone mass and calcium balance. Washington, DC, National Aeronautics and Space Administration, Publ. No. CR-182.

125. Wahl, S., and Renstrom R. (1991). Fibrosis in soft-tissue injuries. In: Leadbetter, W., Buckwalter, J., and Gordon, S. (eds.): Sports-induced Inflammation: Clinical and Basic Science Concepts. Park Ridge, IL, American Academy of Orthopaedic Surgeons, pp. 63–82.

126. Weiss, C. (1979): Normal and osteoarthritic articular cartilage. Orthop. Clin. North Am., 10:175–189.

127. Westers, B.M. (1982): Review of the repair of defects in articular cartilage: Part I. J. Orthop. Sports Phys. Ther., 3:186–192.

128. Williams, P.E., and Goldspink, G. (1978): Changes in sarcomere length and physiological properties in immobilized muscle. J. Anat., 127:459–468.

129. Witzmann, F.A., Kim, D.H., and Fitts, R.H. (1982): Recovery time course in contractile function of fast and slow skeletal muscle after hindlimb immobilization. J. Appl. Physiol., 52:677–682.

130. Wolff, J. (1982): Das Gesetz der Transformation der Knochen. Berlin, A. Hirschwald.

131. Woo, S., Gomez, M.A., Sites, T.J., et al. (1987): The biomechanical and morphological changes in the medial collateral ligament of the rabbit after immobilization and remobilization. J. Bone Joint Surg. [Am.], 69:1200–1211.

132. Woo, S., Inoue, D.M., McGurk-Burleson, E., and Gomez, M.A. (1987): Treatment of the medial collateral ligament injury. II: Structure and function of canine knees in response to differing treatment regimes. Am. J. Sports Med., 15:22–29.

133. Woo, S., Matthew, J.V., Akeson, W.H., et al. (1975): Connective tissue response to immobility. Arthritis Rheum., 18:257–264.

134. Wright, V., Dowson, D., and Kerr, J. (1973): The structure of joints. Int. Rev. Connect. Tissue Res., 6:105–125.

135. Wronski, T.J., and Morey, E.R. (1982): Skeletal abnormalities in rats induced by simulated weightlessness. Metab. Bone Dis., 4:69–74.

136. Yates, C.K., McCarthy, M.R., Hirsch, H.S., and Pascale, M.S. (1992): Effects of continuous passive motion following ACL reconstruction with autogenous patellar tendon grafts. J. Sports Rehab., 1:121–131.

137. Young, A., Hughes, I., Round, J.M., and Edwards, R.H.T. (1982): The effect of knee injury on the number of muscle fibers in the human quadriceps femoris. Clin. Sci., 62:227–234.

138. Young, A., Stokes, M., and Iles, J.F. (1987): Effects of joint pathology on muscle. Clin. Orthop., 219:21–27.

139. Young, A., Stokes, M., Shakespeare, D.T., and Sherman, K.P. (1983): The effect of intra-articular bupivacaine on quadriceps inhibition after meniscectomy. Med. Sci. Sports Exerc., 15:154.

140. Young, D.R., Niklowitz, W.J., and Steele, C.R. (1983): Tibial changes in experimental disuse osteoporosis in the monkey. Calcif. Tissue Int., 35:304–308.

141. Zarins, B. (1982): Soft tissue injury and repair: Biomechanical aspects. Int. J. Sports Med., 3:19–25.

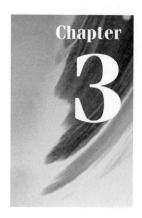

Role of Evaluation in the Rehabilitation Program

Ron Courson, A.T.,C., P.T.

One of the most challenging areas in the field of sports medicine is rehabilitation following athletic injury. The goals of any rehabilitation program include returning the athlete to optimal preinjury status and developing a preventive maintenance program to minimize the possibility of injury recurrence. The clinician should strive to return athletes to their activity without restriction as soon as possible but within safe guidelines. Rehabilitation is challenging in that all athletes are different, as is every athletic injury, and each athlete has unique characteristics. Therefore, each athlete responds to injury in a unique manner. Similarly, every sport and every playing position has special demands and characteristics and, accordingly, places different stresses on the body.

Rehabilitation protocols are frequently used by sports medicine practitioners for guidance in treating specific pathologies. Although these protocols help provide consistency and continuity throughout the rehabilitation process, it must be remembered that they are only guidelines. The optimal rehabilitation program should be individualized to the athlete, the specific pathology, and the resultant problems that the athlete is experiencing. The initial injury evaluation and subsequent re-evaluations are therefore critical. A thorough evaluation provides the information needed to structure a rehabilitation program tailored to address identified problems.

The problem-solving approach best addresses the challenge of rehabilitation after an athletic injury. The evaluation provides the foundation on which the problem-solving approach is constructed. A proper evaluation depends on a detailed and accurate athletic history; knowledge of anatomy, kinesiology, and applied biomechanics; diligent observation; and a thorough physical examination. The examiner should establish an orderly and sequential method for ensuring that nothing is overlooked (Table 3–1). On completion of the evaluation, a list of specific problems should be identified. A plan of care should be developed to address each problem, and with implementation, regular re-evaluations

Table 3–1. Evaluation of Athletic Injuries

By following an orderly sequence, the evaluator performs a comprehensive evaluation and ensures that no affected area is overlooked.

• History	• Muscle performance assessment
• Observation	• Neurovascular assessment
• Inspection	• Special testing
• Palpation	• Functional testing
• Range-of-motion testing	• Sport-specific testing

should be performed to gauge progress and ascertain the effectiveness and efficiency of administered treatments. The problem-solving approach can be summarized as follows:

1. Evaluation: subjective history, objective findings
2. Identification of specific problems
3. Development of plan of care for addressing specific problems, short- and long-term goals, and criteria for return to functional activity
4. Initiation of plan of care
5. Periodic re-evaluation and adaptation of plan of care, as appropriate
6. Return to functional activity after successful completion of identified rehabilitation goals and discharge parameters
7. Development of preventive maintenance rehabilitation program and use of prophylactic devices, as needed, to reduce the incidence of injury recurrence

EVALUATION FORMAT

Subjective History

It is important to obtain a detailed and complete history from the athlete during the evaluation (Fig. 3–1). The evaluator seeks the answers to a number of questions and should obtain the following information:

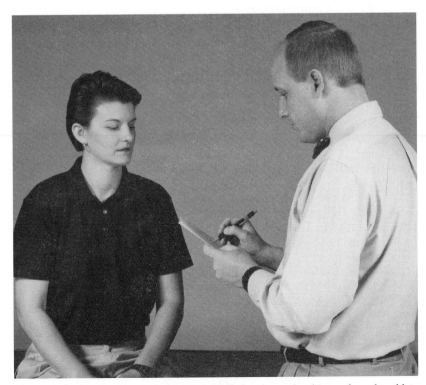

Figure 3–1. The examiner must obtain a detailed and complete history from the athlete.

1. *What is the age, gender, ethnicity, and general body type or build of the athlete?* Research has shown that certain populations may be predisposed to specific pathologies or conditions. The evaluator should be cognizant of these and observe for findings in the evaluation that may correlate with these factors (e.g., increased incidence of epiphyseal fractures in young, skeletally immature athletes; increased incidence of patellofemoral pathology in female athletes secondary to a larger Q angle).

2. *What is the athlete's activity or sport? What position does the athlete play?* This information assists the evaluator in determining the stresses placed on the athlete during participation and in determining functional activity parameters for discharge and return to activity.

3. *What is the athlete's chief complaint?*

4. *What was the mechanism of injury?* Knowledge of the mechanism of injury provides information about what type of trauma was incurred and what anatomic structures may be involved. In addition to the athlete's description, information obtained from witnesses, film, or videotape, if available, can help ascertain the exact injury mechanism.

5. *Does the athlete have a history of related previous injury?* Muscle atrophy, ligamentous laxity, crepitus, or other pathologic findings can be a result of previous injury.

6. *Is the injury of an acute nature or of insidious onset?*

7. *Did the athlete hear or feel an abnormal sound or sensation as the injury occurred?*

8. *Is the athlete experiencing pain, swelling, crepitus, change in sensation, loss of strength, loss of range of motion, instability, or any other reportable abnormality?*

9. *Was the athlete able to continue the activity after injury?*

10. *Does activity or rest change the athlete's perception of the pain?*

11. *Are the symptoms improving, worsening, or remaining the same?* It is important to know the time of onset as well as the duration and intensity of the symptoms.

12. *What are the sites and boundaries of pain or abnormal sensation?* The evaluator may elect to have the athlete complete a subjective pain survey or pain scale rating test such as the McGill-Melzack Pain Questionnaire.

13. *Has the athlete attempted to treat the injury (e.g., with rest, support, assistive ambulation devices, therapeutic heat or cold, or exercise)? If so, what has been the outcome?*

14. *Does the athlete have a history of any unrelated previous or current injuries or illnesses?*

15. *Is the athlete currently taking any type of prescription or over-the-counter medication?*

16. *Are there any etiologic considerations or precipitating factors that may predispose the athlete to an injury or to the exacerbation of an injury?*

Obtaining an accurate and detailed history is important in the evaluation process. With experience, the evaluator can often make a preliminary assessment of the injury from the history. The information obtained from the athlete's history provides guidance and direction to the evaluator in proceeding with the evaluation. Knowledge of the mechanism of injury may provide a biomechanical correlation to the clinical examination. The evaluator should be careful, however, not to jump to conclusions. The adage "You see what you look for, you recognize what you know" should remind the evaluator to always proceed with an open mind and to be aware of all possible scenarios.

Objective Evaluation

The objective evaluation consists of documentable physical findings that the evaluator discovers through observation, inspection, palpation, range-of-motion assessment, muscle performance, neurovascular status, special testing, and functional and sport-specific testing.

OBSERVATION

The observation process begins when the evaluator first encounters the athlete. In an acute on-the-field injury, this involves noting the mechanism of injury and observing the athlete after injury. In a nonacute injury setting, the observation process begins when the athlete presents for evaluation. The evaluator should observe the athlete's general appearance. How does the athlete stand or walk? Does the athlete use crutches, a cane, or other assistive devices? Does the athlete use a support, such as a brace or sling? Does the athlete experience difficulty in removing clothing or taking a place on the evaluation table?

With a lower extremity injury, the examiner should remember to compare the weight-bearing and non–weight-bearing postures. The weight-bearing posture reveals how the body compensates for structural abnormalities. The non–weight-bearing posture illustrates functional and structural ability without compensation.

Photography may provide some degree of objectivity to the observation process. Utilization of a camera to record data, such as photographing a wound with Polaroid grid film to quantify the size and shape of the wound or photographic documentation of trunk range of motion at various points throughout the course of rehabilitation to demonstrate improvement, may be helpful. Developments in technology with the digital camera now allow photographic documentation to be entered into the patient's computer medical record.

INSPECTION

After observation of the athlete's general appearance, the examiner should perform a closer inspection, noting the following (Fig. 3–2): (1) discoloration or ecchymosis; (2) symmetry, using bilateral comparison where available; (3) skin appearance, noting color, texture, and temperature; (4) signs of trauma; (5) obvious deformity; (6) pain; (7) swelling; and (8) bleeding.

PALPATION

Palpation is the process by which the evaluator applies his or her hands to the athlete's body surface to detect evidence of injury or tenderness (Fig. 3–3).

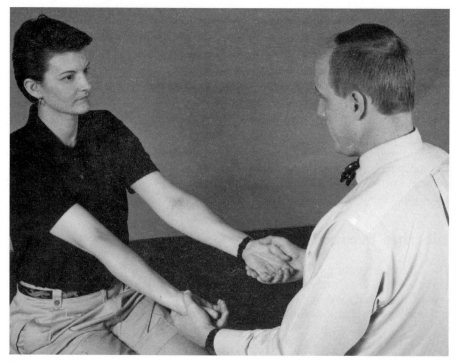

Figure 3–2. During the observation and inspection phases of the evaluation, the examiner should make bilateral comparisons and note ecchymosis, symmetry, effusion, bleeding, and skin temperature.

Palpation should be carried out systematically to ensure that all anatomic structures are examined. This procedure involves determining a starting point and working from that point to the surrounding tissues. The examiner should begin slowly and carefully, applying light pressure initially and gradually working into a deeper palpation pressure. Bilateral comparison should be used, if available. Palpable deformities, elicitation of pain or tenderness, crepitus, and any other differences or abnormalities should be noted.

RANGE-OF-MOTION TESTING

As applicable to the injury situation, the evaluator should measure range of motion, both passively and actively (Fig. 3–4). Passive range of motion is the amount of motion obtained by the evaluator without assistance from the athlete. Passive range-of-motion testing provides information regarding joint arthrokinematics, articular surface integrity, and extensibility of the joint capsule, associated ligaments, and muscles. Active range of motion is the amount of joint motion obtained by the athlete while performing unassisted, voluntary joint motion. Active range-of-motion testing provides additional information regarding a joint, including muscle strength and movement coordination. Assessment of active range of motion is important for providing information regarding the athlete's functional ability.

Range-of-motion deficits can have a number of causes, including the following: (1) mechanical block within the joint caused by a loose body or by osteophyte formation; (2) muscular tightness; (3) adaptive shortening of the capsular or ligamentous structures; (4) swelling; (5) pain inhibition; or (6) a combination of two or more of these factors. It is important to determine the reason for the range-of-motion deficiency in order to plan the appropriate course of treatment in the rehabilitation program.

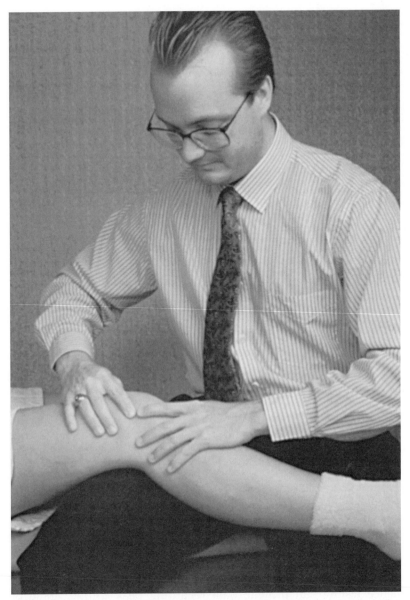

Figure 3-3. During palpation the examiner's hands are applied to the body's external surface to detect evidence of injury or tenderness. (From Mulligan, E.P. [1989]: Etiological considerations in the evaluation of patellofemoral dysfunction. Sports Med. Update, 4:3–6.)

A goniometer should be used to obtain objective range-of-motion measurements (see Chap. 4). Goniometric measurements of active and passive ranges of motion obtained on a regular basis provide objective data regarding the effectiveness of rehabilitation treatment and the athlete's progress.

MUSCLE PERFORMANCE ASSESSMENT

The evaluator should also assess muscle performance as applicable to the injury situation. This can include assessment of the quality, recruitment, and isolation of an isometric contraction in a muscle group with an acute musculoskeletal injury; a postsurgical evaluation; and use of specific manual muscle

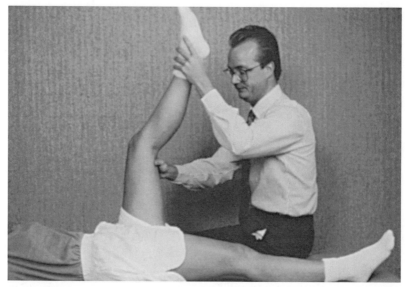

Figure 3–4. Range of motion should be assessed passively and actively to determine the reasons for its loss. (From Mulligan, E.P. [1989]: Etiological considerations in the evaluation of patellofemoral dysfunction. Sports Med. Update, 4:3–6.)

testing techniques or isokinetic testing. Muscle performance tests provide the evaluator with information regarding integrity of the contractile tissues, neuromuscular status, and movement coordination. Isometric muscle testing may be performed either manually, using the traditional five-point rating scale, or using one of the electronic muscle testing devices that provide numeric readings.

Resistive isometric tests can be performed to assess the status of musculoskeletal tissues (Fig. 3–5). Isometric contractions are performed to stress muscle and tendon without stressing accessory tissues. Careful observation, palpation, and correct positioning are essential for the tests to be valid. A knowledge of functional anatomy and kinesiology is paramount. When performing resistive tests, the evaluator should note the strength of the muscle contraction, symmetry to the contralateral side, and whether the contraction elicits pain and should observe for crepitus, muscle deformation, and any other abnormalities.

With nonacute athletic injuries, isokinetic testing, if applicable, may provide a more objective analysis of muscle performance (Fig. 3–6). Isokinetic muscle performance testing can provide data regarding peak torque, angle of peak torque, agonist-to-antagonist muscle ratio, rate of tension development, reciprocal innervation time, and a power, work, and torque curve analysis. Isokinetic testing allows the examiner to load the muscle throughout the entire range of motion at speeds that are more comparable to those attained in athletic activities than are isometric or isotonic contractions.

Regularly performed strength testing, whether manual muscle testing or isokinetic testing, provides objective data regarding the effectiveness of the rehabilitation program and the athlete's progress.

NEUROVASCULAR ASSESSMENT

Neurovascular screening should be performed by the evaluator using tests that the evaluator believes are relevant to the suspected pathology. These may include assessment of balance; testing of motor function, deep tendon reflex, and dermatome sensation; monitoring of pulse and blood pressure; and determination of capillary refilling.

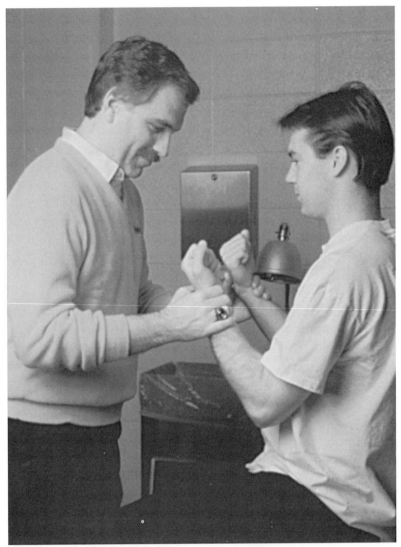

Figure 3–5. Muscle performance testing provides information about the integrity of the contractile tissues, neuromuscular status, and movement coordination. (Photo courtesy of Sports Medicine Update. Birmingham, Alabama, HealthSouth Rehabilitation Corporation.)

SPECIAL TESTING

Once the evaluator has completed the subjective history and preliminary objective evaluation, special testing pertinent to the suspected pathology may be undertaken. This may include joint stability testing, circumferential measurements, and specific pathology tests.

Stability testing is performed to determine the integrity of ligamentous structures by placing a mechanical stress on the structure. The examiner should possess a thorough knowledge of anatomy to be able to visualize each structure tested (Fig. 3–7). The evaluator should first perform stability testing of the uninvolved joint to obtain baseline data for comparison with the involved joint. In addition, allowing the athlete to experience the testing on the uninvolved joint first helps develop confidence and trust in the examiner and decrease apprehension. Correct positioning is essential for ensuring the validity of the stability tests. The athlete should be encouraged to relax, because muscle spasm could negate the validity of the test results. The evaluator should note any

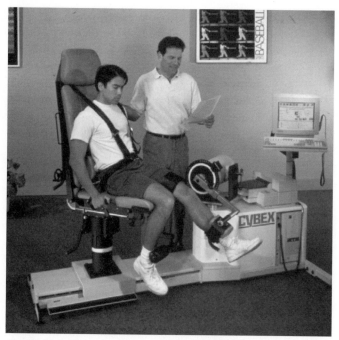

Figure 3–6. Isokinetic testing allows the examiner to load the muscle throughout the entire range of motion at speeds that are more comparable to those of athletic activities than are isotonic contractions. (Photo courtesy of Cybex, Medway, MA.)

degree of instability, elicitation of pain or tenderness, crepitus, or evidence of other abnormalities during the stability testing.

Circumferential measurements can provide objective documentation of such problems as muscle atrophy or effusion. The evaluator should use anatomic landmarks and standard measurements to establish continuity and consistency.

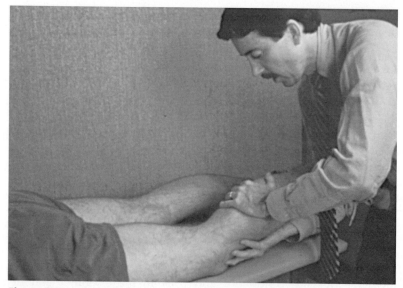

Figure 3–7. Stability testing helps determine the integrity of ligamentous structures by placing a mechanical stress on the structure. (From Moran, D.J., and Floyd, R.T. [1990]: The Lachman test: Alternative techniques and applications for anterior cruciate ligament evaluation. Sports Med. Update, 5:3–5.)

For example, the medial joint line is preferable to the patella as a landmark for measuring the knee because a change in effusion of the knee may cause the patella to shift, affecting the validity and reliability of the measurements.

Special tests can be performed, as indicated, to confirm or rule out suspected pathology (Fig. 3–8). Examples include testing for the rotator cuff impingement sign, the "labral clunk test" for a glenoid labrum tear, the Thompson test for a ruptured Achilles tendon, and the Finklestein test for de Quervain's syndrome.

FUNCTIONAL TESTING AND SPORT-SPECIFIC TESTING

The evaluator may elect to use a functional testing program, as applicable, to determine whether these sequential activities produce pain or other symptoms. For example, a functional testing program for an injured ankle may include the following: (1) squatting (both ankles should dorsiflex symmetrically); (2) standing on toes (both ankles should plantar flex symmetrically); (3) standing on one foot; (4) standing on the toes of one foot; (5) walking on the toes; (6) running straight ahead; (7) running with cutting movements; and (8) jumping. Also, a commercial system such as the Cybex Reactor* can be used to collect objective data on dynamic movement (Fig. 3–9).

If the athlete can perform functional tests without difficulty, the evaluator may elect to proceed with more advanced sports testing specific to the athlete's sport. For instance, the evaluator may ask a quarterback to simulate taking a snap and dropping back to pass or may ask a baseball pitcher returning from a rotator cuff injury to pitch a simulated game.

Additional Considerations

The thorough evaluator must not only consider the pathology but go beyond it to uncover the possible cause. The evaluator must not only examine the

*Available from Cybex, Ronkonkoma, New York

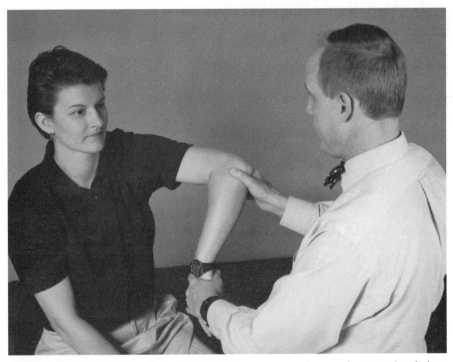

Figure 3–8. Special tests can help determine the presence or absence of suspected pathology.

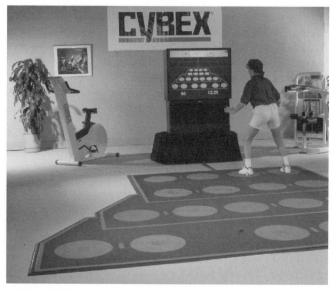

Figure 3–9. Commercial functional testing systems such as the Cybex Reactor may provide a more objective means of assessing components of dynamic movement. (Photo courtesy of Cybex, Medway, MA.)

specific site of pathology but also visualize the entire kinetic chain and examine adjacent joints and other related structures. Biomechanics and kinesiology of the sport-specific skills that the athlete performs should be taken into consideration. On completion of the evaluation, the clinician should develop a plan of care that encompasses rehabilitation of the primary pathology and correction of any underlying problems that may have predisposed the athlete to the pathology.

IDENTIFICATION OF SPECIFIC PROBLEMS

After completion of the evaluation process, the evaluator should compile a list of specific problems related to the athletic injury. For example, evaluation of a college football running back after an acute inversion ankle sprain might reveal the following problems:

1. Physiologic healing constraints with grade I injury to the anterior talofibular and calcaneofibular ligaments (recognizing a 3- to 5-week normal time frame for healing of ligamentous injury)
2. Negative lateral ankle instability but increased pain with mechanical stress placed on the ligaments with stress testing
3. Point tenderness over the lateral aspect of the ankle, specifically centered over the involved ligamentous structures
4. Inability to bear weight fully
5. Moderate effusion and ecchymosis of the ankle and forefoot
6. Decreased range of motion in plantar flexion, dorsiflexion, inversion, and eversion

7. Decreased muscular strength in plantar flexion, dorsiflexion, inversion, and eversion
8. Decreased proprioception and kinesthetic awareness
9. Loss of function; decrease in athletic activities and activities of daily living secondary to pathology
10. Need for cardiovascular and well-limb maintenance program during rehabilitation and recovery process

DEVELOPMENT OF A PLAN OF CARE

After identification of specific problems, a plan of care should be developed to address each problem. For example, in developing a plan of care for the athlete with the injury described above, the clinician might use the following:

1. Partial weight bearing on two crutches, with the ankle placed in a prophylactic brace or strapping to relieve the weight-bearing problem, protect injured ligamentous structures during the recovery phase, and minimize pain and discomfort
2. Cryotherapy, compression (through elastic bandaging or compression sleeve), elevation, intermittent compression, electrical muscle stimulation set at muscle pump-contraction parameters, centripetal massage, and active or active-assisted range of motion to relieve effusion and ecchymosis
3. Cryotherapy and electrical muscle stimulation set at pain modulation parameters to relieve pain
4. Active, active-assisted, and passive range-of-motion program to deal with range-of-motion deficits
5. Submaximal progression to maximal multiple angle isometrics, manual resistance, proprioceptive neuromuscular facilitation diagonal patterns, and submaximal progression to maximal isotonic exercise implemented, as applicable, to treat strength deficits
6. Balance, proprioception, and kinesthetic awareness activities implemented, as appropriate, to manage deficits
7. Implementation of well-limb maintenance program
8. Implementation of upper body ergometer, stationary cycle, and aquatic rehabilitation exercises for cardiovascular maintenance

The components of the rehabilitation program should be directed toward achieving modulation of pain, normal range of motion and joint arthrokinematics, normal muscular flexibility and strength, and the balance, power, coordination, endurance, accuracy, and timing necessary to return to the preinjury activity level without restriction. Through therapeutic exercise, therapeutic modalities, and patient education, a structured rehabilitation program can be designed and individualized to the athlete's specific pathology, and problems can be identified. When a plan of care is being established, two questions should be asked:

1. *What goals and types of treatment constitute a well-designed program?* The clinician should have a scientific rationale for each treatment technique.
2. *Do the proposed treatments safely and effectively accomplish the intended goals?* Objective measurements recorded periodically can assist the clinician in monitoring the progress of the rehabilitation program.

GOAL SETTING AND ESTABLISHMENT OF DISCHARGE PARAMETERS

Along with the plan of care, specific rehabilitation goals should be developed. As with any project, goals help provide a sense of purpose and direction. Goals should be set on both a short-term (7 to 10 days) and a long-term basis. Discharge parameters and criteria for return to athletic activity should also be established. Consideration must be given to the nature of the pathology, the athlete's sport and playing position, and the physical demands placed on the athlete.

The decision to release an athlete recovering from injury for a progressive return to athletic activity is the final stage of the rehabilitation and recovery process. The decision should be carefully considered by each member of the sports medicine team involved in the rehabilitation process. In considering return to activity, the following concerns should be addressed: recognition by the team of physiologic healing constraints; pain; swelling; range of motion; strength; balance, timing, proprioception, and kinesthetic awareness; sport-specific demands; conditioning; prophylactic strapping, bracing, or padding; responsibility of the athlete; predisposition to injury; psychologic factors; gradual, progressive return to activity; athlete education and preventive maintenance program; and functional testing.

PERIODIC RE-EVALUATION

The athlete should be periodically re-evaluated to monitor the effectiveness of the rehabilitation program. Objective data recorded on a regular basis, such as range-of-motion measurements, manual muscle testing grades, and circumferential measurements, provide information about the effectiveness and efficiency of treatment. Following re-evaluation, the original goals of treatment should be re-examined and modified as needed, and the plan of care should be adapted accordingly.

The area of athletic rehabilitation is among the most challenging and exciting in the field of sports medicine. The clinician works with the other members of the sports medicine team to achieve a common goal: return of the injured athlete to the preinjury athletic activity level as soon as possible, within safe guidelines. The success of rehabilitation depends directly on the evaluation process. By performing a thorough evaluation, identifying specific problems, developing a plan of care, and performing subsequent re-evaluations to determine the efficiency and effectiveness of treatments, the clinician can help the injured athlete return to the playing arena.

The following forms represent the steps in a hypothetical evaluation and rehabilitation process for a right ankle sprain.

REHABILITATION: INITIAL EVALUATION

Name: Smith, John   Sport: Football   Date: 9/10/90

Identification # 41024   Age: 20   D.O.B. 7/14/70   Sex: M   Physician: Jones

SUBJECTIVE	¹Present History/Chief Complaint/Mechanism of Injury Athlete presents c/o Rt. ankle pain, swelling, LOF, inability to bear weight. Athlete leapt to catch pass, landing on and forcibly inverting Rt. ankle. Evaluated on football practice field; assisted to T.R.

Past Medical History Athlete states Rt. ankle sprain approximately 2 yrs. ago. Neg. Fx. Returned to athletic activity without further problems until present. PMH otherwise unremarkable.

Medical Tests Rt. ankle x-rays by Dr. Jones at Medical Center, Neg.

Medications None

Treatment to Date I.C.E. NWB with 2 crutches.

OBJECTIVE	Presentation NWB with 2 crutches. Compress. wrap Rt. ankle

Observation Moderate effusion/ecchymosis Rt. ankle, localized over lateral ankle and forefoot.

Palpation Point tenderness elicited over ant. talofibular & calcaneofibular lig. Neg. palpable deformity or crepitus

Range of Motion PF 25°, DF -10°, Inv. 8°, Ever. 2° Toe ext./flex. WNL

Muscle Performance MMT deferred at present 2° to ↑pain with active movement, inability to perform normal active movement patterns.

Neurovascular Bilateral achilles DTR WNL. Intact sensation to light touch. Distal foot pulses WNL.

Special Testing Neg. ligamentous instability, however,↑ pain with inversion stress and anterior drawer tests.

Area of Injury

Circumferential Measurements

Left	Right	Reference Landmarks
26	29	Med. Mall (MM)
23	24.5	5cm prox. MM
25	27	5cm distal MM

Initial Rehabilitation Program:	1) I.C.E. 2)EMS, pain modulation parameters, 3)Intermittent compression @ 80mmHg 60 sec. on/15sec. off x 20 min 4)Application of felt over forefoot & felt horseshoe pad over lat. mall., lat. aspect of ankle with elastic wrap from base of toes to mid-calf. Fitted with crutches & review NWB gait on level surface & ↓↑stairs.

ASSESSMENT	Clinical Impression: Grade I inversion ankle sprain: ant. talofibular and calcaneofibular ligaments.

Tolerated initial Rx. well.

Rehabilitation Problems Identified: ☒ Physiological Healing Constraints ☒ Pain ☒ Swelling ☒↓ ROM   ☒↓ Muscle Performance ☒↓ Balance/Proprioception ☒ Loss of Function ☒ Other Inability to FWB

Rehabilitation Potential Good

Rehabilitation Goals STG (7-10 days): 1)FWB without assistive device, 2)ROM WNL, 3)Minimal effusion, 4)No pain. LTG: Return to previous athletic activity level without restriction. ROM & strength WNL.

PLAN	Continue to monitor progress B.I.D. Advance weight bearing status as tolerable.

REHABILITATION PROGRAM

Name: Smith, John Injury: Rt. Ankle Sprain Sport: Football

	Date of Rehabilitation Session	9/10	9/11	9/12	9/13	9/14	9/15	9/16	9/17	9/18	9/19	9/20	9/21	9/22
THERAPEUTIC EXERCISE	Range of Motion (A AA P)	P/AA	P/AA	P/AA	AA/A									→
	Flexibility	Passive DF with towel	→			Achilles Stretching	Slant Board							→
	Towel Toe Curls			X	X	X	X							
	Marble Pick-ups			X	X	X	X							
	Isometric PF/DF			X	X	X	X							
	Isom. Inv/Ever					X	X							
	TheraBand PF			Blue 2x10	3x10	4x10	Black 3x10	→	5x10	Grey 3x10	→	5x10	—	→
	TheraBand DF			Blue 2x10	3x10	4x10	Black 3x10	→	5x10	Grey 3x10	→	5x10	—	→
	TheraBand Inv.					Blue 2x10	3x10	5x10	Black 3x10	5x10	Grey 3x10	5x10	—	→
	TheraBand Ever.					Blue 2x10	3x10	5x10	Black 3x10	5x10	Grey 3x10	5x10	—	→
	Pro-Fitter								X	X	X	X	X	X
	One Foot Balance				X	X	X	X	X	X	X	X	X	X
	Isokinetic PF/DF						VSRP X	X	X	X	X	X	X	X
	Isokinetic Inv/Ever							VSRP X	X	X	X	X	X	X
	Mini-Trampoline								X	X	X	X	X	X
	PNF					X	X	X	X	X	X	X	X	X
	Balance/Proprioception Activities		NWB BAPS	NWB BAPS	PWB BAPS	PWB BAPS	PWB BAPS	FWB BAPS	FWB BAPS	FWB BAPS	FWB BAPS	FWB BAPS	FWB BAPS	FWB BAPS
	Cardiovascular Training													→
	Well Limb Maintenance	Continue well-leg, U.E. strength training under strength coach supervision	UBE	UBE	Fitron									→
	Aquatic Exercise			Wet-Vest	Wet-Vest	Wet-Vest	Wet-Vest	Pool Run	Pool Run	Pool Run	Pool Run	Spt. Skill	Spt. Skill	Spt. Skill
THERAPEUTIC MODALITIES	Cryotherapy	with elev	with elev	with elev	with elev	with elev	with elev	X	X	X	X	X	X	X
	Diathermy													
	Elec. Stim. Current *	6	6	2	2	2	2							
	Iontophoresis c̄___													
	Intermittent Compression	c elev X	X	X	X	X								
	Massage (centripetal)	X	X	X	X	X								
	Mobilization													
	Phonophoresis c̄___													
	Thermotherapy													
	Traction													
	Ultrasound					Pulse 25%	Pulse 50%	Pulse 75%	Cont. 1.0W	Cont. 1.0W	Cont. 1.25W	Cont. 1.25W	Cont. 1.5W	Cont. 1.5W
	Whirlpool (Contrast)				X	X	X							
	Warm WP @ 100°F							X	X	X	X	X	X	X

* Electrical Stimulating Current Parameters:
1. Mm. re-ed.
2. Mm. pump contractions
3. Retard. of atrophy
4. Mm. Strengthening
5. Increase ROM
6. Pain Modulation

REHABILITATION: RE-EVALUATION

Name: Smith, John   Sport: Football   Date: 9/16/90

Identification # 41024   Age: 20   D.O.B. 7/14/70   Sex: M   Physician: Jones

SUBJECTIVE

Present Injury History S/P 1 wk. Rt. Grade I inversion ankle sprain. Athlete presents without c/o. States "Fell I'm progressing well with rehab... when do you think I'll be ready to go back to football practice.

OBJECTIVE

Presentation FWB with Air-Cast Ankle Brace, Rt.
Observation Minimal effusion Rt. ankle. Neg. effusion in foot. Pocket of swelling localized over anterior lateral aspect of ankle. Ecchymosis breaking up.

Palpation Minimal point tenderness elicited over anterior talofibular & calcaneofibular lig. Neg. deformity, crepitus
Range of Motion PF, Inv., Ever. = WNL.
DF = 5°

Muscle Performance MMT Grades:
PF = 4+/5   DF := 4+/5
Inv. = 4/5   Ever. = 4/5
Neurovascular NVI

Special Testing Neg. instability. Neg. pain with ligamentous stress testing

Area of Injury

Circumferential Measurements

Left	Right	Reference Landmarks
26	27	Med. Mall. (MM)
23	23.5	5cm prox. MM
25	26	5cm distal MM

Overview: Rehabilitation Program To Date:

Progressed from NWB --- TDWB --- PWB --- FWB over past week. Initial rehab. concentrated on pain modulation, effusion, and strength & ROM. Working with strength & conditioning coach with wll-limb maintenance program & cont'd cardio-vascular maintenance program with UBE, Fitron, & aquatic rehab. Pt. has progressed well with initiation of proprioception & balance activities.

ASSESSMENT

Clinical Impression/Rehabilitation Progress: Progressing well at this time-frame with injury.

Rehabilitation Problems Identified: ☒ Physiological Healing Constraints ☒ Pain ☒ Swelling ☒↓ROM ☒↓ Muscle Performance ☒↓ Balance/Proprioception ☒ Loss of Function ☐ Other

Rehabilitation Goals STG: 1) DF ROM WNL, 2)Neg. effusion, 3) Neg. pain, 4)MMT ankle strength levels WNL. LTG: Return to athletic activity level without restrictions. ROM/strength WNL. Prevenative maintenance program.

PLAN

Continue to monitor progress B.I.D. Advance strength, balance, proprioception activities as appropriate. Begin preparation for gradual return to functional activity.

REHABILITATION: DISCHARGE SUMMARY

Name: Smith, John   Sport: Football   Date: 9/22/90

Identification # 41024   Age: 20   D.O.B. 7/14/70   Sex: M   Physician: Jones

SUBJECTIVE

Present Injury History S/P 2 wks. Rt. Grade I inversion ankle sprain. Athlete presents without c/o. "I'm ready to go full-speed now".

OBJECTIVE

Presentation FWB

Observation Neg. effusion Rt. ankle/foot
Neg. ecchymosis.

Palpation Neg. point tenderness.
Neg. deformity, crepitus.

Range of Motion PF, Inv., Ever. = WNL
DF = 10°

Muscle Performance MMT reveals 5/5 PF/DF/Inv/Ever.
Isokinetic testing reveals peak torque & total
work WNL in PF/DF & Inv/Ever (enclosed in chart)

Neurovascular NVI

Special Testing Neg. ligamentous instability. Neg. pain
with ligamentous stress testing.

Area of Injury

Circumferential Measurements

Left	Right	Reference Landmarks
26	26	Med Mall (MM)
23	23	5cm prox MM
25	25	5cm distal MM

Functional Testing/
Sports Specific
Skills
Perfromed following under supervision without pain, instability, or
other symptoms, full squat, standing on toes, one foot balance, one
foot hopping, forward/reverse running, cutting, figure 8 run, carioca, 5-10-5
lateral mobility run, sport simulated movemtnets (cuts, pass paterns).

ASSESSMENT

Clinical Impression: Progressing well at this time-frame since injury. Participating in 1/2
and 3/4 speed drills and non-contact activities over past 3 days without
difficulty.

PLAN

☐ Return to athletic activity without restrictions

☒ Return to athletic activity with the following restrictions: Continue maintenance rehab. program & use of
protective bracing.

☒ Performance of preventative maintenance program as follows: Achilles flexibility pre/post athletic activity
Ankle PF/DF/Inv/Ever resistive ex. with Thera-Band 3x10 ea QD; proprioceptive/
balance activities with BAPS, Pro-Fitter, one foot balance QD; cryotherapy after
athletic activity.

☒ Prophylactic strapping/bracing as follows: Taping, Air-Cast stirrup ankle brace for athletic
activities.

☒ Other: Fitted with high top athletic shoes by equipment manager.

Bibliography

Arnheim, D. (1997): Modern Principles of Athletic Training, 9th ed. St. Louis, Times Mirror/Mosby.

Gould, J., and Davies, G. (1985): Orthopaedic and Sports Physical Therapy. St. Louis, C.V. Mosby.

Kessler, R.M., and Hertling, D. (1985): Management of Common Musculoskeletal Disorders. Philadelphia, Harper & Row.

Kisner, C., and Colby, L.A. (1985): Therapeutic Exercises: Foundations and Techniques. Philadelphia, F.A. Davis.

Magee, D.J. (1997): Orthopedic Physical Assessment, 3rd ed. Philadelphia, W.B. Saunders.

Prentice, W.E. (1994): Rehabilitation Techniques in Sports Medicine, 2nd ed. St. Louis, Times Mirror/Mosby.

Roy, S., and Irvin, R. (1983): Sports Medicine: Prevention, Evaluation, Management, and Rehabilitation. Englewood Cliffs, NJ, Prentice-Hall.

Torg, J.S., Vesgo, J.J., and Torg, E. (1987): Rehabilitation of Athletic Injuries. Chicago, Year Book Medical Publishers.

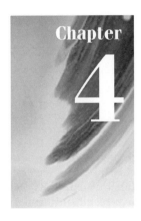

Measurement in Rehabilitation

Gary L. Harrelson, Ed.D., A.T.,C.

Measurement has long been used to chart progress during the rehabilitation process. Therefore, it is important for all clinicians to be competent in performing and interpreting objective measurements of girth and joint motion. This chapter addresses the reliability and validity of these measurements, ensuring reliable measurements, and various techniques for performing girth and joint motion assessments.

GIRTH MEASUREMENTS

The use of a flexible tape measure to measure girth is probably the most common clinical method to document muscle bulk and swelling. Girth assessment by use of a tape measure is also referred to as girth measurement, circumferential measurement, or anthropometric measurement. Not only is this assessment technique used before implementing a weight-training program to assess its impact on muscle hypertrophy, but it is also used to assess muscle atrophy or joint swelling after injury or surgery and to determine the subsequent effect of a rehabilitation program on muscle hypertrophy and joint swelling. Girth measurements have been reported in the literature for documenting the effects of a rehabilitation program on muscle atrophy or hypertrophy and joint swelling[36] after injury,[10, 18, 46] surgery, or implementation of a rehabilitation program.[26, 28, 31, 33]

The increase or decrease in girth measurement is thought to indicate a direct relationship between an increase or decrease in muscle strength. For example, as a muscle atrophies, the loss of strength is directly related to muscle size because the muscle fibers themselves reduce in size; the outcome, therefore, is a reduction in strength. However, there is evidence to support the absence of a direct relationship between girth measurement and muscle size.[6]

Most of the variability in obtaining girth measurements arises from use of different anatomic landmarks, tension placed on the tape measure by the clinician, and whether the muscle is contracted. The tension placed on the tape measure when assessing girth does not appear to be as big an issue as previously thought.[16, 41] The following recommendations are made to improve intra- and interclinician reliability during girth assessments:

- Attempt to place the same amount of tension on the tape measure with each measurement.

- All clinicians should use the same anatomic land-marks when determining the site of the girth measurements.
- If possible, take the girth measurement with the muscle contracted.

Several investigations[16, 41] have assessed the reliability of lower extremity girth measurements in healthy young athletes. The data suggest that these measurements are reliable and can be reproduced with a high degree of accuracy both within and between clinicians, with a standard error of measurement of less than 1 cm. Also, many times clinicians often use a healthy extremity to determine the amount of atrophy that may have occurred as a result of trauma. Healthy right and left lower extremities appear to have similar circumferences and should not vary more than 1.5 cm between right and left sides.[41] Additionally, comparisons between a standard flexible tape measure and a Lufkin tape measure with a Gulick spring-loaded end indicate that there is no significant difference between the two (Fig. 4–1).[16]

Although girth measurements appear to be reproducible, the validity of the measurement has been questioned with regard to thigh bulk. Stokes and Young[37] were concerned that the tape measure was not sensitive and accurate enough for measuring the selective wasting of the quadriceps. Doxey[5] reports that detecting changes in muscle bulk in nonsurgical subjects probably requires more sensitive methods than girth measurements, such as ultrasonography or computed tomography. Furthermore, a small decrease (1%) in thigh measurement may be an indicator of a significant reduction (13%) in muscle bulk.[5] Research using ultrasonography[5, 47] and computed tomography[6] has shown that muscle fiber atrophy is not adequately reflected by circumference measurements. Rather, extremity fat can mask this muscle atrophy. Thus, caution should be used in interpreting the results of girth measurements with regard to muscle strength and progressing individuals along a plan of care.

GONIOMETRY

Goniometry is the use of instruments for measuring the range of motion in body joints. All clinicians should be competent in performing and interpreting objective measurements of joint motion. Initial range-of-motion measurements provide a basis for developing a treatment plan, and repeated measurements

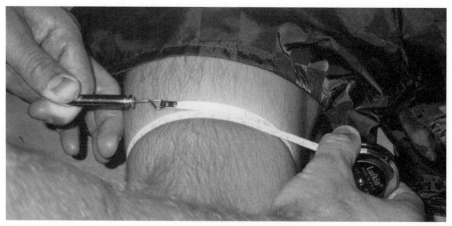

Figure 4–1. Lufkin tape measure with a Gulick spring-loaded end.

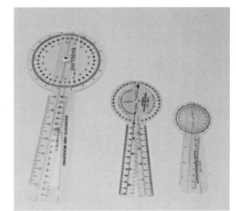

Figure 4–2. Full-circle manual universal goniometer.

throughout the course of rehabilitation help determine whether improvement has been made and goals achieved.

Historical Considerations

The literature on goniometry is extensive and describes many aspects of goniometric measuring. Gifford,[12] in 1914, was probably the first to have reported on goniometric devices in the United States. Historically, many articles have described and recommended various instruments and methods of measurement.[4, 19, 24, 25, 30, 40, 42, 43] These instruments are generally of two types: (1) devices of universal application (e.g., full-circle universal goniometer), which remain the most versatile and popular (Fig. 4–2); and (2) goniometers designed to measure a single range of motion for a specific joint (Fig. 4–3). Although not as common as universal goniometers, gravity-dependent goniometers or inclinometers use gravity's effect on pointers or fluid levels to measure joint position and motion.[27] These are either (1) pendulum goniometers that consist of a 360° protractor with a weighted pointer hanging from the center of the protractor; or (2) fluid goniometers that have a fluid-filled circular chamber containing an air bubble, similar to a carpenter's level (Fig. 4–4).

As goniometry evolved, efforts were directed toward standardizing methods of measurement, including developing common nomenclature and definitions

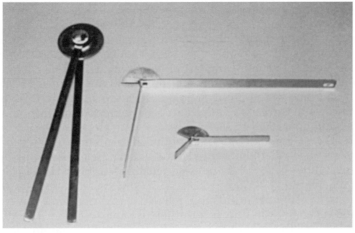

Figure 4–3. Goniometers for measuring a single joint motion.

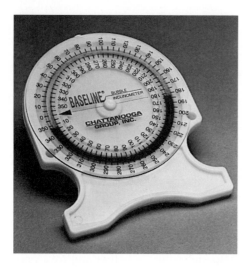

Figure 4–4. Bubble inclinometer. (Photo courtesy of the Chattanooga Group, Chattanooga, Tennessee.)

of terms, clearly defining movements to be measured, and establishing normal ranges of motion. In 1965, the American Academy of Orthopaedic Surgeons published a manual of standardized methods of measuring and recording joint motion; since then, there have been numerous reprints.[2] Norkin and White[27] have also provided a thorough description of goniometry.

Goniometric Assessment

ANATOMIC ZERO POSITION

The anatomic zero position is the starting 0° orientation for most measurements.[24] The exceptions are shoulder rotation, hip rotation, and forearm pronation-supination, in which the starting position is between the two extremes of motion. If the individual to be measured cannot assume the starting position, the position of improvisation should be noted when recording joint motion. The degrees of joint motion are added in the direction of joint movement. Average ranges of motion for the upper and lower extremities are outlined in Table 4–1.[2]

VALIDITY AND RELIABILITY OF GONIOMETRIC MEASUREMENT

The purpose of goniometry is to measure the joint angle or range of motion.[27] It is assumed that the angle created by aligning the arms of a universal goniometer with bony landmarks truly represents the angle created by the proximal and distal bones composing the joint.[27] One infers that changes in goniometer alignment reflect changes in joint angle and represent a range of joint motion.[27] Additionally, goniometer measurements are generally compared with radiographs, which represent the "gold standard" for measurements. Several studies[1, 8, 13] have indicated a degree of relationship between measurements obtained with radiography and goniometry.

The reliability of goniometric joint motion measurements has been studied. Several reports noted that joint range of motion can be measured with good-to-excellent reliability.[7, 11, 13, 20, 21] Intratester reliability appears to be higher than intertester reliability.[3, 7, 14, 15, 17, 21–23, 29, 32, 34, 35] Additionally, it appears that upper extremity joint measurements are more reliable than those of the lower extremity joints,[3, 29] and reliability can be less for different joints.[9, 20, 21, 38, 45] This may be due to the complexity of the joint or the difficulty in palpating anatomic landmarks.[27] Because reliability is different for each joint, the standard error of measurement

Table 4–1. Average Ranges of Motion for the Upper and Lower Extremities

JOINT	MOTION	RANGE OF MOTION (degrees) AMERICAN ACADEMY OF ORTHOPAEDIC SURGEONS[2]	KENDALL AND McCREARY[17a]
Shoulder	Flexion	0–180	0–180
	Extension	0–60	0–45
	Abduction	0–180	0–180
	Internal rotation	0–70	0–70
	External rotation	0–90	0–90
Elbow	Flexion	0–150	0–145
Forearm	Pronation	0–80	0–90
	Supination	0–80	0–90
Wrist	Extension	0–70	0–70
	Flexion	0–80	0–80
	Radial deviation	0–20	0–20
	Ulnar deviation	0–30	0–35
Thumb			
CMC	Abduction	0–70	0–80
	Flexion	0–15	0–45
	Extension	0–20	0
MCP	Flexion	0–50	0–60
IP	Flexion	0–80	0–80
Digits 2 to 5			
MCP	Flexion	0–90	0–90
	Extension	0–45	
PIP			
DIP	Flexion		
	Extension		
Hip	Flexion	0–120	0–125
	Extension	0–30	0–10
	Abduction	0–45	0–45
	Adduction	0–30	0–10
	External rotation	0–45	0–45
	Internal rotation	0–45	0–45
Knee	Flexion	0–135	0–140
Ankle	Dorsiflexion	0–20	0 20
	Plantar flexion	0–50	0–45
	Inversion	0–35	0–35
	Eversion	0–15	0–20
Subtalar	Inversion	0–5	
	Eversion	0–5	

Adapted from Norkin, C.C., and White, D.J. (1985): Measurement of Joint Motion: A Guide to Goniometry, Philadelphia, F.A. Davis.
CMC, Carpometacarpal; DIP, distal interphalangeal; IP, interphalangeal; MCP, metacarpophalangeal; PIP, proximal interphalangeal.

can also differ for each joint. Norkin and White[27] have documented the standard deviation and standard error of measurement for each joint in their book on goniometry. Boone and colleagues[3] have indicated that the same individual should perform goniometric measurements when the effects of treatment are evaluated. Visual estimation is used by some clinicians to assess joint positions. Investigations assessing the accuracy and reliability of visual estimation versus goniometer measurements report the latter to be more accurate and reliable.[9, 17, 21, 23, 39, 44, 45]

TECHNICAL CONSIDERATIONS

The positioning of the athlete should be consistent. The prone or supine position provides greater stabilization through the athlete's body weight. Measurements should be acquired as passive range of motion when possible, and the body part should be uncovered for better accuracy. The goniometer is placed next to or on top of the joint, whenever possible, and the goniometer arms are placed along the longitudinal axis of the bones of the joint after the motion has occurred. In evaluating the joint and assessing range of motion, the clinician should view the affected joint from above and below to determine whether any additional limitations are present in the involved extremity. The opposite extremity must also be assessed to determine normal motion for that athlete.

Norkin and White[27] suggest the following guidelines to increase goniometry reliability:

- Use consistent, well-defined testing positions and anatomic landmarks to align the arms of the goniometer.
- Take repeated measurements on a subject with the same type of measurement device.
- Use large universal goniometers when measuring joints with large body segments.
- Inexperienced examiners should take several measurements and record the average of those measurements to improve reliability, but one measurement is usually sufficient for more experienced examiners using good technique.
- Successive measurements are more reliable if taken by the same examiner rather than by different examiners.

Applications

UPPER EXTREMITIES
Shoulder
Flexion
Suggested Testing Position. The athlete is in the anatomic supine position (Fig. 4–5), with the forearm in midposition between supination and pronation.

Goniometer Alignment. The goniometer is aligned along (1) the midline of the humerus and (2) the midaxillary line of the trunk (Fig. 4–6).

Extension
Suggested Testing Position. The athlete is in the anatomic prone position (Fig. 4–7), with the forearm in midposition between supination and pronation.

Goniometer Alignment. The goniometer is aligned along (1) the midline of the humerus and (2) the midaxillary line of the trunk (Fig. 4–8).

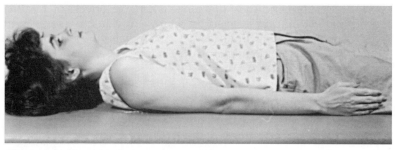

Figure 4–5. Shoulder flexion: testing position.

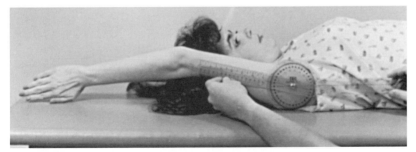

Figure 4–6. Shoulder flexion: goniometer alignment.

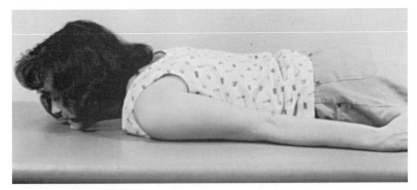

Figure 4–7. Shoulder extension: suggested testing position.

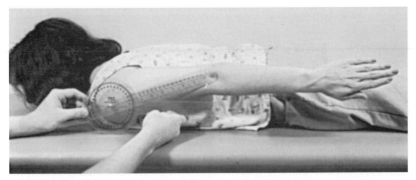

Figure 4–8. Shoulder extension: goniometer alignment.

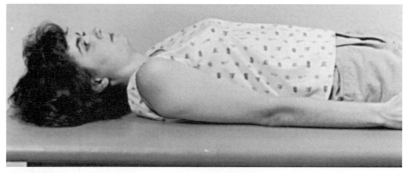

Figure 4–9. Shoulder abduction: suggested testing position.

Abduction

Suggested Testing Position. The athlete is in the anatomic supine position (Fig. 4–9), with the forearm in midposition between supination and pronation.

Goniometer Alignment. The goniometer is aligned (1) along the anterior longitudinal axis of the humerus and (2) parallel to the midline of the body (Fig. 4–10).

Adduction

Suggested Testing Position. The athlete is in the anatomic supine position, with the forearm in midposition between supination and pronation (see Fig. 4–9).

Goniometer Alignment. The goniometer is aligned (1) along the anterior longitudinal axis of the humerus and (2) parallel to the midline of the body (Fig. 4–11).

External Rotation

Suggested Testing Position. The athlete is supine, with the arm abducted to 90°, the elbow flexed to 90°, and the forearm pronated and perpendicular to the table (Fig. 4–12).

Goniometer Alignment. The goniometer is aligned (1) along the ulna to the ulnar styloid process and (2) perpendicular to the table (Fig. 4–13).

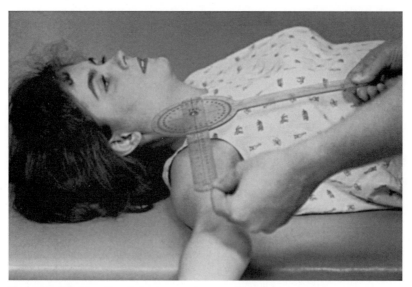

Figure 4–10. Shoulder abduction: goniometer alignment.

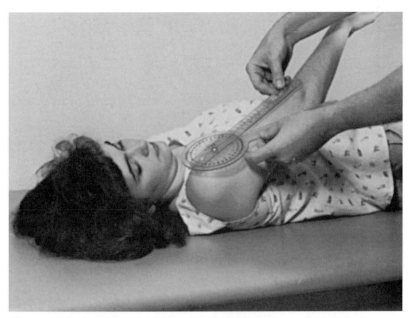

Figure 4–11. Shoulder adduction: goniometer alignment.

Internal Rotation
Suggested Testing Position. The athlete is supine, with the arm abducted to 90°, the elbow flexed to 90°, and the forearm pronated and perpendicular to the table (see Fig. 4–12).

Goniometer Alignment. The goniometer is aligned (1) along the ulnar styloid process and (2) perpendicular to the table (Fig. 4–14).

Elbow
Flexion
Suggested Testing Position. The athlete is in the anatomic supine position (see Fig. 4–9).

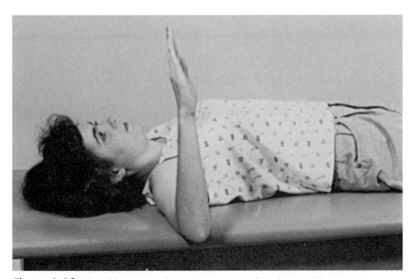

Figure 4–12. Shoulder external rotation: suggested testing position.

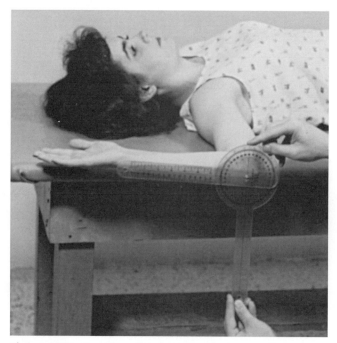

Figure 4-13. Shoulder external rotation: goniometer alignment.

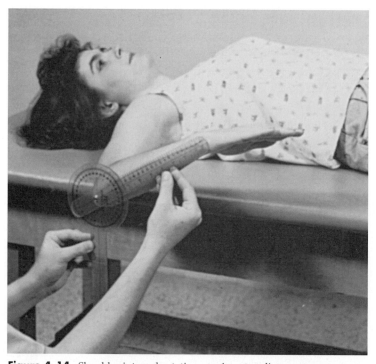

Figure 4-14. Shoulder internal rotation: goniometer alignment.

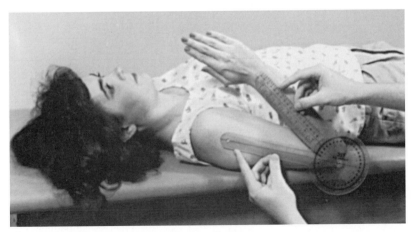

Figure 4–15. Elbow flexion: goniometer alignment.

Goniometer Alignment. The goniometer is aligned along (1) the lateral midline of the humerus, humeral head to lateral condyle, and (2) the midline of the radius to the radial styloid process (Fig. 4–15).

Extension
Suggested Testing Position. The athlete is in the anatomic supine position (see Fig. 4–9).
Goniometer Alignment. The goniometer is aligned along (1) the lateral midline of the humerus, humeral head to lateral condyle, and (2) the midline of the radius to the radial styloid process (Fig. 4–16).

Forearm
Pronation
Suggested Testing Position. The athlete is seated, with the elbow flexed to 90° and the forearm midway between supination and pronation (Fig. 4–17).
Goniometer Alignment. (1) With the fingers straight, the goniometer is lined up with the line formed by the fingertips or, with the fingers flexed, lined up with the line formed by the proximal interphalangeal joints and (2) parallel to the table (Fig. 4–18).

Supination
Suggested Testing Position. The athlete is seated, with the elbow flexed to 90° and the forearm midway between supination and pronation (see Fig. 4–17).

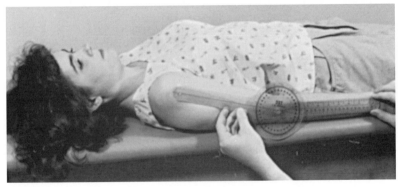

Figure 4–16. Elbow extension: goniometer alignment.

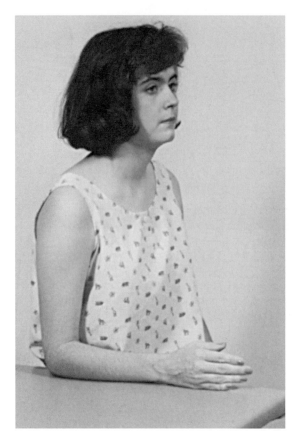

Figure 4–17. Forearm pronation: suggested testing position.

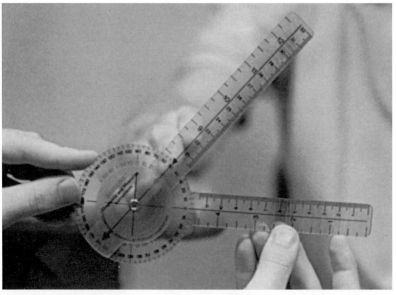

Figure 4–18. Forearm pronation: goniometer alignment.

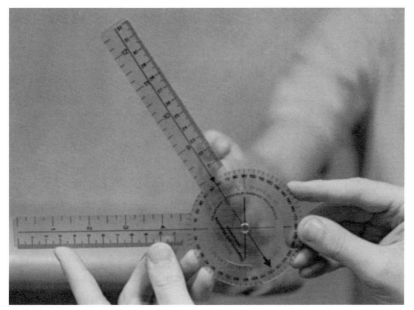

Figure 4–19. Forearm supination: goniometer alignment.

Goniometer Alignment. (1) With the fingers straight, the goniometer is lined up with the line formed by the fingertips or, with the fingers flexed, lined up with the line formed by the proximal interphalangeal joints and (2) parallel to the table (Fig. 4–19).

Wrist
Flexion
Suggested Testing Position. The athlete is supine, with the arm abducted to 90° and internally rotated, the elbow flexed to 90°, and the forearm pronated (Fig. 4–20).

Goniometer Alignment. The goniometer is aligned with (1) the midline of the ulna and (2) the fifth metacarpal (Fig. 4–21).

Extension
Suggested Testing Position. The athlete is supine, with the arm abducted to 90° and internally rotated, the elbow flexed to 90°, and the forearm pronated (see Fig. 4–20).

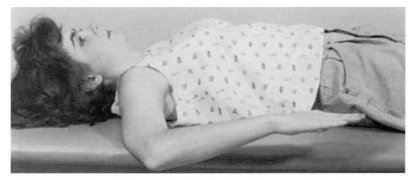

Figure 4–20. Wrist flexion: suggested testing position.

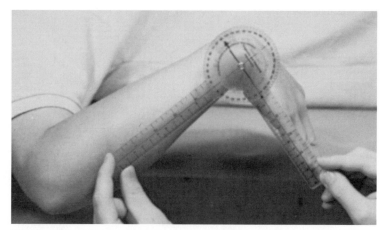

Figure 4–21. Wrist flexion: goniometer alignment.

Goniometer Alignment. The goniometer is aligned with (1) the midline of the ulna and (2) the fifth metacarpal (Fig. 4–22).

Radius and Ulna
Radial Deviation
Suggested Testing Position. The athlete is in the supine position, with the arm abducted to 90° and internally rotated, the elbow flexed to 90°, and the forearm pronated (see Fig. 4–20).

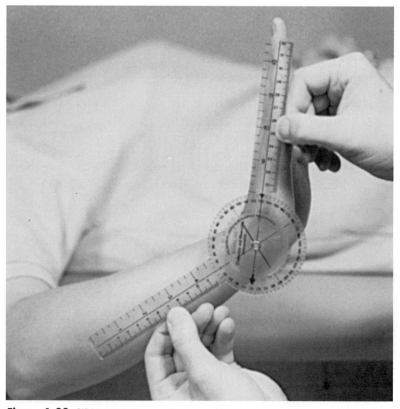

Figure 4–22. Wrist extension: goniometer alignment.

Goniometer Alignment. The goniometer is aligned (1) over the ulnar styloid process and parallel to the third metacarpal and (2) perpendicular to the third metacarpal (Fig. 4–23).

Ulnar Deviation
Suggested Testing Position. The athlete is supine, with the arm abducted to 90° and internally rotated, the elbow flexed to 90°, and the forearm pronated (see Fig. 4–20).
Goniometer Alignment. The goniometer is aligned (1) over the radial styloid process and parallel to the third metacarpal and (2) perpendicular to the third metacarpal (Fig. 4–24).

Fingers
Flexion
Goniometer Alignment. The goniometer is aligned along (1) the medial side of the proximal phalanx and (2) the medial side of the distal phalanx (Fig. 4–25).

Extension
Goniometer Alignment. The goniometer is aligned along (1) the medial side of the proximal phalanx and (2) the medial side of the distal phalanx (Fig. 4–26).

LOWER EXTREMITIES
Hip
Flexion
Suggested Testing Position. The athlete is in the anatomic supine position, with the knee bent to 90° when going through the motion (Fig. 4–27).
Goniometer Alignment. The goniometer is aligned (1) laterally along the long axis of the trunk and (2) on the lateral side, along the longitudinal axis of the femur, from greater trochanter to lateral femoral condyle (Fig. 4–28).

Extension
Suggested Testing Position. The athlete is in the anatomic prone position (Fig. 4–29).

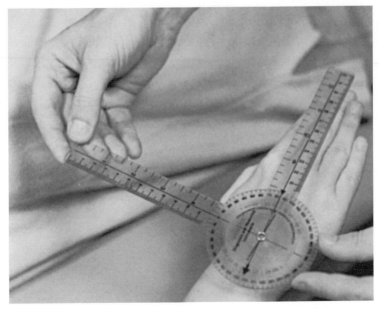

Figure 4–23. Radial deviation: goniometer alignment.

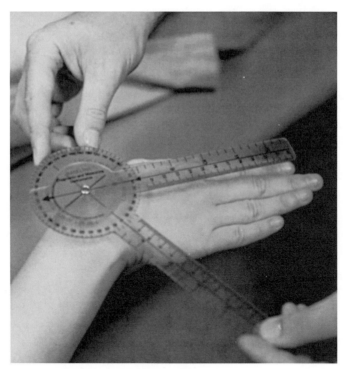

Figure 4–24. Ulnar deviation: goniometer alignment.

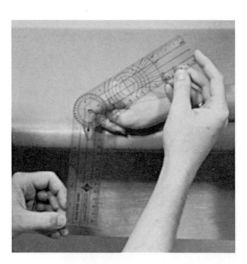

Figure 4–25. Finger flexion: goniometer alignment.

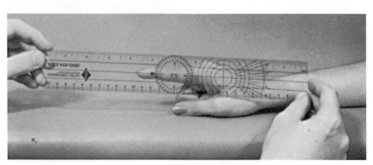

Figure 4–26. Finger extension: goniometer alignment.

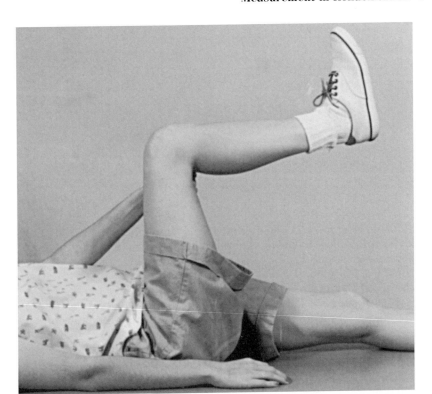

Figure 4–27. Hip flexion: suggested testing position.

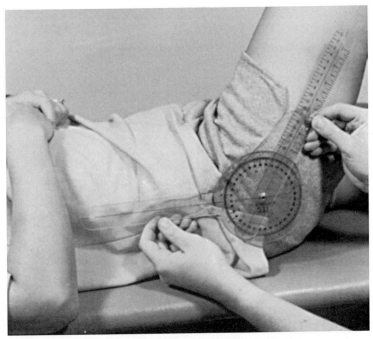

Figure 4–28. Hip flexion: goniometer alignment.

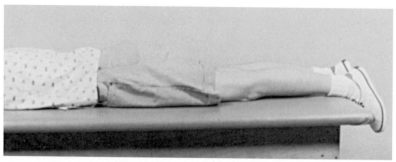

Figure 4–29. Hip extension: suggested testing position.

Goniometer Alignment. The goniometer is aligned (1) laterally along the long axis of the trunk and (2) on the lateral side, along the longitudinal axis of the femur, from greater trochanter to lateral femoral condyle (Fig. 4–30).

Straight Leg Raising
Suggested Testing Position. The athlete is in the anatomic supine position, with the knee straight through the motion, and the ankle dorsiflexed.
Goniometer Alignment. The goniometer is aligned (1) laterally along the axis of the femur, from greater trochanter to lateral femoral condyle, and (2) parallel to the fibula and lateral malleolus (Fig. 4–31).

Abduction
Suggested Testing Position. The athlete is in the anatomic supine position (Fig. 4–32).
Goniometer Alignment. The goniometer is aligned (1) over the two anterior superior iliac spines and (2) along the anterior thigh, from the midline of the thigh to the midline of the patella (Fig. 4–33).

Adduction
Suggested Testing Position. The athlete flexes the hip and knee in a supported position, with the extremity to be tested brought under the other extremity.
Goniometer Alignment. The goniometer is aligned (1) over the two anterior superior iliac spines and (2) along the anterior thigh, from the midline of the thigh to the midline of the patella (Fig. 4–34).

Internal Rotation
Suggested Testing Position. The athlete is seated, with the hip flexed to 90° and the knee flexed to 90° over the edge of the table (Fig. 4–35).
Goniometer Alignment. The goniometer is aligned (1) parallel to the table

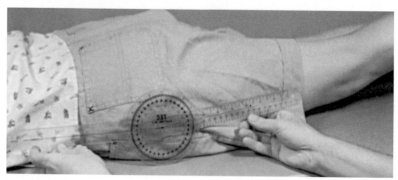

Figure 4–30. Hip extension: goniometer alignment.

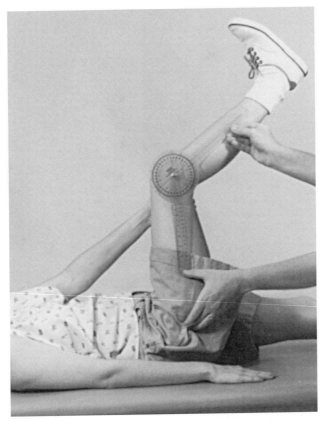

Figure 4–31. Straight leg raising: goniometer alignment.

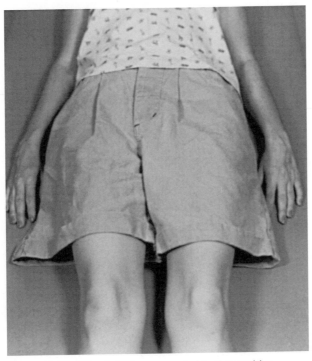

Figure 4–32. Hip abduction: suggested testing position.

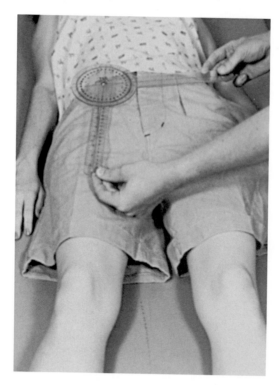

Figure 4–33. Hip abduction: goniometer alignment.

Figure 4–34. Hip adduction: goniometer alignment.

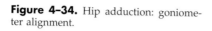

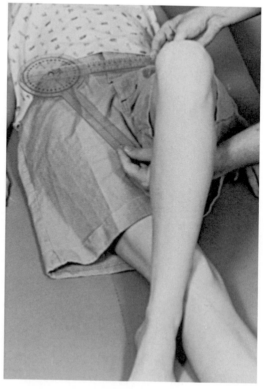

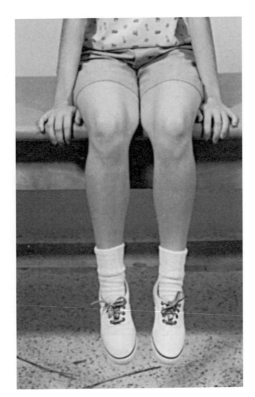

Figure 4-35. Hip internal rotation: suggested testing position.

and (2) along the midline of the anterior tibia, from the patella to midposition between the malleoli (Fig. 4–36).

External Rotation

Suggested Testing Position. The athlete is seated, with the hip flexed to 90° and the knee flexed to 90° over the edge of the table (see Fig. 4–35).

Goniometer Alignment. The goniometer is aligned (1) parallel to the table and (2) along the midline of the anterior tibia, from the patella to midposition between the malleoli (Fig. 4–37).

Knee

Flexion

Suggested Testing Position. The athlete is in the supine position, with the hip flexed.

Goniometer Alignment. The goniometer is aligned along (1) the lateral femur, from the greater trochanter to the lateral femoral condyle and (2) the fibular head to the lateral malleolus (Fig. 4–38).

Extension

Suggested Testing Position. The athlete is in the anatomic supine position.

Goniometer Alignment. The goniometer is aligned along (1) the lateral femur, from the greater trochanter to the lateral femoral condyle and (2) the fibular head to the lateral malleolus (Fig. 4–39).

Ankle

Plantar Flexion

Suggested Testing Position. The athlete is in the anatomic supine position, with the knee straight, or is seated, with the knee flexed.

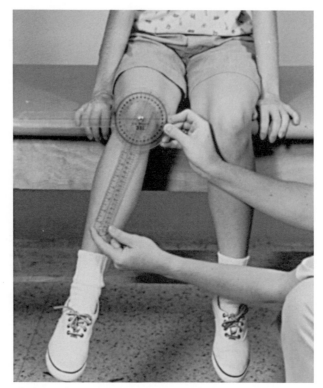

Figure 4–36. Hip internal rotation: goniometer alignment.

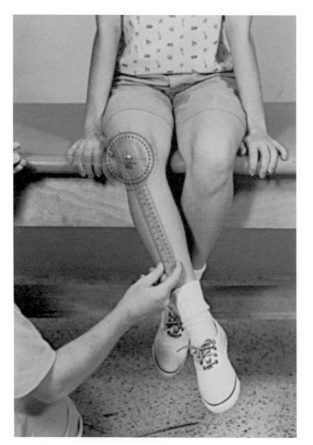

Figure 4–37. Hip external rotation: goniometer alignment.

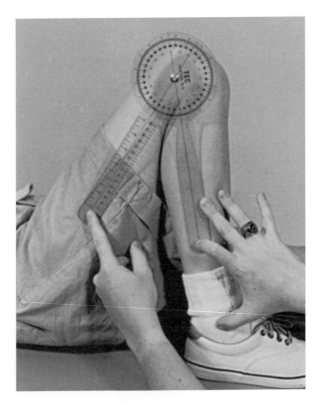

Figure 4–38. Knee flexion: goniometer alignment.

Goniometer Alignment. The goniometer is aligned (1) along the midline of the fibula, fibula head to lateral malleolus, and (2) along the midline of the fifth metatarsal (Fig. 4–40).

Dorsiflexion

Suggested Testing Position. The athlete is in the anatomic supine position, with the knee straight, or is seated, with the knee flexed.

Goniometer Alignment. The goniometer is aligned (1) along the midline of the fibula, fibula head to lateral malleolus, and (2) along the midline of the fifth metatarsal (Fig. 4–41).

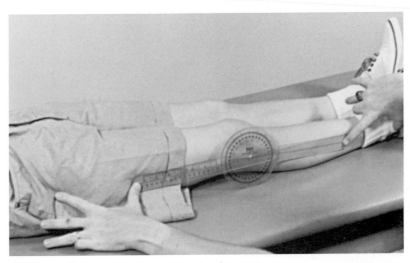

Figure 4–39. Knee extension: goniometer alignment.

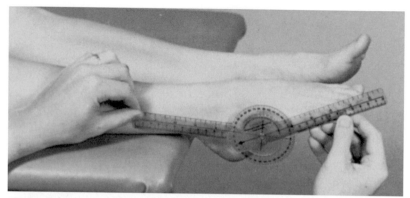

Figure 4–40. Ankle plantar flexion: goniometer alignment.

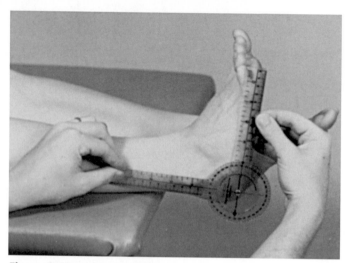

Figure 4–41. Ankle dorsiflexion: goniometer alignment.

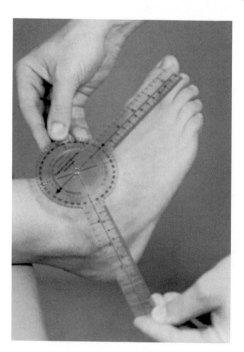

Figure 4–42. Ankle inversion: goniometer alignment.

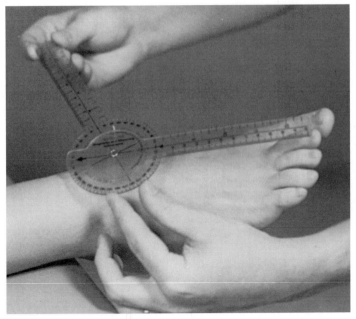

Figure 4–43. Ankle eversion: goniometer alignment.

Inversion
Suggested Testing Position. The athlete is in the anatomic supine position.
Goniometer Alignment. The goniometer is aligned (1) across the two malleoli and (2) parallel to the second metatarsal (Fig. 4–42).

Eversion
Suggested Testing Position. The athlete is in the anatomic supine position.
Goniometer Alignment. The goniometer is aligned (1) across the two malleoli and (2) parallel to the second metatarsal (Fig. 4–43).

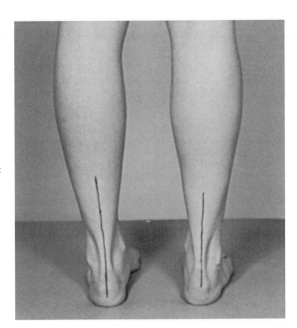

Figure 4–44. Rearfoot varus/valgus: suggested testing position.

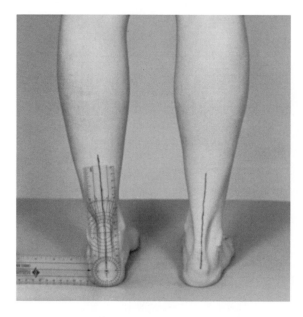

Figure 4–45. Rearfoot varus/valgus: goniometer alignment.

Rearfoot

Varus/Valgus

Suggested Testing Position. The athlete is in the standing position (Fig. 4–44).
Goniometer Alignment. The goniometer is aligned (1) parallel to the floor and (2) bisecting the calcaneus and Achilles tendon (Fig. 4–45).

References

1. Ahlback, S.O., and Lindahl, O. (1964): Sagittal mobility of the hip-joint. Acta Orthop. Scand., 34:310–314.
2. American Academy of Orthopaedic Surgeons (1965): Joint Motion: Methods of Measuring and Recording. Chicago, American Academy of Orthopaedic Surgeons.
3. Boone, D.C., Azen, S.P., Linn, C.N., et al. (1978): Reliability of goniometric measurements. Phys. Ther., 58:1355–1360.
4. Clark, W.A. (1921): A protractor for measuring rotation of joint. J. Orthop. Surg., 3:154–155.
5. Doxey, G. (1987): The association of anthropometric measurement of thigh size and B-mode ultrasound scanning of muscle thickness. J. Orthop. Sports Phys. Ther., 8:462–468.
6. Doxey, G. (1987): Assessing quadriceps femoris muscle bulk with girth measurements in subjects with patellofemoral pain. J. Othop. Sports Phys. Ther., 9:177–183.
7. Ekstuand, J., Wiktorsson, M., and Oberg, B. (1982): Lower extremity goniometric measurements: A study to determine their reliability. Arch. Phys. Med., 63:171–175.
8. Enwemeka, C.S. (1986): Radiographic verification of knee goniometry. Scand. J. Rehabil. Med., 18:47–50.
9. Fitzgerald, G.K., Wynveen, K.J., Rheault, W., and Rothschild, B. (1983). Objective assessment with establishment of normal values for lumbar spine range of motion. Phys. Ther., 63:1776–1781.
10. Fowler, P.J., and Regan, W.D. (1987): The patient with symptomatic chronic anterior cruciate ligament insufficiency. Am. J. Sports Med., 15:321–325.
11. Gajdosik, R.L., and Bohannon, R.W. (1987): Clinical measurement of range of motion: Review of goniometry emphasizing reliability and validity. Phys. Ther., 67:1867–1872.
12. Gifford, H.D. (1914): Instruments for measuring joint movements and deformities in fracture treatment. Am. J. Surg., 28:237–238.
13. Gogia, P.P., Braatz, J.H., Rose, S.J., and Norton, B. (1987): Reliability and validity of goniometric measurements of the knee. Phys. Ther., 67:192–195.
14. Grohmann, J.L. (1983): Comparison of two methods of goniometry. Phys. Ther., 63:922–926.
15. Hamilton, G.F., and Lachenbruch, P.A. (1969): Reliability of goniometers in assessing finger joint angle. Phys. Ther., 49:465–469.
16. Harrelson, G.L., Fincher, A.L., and Harrelson, L.M. (1995): Inter- and intratester reliability of lower extremity circumference measurements. 1995 National Athletic Trainers Association Clinical Meeting and Symposium, Indianapolis, IN.
17. Hellebradt, F.A., Duvall, E.N., and Moore, M.L. (1949): The measurement of joint motion. Part III. Reliability of goniometry. Phys. Ther. Rev., 29:302–307.

17a. Kendall, F.P., and McCreary, E.K. (1983): Muscle Testing and Function, 3rd ed. Baltimore, Williams & Wilkins.

18. Kirwan, J.R., Byron, M.A., Winfield, J., et al. (1979): Circumferential measurements in the assessment of synovitis of the knee. Rheumatol. Rehabil., 18:78–84.

19. Leighton, J.R. (1955): An instrument and technic for the measurement of range of joint motion. Arch. Phys. Med., 36:571–577.

20. Lovell, F.W., Rothstein, J.M., and Personius, W.J. (1989): Reliability of clinical measurement of lumbar lordosis taken with a flexible rule. Phys. Ther., 69:96–101.

21. Low, J.L. (1976): The reliability of joint measurement. Physiotherapy, 62:227–229.

22. Reference deleted.

23. Mayerson, N.H. and Milano, R.A. (1984): Goniometric measurement reliability in physical medicine. Arch. Phys. Med. Rehabil., 65:92–97.

24. Moore, M.L. (1949): The measurement of joint motion. Part I. Introductory review of the literature. Phys. Ther. Rev., 29:195–205.

25. Moore, M.L. (1949): The measurement of joint motion. Part II. The technic of goniometry. Phys. Ther. Rev., 29:256–264.

26. Morrissey, M.C., Brewster, C.E., Shields, C.L., and Brown, M. (1985): The effects of electrical stimulation on the quadriceps during postoperative knee immobilization. J. Sports Med., 12:40–45.

27. Norkin, C.C., and White, D.J. (1995): Measurement of Joint Motion: Guide to Goniometry, 2nd ed. Philadelphia, F.A. Davis.

28. Noyes, F.R., Mangine, R.E., and Barber, S. (1987): Early knee motion after open and arthroscopic anterior cruciate ligament reconstruction. Am. J. Sports Med., 15:149–160.

29. Pandya, S., Florence, J.M., King, W.M., et al. (1985): Reliability of goniometric measurement in patients with Duchenne muscular dystrophy. Phys. Ther., 65:1339–1345.

30. Parker, J.S. (1929): Recording arthroflexometer. J. Bone Joint Surg., 11:126–127.

31. Reynolds, N.L., Worrell, T.W., and Perrin D.H. (1992): Effect of a lateral step-up exercise protocol on quadriceps isokinetic peak torque values and thigh girth. J. Orthop. Sports Phys. Ther., 15:151–155.

32. Riddle, D.L., Rothstein, J.M., Lamb, R.L. (1987): Goniometric reliability in a clinical setting: Shoulder measurements. Phys. Ther., 67:668–673.

33. Romero, J.A., Sanford, T.L., Schroeder, and R.V., Fahey, T.D. (1982): The effects of electrical stimulation of normal quadriceps on strength and girth. Med. Sci. Sports Exerc., 14:194–197.

34. Rothstein, J.M., Miller, P.J., Roettger, R.F. (1983): Goniometric reliability in a clinical setting: Elbow and knee measurement. Phys. Ther., 63:1611–1615.

35. Solgaard, S., Carlsen, A., Krauhoft, M., and Petersen, V.S. (1986): Reproducibility of goniometry of the wrist. Scand. J. Rehabil. Med., 18:5–7.

36. Spencer, J.D., Hayes, K.C., and Alexander, I.J. (1984): Knee joint effusion and quadriceps reflex inhibition in man. Arch. Phys. Med. Rehabil., 65:171–177.

37. Stokes, M., and Young, A. (1984): The contribution of reflex inhibition to arthrogenous muscle weakness. Clin. Sci., 67:7–14.

38. Tucci, S.M., Hicks, J.E., Gross, E.G., Campbell, W., et al. (1986): Cervical motion assessment: A new, simple and accurate method. Arch. Phys. Med. Rehabil., 67:225–230.

39. Watkins, M.A., Riddle, D.L., Lamb, R.L., and Personius, W.J. (1991): Reliability of goniometric measurements and visual estimates of knee range of motion obtained in a clinical setting. Phys. Ther., 71: 90–96.

40. West, C.C. (1945): Measurement of joint motion. Arch. Phys. Med., 26:414–425.

41. Whitney, S.L., Matttocks, L., Irrgang, J.J., et al. (1995): Reliability of lower extremity girth measurements and right- and left-side differences. J. Sports Rehabil., 4:108–115.

42. Wiechec, F.J., and Krusen, F.H. (1939): A new method of joint measurement and a review of the literature. Am. J. Surg., 43:659–668.

43. Wilson, J.D., and Stasch, W.H. (1945): Photographic record of joint motion. Arch. Phys. Med., 27:361–362.

44. Youdas, J.W., Bogard, C.L., and Suman, V.J. (1993): Reliability of goniometric measurements and visual estimates of ankle joint active range of motion obtained in a clinical setting. Arch. Phys. Med. Rehabil., 74:1113–1118.

45. Youdas, J.W., Carey, J.R., and Garrett, T.R. (1991): Reliability of measurements of cervical spine range of motion: Comparison of three methods. Phys. Ther., 71:2–7.

46. Young, A., Stokes, M., and Iles, J.F. (1987): Effects of joint pathology on muscle. Clin. Orthop., 219:21–27.

47. Young, A., Hughes, I., Russell, P., et al. (1980): Measurement of quadriceps muscles wasting by ultrasonography. Rheumatol. Rehabil., 19:141–148.

Chapter 5

Use of Modalities in Rehabilitation

Gary L. Harrelson, Ed.D., A.T.,C.,
Mark D. Weber, M.S., A.T.,C., P.T., S.C.S., and
Deidre Leaver-Dunn, M.Ed., A.T.,C.

Because athletic trainers and physical therapists are frequently the first of the health care team to treat the injured athlete, they can be either extremely effective or damaging in the treatment of that athlete. A thorough evaluation, with proper consideration of important clinical signs and symptoms, enables the clinician to detect serious injuries in the early stages before the full extent of damage is evident, to prevent minor problems from developing into more serious injury, and to treat more chronic conditions that have not yet progressed to the point of interfering with performance and causing debilitation. Athletic trainers and physical therapists can be extremely effective in helping modify the course of an athlete's injury. The judicious and timely use of therapeutic techniques, tailored specifically to the individual athlete's condition, can radically alter the events that follow. For example, athletic trainers and physical therapists are in an excellent position to prevent the development of chronic edema, which can markedly interfere with later attempts at treatment, and to help prevent additional injury in an athlete who has attempted too much activity after prolonged immobilization.

Some powerful therapeutic tools available to clinicians include cold, heat, electricity, biofeedback, compression, and massage, commonly known as therapeutic modalities. Application of the appropriate modality at a particular stage of the healing process can prevent undue complications and can save time by preventing an unnecessarily prolonged period of convalescence. This chapter describes these therapeutic modalities: how they act on the human body, their methods of application, and considerations for their clinical use.

THERAPEUTIC COLD

Physiologic Effects

Therapeutic cold, or cryotherapy, is used in the management of acute and chronic athletic injuries. When applied to the human body, cryotherapy elicits a number of physiologic responses. These responses vary somewhat according to the situation in which cryotherapy is used, but they can be summarized as follows: decreased temperature, decreased cellular metabolism, decreased pain, decreased muscle spasm, increased tissue stiffness, increased or decreased inflammatory effects, and increased or decreased circulatory effects.[63] Additional effects of cryotherapy relate to muscle strength and proprioception.

CELLULAR METABOLISM

Cellular processes proceed more slowly at lower temperatures. Therefore, cryotherapy acts to slow the rate of the chemical reactions that occur as part of tissue metabolism.[63] In addition, cold acts to inhibit the release of histamine.[55] After an injury, damaged cells stimulate the release of histamine, a potent vasodilator that dramatically increases blood flow to an area. The histamine response is then maintained by mast cells.[44] The net effect of this process is the development and maintenance of large amounts of edematous fluid. Although edema itself is not harmful to the body, it can slow the exchange of nutrients and cellular waste. Increases in intracellular pressure caused by edema can also contribute to cellular anoxia.

PAIN

Cryotherapy is the modality of choice in the initial treatment of an acute injury primarily because of its role in decreasing cellular metabolism. In addition, cold is an effective pain reliever, a property that is of clinical importance in the treatment of acute injury and in injury rehabilitation. Although the precise mechanism by which the application of cold reduces pain is not known, speculation implicates one of two processes or, possibly, a combination of these.

A decrease in nerve conduction velocity after the application of cryotherapy is well documented.[42, 63, 134] Transmission can be slowed by as much as 29.4% after a 20-minute cold application, with conduction continuing to be impaired to some degree for up to 30 minutes after the cold modality is removed.[86] It has also been speculated that cold relieves pain through the gate control mechanism by interfering with the transmission of pain impulses at the second-order neurons located in the dorsal root ganglion of the spinal cord.[60] Thus, cold modalities are believed to relieve pain by slowing and reducing the number of pain impulses sent by the peripheral nerves and by interfering with the transmission of those impulses to the brain.

MUSCLE SPASM

As with pain relief mechanisms, several theories have been proposed to explain the reduction of muscle spasm through the application of cryotherapy. One explanation holds that because of a decrease in nerve conduction velocity, cryotherapy reduces the amount of sensory nerve activity and, hence, the resultant motor nerve activity that triggers and maintains spasm. However, a more complex spasm reduction mechanism that involves reflexes also appears to be at work.[63] This reflex theory is based on (1) the decrease in reflex responses soon after the application of cryotherapy, (2) the relationship between cutaneous cooling and decreased tonic stretch reflexes, and (3) the decrease in muscle spindle activity during stretching after sympathetic stimulation.[63] Finally, breaking of the pain-spasm-pain cycle is hypothesized to relieve muscle spasm. The inhibitory effects of cryotherapy on pain result in an interruption of this cycle, thereby allowing muscle relaxation and a reduction in the excitatory state.[63]

TISSUE STIFFNESS

The stiffness of the soft tissues of the body is increased with the application of cryotherapy. As a result, these tissues are less elastic and more resistant to movement. Although the exact mechanisms for these changes are not well understood,[63] the consequences of the explosive movement of cooled tissues are clear. Cryotherapy in combination with stretching assists in the reduction of muscle spasm, but attempts to increase the length of a cooled muscle could result in tearing of tissue.

INFLAMMATION

In his research on cryotherapy, Knight[63] discovered that the effects of cold application on inflammation after traumatic injury are not well investigated. Studies on inflammation have shown cryotherapy to mitigate, activate, or hamper the process in different situations.[63, 107] Cold can stimulate prostaglandin-mediated inflammation and inhibit inflammation that is thought to be similar to traumatically induced inflammation.[107]

CIRCULATION

Although cryotherapy leads to vasoconstriction, in the setting of acute injury, ice is usually not applied until vasoconstriction has been initiated in the body as part of the acute inflammatory response. Therefore, the circulatory effects of cryotherapy on acute injuries are not significant.[63]

In considering the application of cold in the acute and nonacute settings, there is much confusion about cold-induced vasodilation (CIVD) and the "hunting response" described by Lewis.[73] CIVD involves the dilation of blood vessels after the application of cold. The confusion resulted in the inference by clinicians that CIVD always occurs with cryotherapy and that this is also translated into increased blood flow, with a resultant increase in swelling.[63] Additional investigation[63] has shown that when CIVD occurs, it does so at the end of applications that are longer in duration than those used in the athletic arena. Furthermore, the net increase in vessel diameter still leaves the vessel in a state of vasoconstriction relative to its original diameter.[63]

PROPRIOCEPTION

A logical assumption from the decrease in nerve conduction velocity as a result of cold application would be that cryotherapy also decreases proprioception. Some recent research has supported this premise,[22] whereas other work has shown this not to be the case.[39, 122] The effect of cryotherapy on knee-joint position sense, as assessed by joint repositioning, was investigated by Thieme and colleagues.[122] Results of this investigation showed that a 20-minute application of ice packs to the anterior and posterior knee had no effect on the ability of the subjects to reproduce a passively demonstrated knee position. As a result of these data, the authors concluded that cooling has no impact on proprioception at the knee.

Work by Cross and colleagues[22] and Evans and colleagues[39] has examined the effect of cryotherapy on functional performance in athletic subjects. The effects of a 20-minute ankle ice immersion at 13° C on the shuttle run, 6-m hop test, and single leg vertical jump were studied by Cross et al.[22] Data from this study show decreases in performance on shuttle run time and vertical jump height in the experimental group after the application of cryotherapy. These results suggest that motor activity is inhibited by cold application. Conversely, research by Evans et al[39] concluded that a 20-minute ankle ice immersion at 1° C had no significant effect on motor activity. Results of a shuttle run, cocontraction test, and carioca maneuver were not affected after the application of cryotherapy in this sample of athletes.

MUSCLE STRENGTH

Cold has been reported to increase isometric muscular strength.[57, 94] Measures of strength taken immediately after a 30-minute submersion of a leg into a cold bath at 10° to 20° C (50° to 68° F) have revealed strength to be significantly diminished (Figs. 5–1 and 5–2). Measures taken after this period, however, showed that muscle strength increased and eventually exceeded pretreatment levels.[94] In both studies, strength of the cooled muscle tissue began to exceed

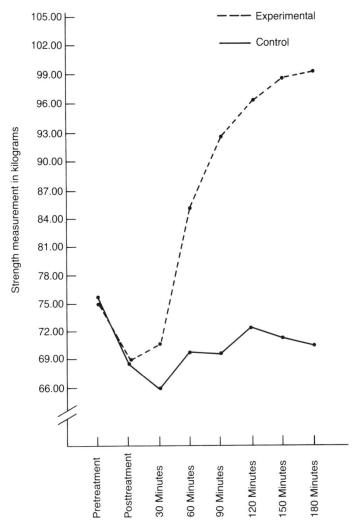

Figure 5-1. Mean plantar flexion strength measurements during and after cold immersion. (From Oliver, R.A., Johnson, D.J., Wheelhouse, W.W., and Griffin, P.P. [1979]: Isometric muscle contraction response during recovery from reduced intramuscular temperature. Arch. Phys. Med. Rehabil., 60:128.)

precooled or normal levels at 60 to 80 minutes after removal from the cold modality, and it was maintained at remarkably high levels for up to 180 minutes.[57, 94] Both studies also noted the accompanying elevation of blood flow to the cooled muscle, with a consequent rise in tissue temperature. Johnson and Leider[57] have speculated that the mechanism by which muscle strength increases is by elevation of tissue temperature. Thus, less strength would be spent in overcoming the innate stiffness of the muscles and tendons that act to produce the movement. From their study of the effect of ice on concentric strength, Oliver and colleagues[94] have suggested that the expanded blood flow to the area disproportionately increases the excitability of muscle membranes, so that in response to a given neuronal stimulus more fibers are recruited.[94]

Similar results with respect to concentric and eccentric muscle strength have been obtained by Ruiz et al.[106] After application of an ice pack to the quadriceps for 25 minutes, subjects' strength levels were significantly decreased. Testing at 20 minutes posttreatment did not demonstrate any significant differences either

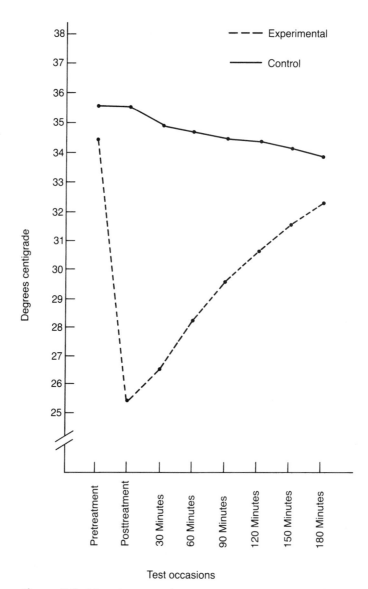

Figure 5–2. Mean intramuscular temperature measurements during and after cold immersion. (From Oliver, R.A., Johnson, D.J., Wheelhouse, W.W., and Griffin, P.P. [1979]: Isometric muscle contraction response during recovery from reduced intramuscular temperature. Arch. Phys. Med. Rehabil., 60:128.)

concentrically or eccentrically. These data suggest that ice does have the immediate effect of decreasing strength. However, these results do not support the position that the application of cryotherapy results in strength increases.

Considerations for Use

In using cold modalities, the clinician must consider ways to avoid undercooling, which does not achieve the desired result, and overcooling, which risks tissue damage. Therapeutic cold modalities produce their effects by conducting higher-energy, warmer molecules out of the body tissues to the lower-energy, colder molecules of the modality, to which they transfer their energy. This removes heat energy from the body tissues, thereby cooling the tissues. To do this effectively, several factors must be taken into account; their interrelationship can be summarized by the following equation:

$$D = \frac{\text{area} \times k \times (T_1 - T_2)}{\text{thickness of tissue}}$$

where D is the rate of energy transfer, area is the amount of surface area to which the cold modality is applied, k is the thermal conductivity of the tissue, $(T_1 - T_2)$ is the temperature difference between the skin and the cold modality, and thickness of tissue is the depth of cooling to be achieved.[86] In other words, to cool a segment of tissue effectively, the modality must be cold enough, must cover a sufficiently large area, and must be located over tissue with a thermal conductivity that allows heat to be transferred to the surface. Therefore, ice packs containing chipped ice are strongly recommended, because they remain at 0° C (32° F) until all the ice has melted, a feature not found in commercial cold packs.[82]

Water, muscle, and bone all have thermal conductivities that allow cooling of tissues after topical cold application. Fat, however, is an excellent insulator, with a thermal conductivity less than half that of muscle or bone and almost one third that of water.[86] Research has shown that the thickness of the subcutaneous fat layer between the skin and muscle being cooled can have a dramatic effect on how cold the underlying muscle tissue becomes (Fig. 5–3).[76] Thus, for a patient with a substantial layer of subcutaneous fat, effective cooling can take a long time.[12]

The application of cold to superficial areas can result in excessive cooling of nerve tissues that are especially vulnerable to the effects of local cooling. Drez and associates[37] have reported five patients with nerve palsy secondary to cryotherapy, one of whom had not spontaneously recovered by 9 months after injury. They recommended that ice not be applied for more than 20 minutes,

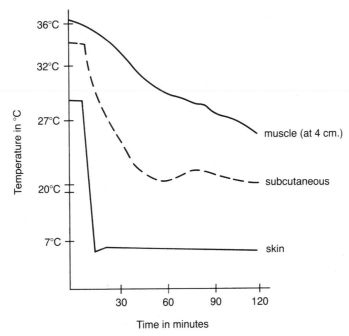

Figure 5–3. Tissue temperature changes during application of ice pack to the calf. (From Michlovitz, S. [1986]: Thermal Agents in Rehabilitation. Philadelphia, F.A. Davis, p. 75.)

with 30 minutes being the absolute maximum length of treatment, and that areas of tissue in which superficial nerves are located be avoided altogether.[37]

Finally, the clinician should exercise caution in applying cold directly over open wounds during the first 2 to 3 weeks of healing because studies have reported that this practice significantly reduces the tensile strength of the wound.[86] Cold diminishes the rate of metabolic processes, thus slowing the rate of scar formation and healing.

Indications and Contraindications

Knowledge of the physiologic effects of cold modalities helps determine the types of conditions for which cryotherapy is indicated. Therapeutic cold is clearly an excellent choice in treating acute trauma. It helps prevent secondary hypoxic injury, controls the formation of edema, and is an outstanding pain reliever. In addition, the analgesic properties of cryotherapy make it useful in the rehabilitation of athletic injuries.

Cryotherapy is contraindicated for Raynaud's disease, in which the application of cold causes peripheral vasoconstriction, with resultant tissue ischemia. It is also contraindicated for athletes with cold allergies, in whom cold modalities produce skin redness, wheal formation, flushing of the face, fainting, decrease in blood pressure, and increase in heart rate.[86] Other contraindications include individuals with multiple myeloma, leukemia, and systemic lupus erythematosus, who should be checked for cryoglobulinemia. The presence of cryoglobulin causes blood to gel or a precipitate to form when cold is applied. The precipitate then shuts off the blood supply to tissues. Finally, athletes who have cold hemoglobinuria should not use cold modalities.[86] In these athletes, cold causes a breakdown of red blood cells, resulting in blood in the urine.

Cryotherapy should be carefully considered and vital signs should be closely monitored in athletes with pre-existing high blood pressure because of the vasopressor response, involving a sudden increase in blood pressure, that most individuals experience when exposed to cold. These conditions are rare, however, and the athlete with Raynaud's phenomenon is most likely aware of the problems posed by the application of cold. Because of the severity of reaction in individuals who may not be aware that they have a cold allergy, cryoglobulinemia, or cold hemoglobinuria, it is strongly recommended that athletes be monitored closely for abnormal reactions during their initial treatment sessions.

Cold should never be applied over areas of tissue that have a compromised circulatory supply or over anesthetic skin. In both these instances, the tissue is not protected from the potential damage of cold injury.

Specific Modalities and Their Application

COLD PACKS

Cold packs used in clinics and training rooms are typically found in one of two forms—conventional packs made by the clinician or those commercially prepared.

Conventional Cold Packs

Conventional cold packs consist of chipped ice placed in a plastic bag, with the size determined by the area to be covered.

Application. A quantity of chipped ice is placed in a plastic bag, which is knotted to keep the ice in the bag (Fig. 5–4). The usual length of application is

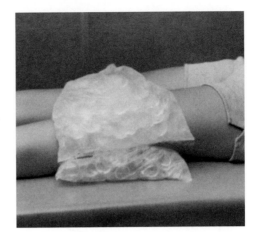

Figure 5-4. Conventional cryotherapy technique.

20 to 30 minutes, with the skin being checked periodically for wheal or blister formation, especially during the first few treatment sessions. When finished, the pack is thrown away. It is strongly recommended that compression be used in conjunction with ice application. Research by Merrick et al[85] has demonstrated significantly greater tissue cooling when ice and compression are jointly used than when ice is used alone.

Advantages and Disadvantages. Probably the greatest advantage of conventional ice packs is their ability to maintain a constant temperature (ice remaining at 0° C or 32° F), which makes them more effective for cooling tissues. In animal studies, McMaster and colleagues[82] have found that compared with other forms of cold packs, ice consistently produces the greatest decrease in tissue temperature over a 60-minute period of cooling (Table 5-1, Fig. 5-5). Additionally, the ice pack can be molded to body parts with difficult configuration, such as the shoulder, elbow, and ankle. Finally, once the initial expense of an on-site ice machine has been met, the individual ice packs are not expensive to make.

Commercial Cold Packs

Typically, commercial cold packs are single-use packs or are reusable. Single-use packs rely on a chemical interaction, after the activation of a catalyst, to produce cold. Conversely, reusable packs usually consist of a silicone gel enclosed in a strong vinyl case (Fig. 5-6). These must be kept frozen at temperatures of at least −5° C (−23° F) for a minimum of 2 hours prior to use.[86]

Application. To protect against cold injury, a wet towel or elastic wrap should be placed between the athlete's skin and the commercial cold pack. The usual length of application is 15 to 20 minutes. With longer application, the pack may

Table 5-1. Mean Decrease in Temperature (°C) with Ice Pack Application

COOLANT DEVICE	LENGTH OF EXPOSURE (MIN)			
	15	30	45	60
Ice	3.4	6.9	9.2	11.3
Gel	1.8	4.4	6.5	8.4
Chemical	1.6	2.9	3.0	3.5
Freon	0.2	0.9	1.2	1.7

From McMaster, W.C., Liddle, S., and Waugh, T.R. (1978): Laboratory evaluation of various cold therapy modalities. Am. J. Sports Med., 6:291–294.

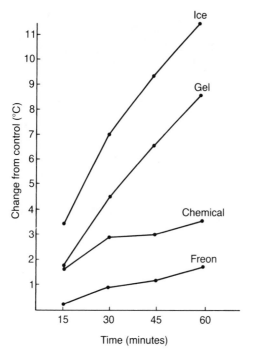

Figure 5–5. Average tissue temperature reduction achieved by the use of various modalities. (From McMaster, W.C., Liddle, S., and Waugh, T.R. [1978]: Laboratory evaluation of various cold therapy modalities. Am. J. Sports Med., 6:291–294.)

become sufficiently warm to require replacement with a colder pack. The pack can be molded to the body and may need to be held in place with elastic straps or bandages. When treatment is complete, the pack may be discarded (if disposable) or refrozen for subsequent use (if reusable).

Advantages and Disadvantages. Commercial cold packs are convenient, and the initial cost of some types is offset by the fact that these are reusable. Also, the initial cost of these packs is much less than that for a chipped ice machine. Although commercial packs do provide adequate cooling, they are not as effective as conventional cold packs (see Fig. 5–5) and must be frozen for a relatively long period (at least 2 hours) before they are cold enough to be used again. The exact temperature of these packs is also difficult to determine. Therefore, cold injury can result from their improper use. Finally, although the silicone gel pack can be reused indefinitely, if the vinyl covering is broken, it leaks gel and cannot be repaired.

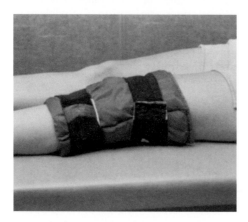

Figure 5–6. A commercial cold pack is convenient, but it does not cool as effectively as a conventional ice pack. Although not pictured, a moist towel can be used under the ice pack for comfort and a dry towel can be placed over the ice pack to slow down warming to room temperature.

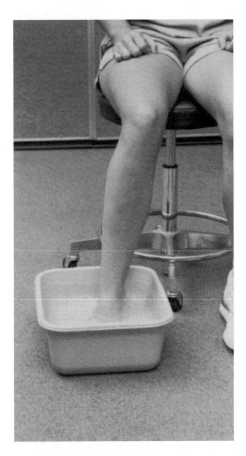

Figure 5–7. An ice bucket or bath is excellent for treating distal portions of extremities but is not indicated for those in whom edema must be reduced.

ICE BUCKET OR BATH

When cooling of the entire surface of a distal extremity such as a hand, forearm, foot, or lower leg is desired, the use of an ice bucket or whirlpool filled with ice and water can be most effective (Fig. 5–7).

Application. The bucket or whirlpool is filled with water, and ice is added until the temperature drops to the desired level. The temperature range is typically 13° to 18° C (55° to 64° F).[86] The limb is then placed in the bucket or bath, usually for 5 to 15 minutes.[99]

Advantages and Disadvantages. This particular method of cold application is ideal for treating the distal portions of the extremities. If the goal is to reduce edema, however, placing the body part in a dependent position can diminish or even overcome the beneficial effects of the cold and, thereby, produce a limb that is more edematous after treatment. In addition, many athletes complain that cold water immersion is very painful. Pain perception can be alleviated through the use of a neoprene toe cap, as shown by Misasi et al.[88]

Advocates of ice buckets and baths claim that this method has an enormous advantage over the application of other forms of cold because the athlete can actively move the body part, performing cryokinetics, while it is submerged. The buoyancy of water can also facilitate the regaining of range of motion. For athletes who cannot harm themselves by excessive motion, exercising under the pain-relieving effects of cold is advantageous. However, for athletes who must use pain as their guideline for safe limits of movement, this method is obviously contraindicated.

ICE MASSAGE

Application. Ice is formed into the proper shape in a small paper or Styrofoam cup. When ready for use, a section of the cup is peeled away, exposing the

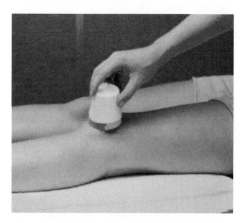

Figure 5–8. Ice massage effectively produces local cooling in discrete areas, making it an excellent treatment choice for overuse syndromes.

portion of ice to be rubbed against the athlete's skin. A portion of the cup is held over the ice to protect the fingers, or a tongue depressor is placed into the cup before freezing to act as a handle. The ice is rubbed in a circular or lengthwise stroking fashion over a relatively small area, usually about a 4-inch square (Fig. 5–8). The athlete should experience several distinct sensations— intense cold, burning, aching, and finally analgesia. When analgesia is reached, the massage is usually discontinued, although some clinicians recommend stopping after 5 to 7 minutes even if analgesia has not occurred.

Advantages and Disadvantages. Although it remains controversial as to how much deep cooling this method of therapeutic cold produces, it clearly accomplishes dramatic cooling of the skin.[60] Thus, in conditions in which pain and muscle spasm are significant, use of this method can be extremely beneficial, resulting in pain relief and muscle relaxation. Additionally, it produces local cooling of discrete areas efficiently, with a large reactive hyperemia to the areas cooled once the treatment has ended. This makes it ideal for treating overuse syndromes, poorly perfused tissues (e.g., the ligaments of the ankle), and areas of local inflammation (e.g., bursitis). Finally, because skin temperature rarely drops below 15° C (59° F), this treatment can be performed with safety at home by the athlete.[86]

The primary disadvantage of ice massage is the discomfort the athlete experiences before analgesia is reached. It may be helpful to inform the athlete that although initial treatment sessions of ice massage are uncomfortable, this perception lessens after continued use and habituation.[74]

THERAPEUTIC HEAT

Specific modalities of therapeutic heat can appropriately be divided into two classes of heating agents: superficial and deep. Because they share many common features, it could be argued that the two groups merely occupy different positions along the same spectrum. This is certainly true in regard to the degree of vasodilation elicited by superficial and deep heating agents. The deep heating agents, however, have some unique differences, both in the effects they produce and in the energy sources they use, and hence represent a separate class. For our purposes, therefore, therapeutic heating agents are presented as two distinct groups.

Superficial Heating Modalities

PHYSIOLOGIC EFFECTS

Most superficial heating agents transfer their energy to the body in the same way as do therapeutic cold modalities—by conduction. Energy in the form of heat is applied externally to the body. The energy is transferred from the object of higher energy (in this case, the modality) to the object of lower energy (in this case, the body), which has the net effect of warming the tissues. Superficial heating agents are similar in certain ways to therapeutic cold modalities. Because both modalities are applied externally, they have similar physiologic effects, although the direction of heat transfer is reversed because the heating agents are warmer than the body. The physiologic responses to superficial heat can be categorized as follows: increased temperature, vasodilation, increased cellular metabolism, decreased pain, diminished muscle tone and spasticity, and decreased joint stiffness.

Tissue Temperature

Superficial heating agents, when applied to the body, produce only mild increases in tissue temperature. Generally, when a superficial heating agent is applied to the body, internal temperatures rise gradually and do not exceed 40° C (104° F), and the duration of temperature elevation at its peak level is relatively short.[66]

Circulation

As expected, an elevation in tissue temperature elicits an increase in local blood flow. This occurs primarily in the vessels of the skin and subcutaneous tissues.[86] Increases in blood flow to deeper tissues such as skeletal muscle usually appear to be produced by the metabolic demands of exercising muscle, and thus blood flow changes little with the application of a superficial heating agent.[86] The vigor of this response is determined by the combined actions of reflexes to local axons and the spinal cord, as well as by the prostaglandins and histamine released by the local tissues whose temperature is elevated.[86] In addition, perspiration leads to the release of kallikrein (a potent vasodilator) from sweat glands, which in turn acts on an intermediary globulin, stimulating bradykinin release. Bradykinin further dilates the blood vessels. The net effect is a mild inflammatory response, with increases in intravascular pressure and permeability of vessel walls resulting in outward fluid filtration and consequent edema formation.[86] For this reason, heating agents are usually contraindicated in the presence of an active inflammatory process or significant amounts of edema.

Vasodilation occurs not only in the area being heated but also in tissues distant from the heating agent through consensual or indirect vasodilation.[1] Thus, an area of the body opposite to that being directly heated shows evidence of vasodilation and increased blood flow, even though neither the temperature of the tissue nor its metabolic demands has changed from the resting state. Because increased blood flow occurs reflexively instead of being demanded by an increase in temperature or metabolism, no damage occurs in tissues with compromised circulation. In fact, for the geriatric athlete or the younger individual recovering from trauma involving the circulatory system, consensual vasodilation is an excellent method for encouraging the development of collateral circulation.

Cellular Metabolism

The increase in blood flow not only cools the tissues by drawing heat away to other areas of the body, where it can be dispersed, but also brings greater than normal amounts of oxygen and nutrients into the area. The rates of chemical reactions, especially those of cell metabolism, are dramatically increased by the rise in temperature.[86, 129] Thus, a sudden and large demand for both oxygen and nutrients is made by the cells. If this demand is not satisfied adequately, the cells die. Heating modalities are therefore always contraindicated for tissues with a restricted blood supply. Damaged tissues in the process of healing also increase the rate of their cellular processes, which, it is hoped, speeds their rate of repair.

Pain and Muscle Spasm

It is thought that superficial heating agents act to relieve pain and diminish muscle spasm in the same ways as do the cold modalities. Both Michlovitz[86] and Licht[74] have cited numerous studies indicating that muscle tone is decreased by the topical application of heat. Although its precise neurologic mechanism remains controversial, the reduction of muscle tone with heat is widely accepted and well known from the muscle-relaxing effects of a hot shower, heating pad, or Jacuzzi. Also, topically applied heating agents stimulate the activity of skin thermoreceptors. According to the gate theory of sensory afferent modulation, the increased input from these receptors is believed to compete with pain impulses for transmission to the central nervous system, with fewer pain impulses making their way to the brain.[60]

Joint Stiffness

Finally, the topical application of heating agents decreases joint stiffness.[133] This effect, in combination with the mild pain-relieving and vasodilatory properties, makes superficial heat an ideal modality to use prior to exercise.

INDICATIONS AND CONTRAINDICATIONS

As might be concluded from this discussion, the use of superficial heating agents is indicated whenever a mild increase in blood flow, increased speed of healing, partial relief of pain, relaxation of muscles, or decreased joint stiffness is desired. In conditions such as relief of painful muscle spasms, nonacute muscle contusions, and tight joint capsules, superficial heating modalities can be useful components of the treatment regimen. The clinical use of hot packs, whirlpools, paraffin baths, contrast baths, and fluidotherapy is usually related to their pain-relieving and joint pliability–inducing properties. Alterations in blood flow by superficial agents are restricted to the skin and subcutaneous tissues.

Superficial heating agents, as is true of all topically applied modalities, are contraindicated for use on anesthetic skin. Because of their vasodilatory and growth-promoting properties, they are contraindicated for use on areas of tissue not adequately supplied with blood and are contraindicated in the presence of internal infections, thrombophlebitis, cancers, rheumatoid arthritis during the active phase, an ongoing inflammatory process, or significant edema. Individuals with bleeding disorders should also avoid the use of heating agents.

SPECIFIC MODALITIES AND THEIR APPLICATION

Hot Packs

Hydrocollator packs consist of a silicone gel in a canvas cover. The packs are stored in a water bath maintained at a temperature of 71° to 79.4° C (160° to 175° F).[66] When in use, the packs are wrapped in dry toweling, with six to eight layers between the athlete's skin and the pack (Fig. 5–9).

Application. The packs can be molded to irregular surfaces and are held in place by small weights or loosely applied elastic wraps. The athlete should never lie on top of a pack, because this could squeeze water out into the protective layers of toweling, possibly causing a skin burn.[66, 86] Packs are usually applied

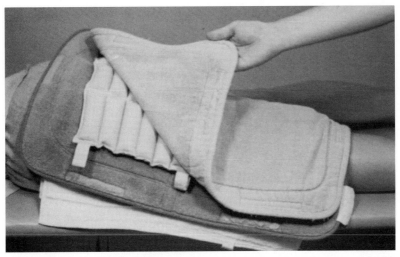

Figure 5–9. A hydrocollator pack transmits heat well and is not associated with a high incidence of overheating or skin burns.

for 20 minutes; they must be reimmersed in the water bath for at least 30 minutes before reuse.[86]

Advantages and Disadvantages. Hot packs are convenient and are not particularly expensive. They usually provide good transmission of heat and are not associated with a high incidence of overheating or skin burns. However, because of their stiffness, they are difficult to apply to curved surfaces, which often prevents total surface contact. Athletes should not lie on top of the hydrocollator pack, and those who are in pain may not be able to tolerate the weight of the pack and toweling as it is placed onto the body part to be heated. Position modifications to allow hot pack placement are common.

Whirlpools

Whirlpool tanks can be of extremity, lowboy, or Hubbard size. They are commonly used to clean open wounds and are used before exercises for the relief of pain and stiffness (Fig. 5–10). If wound healing is the purpose of the treatment, various antibacterial agents can be added to the whirlpool; the most common additives are povidone-iodine solution (Betadine) and 5% bleach solution (Dakin's solution). Whirlpools are especially useful in the treatment of athletes who have just resumed activity after casting or prolonged immobilization and whose primary problem is restricted range of motion. The heat diminishes joint and tissue stiffness while the body part is moved and stretched.

Application. Water for the tank is usually at a temperature between 36.5° and 40° C (98° to 104° F) and can be agitated by turbines, which mix air and water. The body part is submerged and can be actively moved during the treatment. The usual length of treatment is 20 minutes.

Advantages and Disadvantages. As a tool in the rehabilitation of athletes, whirlpools have several advantages for both the acute and long-term phases of care. Whirlpools are ideal for cleaning large, open wounds that might have grass, soil, or surface particles embedded in them. The water cleans the wounds mechanically and introduces antibacterial agents into the tissues. Both the warmth of the water and the buffeting of the agitator relieve pain according to the gate theory of pain modulation. In addition, the buoyancy of the water facilitates regaining of motion.

Warm whirlpools should not be used when edema is present. The heat of the water causes vasodilation and creates an outward fluid filtration; when com-

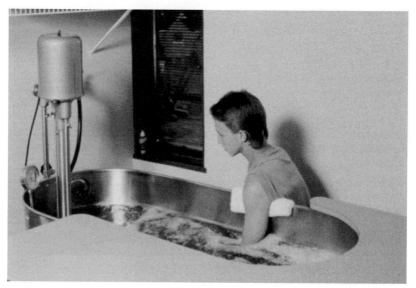

Figure 5–10. A whirlpool bath is ideal for wound cleaning. The warmth of the water and buffeting of the agitator help relieve pain. (Photo courtesy of Sports Medicine Update. Birmingham, Alabama, HealthSouth Rehabilitation Corporation.)

bined with the dependent position of the body part or extremity, this brings about a definite increase in edema. Active movement of the body part during the whirlpool treatment facilitates venous and lymphatic return, which helps to reduce the edema but does not eliminate it.

Contrast Baths

Contrast baths are a special form of therapeutic heat and cold that can be applied to distal extremities. They are frequently used in the treatment of ligament and joint capsule sprains as well as for stasis edema because of the vigorous hyperemia they elicit. They can also be used in individuals with peripheral vascular disease to improve circulation in the contralateral extremity by consensual vasodilation and to improve range of motion in arthritic joints.

Application. Two tubs are used, one containing warm water (approximately 38° to 44° C [100° to 111° F]) and one containing cold water (approximately 10° to 18° C [50° to 66° F]). Although protocols for contrast therapy vary among clinicians, an example of a typical protocol is as follows. The extremity is initially submerged in the warm bath for 10 minutes. It is then alternated between the cold bath for 1 minute and the warm bath for 4 minutes, ending in the warm bath. The cycle is repeated four times, with the total treatment time usually being 30 minutes.

Advantages and Disadvantages. Contrast baths do elicit a vigorous hyperemia, as judged by the skin color changes seen in treated individuals. Hyperemia is not a common feature of superficial heating agents, and studies reporting this physiologic effect are scarce. The cold cycle can be uncomfortable for the athlete and may create a problem of compliance. The pumping effect that is believed to be created by successive episodes of vasoconstriction and vasodilation is not as great as that achieved by exercise.

Paraffin Baths

Paraffin baths are liquid mixtures of paraffin wax and mineral oil. Body parts are either dipped into the bath or painted with the mixture. Use of this modality is usually followed by stretching exercises in the treatment of painful, arthritic joints, because the heat diminishes pain and joint stiffness. When applied to joints covered by subcutaneous soft tissue, paraffin baths produce only mild heating, but when they are applied to the joints of the hands, wrist, foot, or ankle, internal temperatures approach 45° C (113° F). Thus, for these joints, paraffin baths are considered to be a deep heating modality.

Application. A commercially available mixture of paraffin wax and mineral oil is heated in a thermostatically controlled bath to temperatures ranging from 47.8° to 54.5° C (117° to 130° F).[86] The athlete's hand or foot is dipped into the bath or, if a larger joint is to be treated, the paraffin is painted onto the body (Fig. 5–11). The skin must be cleaned thoroughly, and all jewelry must be removed prior to application. Treatment of the hand or foot can be accomplished by repeatedly dipping the body part into the bath, gradually producing a thick layer of paraffin. The paraffin-coated body part is wrapped in plastic and five or six layers of toweling for 20 minutes. More vigorous heating can be obtained if the body part is dipped several times to form a protective layer and is then immersed for 20 minutes.[66] Paraffin is contraindicated if the athlete has an open wound.

Advantages and Disadvantages. Paraffin baths are effective for heating small joints of the upper and lower extremities. Coupled with range-of-motion stretching, this can be an excellent method for regaining mobility. However, because significant heating and vigorous vasodilation occur, the clinician should expect edema formation. If edema is a problem prior to treatment, this modality should not be used.

Fluidotherapy

Fluidotherapy treatments consist of warm air (37.8° to 48.9° C [99° to 119° F]) blown through fine glass beads or, more commonly, through cellulose particles.[53]

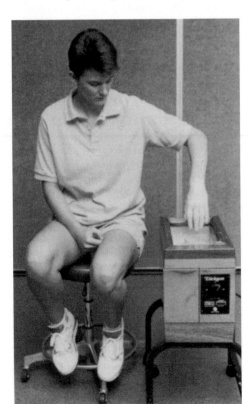

Figure 5–11. A paraffin bath is effective for heating small joints.

The air-particle mixture is housed in containers. Fluidotherapy tanks are available in various sizes, allowing treatment of all body parts. Nylon mesh sleeves are attached to the body part being treated, and these help prevent escape of the particles.

Application. The machine must be warmed up and should be turned on in advance (exact times vary among machines). The athlete places the body part to be treated into the tank, with the nylon sleeve securely fastened. The athlete can easily move within the tank, as the concentration of particles and size of the tank allow active movement. The skin should be cleaned thoroughly prior to treatment, and any open wound should be protected with a plastic dressing to prevent particles from being embedded in the wound or from being contaminated.

Advantages and Disadvantages. According to the gate theory of pain control, the combination of heat, movement of the body part, and mechanical stimulation of the skin (bombardment by the particles) should prove to be a potent pain reliever. Because this modality relieves pain and allows the athlete to move during treatment, it is an outstanding method for regaining mobility lost to restricted range of motion. As with a paraffin bath, vigorous heating of the hands and feet occurs, and therefore, an athlete who still has significant edema in an extremity should avoid use of this modality.

Deep Heating Modalities

PHYSIOLOGIC EFFECTS

In contrast to the superficial heating agents, deep heating modalities can produce much higher temperatures in tissues and, therefore, a more vigorous response. Deep heating agents typically raise temperatures at a fairly rapid rate, elevate tissue temperatures close to tolerance levels (45° C [113° F]), and maintain peak temperatures for a relatively long period.[66] Deep heating agents transmit their energy into the body through sound waves and electromagnetic energy to bring about tissue heating.

SPECIFIC MODALITIES AND THEIR APPLICATION

Shortwave Diathermy

Shortwave diathermy machines create high-frequency alternating currents that produce a magnetic field when applied to electrical wires. A more intense magnetic field is created if the coils are formed into a solenoid shape. Diathermy machines available for clinical use operate at a frequency of 27.12 MHz. Application of a high-frequency alternating current (AC) to electrical wires yields electromagnetic waves composed of transverse electrical and magnetic fields.[86] Although both capacitance and inductance electrodes are capable of delivering both types of fields concurrently, each favors delivery of one type over the other.[86] Capacitance electrodes build up electrical charges on two plates separated in space. Because of the separation of opposite charges, a strong electrical field develops between the two plates. In an electrical field, tissues that are poor conductors (e.g., fat and skin) act to resist current flow, and they can thus be overheated by the diathermy wave.[29]

Inductance electrodes create a magnetic field that envelops the body part. The electromagnetic wave affects biologic tissues differently, depending on their fluid content and consequent electrical conductivity. In a magnetic field, tissues with a high fluid content (e.g., skeletal muscle and fluid-filled cavities) absorb more of the electromagnetic wave and are heated to a greater extent.[29] Fat tissue does not produce as great a resistance in a magnetic field as in an electric field and thus is not heated as much.[29]

Therapeutic Actions. The chief therapeutic action of shortwave diathermy is derived from its ability to elevate temperatures in deep tissues, specifically skeletal muscle and joints. Regardless of the type of electrode used, shortwave diathermy has been shown to bring skeletal muscle tissue at depths of 2 to 3 cm to therapeutic levels of temperature (40° to 50° C [104° to 122° F]). As tissue temperatures increase, vasodilation occurs, bringing large amounts of relatively cool blood in an attempt to reduce temperatures to homeostatic levels.[68] As discussed earlier, increased blood flow provides tissues with greater than normal quantities of oxygen and nutrients; in combination with an increased rate of chemical reaction, this speeds healing of stretched or torn tissues. This increased blood flow also aids in the resolution of inflammatory infiltrates and exudates.[86] As with other heating modalities, joint stiffness decreases, and both pain and muscle spasm are relieved.[86]

Knowledge of its physiologic effects helps provide indications for using shortwave diathermy. Of all the therapeutic modalities currently available, shortwave diathermy is probably the most effective for heating skeletal muscle.[60] Thus, if an increased rate of healing or resolution of inflammatory by-products of skeletal muscle is desired, shortwave diathermy is recommended. It is also excellent for relieving muscle spasms that encompass a large area.

There are many contraindications to the use of shortwave diathermy. As Dowling[29] has noted, shortwave diathermy, in common with other heating modalities, is contraindicated in the following conditions: for tissue not adequately perfused with blood, pregnancy, cancer, infections, inflammation of any tissue, edema, and effusion. This modality, however, has additional contraindications that are not usually considered. These include the presence of any metal in the field, whether internal (surgical implants), worn by the individual (jewelry, watches), or environmental (stools, tables).[29] Shortwave diathermy interferes with the usual function of devices such as pacemakers and urinary stimulators, and therefore, any individual with such a device should avoid the area in which shortwave diathermy treatments are being given.[29] Shortwave diathermy is contraindicated on bony prominences and in any fluid-filled cavity, so application to the eyes, testes, or brain is not recommended. Finally, because the clinician must rely on the subjective report from the athlete to determine adequate or excessive dosage, this modality is not recommended for individuals with anesthetic skin.

Application. When using capacitance electrodes, physical contact between the plate surface and the athlete's body is prevented by interposing layers of towels or air spaces. Inductance electrodes have coils or wire placed close together, with electrical currents running through them, and they can be wrapped around the body part or be housed in a drum. A layer of towels 1 to 2 cm thick must separate the wrapped coil from the skin. For both forms of electrodes, at least one layer of toweling must be placed over the athlete's skin to absorb perspiration, which, because of its high water content, is selectively heated and could cause a skin burn. Care must be taken to prevent the wires from touching each other, the athlete, or the furniture to avoid burns. Dosage is determined by reports from the athlete. A warm, toasty feeling that is not excessively hot should be described. The usual treatment length is 20 minutes.

Advantages and Disadvantages. As noted previously, shortwave diathermy is probably the most effective modality for heating skeletal muscle.[60] Because heating is accomplished without physical contact between the modality and skin, it can be used even if the skin is abraded, provided there is no significant edema. The inconvenience of diathermy is its primary disadvantage. The equipment is large, bulky, and difficult to maneuver and set up. The treatment area must be cleared of all metal, and anyone possessing a pacemaker must be at least 4.5 m (15 feet) away.[86]

Ultrasound

Therapeutic ultrasound is a deep heating modality that produces a sound wave of 0.8 to 3.0 MHz. The sound wave is produced by applying a high-frequency, alternating electrical current to a natural quartz or synthetic crystal. This converts the electrical current to a mechanical vibration,[74] a reversal of the piezoelectric effect. In piezoelectricity, compression and elongation of a neutral crystal alter its configuration (Fig. 5–12). This relative change in the mechanical orientation of the crystal produces a dipole. When the process is repeated rapidly, the dipole alternates its charges, and an alternating current to the crystal causes it to distort into its compressed and elongated forms. Molecules next to the crystal are moved forward by the longitudinal compression wave created by movement of the crystal. The frequency of the compression wave is identical to that of the electrical current applied to the crystal.

Therapeutic Actions. In the human body, ultrasound has several pronounced effects on biologic tissues. It is attenuated by certain tissues and reflected by bone. Ultrasound has been shown to penetrate subcutaneous fat of varying thicknesses, with a resultant therapeutic rise in muscle tissue termperature.[34] Thus, tissues lying immediately next to bone can receive an even greater dosage of ultrasound, as much as 30% more.[35, 67, 71] For ultrasound to achieve its thermal effects, the tissue temperature must be raised by 1° C to more than 4° C, depending on the desired outcome of the treatment.[35] The frequency of the ultrasound determines its depth of penetration. Typically, a 1-MHz ultrasound unit in the continuous mode is used for heating tissues 2.5 to 5.0 cm deep, whereas 3 MHz are used to heat tissues less than 2.5 cm deep.[43] Thus, a 3-MHz ultrasound unit should be used to sonate superficial tissues. If a 1-MHz ultra-sound unit is used to sonate superficial tissues, the sound wave will be reflected off the bone, causing periosteal pain; the clinician often responds by turning down the intensity, thereby losing the therapeutic effect. Thus, a higher intensity can be used with a 3-MHz mode to bring about the desired temperature increase when the target tissue is superficial.[35]

The increased extensibility that ultrasound produces in tissues of high collagen content, combined with the proximity of joint capsules, tendons, and ligaments to cortical bone, where they receive a more intense irradiation, makes ultrasound an ideal modality for increasing mobility in those tissues with restricted range of motion. Sonation of tissues must be combined with passive stretching to gain permanent motion in tight tissues, with stretch applied during and for a time after the treatment has ended.[70] Long-duration, low-load stretching has been

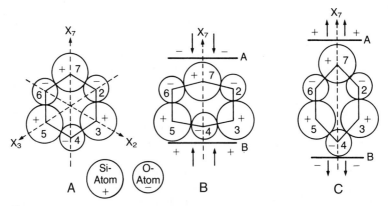

Figure 5–12. Schematic representation of the piezoelectric effect. *A,* Neural piezoelectric crystal. *B* through *C,* Change in the crystals' polarity as a result of the expansion and contraction of the crystal from passing an alternating current through the crystals. (From Licht, S. [1965]: Therapeutic Heat and Cold, 2nd ed. Baltimore, Williams & Wilkins, p. 331.)

found to produce effective elongation while causing the least tissue damage.[126] Wessling et al[128] found that static stretching after ultrasound treatment increased muscle extensibility by 20% compared with stretching alone. Draper[33] and Rose[105] have described what they believe to be a therapeutic "stretching window" after application of 1-MHz and 3-MHz ultrasound. These authors reported ultrasound to increase muscle temperature 3° C above the baseline temperature and recommended that patients begin stretching during the last few minutes of the ultrasound treatment and continue stretching through the next 2 to 3 minutes after the conclusion of the treatment. Additionally, thermal decay of 1-MHz ultrasound was slower than that of 3-MHz ultrasound, and the deeper tissue cooled at a slower rate than did superficial tissue after treatment with 1-MHz ultrasound. Thus, the stretching window was open longer for deep-seated structures than for superficial ones.

The effect of heating or cooling of tissues before applying ultrasound has also been investigated. From these investigations it appears that preheating of the tissues has no significant effect on enhancing the effect of ultrasound on raising tissue temperature.[5, 71] Moreover, when the tissues are precooled, the application of ultrasound does not raise the tissue temperature to the precooled level, and ultrasound alone will provide a greater heating effect than ultrasound preceded by ice application.[101] The rationale for cooling the tissue before applying ultrasound is based on the premise that the ultrasound is more effectively transmitted through dense materials.[71, 86, 99] The denser the medium, the greater the wave propagation. Thus, the application of cold to a treatment area should increase tissue density because the tissue temperature is decreased.

In addition to increasing collagen tissue extensibility, ultrasound also increases blood flow to an area as the body attempts to cool overheated tissue through reactive vasodilation.[2, 5, 11, 75, 96] Blood flow remains elevated for 45 to 60 minutes after ultrasound application.[5, 75] This action is thought to be useful in the resolution of inflammatory exudates and of calcium deposits in bursae and tendon sheaths.[21] Ultrasound is an accepted and recommended clinical treatment for bursitis, although research has failed to substantiate this.[30] Heating of tissues is thought to be responsible for the temporary increase in nerve conduction velocity seen in sonated peripheral nerves.[64]

Phonophoresis. A final effect of ultrasound is the stirring and streaming of molecules in the path of the sound wave. This nonthermal effect is believed to be partly responsible for the positive effect of ultrasound on chronic wounds and is the basis for phonophoresis. With phonophoresis, it is believed that drug molecules are propelled forward into the body. A cream emulsion containing the medication is placed on the skin and is used as a coupling agent while molecules of the medicine are propelled into the body. The most common pharmacologic agents introduced in this fashion include hydrocortisone, dexamethasone, salicylates, and lidocaine.[8] Studies supporting the efficacy of phonophoresis are conflicting. The reasons for the conflicting data are use of poor experimental controls, subjective reports of improvement in pain and dysfunction by patients rather than direct tissue or serum analysis, and extrapolation of data from animal models to humans.[8] Animal studies[16, 23, 47, 48, 50, 72] have documented drug penetration with phonophoresis. Additionally, in animal studies, medication introduced by phonophoresis has been detected in tissue at depths of 5 to 6 cm.[86] However, Brown[15] urges caution when extrapolating these animal studies to humans because of the anatomic and physiologic differences. Also, many of the ultrasound protocols used on animals would generally not have been tolerated by humans.[15]

Only recently have clinical trials involved human subjects to study the efficacy of phonophoresis with regard to depth of penetration of specifc pharmacologic agents. Studies involving human subjects using 10% hydrocortisone acetate,[8] benzydamine,[10] salicylates,[95] and an anesthetic[81] concluded that ultrasound did not enhance the percutaneous absorption of these medications. Bare and colleagues[8] investigated one of the most frequently used phonophoresis preparations—10% hydrocortisone combined with a gel base. A control treatment (ultrasound alone) and an experimental treatment (hydrocortisone phonophoresis) were applied on each subject to the volar aspect of the forearm 1 week apart. Ultrasound was delivered over a 50 cm² area for 5 minutes at an intensity of 1.0 W/cm² and a frequency of 1 MHz. Blood was drawn from the cubital vein from subjects in both the control and the experimental groups at 0, 5, and 15 minutes posttreatment, and serum cortisol concentrations were measured. No rise in serum cortisol concentrations after hydrocortisone phonophoresis was detected.

There has been some concern regarding the transmissibility of the media containing the medication. Warren et al[125] reported a 50% loss of transmissibility with hydrocortisone phonophoresis, and Cameron and Monroe[18] reported zero transmissibility of ultrasonic energy, using a 10% hydrocortisone preparation, through a 5-mm-thick layer of coupling medium. Table 5–2 represents the work of Cameron and Monroe,[18] who investigated the transmissibility of various phonophoresis media. They reported that most clinicians use 10% or 1% hydro-

Table 5–2. Ultrasound Transmission by Phonophoresis Media

PRODUCT	TRANSMISSION RELATIVE TO WATER (%)
Media that transmit US (ultrasound) well	
Lidex gel, fluocinonide 0.05%[a]	97
Thera-Gesic cream, methyl salicylate 15%[b]	97
Mineral oil[c]	97
US gel[d]	96
US lotion[e]	90
Betamethasone 0.05%[f] in US gel[d]	88
Media that transmit US poorly	
Diprolene ointment, betamethasone 0.05%[g]	36
Hydrocortisone (HC) powder 1%[h] in US gel[d]	29
HC powder 10%[h] in US gel[d]	7
Cortril ointment, HC 1%[i]	0
Eucerin cream[j]	0
HC cream 1%[k]	0
HC cream 10%[k]	0
HC cream 10%[k] mixed with equal weight US gel[d]	0
Myoflex cream, trolamine salicylate 10%[l]	0
Triamcinolone acetonide cream 0.1%[k]	0
Velva HC cream 10%[h]	0
Velva HC cream 10%[h] with equal weight US gel[d]	0
White petrolatum[m]	0
Other	
Chempad-L[n]	68
Polyethylene wrap[o]	98

Reprinted from Cameron, M.H., and Monroe, L.G. (1992): Relative transmission of ultrasound by media customarily used for phonophoresis. Phys. Ther., 72:147. With the permission of the APTA.
[a]Syntex Laboratories Inc, 3401 Hillview Ave, PO Box 10850, Palo Alto, CA 94303.
[b]Mission Pharmacal Co, 1325 E Durango, San Antonio, TX 78210.
[c]Pennex Corp, Eastern Ave at Pennex Dr, Verona, PA 15147.
[d]Ultraphonic, Pharmaceutical Innovations Inc, 897 Frelinghuysen Dr, Newark, NJ 07114.
[e]Polysonic, Parker Laboratories Inc, 307 Washington St, Orange, NJ 07050.
[f]Pharmfair Inc, 100 Kennedy Dr, Hauppauge, NY 11788.
[g]Schering Corp, Galloping Hill Rd, Kenilworth, NJ 07033.
[h]Purepac Pharmaceutical Co, 200 Elmora Ave, Elizabeth, NJ 07207.
[i]Pfizer Labs Division, Pfizer Inc, 253 E 42nd St, New York, NY 10017.
[j]Beiersdorf Inc, PO Box 5529, Norwalk, CT 06856-5529.
[k]E Fougera & Co, 60 Baylis Rd, Melville, NY 11747.
[l]Rorer Consumer Pharmaceuticals, Div of Rhône-Poulenc Rorer Pharmaceuticals Inc, 500 Virginia Dr, Fort Washington, PA 19034.
[m]Universal Cooperatives Inc, 7801 Metro Pkwy, Minneapolis, MN 55420.
[n]Henley International, 104 Industrial Blvd, Sugar Land, TX 77478.
[o]Saran Wrap, Dow Brands Inc, 9550 Zionsville Rd, Indianapolis, IN 46268.

cortisone in a thick white cream base. Their findings showed that all thick white corticosteroid creams tested transmitted ultrasound poorly. Additionally, ultrasound gel mixed with micronized hydrocortisone acetate powder also yielded a poorly transmitting medium. The three drug-containing media that were found to transmit ultrasound well were Lidex gel*, betamethasone gel, and Thera-Gesic cream†. Several studies[49, 61] with human subjects support the use of hydrocortisone. However, these studies are based on patient-reported decrease in pain and improved range of motion, rather than on empiric evidence of penetration of the hydrocortisone.

Indications and Contraindications. Ultrasound is the modality of choice for heating to the deepest level possible or when increased extensibility of joint, ligament, or scar tissue is desired. The exact mechanism by which ultrasound acts as an analgesic is still not understood.[52] However, it has been reported to temporarily alleviate pain, possibly by the alteration of threshold stimulation in free nerve endings.[86]

Because ultrasound causes an increase in local blood flow and enzymatic activity, it should not be applied to edematous or ischemic tissues. Similarly, joints that are hypermobile should not receive ultrasound unless any stretching movement, which would increase the pre-existing hypermobility, can be controlled. Athletes with anesthetic skin or bleeding disorders should also not receive ultrasound therapy.[74] Because of the damaging effect of increasing tissue temperature on a fetus, therapeutic ultrasound to the uterus of a pregnant woman is contraindicated; also, ultrasound should not be applied to the abdomen or low back area of a woman unless she is certain she is not pregnant. The possibility of cavitation prevents clinicians from applying ultrasound to fluid-filled cavities such as the eyes, brain, and heart. Ultrasound applied directly to cardiac pacemakers can interfere with their functioning, so individuals with pacemakers need to be protected from any stray sound waves.[86] Stirring effects have been implicated in increased detachment of cancer cells, with an increased possibility of metastasis, and therefore, no cancer patient should receive ultrasound except for special hyperthermic treatment of the cancer.[78, 86] The vibrational qualities of ultrasound dictate that it should not be applied to the epiphyseal plates of children or to unhealed surgical sites, in which the movement of adjacent molecules would retard or damage ongoing healing processes.

Application. In order for the sound wave to be propagated forward, it must pass through a medium that can be compressed. It cannot move through air, so a coupling agent is used to make a connection between the sound head, or applicator, and the athlete's skin (Fig. 5–13). The most commonly used coupling

---

*Available from Syntex Laboratories Inc., Palo Alto, California
†Available from Mission Pharmacal Co., San Antonio, Texas

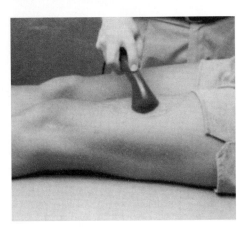

Figure 5–13. Ultrasound is effective for increasing collagen extensibility and blood flow in an area. A coupling agent such as commercial gel is required to transmit the sound waves from the applicator to the skin.

agents are commercially prepared gels, water, and mineral oil. Various studies have examined their efficacy. Commercially prepared gels have consistently been found to be the most efficient in transmitting sound waves and in raising the tissue temperature to therapeutic levels.[6, 36, 40, 41, 123, 125] Water is less efficient[36, 40, 41, 124] but is advocated for body surfaces too irregular to ensure transmission when using gel (e.g., hand, elbow, ankle). Although the reasons for the immersion technique being less efficient at raising tissue temperature are multiple, it appears that the sound wave is significantly attenuated, even at a distance of 1 to 2 cm from the body part being sonated.[124] When this technique is used, the body part is immersed in a water bath made of plastic, ceramic, or rubber. Care must be taken to remove air bubbles when sonating underwater, because they interfere markedly with sound wave transmission.[125] Because of formation of air bubbles during underwater sonation, degassed water has been recommended as a medium. At present, it appears that degassed water is no better than tap water, and neither is as effective as commercially prepared gels in transmitting the sound wave.[36, 41, 101] For small areas or for body parts on which gel would be unpleasant, such as the face, transmission can be accomplished by the bladder method. A balloon, condom, or plastic bag is filled with water, air pockets are removed, and the bladder is coated with a coupling medium (Fig. 5–14). If a balloon is used, the neck of the balloon is placed over the sound head with a thin layer of gel placed between the balloon and the skin. Otherwise, the bladder is held against the body part and the sound head is moved over the bladder.

Newer models of ultrasound units use small-diameter applicators. They have an extremely small depth of penetration because of the problem of beam divergence.[74] Customary use of ultrasound for target tissues at a depth of 3 to 5 cm requires a sound head no smaller than 5 cm².[74] Usual dosages range from 0.5 to 3.0 W/cm², with the specific dosage for each individual being determined by the depth of the target tissue, the degree of heating desired, and the athlete's response. If an even lower level of heating or nonthermal effects is desired, the sound wave can be pulsed, although few studies have demonstrated the efficacy of this method.

Using an adequate layer of coupling medium, the clinician moves the sound head in circular, overlapping strokes. It has been suggested that the size of the

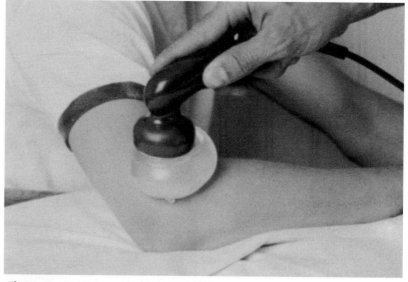

Figure 5–14. Ultrasound. A balloon filled with water can be used for sonation over very small areas or over body parts on which gel would be unpleasant or over bony prominences on which good surface contact cannot be made.

area to be sonated be limited to an area twice the size of the effective radiating area of the transducer.[100] If tissue temperatures exceed tolerance levels, such that tissue damage is imminent, the athlete experiences periosteal pain. This is usually reported as a deep aching or soreness. The clinician should immediately reduce the intensity by 10% to 15% or expand the field size.[60] Periosteal pain should quickly subside. If it does not, the intensity should be reduced further. A note should be made for future treatment sessions about the proper dosage for each athlete.

Stationary application of ultrasound (the sound head is simply held in position over the target structure) is discouraged because the rapid rise in temperature creates "hot spots"[74] and increases the possibility of blood clot formation.[93] To ensure temperature elevation to therapeutic levels, sonation needs to last from 3 to 10 minutes, depending on the depth of the target tissue, size of the area sonated, frequency and intensity of the ultrasound, and medium used to transmit the sound wave.[33, 36, 69, 105] Draper[31, 35] reports that at an intensity of 1.5 W/cm^2 it takes 3 to 4 minutes to reach a therapeutic level of heating with 3-MHz ultrasound and 10 minutes to heat tissue using a 1-MHz ultrasound unit. Also, a guideline of 1 to 2 minutes for each area 1.5 times the size of the transducer face has been suggested.[80] Thus, it is clear that the typical approach of using an ultrasound output of 1.5 W/cm^2 over a nondefined area for a 5-minute treatment is not acceptable if consistent thermal results are to be obtained.[5, 35, 80]

Advantages and Disadvantages. Ultrasound is an extremely useful clinical tool, especially for stretching tight ligaments, tendons, and capsular tissues. It effectively induces therapeutic temperatures in deep tissues to speed healing, is relatively easy to apply, and is comfortable for the athlete to experience. However, it is not the panacea many clinicians seem to expect, and it successfully executes only those functions for which it is designed. Several potentially serious complications can arise if ultrasound is applied improperly.

Considerations for Use

After a thorough history and physical examination have identified the target tissue, the clinician must decide which heating modality is most likely to accomplish the desired goal (e.g., increased blood flow, relief of pain, resolution of inflammatory exudates, or increased extensibility of collagen tissue) without bringing about unwanted side effects. Of primary consideration is the type of heat energy that the target tissue selectively absorbs. Shortwave diathermy, especially as delivered by the induction method, is selectively absorbed by skeletal muscle, whereas ultrasound is effective on connective tissues. Of equal importance is the depth of the tissue to be heated. Superficial heating agents rarely penetrate to a depth greater than 1 to 2 cm unless soft-tissue covering is minimal (e.g., on the hand), whereas ultrasound effectively penetrates up to a tissue depth of 5 cm. Inherent in this consideration is the thickness of the subcutaneous fat layer, especially for the superficial heating agents, which transmit their energy through conduction. For obese athletes, superficial heating agents may require longer times than the usual application periods, or they may produce only slight temperature changes in tissue below the skin. Finally, the expected vascular response must be considered. If tissue heating is slight, the increased homeostatic blood flow to the area may prevent any change in cellular metabolic rate, nerve conduction velocity, or joint stiffness, and therefore, the goal of treatment will not be reached. If tissue heating approaches tolerance levels, however, vasodilation is vigorous. Blood flow to the area increases dramatically, rates of chemical reactions increase, and stiffness of involved joints diminishes. The clinician should also expect an increase in edema. In a tissue in which healing is already impeded by excessive edema, this can further compromise the healing process.

THERAPEUTIC ELECTRICITY

The use of electrical stimulation in the training room and clinic has increased in popularity in recent years, in part because stimulators have become more user-friendly. However, along with this improvement, it has become easier to punch the manufacturer's preset buttons, losing sight of what the modality is actually capable of treating. For example, most manufacturers have preset values for treating swelling, yet scientific evidence that electrical stimulation has any impact on acute swelling in the clinical setting is essentially nonexistent.[84, 87] The plethora of instrumentation available has also led to confusion among clinicians, especially in the associated terminology. For instance, is there a difference in using one manufacturer's "4 pad" interferential current (IFC) and another's "quadripolar" IFC?

This section will provide the clinician with the basic knowledge needed to effectively use electrical stimulation in the rehabilitation of the injured athlete, with emphasis on the uses aimed at influencing excitable tissue (i.e., nerves and muscle). The reason for this emphasis is that although knowledge is far from complete with regard to the impact of electrical stimulation on excitable tissue, our understanding of its effects on nonexcitable tissue is lacking even more. In dealing with excitable tissue there is essentially one major goal, and that is to create an action potential in a particular type of nerve that in turn will activate a desired response. Before discussing the physiologic responses, a review of basic electricity is necessary.

Basic Considerations

Atoms are composed of protons, neutrons, and electrons. Protons are positively charged, electrons are negatively charged, and neutrons have no charge (neutral). Protons and neutrons are clustered in the nucleus of the atom, with electrons orbiting around them. Protons and electrons are electrically equivalent, so that equal numbers of each produce an overall electrical neutrality of the atom. To transfer a charge from one atom to another, only electrons are moved—protons are never removed from the nucleus.

Subtraction of electrons from or addition of electrons to the orbit of an atom creates an electrical imbalance, so that the atom becomes electrically charged. An atom that is electrically charged is known as an ion. Ions with a deficiency of electrons (more protons than electrons) are positively charged and are known as cations, whereas ions with an excess of electrons (more electrons than protons) are negatively charged and are known as anions. Ions of similar charge repel one another, whereas ions of dissimilar charge attract each other. This force of attraction or repulsion is directly proportional to the strength of the charges on the two ions and inversely proportional to the distance between them. It causes ions to move toward or away from one another, depending on the strength and direction (attraction or repulsion) of the force. The force that causes ions to move is known as voltage. Whereas voltage is the force that causes ions to move, the actual movement of the ions is known as current. Current can be defined as "the movement of charged particles in a conductor in response to an applied electrical force," with the applied electrical force being the voltage.[102] Current is measured in amperes (A), with 1 ampere being equal to 1 coulomb of electrons moving past a defined point in 1 second. Current and voltage are thus proportional. High voltage (all other factors being equal) produces a movement of many ions, which represents a high level of current flow. In the body, current flow is accomplished by the movement of ions.

As might be expected, however, all considerations are rarely equal. The media through which ions are moving and whether these media facilitate or inhibit this movement must be considered. Media that facilitate movement are known as conductors. Biologic conductors are water, blood, and electrolyte solutions such as perspiration. Media that inhibit movement of ions are known as resistors. Biologic resistors include skin, fat cells, and bone.

The relationship among voltage, current, and resistance of the medium to the movement of ions is described by Ohm's law:

$$I = V/R$$

where I is current, V is voltage, and R is resistance. The law states that the current (I) induced in a conductor increases as the applied driving force is increased (V becomes larger) or as opposition to the movement of ions is decreased (R becomes smaller).

Despite the plenitude of names, only three types of electrical current are applied to biologic tissues: direct, alternating, and pulsed (Fig. 5–15). Direct current (DC) is a continuous, one-directional flow of charged ions and is sometimes known as galvanic current. AC is a continuous, two-directional flow of charged ions and may be referred to as faradic current. Pulsed current is a flow of ions that is periodically discontinued for a finite period of time, and the flow can be unidirectional or bidirectional. Most clinical stimulators produce some form of pulsed current. The key to understanding how pulsed current is different from DC or AC lies in the periodic interruption (interpulse interval) of the current flow. The interval allows for independent adjustment of frequency and phase duration in pulsatile units that is not possible in AC and DC generators because they lack this interval. The importance of these adjustments will be addressed later in the chapter.

As can be seen from Figure 5–15, pulsed current actually looks the same as DC or AC, except that it is cyclically interrupted. Pulsed currents are described by their waveforms. They can be monophasic (each pulse contains one phase), in which the deviation from the baseline occurs in one direction only, or biphasic (each pulse contains two phases), in which the deviation from the baseline occurs in two directions. The phase can be symmetric or asymmetric depending on whether the sizes of the two phases are equal. A third type of pulsed current is polyphasic, in which each pulse contains three or more phases. This waveform is referred to by many different names, some of which include burst AC, medium-frequency stimulation, and carrier-frequency stimulation. Once a specific current has been identified as direct, alternating, or pulsed, with monophasic, biphasic, or polyphasic waveforms, symmetric or asymmetric, additional terms can be used to describe the phases of a pulse and the pulses themselves (Fig. 5–16):

1. Peak amplitude: the maximum value a current can reach in a monophasic current or in either phase of a biphasic current
2. Phase duration: the length of time during which a single phase of the current is applied
3. Pulse duration: the time from the beginning to the end of a single pulse (the term "pulse width" is sometimes used to denote this; it is also used sometimes to denote phase duration, which can lead to added confusion)
4. Intrapulse interval: the time elapsed from one phase of a pulse to the next (also described as the interphase interval)
5. Interpulse interval: the time between pulses
6. Frequency: the number of pulses that occur in 1 second

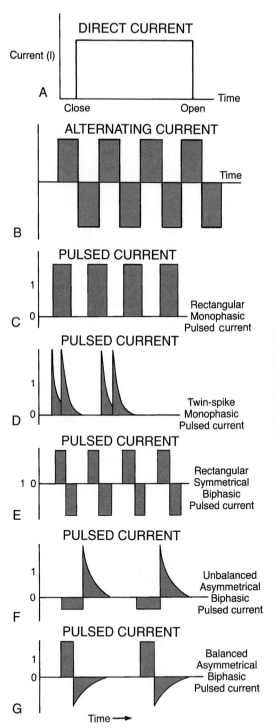

Figure 5–15. Graphic representation of the three types of electrical current. *A,* Direct current. *B,* Alternating current. *C* through *G,* Pulsed currents. (Modified from Robinson, A.J. [1989]: Basic concepts and terminology in electricity. *In:* Snyder-Mackler, L., and Robinson, A.J. [eds.]: Clinical Electrophysiology. Baltimore, Williams & Wilkins, pp. 9, 11, 13.)

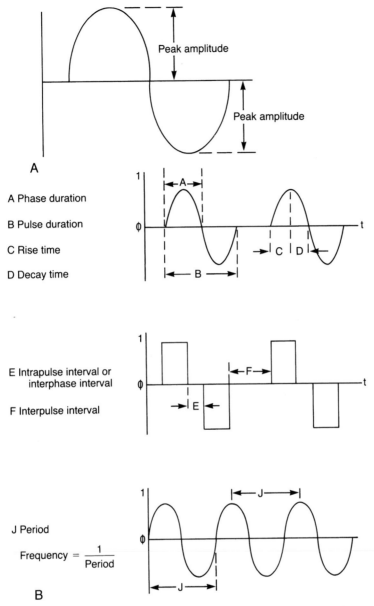

A

A Phase duration

B Pulse duration

C Rise time

D Decay time

E Intrapulse interval or
   interphase interval

F Interpulse interval

J Period

Frequency = $\dfrac{1}{Period}$

B

Figure 5–16. Electricity characteristics. (From Robinson, A.J. [1989]: Basic concepts and terminology in electricity. *In:* Snyder-Mackler, L., and Robinson, A.J. [eds.]: Clinical Electrophysiology. Baltimore, Williams & Wilkins, p. 15.)

Phases can also be modified so that the full strength of the current is not applied all at once or turned off abruptly. Rise time (the time during which the current of a phase increases from zero at the baseline to the peak amplitude) and decay time (the time during which the current of a phase decreases from peak amplitude to zero) denote these modifications. Similarly, the current itself can be altered in this manner through ramping (Fig. 5–17). Current can be ramped up or down by increasing or decreasing current intensity, length of the pulse duration, or pulse frequency.

Electrical current is passed into the body through electrodes and a conducting medium. Water, an electrolyte gel, or conductive polymers are common conducting media. To make a circuit for current to flow through the body, at least one

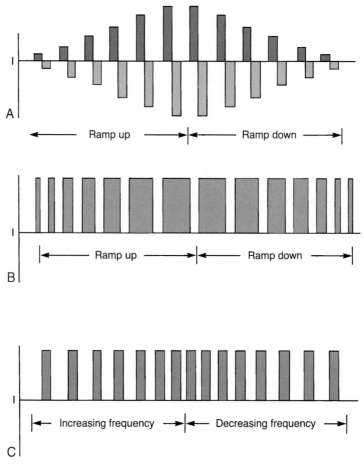

Figure 5–17. Methods of ramping current. *A*, Amplitude modulation. *B*, Pulse duration modulation. *C*, Frequency modulation. (From Robinson, A.J. [1989]: Basic concepts and terminology in electricity. *In:* Snyder-Mackler, L., and Robinson, A.J. [eds.]: Clinical Electrophysiology, Baltimore, Williams & Wilkins, p. 18.)

electrode from each of the two leads must be in contact with the body. Each channel of a stimulator has two leads, both of which are essential to current flow. A common mistake is to call one lead a ground. A ground is used to safely remove excess current from a stimulator; no such mechanism is attached to the patient. A way to illustrate this concept is to consider a three-prong electrical outlet. Current will flow as long as a circuit is created between the flat outer slots, with no need to have anything in the round center slot (the ground). Current will not flow if a circuit is made between one of the flat slots and the ground. When electrical stimulation is applied to an athlete, both leads must be attached to the athlete; if one lead were a ground, it would not need to be attached to the athlete for current to flow. Although electrodes can be arranged in numerous configurations, they can be categorized as one of two electrode placement techniques: monopolar and bipolar.

In a monopolar arrangement (Fig. 5–18*A*), one lead with its electrode or electrodes is placed in the target region (the region in which the athlete should perceive the strongest sensation of current). The electrode or electrodes from the other lead are placed in a non–target area (an area in which the athlete will perceive little or no sensation of current). The way the current perception is modified to allow for strong sensation at the target site and little or no sensation at the non–target site is through the manipulation of current density.

Current density is defined mathematically as the amount of current divided by the contact surface area of the skin-electrode interface. The higher the current density, the greater the perception of current. Therefore, in the typical monopolar electrode technique, one lead is usually attached to a rather large electrode (often inappropriately referred to as the ground), whereas the other lead is attached to one or two electrodes that are significantly smaller. The large electrode with its large skin-electrode interface area has a relatively low current density and thus provides little if any sensation of current compared with the smaller electrode

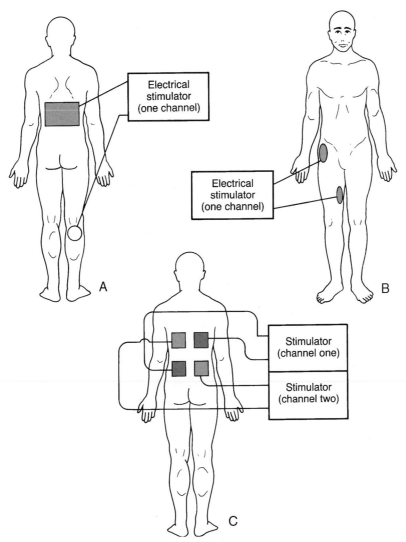

Figure 5–18. Electrode placement configurations in clinical electrical stimulation. *A*, Monopolar orientation, with a small "active" electrode over the posterior calf target region and a large "dispersive" or "indifferent" electrode in the low back region. *B*, Bipolar orientation, with two electrodes placed over the anterior thigh musculature target area; electrodes might not be the same size in all applications. *C*, Quadripolar orientation of electrodes, with two electrodes from each of two separate stimulation "channels" placed in the low back target region. (From Myklebust, B.M., and Robinson, A.J. [1989]: Instrumentation. *In:* Snyder-Mackler, L., and Robinson, A.J. [eds.]: Clinical Electrophysiology, Baltimore, Williams & Wilkins, p. 31.)

or electrodes on the other lead. The smaller electrodes have a larger current density, and therefore, the current is perceived as being much more intense under them.

Bipolar arrangements (Fig. 5–18B) involve the use of electrodes of the same or similar size on both leads. Electrodes from both leads are typically placed in target areas. With the multichannel stimulator units available currently, the term "quadripolar electrode arrangements" is often used (Fig. 5–18C). As can be seen from the figure, this arrangement is nothing but the use of two channels, each with a bipolar electrode technique.

Guidelines for Various Input Parameters

Because the most frequent use of electrical stimulation is for stimulation of excitable tissue, the following section will provide some basic guidelines for choosing parameters on the basis of the treatment goal. This section is designed as a generic guide to the various settings and parameter choices that may be found on commercial stimulator units.

POLARITY

The ability to make polarity choices is found on stimulators that produce monophasic pulsed current, asymmetric unbalanced biphasic pulsed current, or DC. Of these, by far the most typical current form generated by clinical units is the monophasic pulsed form. When electrical stimulation is being used for pain control, polarity of the electrodes has little impact on the effectiveness of the stimulation.

If muscle stimulation is the desired goal, the importance of the polarity depends on the chosen electrode technique. If a bipolar electrode technique is used with the electrodes placed on proximal and distal ends of the muscle belly, polarity is not a factor in the strength of the stimulated contraction.[132] However, if a monopolar electrode technique is used, the electrodes in the target area should be made negative. This will allow for a stronger contraction at any given current amplitude compared with the contraction strength obtained with positive target area electrodes.[127]

DC is primarily used for iontophoresis. The polarity chosen for the medication-containing electrode will depend on whether the medication is a positive or a negative ion.

WAVEFORM

Some pulsed current stimulators allow the clinician to choose among monophasic, biphasic, or polyphasic waveforms as well as among different shapes of these forms. Contrary to many manufacturer claims, the choice of waveform and shape is directed more by individual patient comfort than by any other element. The generation of an action potential is an all-or-none response, and the occurrence of this response is governed by three factors that include current amplitude (intensity), phase duration, and rate of current rise from baseline. As long as these three criteria are met, an action potential will be generated, regardless of the type of waveform (monophasic, biphasic, or polyphasic) and shape of wave (e.g., square or rectangular) used.

Why, then, is the clinician given such a choice? Patients will typically find one particular waveform more comfortable; however, there is no single waveform that all patients will find the most comfortable.[25, 28] The ability to try different waveforms allows the clinician to find one that is most comfortable, which can facilitate achieving the desired treatment response.

STRENGTH (INTENSITY) AND DURATION PARAMETERS

The intensity is one of the most important parameters that control whether the desired response is achieved. As stated earlier, it is one of the three criteria that determine the production of an action potential by excitable tissue. Except for iontophoresis, it is not necessary to record the actual numeric setting on the stimulator. Clinically, intensity is measured by the athlete's response. Does the athlete feel any current at all? If not, it is considered subsensory. Does the athlete feel a strong but comfortable tingling sensation? If so, this is considered the sensory level. Is the stimulation producing a visible muscle contraction or motor response? Motor responses can be categorized as minimal motor, moderate motor, or maximally tolerated motor response. Finally, is the stimulation causing an uncomfortable or painful response? If this is the case, this is considered the noxious level. The reason for recording the intensity in this manner is that the numeric intensity that elicits the desired response will differ somewhat on different treatment days.

Sensory, moderate motor, and noxious intensities are typically used for pain control. Minimal to moderate motor intensity levels can be used in much the same way a biofeedback unit can be used for muscle re-education. Maximally tolerated motor intensity level is used if the desired response is muscle strengthening.

Phase duration is another of the three criteria that determine the generation of an action potential. The interaction between intensity and phase duration can be described best by the strength-duration graph (Fig. 5–19). As can be seen from the graph, if sensory level stimulation is the desired response, keeping the phase durations shorter makes it easier to avoid a motor or noxious response. If the desired response is motor or noxious level stimulation, use of a longer phase duration will allow either of these responses to be obtained with a lower intensity. This allows fine-tuning of the response. In summary, shorter phase durations are typically used for sensory level pain control, whereas longer phase durations are used for muscle contractions and for noxious level pain control.

FREQUENCY

Frequency does not determine whether an action potential is generated in an excitable tissue. The purpose for adjusting frequency is to control how many times per second the action potential is generated, once the intensity and phase duration are sufficient to cause an action potential. For example, if the frequency is set at 100 Hz and the intensity and phase duration are sufficient to depolarize the nerve, that nerve will produce 100 action potentials each second. The choice of treatment frequency is then determined by how many action potentials are desired every second, which in turn is guided by the treatment goal.

At motor level stimulation, a frequency of 1 pulse per second will produce a muscle twitch. As frequency is increased, the twitches will occur closer together until they fuse into a smooth, tetanized contraction. The frequency at which this fusion occurs in most cases will be between 15 and 30 pulses per second, varying with the muscle selected. Once tetany is reached, further increases in frequency will cause increases in force production. The increase in force production is not without cost, because as the frequency increases, so does the rate of muscle fatigue (Fig. 5–20).

Finally, the electrical action of skeletal muscle motor units is guided by the absolute refractory period of the motor units. The absolute refractory period for normal subjects is such that motor units can be stimulated only approximately 1000 times per second.[102] A higher frequency of stimulation does not produce a greater strength of contraction.

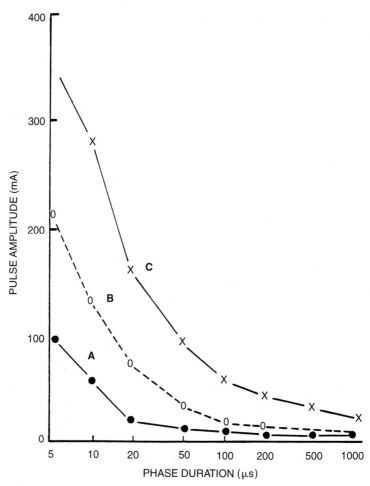

Figure 5-19. Strength-duration curves of the three excitatory responses. A, sensory; B, motor; C, noxious. (Modified from Alon, G. [1987]: Principles of electrical stimulation. *In:* Nelson, R.M., and Currier, D.P. [eds.]: Clinical Electrotherapy. Norwalk, CT, Appleton & Lange, p. 58.)

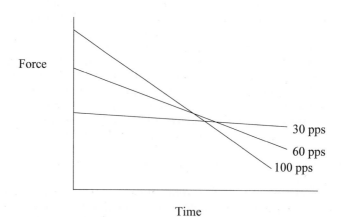

Figure 5-20. Frequency-force-fatigue relationships. Higher frequencies generate greater forces, but rates of fatigue are accelerated. pps, pulse per second.

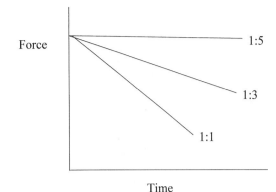

Figure 5–21. On/off cycle–fatigue relationship. As depicted graphically, longer rest (off) times reduce fatigue.

ON/OFF CYCLE

The on/off cycle settings on stimulators are used to determine the length of time during the treatment period that the stimulation is perceived. The cycle can be set on "continuous," which means that the unit will deliver the set current throughout the entire treatment time. "Continuous" does not mean that current is flowing continuously as in AC or DC. It should be kept in mind that in pulsatile stimulators there is an interpulse interval in which no current is flowing. To illustrate this concept, consider a monophasic waveform stimulator set at a moderate motor intensity, a 90-microsecond phase duration, a 1-pulse-per-second frequency, a continuous on/off cycle, and a 20-minute treatment time. The athlete will receive a single pulse, 90 microseconds in duration, one time each second, every second for 20 minutes. The response observed will be that of a one-muscle twitch every second for 20 minutes.

The on/off cycle can also be set for a certain number of seconds on, followed by a certain number of seconds off. This type of setting is used to break up tetanized motor responses. It would be extremely uncomfortable to be subjected to an electrically elicited muscle contraction for extended periods of time. Figure 5–21 illustrates the role the on/off cycle plays in controlling muscle fatigue during strengthening stimulation. If strengthening is the goal, it is important to set the on time long enough to achieve a good contraction. Times less than 5 seconds, even with a zero ramp time, are usually not sufficient to accomplish a complete contraction of the muscle.

General Indications, Contraindications, and Precautions

Tables 5–3 to 5–6 outline the general indications, contraindications, and precautions to consider when applying electrical stimulation. Not all of the indicated uses can be performed by any one class of commercial stimulators. Specific classes of units and their capabilities are discussed later.

Physiologic Effects

Generally, therapeutic electricity has been used for the maintenance or gain of muscular strength, relief of pain, reduction of edema, delivery of medication transcutaneously, and healing of chronic wounds and nonunion fractures. Electricity is not as well understood as are therapeutic cold and heat; despite many

Table 5–3. Suggested Uses of Electrical Stimulation*

Re-education of muscle
Strengthening of muscle after injury
Control of pain in numerous acute and chronic syndromes
Control of postoperative pain
Control of labor pain
Treatment of urinary incontinence
Control of edema
Healing of wound
Healing of delayed or nonunion fractures
Functional electrical stimulation (orthotic)
Introduction of medications transcutaneously
Improvement or maintenance of range of motion
Stimulation of denervated muscle
Inhibition of spasticity
Relief of muscle spasms
Temporary increase of blood flow to an area
Treatment of neurovascular disorders involving
    vasospastic and pseudovasospastic disorders

*Not all of the above uses have been substantiated by clinical or basic science research.

Table 5–4. Contraindications for Electrical Stimulation

Stimulation over carotid sinus
Stimulation across heart
Operating unit within 15 feet of an operating diathermy unit
Stimulation over abdomen or low back during pregnancy
Stimulation over acute thrombophlebitis
Active hemorrhage
Pain of unknown origin
Active cancer in the area being treated
Individuals with a synchronized or demand form of pacemaker
Bleeding disorders
Tuberculosis

Table 5–5. Patients Requiring Precaution During Electrical Stimulation

Patients prone to seizures
Patients with peripheral occlusive arterial disease
Patients with severe hypotension or hypertension
Patients with areas of excessive adipose tissue
Patients who are unable to give clear appropriate feedback
Patients with regions without sensation

Table 5–6. Signs of Possible Overstimulation or Lack of Tolerance to Stimulation

Increased nervousness
Increased pain or symptoms
Worsening of signs

Skin burns
Muscle soreness

studies of the various electrical modalities, the precise mechanisms for many of its effects remain mostly unknown.

MUSCLE STRENGTHENING

Electrical stimulation for strength training is commonly referred to as neuromuscular electrical stimulation (NMES) (Fig. 5–22). The findings from research on the effects of therapeutic electricity on muscle strength are confusing and controversial, in part because of significant differences in research methodology, as well as in choice of subjects. There appears to be less consensus among studies using electrical stimulation for strength training in healthy subjects than among studies on patient populations. The consistency of conclusions is better in studies on patient populations when the results from designs using AC-powered clinical model stimulators are separated from results obtained with battery-operated portable units. In summary, the use of NMES as a mode of strength training can be beneficial,[26, 116, 118, 119] particularly early in rehabilitation, for the injured athlete as long as it is performed with an AC-powered clinical stimulator capable of producing a muscle contraction that is at least 10% of the maximal voluntary contraction of the corresponding muscle on the uninvolved side.[119] Battery-operated units and some clinical models are not capable of producing this minimal dose response, and therefore, in studies using these units, strengthening has not been shown.[89, 111, 119] Obtaining mixed results from studies of NMES in normal subjects is, in reality, of little consequence to the rehabilitation professional because it is not time- or cost-effective to attempt to train healthy athletes with electrical stimulation.

A recent study by Snyder-Mackler and associates[116] best illustrates the benefits of using electrical stimulation early in the rehabilitation process. The study was a multicenter, randomized clinical trial examining the effect of NMES on quadriceps strength after anterior cruciate ligament reconstruction. Patients were randomly assigned to one of four groups: a high-intensity clinical NMES, a portable stimulator NMES, a high-intensity clinical plus portable unit NMES, and a control group. All four groups participated in the same accelerated exercise rehabilitation program described by Shelbourne and Nitz.[110] The patient groups receiving the high-intensity clinical NMES were treated as follows: The patient's knee was stabilized in 65° of flexion. Using a polyphasic waveform generator,

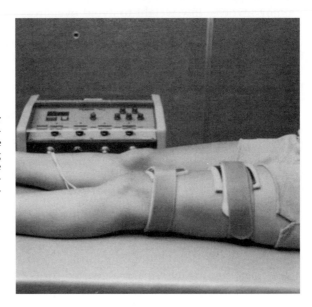

Figure 5–22. Example of bipolar electrode placement for neuromuscular electrical stimulation of the quadriceps femoris. After securing the electrodes, the knee should be stabilized in the appropriate midrange position if muscle strengthening is the goal.

the patient performed 15 maximally tolerated training contractions, three times a week for 4 weeks, beginning 2 weeks postsurgery.

All four groups of patients were tested for quadriceps strength recovery and functional status 6 weeks postsurgery. The groups receiving high-intensity NMES showed a 70% recovery of quadriceps strength compared with 51% to 57% recovery in the groups not receiving high-intensity NMES. Functional status was evaluated as knee control during the stance phase of gait, with use of two-dimensional video motion analysis equipment. The high-intensity NMES groups showed significantly better control of knee flexion-excursion compared with the other groups. Of great interest in this study was the ability of open-chain, electrical stimulation training at 65° of knee flexion to have a significant impact on a closed-chain, volitional activity taking place between 0° and 25° of knee flexion.

One explanation for why NMES is more effective for patients than exercise alone lies in the difference in recruitment and firing patterns between NMES and volitional muscle contractions. In a volitional contraction the recruitment of motor units in skeletal muscle follows a consistent and orderly pattern. When central nervous system input demands initiation of contraction in a muscle, the smallest alpha motoneurons are recruited first. As the central nervous system's demand for a greater strength of contraction continues, larger and larger motoneurons are recruited, with the largest being enlisted last. This recruitment pattern is known as the size principle. The smallest alpha motoneurons innervate slow-twitch muscle fibers, whereas the largest alpha motoneurons innervate fast-twitch glycolytic fibers.

Another way in which the human body can produce a greater strength in a volitional contraction is through a change in the motoneuron discharge rate, a process known as rate coding. Increasing the discharge frequency from the alpha motoneurons that are already firing acts to increase the tension developed by individual muscle fibers and may fuse the twitches into a tetanic contraction. Thus, greater torque is developed by the muscle. Discharge rates developed in this way from healthy motoneurons are rarely higher than 30 pulses per second.[102]

Recruitment of motor units during an electrically stimulated contraction follows the opposite pattern from that of a volitional contraction. Because a larger nerve will depolarize at lower intensity–phase duration combinations than will a smaller nerve, the larger alpha motoneurons innervating fast-twitch glycolytic fibers are preferentially recruited first.[27] In early rehabilitation, typical exercise training involves low weight to avoid overstress to the injured joint. Therefore, fast-twitch fibers would be recruited rarely and hence would receive little training effect from such exercise. With NMES, the joint can be stabilized and the fast-twitch fibers can be recruited with each contraction. Because fast-twitch fibers can produce more force, it makes sense that with such a training stimulus early in rehabilitation, greater strength gains are made with NMES training than with exercise alone.

Training stimulus with NMES may also be impacted by the firing rate. Any motor unit recruited by NMES will be firing at the frequency set on the machine. For strengthening, the use of frequencies from 35 to 80 Hz is typically recommended. As stated earlier, in a volitional muscle contraction, the rate coding rarely exceeds 30 discharges per second, and therefore, in addition to an intensity overload, the muscle may also be responding to a frequency overload.[27]

Another possible explanation for the benefits of training with NMES in early rehabilitation is that the clinician can override the neurologic inhibition of the muscle.[117] Because the stimulator is controlling the motor axon firing it would seem plausible that the normal nervous system feedback mechanisms would not have much effect on inhibiting the muscle contraction.

The following guidelines are suggested for NMES application.

1. Place the negative electrodes over the motor point of the muscle if using a monophasic waveform generator in a monopolar electrode technique.[83, 127] If using a bipolar electrode technique, make sure the electrodes are placed on muscle tissue and not over tendons. Also, place the electrodes in such a way that current will flow parallel to the muscle fibers.[14]

2. Use the largest electrodes that fit the area being stimulated. This will improve patient comfort.

3. Stabilize the joints affected by the muscle contraction in a safe non–end-range position to improve patient tolerance and comfort and allow for higher-intensity stimulation. Results from the study of Synder-Mackler et al[116] suggest that there is little, if any, reason to position a joint near its end range during high intensity NMES.

4. Have the athlete contract the muscle with the stimulation. In most instances this will improve tolerance.

5. Encourage the athlete to use the highest tolerable intensity because there is a linear relationship between the strength gained and the intensity of the stimulated contraction.[119] The intensity of the contraction should be at least 10% of the uninvolved maximal isometric contraction. If the athlete has difficulty tolerating stimulation, it may be beneficial to begin with low-level stimulation (even as low as sensory level) and to gradually increase the intensity over several treatment visits.

6. Use the longest phase duration available on the stimulator, which will make it easier to get a strong contraction.

7. Keep in mind the relationship between frequency, strength of contraction, and fatigue. Frequency is typically set between 35 and 80 Hz. During initial training periods it may be beneficial to use frequencies on the lower end (35 to 50 Hz) to avoid excessive fatigue. As the athlete progresses, the frequency should be increased to at least 60 pulses per second, because these frequencies are most appropriate for maximum force generation to continue an overload stimulus.[13]

8. Set the on/off cycle initially at a 1:4 or 1:5 ratio to avoid excessive fatigue. It can be reduced toward a 1:1 ratio, as needed, to continue the overload stimulus. In order to attain a good, full contraction, it is suggested that the on time be between 10 and 15 seconds, with the off cycle adjusted accordingly.

9. Have the athlete complete 15 training-level isometric contractions.[116]

PAIN RELIEF

Use of various electrical modalities for pain relief was a generally accepted practice for years, long before Melzack and Wall presented their gate theory of pain modulation in 1965. Since then the number and variety of electrical modalities used to provide analgesia for the relief of all types of pain have proliferated at an astounding rate. Relief of pain has been cited as an indication for the use of high-voltage stimulators, interferential stimulators, transcutaneous electrical nerve stimulators (TENS units), Medcosonolators, and low-voltage stimulators.

It is commonly thought that these devices relieve pain by two methods. Electrical stimulation of the skin and mild contraction of muscles act on receptors within tissues that transmit their message to the central nervous system, closing the "pain gate" at the spinal cord level. This process is commonly known as counter-irritation.[60] More intense stimulation, which elicits strong muscular contractions and is reported to be a painful sensation, is believed to stimulate release of endogenous opiates into the general circulation, producing a more general analgesia throughout the body.[112]

It has been suggested that the different forms and levels of stimulation are more effective for the relief of the varying types and intensities of pain that confront the average clinician. These modes of stimulation are usually described as sensory level, motor level, and noxious level stimulation (Table 5–7).[112]

Sensory level stimulation, also known as conventional stimulation, uses a relatively high-frequency, low-level current (enough to produce a skin sensation of buzzing or tingling), and the pain relief provided lasts only as long as the stimulation is applied.[112] No muscular contraction should be evident, either visually or through palpation.[112] It is thought that this form of stimulation produces analgesia by interference with pain message transmission, as described by the gate theory of pain. It is the most comfortable and least frightening of all the levels of stimulation and therefore is an excellent choice for the athlete who is apprehensive about receiving electroanalgesia treatment.

By comparison, motor level or acupuncture-type stimulation has a lower frequency of stimulation and a longer pulse duration and uses a current strong enough to elicit a regular motor response.[112] The relief obtained through this stimulation method does not immediately follow initiation of treatment but lasts for a period after stimulation ceases.[112] Thus, it is believed to relieve pain by stimulating the release of endogenous opiates.[112]

Noxious level stimulation (as may be expected from its name) is the least comfortable of all the stimulation modes. It has a relatively low frequency of stimulation and uses sufficient current to be painful to the athlete. This current can produce a muscle contraction if the electrodes are placed close enough to a motor point.[112] The usual length of treatment is relatively short, lasting from only seconds to several minutes. The discomfort from this form of stimulation is related to the long phase duration (up to 1 second),[112] as well as to the small electrodes often used to elicit the response. It produces a generalized analgesia that endures long after treatment has ceased.

Although these general guidelines are widely accepted, more specific recommendations are a subject of much controversy. In an outstanding review of studies of TENS for pain relief, Gersh and Wolf[45] noted extensive variations in recommendations for clinical use with regard to pulse duration, pulse frequency, current intensity, and frequency and duration of treatments, even for patients with similar diagnoses. By comparison, Jette[56] induced pain in the form of an electrically induced pinprick sensation in healthy subjects and then treated them with one of five commonly used TENS protocols: low frequency, burst frequency, hyperstimulation, high frequency with low-voltage galvanic stimulation, and high frequency with high-voltage galvanic stimulation. No significant difference was found in measured pain threshold or tolerance to pain among those receiving differing protocols. These results contrast with those of other studies, which showed definitive relief of pain with specific protocols.[45]

The most accurate conclusion may be that although many forms of electrical stimulation produce significant reductions in pain, research results are both confusing and contradictory. This lack of consistency, despite widespread study, was probably stated best by Mayer and Price[79]:

Table 5-7. Common Stimulation Characteristics of Electroanalgesia

MODE OF STIMULATION	PHASE DURATION (μsec)	FREQUENCY (PPS)	AMPLITUDE	DURATION OF TREATMENT	DURATION OF ANALGESIA	ELECTRODE PLACEMENT
Sensory level	2–50	50–100	Perceptible tingling	20–30 min	Little, residual postreatment	In the area of pain
Motor level	>150	2–4	Strong, visible muscle contraction	30–45 min	Hours	Remote, usually in the same sclerotome
Noxious level	<1 sec	1–5 or >100	Noxious; below motor threshold	Seconds to minutes	Hours	Close or remote; widely varied

Adapted from Snyder-Mackler, L. (1989): Electrical stimulation for pain modulation. *In*: Snyder-Mackler, L., and Robinson, A.J. (eds.): Clinical Electrophysiology, p. 208. © 1989, the Williams & Wilkins Co., Baltimore.

In conclusion, acupuncture and transcutaneous electrical nerve stimulation appear to be forms of counter-irritation which activate both opiate and non-opiate systems. The variable clinical outcomes observed following these treatments probably result from differential recruitment of segmental, extrasegmental, opiate, and non-opiate pain inhibitory systems, all of which are now known to be activated by these types of stimulation in animals.

The following guidelines are suggested for sensory pain control application.

1. Use of sensory level stimulation is probably best for acute conditions when the stimulation is applied over the region of injury. It is probably less effective in chronic conditions than are motor level or noxious level stimulation.
2. Use the largest electrodes that fit the area being stimulated. This will improve patient comfort.
3. Use short phase durations to minimize the possibility of causing muscle contractions.
4. Set the frequency between 20 and 150 Hz. There is some evidence that frequencies between 20 and 80 Hz may be most effective for pain relief.[58]
5. Modulate the stimulation to reduce adaptation to the stimulus. Clinical units typically offer only frequency modulations, whereas portable units for home use often offer amplitude, phase duration, frequency, and combination modulations. Use the modulation that the athlete finds most comfortable.
6. Although electrodes are typically placed directly over the site of pain, try placements over dermatomes, nerve roots, or peripheral nerves if the stimulation is not effective.
7. Set the on/off cycle on continuous.
8. Provide the athlete with a portable home unit (TENS unit) to continue the pain relief gained in the clinic because there is little carryover of pain relief once the stimulator is removed.

The following guidelines are suggested for motor or noxious level pain control application.

1. Do not apply these forms of pain control directly over the site of injury in the acute phase. They can be used for pain control after acute injury if applied to distant sites that are associated with the area of injury, for example, dermatomes, nerve roots, or acupuncture sites.
2. For noxious level pain control, use the smallest electrodes provided with the stimulator. Smaller electrodes will cause a noxious sensation at a lower intensity.
3. With either protocol, use long phase durations to allow the appropriate response to be achieved at lower current amplitudes.
4. If a motor response is occurring with the chosen electrode placement, set the frequency below that

for tetany. Frequencies between 1 and 12 Hz will typically meet this criterion. This should be done to avoid a prolonged tetanized contraction.

5. Stimulation modulations are not as necessary for either of these protocols because adaptation to the stimulus is much less common.
6. Set the on/off cycle to continuous.
7. If the athlete has difficulty tolerating either of these protocols, set the stimulation at a sensory level for the first 5 minutes of treatment and complete the treatment with the motor or noxious protocol after the athlete is "numb."
8. Patient tolerance usually limits treatment time for either of these protocols to 30 to 45 minutes.

EDEMA REDUCTION

Two electrical stimulation protocols for edema reduction have been historically advocated, a low-frequency motor level stimulation for muscle pump and a sensory level stimulation for electrical field effects. Neither of these protocols has proven to be effective in humans for accelerating the resolution of edema in the acute phase of injury.

There is some promising research using animal models, but to date, human trials are lacking.[84] In animal models, the protocol that has been successful was applied using a high-voltage pulsed stimulation (HVPS) unit.[84] The negative electrode was placed over the site of injury, and the sensory level (120 Hz) treatment was applied for 30 minutes. In the animal model, to curb edema formation for up to 24 hours, it appears that the treatment must be initiated within the first 4.5 hours after injury and must be applied four times with 60-minute rest intervals between applications. The reader is referred to an excellent discussion and review of these studies by Mendel and Fish.[84] They suggest a tentative protocol for acute edema management, which uses HVPS, with the negative electrode stimulation to the site of edema starting immediately after injury and being applied at an intensity 90% of visible motor threshold and at a frequency of 120 Hz every 4 hours for as long as edema is likely to be occurring.

It is interesting that for several years most manufacturers of electrical stimulation units have provided automated protocols for treating swelling, even with no scientific evidence to support such use. This suggests that the clinician should rely less on the manufacturer's suggested protocols and trade publications and more on the results of published studies in peer-reviewed journals.

WOUND HEALING

In recent years the use of electrical stimulation for wound healing has increased on the basis of positive research findings. Of the types of stimulators studied, microamperage DC stimulators and HVPS units appear to produce the most predictable responses.[62, 115] The type of stimulator needed to produce microamperage DC is not currently available commercially.[62] This leaves the HVPS unit as the unit of choice for the clinician. Fortunately, HVPS appears to be as effective as microamperage DC stimulation in wound healing.[62] Human studies assessing the effectiveness of HVPS have centered on the treatment of chronic dermal ulcers. The stimulation parameters that have been effective include 45 to 60 minutes of stimulation daily, an intensity less than 200 volts (sensory level), and a frequency of 100 to 105 pulses per second. Success has been reported with use of either positive or negative polarity of the electrode placed over the wound.[62] Because of this and on the basis of studies using microamperage DC, many clinicians are using protocols that change the polarity either every 3 days or when signs of healing plateau. There is literature to suggest a bactericidal effect from the negative electrode and an enhancement of re-epithelialization from the positive electrode.[62]

Specific Modalities and Their Application

HIGH-VOLTAGE PULSED STIMULATION

HVPS units deliver a monophasic pulse with, typically, a double-peak configuration (Fig. 5–23). There is no physiologic reason for this particular wave configuration, and in fact some manufacturers are now making HVPS units that do not produce the twin-peak waveform. Some sources suggest that the twin peak is used because the duration of each individual peak does not deliver enough current to the electrically excitable tissues to ensure a response, especially if a muscle contraction is desired.[90] However, there are other equally effective ways of ensuring the delivery of enough charge to obtain the desired response.

An HVPS unit is a stimulator having an output greater than 100 to 150 volts. For most stimulators now in use, this range is usually about 300 to 500 volts.[3] Their pulse duration is approximately 5 to 75 microseconds per peak.[3, 90] The pulse frequency can be varied, ranging from 1 to 120 pulses per second. HVPS units were once referred to as high-voltage "galvanic" pulsed stimulators. They are not actually galvanic stimulators, because they do not produce continuous DC.[3] HVPS units generate a pulsed current and therefore should not be referred to as galvanic. The old designation has led many clinicians to assume that the units may be capable of stimulating denervated muscle or performing iontophoresis, both of which require DC generators.

Because the phase durations of HVPS are so short, they must produce high peak currents in order to elicit a response from excitable tissue. However, because the phase duration is so short and interpulse interval so long, the total current (amount of current flow per second[4]) delivered by these units is very low. For example, if the unit has a duration of 25 microseconds per peak (50 microseconds total pulse duration) and is set at a frequency of 100 pulses per second and a treatment time of 20 minutes, it actually delivers current for a total of 6 seconds, distributed over the 20-minute treatment time. The clinical impact of this is that these stimulators tend to be perceived as being comfortable.

As can be noted in Figure 5–23, because the pulses are monophasic, the current leaves a charge in the tissues.[3] However, because of the combination of the very short phase duration and very long interpulse interval there is no measurable change in skin pH under the electrodes during stimulation.[91] This virtually eliminates the possibility of producing burns when using these units, even though there is a net deposit of charge on the skin.

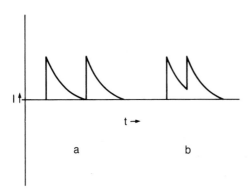

Figure 5–23. Schematic representation of a high-voltage pulsed galvanic waveform. I, current amplitude; t, time (microseconds); a, representative of a wave with a long intrapulse interval; b, representative of a wave with a short intrapulse interval. (From Newton, R. [1987]: High-voltage pulsed galvanic stimulation: Theoretical bases and clinical applications. In: Nelson, R.M., and Currier, D.P. [eds.]: Clinical Electrotherapy. Norwalk, CT, Appleton and Lange, p. 166.)

Application. Because of the characteristics of the current, HVPS can be used safely with a variety of electrode sizes, making it a flexible clinical tool for pain control. Larger electrodes can be used to produce very comfortable sensory or motor level pain control, whereas very small electrodes can be used safely to produce noxious level pain control. The HVPS unit is currently the only commercially available stimulator with research supporting its use for healing chronic wounds. On the horizon is the development of clinical protocols for use of HVPS in the control of acute edema.

HVPS can be used for attaining a motor level contraction, but not all units can produce contractions that elicit a strength-training response.[7, 89] Unfortunately, there is no list that categorizes the capability of current units to augment muscle strength. If the athlete is able to tolerate the maximum intensity level produced by the machine within a few treatments or if the contraction is less than 10% of the uninvolved side, the unit is probably not powerful enough to use for strengthening.

HVPS cannot be used to stimulate denervated muscle because the phase duration is too short. For the same reason, HVPS cannot be used for iontophoresis.

LOW-VOLTAGE PULSED STIMULATION

All stimulators discussed in the remainder of this chapter can be categorized as low-voltage pulsed stimulators. Specific types of units are discussed in subsequent subsections because of their individual differences within the low-voltage class. The "standard" low-voltage stimulator has a maximum output of 100 mA. The waveform produced is generally biphasic or polyphasic, and the unit often provides the clinician with a choice of the two waveforms or between different waveform shapes, such as square or sinusoidal. The frequency commonly ranges from 1 to 100 pulses per second; however, it is not uncommon to find a unit with a maximum frequency of 250 pulses per second. Most clinical models allow the user to set an on/off cycle.

If the unit produces a biphasic waveform, the phase duration is set in the usual way with the phase duration control. If the unit produces a polyphasic waveform, the phase duration is often set by selecting the "carrier" frequency for the polyphasic pulse. The clue to distinguishing whether the unit adjusts in this manner is to determine whether the unit has a frequency adjustment in the standard treatment frequency range of 1 to 100 pulses per second, as well as a frequency adjustment that ranges from 2000 to 10,000 Hz. The frequency adjustment from 2000 to 10,000 Hz selects the carrier frequency. For example, if the unit is set at a treatment frequency of 50 pulses per second and a carrier frequency of 2500 Hz, it behaves as 2500-Hz AC that is interrupted 50 times each second. In AC, the phase duration is determined by the frequency; therefore, if in this case there are 2500 cycles each second, and each cycle is made up of two phases, the number of phases delivered each second is 5000. Dividing 1 second by 5000 gives the length of each phase, which in this example is 0.0002 second. After converting seconds to microseconds one determines that the 2500-Hz carrier frequency produces a phase duration of 200 microseconds. Carrier frequencies greater than 2500 Hz lead to shorter phase durations, whereas those less than 2500 Hz result in longer phase durations.

Application. The most common clinical applications for "standard" low-voltage units are pain control and muscle strengthening or re-education. The flexibility of these units allows them to be set up in any of the pain control protocols. Most of the clinical research concerned with electrical stimulation and muscle strengthening has been performed using these units, in particular the polyphasic waveform generators. To date these units have not been shown to have an impact on edema[84] or accelerate wound healing. Because they are pulsatile units, they are not capable of performing iontophoresis or stimulating denervated muscle.

TRANSCUTANEOUS ELECTRICAL NERVE STIMULATION

TENS units are small, hand-held electrical simulators whose energy source is a disposable or rechargeable battery. Most TENS units are small enough to be worn clipped to the athlete's belt or clothing and produce either a monophasic rectangular or balanced, asymmetric, biphasic pulse (Fig. 5–24).[103, 104]

Application. Electrodes for TENS units are typically small, about 4 to 5 cm², and are commercially available in various shapes. They come in two basic forms, single-use and multiuse electrodes. The single-use electrodes typically have a layer of conductive polymer over a thin carbon or foil layer and are held in place by a nonconductive cloth or foam adhesive backing. These easy-to-apply electrodes are relatively inexpensive and can often be left on the skin for 3 to 5 days, depending on the manufacturer's suggested length of use. This style of electrode will typically stay in place even when the athlete sweats. The disadvantages of the single-use electrodes include skin reactions and irritation, and once removed, they will not stick again.

The multiuse electrodes have a self-adhesive conductive polymer layer and a variety of thin carbon, foil, or foam backings. The advantages to using these electrodes include ease of application, ability to remove and reuse them, and lower incidence of skin irritation. The two disadvantages of this type of electrode system are cost and inability to stick well when the athlete sweats.

In general, both of these electrodes provide a higher resistance to current flow when compared with the standard carbon electrode used with conductive gel.[92] However, the ease of application of the single- and multiuse electrodes described above far outweighs the problem of a higher resistance.

Opinions regarding effective or optimal placement of electrodes in TENS are divided. Most clinicians appear to agree that placing electrodes around the painful area, in the relevant dermatome, or along the spinal segment of the relevant sclerotome is efficacious. Placement over acupuncture or trigger points, along peripheral nerves, or on the contralateral dermatome is also advocated.[90]

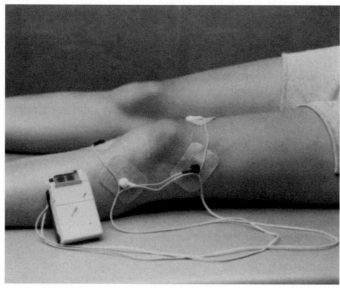

Figure 5–24. Transcutaneous electrical nerve stimulation is advocated for relief of almost all levels of pain.

Placement of electrodes over the contralateral dermatome is particularly useful in the treatment of conditions too painful to allow direct placement of an electrode, such as reflex sympathetic dystrophy or postherpetic neuralgia.[90]

Ideally, a TENS unit allows the clinician to modify the stimulation delivered to the patient by adjustment of the stimulation frequency, pulse duration, and intensity of the stimulating current. By adjusting these parameters, TENS units are commonly set according to the guidelines of the various modes of stimulation presented earlier.

Conventional or high-frequency TENS units use a short-duration pulse (20 to 60 microseconds) combined with a 50- to 100-Hz frequency of stimulation.[90] The current is adjusted to sensory level stimulation only, delivering a slight tingling or buzzing to the athlete's skin. This form of TENS is most commonly used for athletes with acute or postsurgical pain[90] or as an introduction to electroanalgesia for the apprehensive athlete.[113] The relief of pain lasts only as long as the stimulus is applied, and considerable accommodation to the stimulus is thought to occur. Therefore, frequent adjustments of the stimulus characteristics are necessary and can be performed by the athlete after instruction by the clinician. The use of current modulations may be helpful in reducing the accommodation. The conventional form of TENS can be used continuously, as is common in the treatment of postsurgical pain, or in a 30- to 60-minute session several times per day.[90]

The acupuncture-type TENS unit has a low frequency (1 to 4 Hz) and a long pulse duration (150 to 200 microseconds). The intensity is adjusted so that a strong muscular contraction is elicited.[90] This form of TENS takes longer to provide pain relief after initiation of treatment, and analgesia lasts for some time after stimulation is ended. It is believed that the acupuncture and noxious forms of TENS act to elicit the release of endogenous opiates. Usually, treatment sessions using this type of TENS units are provided daily, lasting for 20 to 30 minutes.

The noxious level or brief, intense TENS is characterized by an extremely long pulse duration that can last up to 1 second.[113] The frequency can be low (1 to 5 Hz) or in excess of 100 Hz.[113] Current amplitude is adjusted to the greatest intensity the athlete can tolerate. This form of TENS produces a long-lasting, profound, and generalized analgesia, believed to be mediated by the endogenous opiates, which are released following brief periods of extreme discomfort.

INTERFERENTIAL CURRENT

The term "interferential" refers to the manner in which the electrical current is generated. Two independent channels are needed to produce two alternating currents that are out of phase with each other. These two currents operate within the medium-frequency range, 1000 to 10,000 Hz. This takes advantage of the dramatically lower skin resistance in this frequency range. In a 100-cm^2 area of tissue, skin resistance to a current of 50 Hz is about 3000 ohms.[24] If the frequency is increased to 4000 Hz, this resistance decreases to approximately 40 ohms. The trade-off for this decrease in skin resistance is a tremendous increase in total current produced by this type of stimulator. In the example from the section on HVPS, the current was actually produced for 6 seconds and was distributed over the 20-minute treatment time. With an interferential current (IFC) unit set at the same frequency and phase duration for 20 minutes, the unit is basically producing a current for almost the entire 20 minutes. Therefore, although the skin resistance may be low, the high total current precludes the use of very small electrodes.

The physiologic response produced by IFC is not simply a response to two independent medium-frequency (1000 to 10,000 Hz) alternating currents. The two current frequencies are known as the carrier frequencies; that is, they "carry" the current into the tissues. Because the two currents are out of phase, they summate or diminish each other to an intensity greater or lesser than either current alone. The resultant current, which is not formed until the two carrier currents meet inside the tissues, is a waveform whose intensity is constantly changing. The number of times that the intensity rises to its maximal level and drops to its minimal level is the beat frequency. The physiologic response (production of an action potential) occurs at the peak intensity of each beat envelope. For example, channel 1 might be operating at a frequency of 4000 Hz and channel 2 operating at 4125 Hz. The beat frequency then is approximately the difference between the two out-of-phase circuits, or as in the example, 125 Hz. Physiologically, therefore, the nerves that are recruited in this example would be depolarizing approximately 125 times per second. In other words, two AC circuits with frequencies of 4000 and 4125 Hz, both frequencies being considerably higher than the number of times a nerve can depolarize per second, are converted to a treatment frequency of 125 pulses per second, which is within the range of the number of times a nerve can depolarize each second. It should be noted that the treatment frequency is within the normal frequency range used with other types of stimulators.

Some manufacturers allow the clinician to choose the carrier frequency. This, in essence, allows the clinician to choose the phase duration. The higher the carrier frequency, the shorter the phase duration, whereas the lower the carrier frequency, the longer the phase duration. The use of a carrier frequency of 4000 Hz is almost equivalent to the use of a 125-microsecond phase duration. A carrier frequency of 10,000 Hz translates to an approximate phase duration of 50 microseconds.

Application. Because the development of the beat frequency requires two channels, a minimum of four electrodes, one for each lead of each channel, is required. A fairly precise knowledge of target tissue location is essential, because the final stimulating current is a synthesis of the two currents delivered from the four electrodes and is formed within the tissues. Typically, the two circuits are arranged to intersect each other in a diagonal pattern, but they can be placed in any manner that allows the two circuits to interfere with each other. For instance, when treating an athlete with low back and leg pain, the electrodes can be placed in a curvilinear formation beginning at the spine and running down the leg, as long as the electrodes from the two circuits are alternated.

The commonly referred to cloverleaf interference pattern depicted in Figure 5–25 occurs only in a homogeneous medium. This type of homogeneous field in no way represents the heterogeneous human body with its muscle-fascia interfaces and skeletal tissues. Because of the heterogeneous nature of the human body, the exact location of the interference cannot be predicted. Therefore, just placing the electrodes in an intersecting diagonal pattern with the intersection directly over the injured tissue does not ensure that the interference pattern will be developed at that site. Fortunately, IFC units typically allow for the adjustment of the balance between the two circuit intensities. By adjusting the balance the clinician can move the interference pattern into the desired area. This is done by adjusting the balance and by receiving verbal feedback about where the stimulation is being perceived.

If the area being treated is large and diffuse, it is probably best to use the manufacturer's automatic scanning mode. In this mode the intensities of the two circuits are automatically modulated by adjusting the balance between them. The resultant interferential current moves closer to the stronger of the two circuits; the balance is then reversed, and the IFC sweeps across an area of tissue to align itself more closely with the more intense circuit (Fig. 5–26). This modulation allows the interference pattern to move throughout the region of the electrodes. The athlete will describe a sensation of the current "rolling" from one electrode to the next.

IFC can be delivered to the skin by using various electrodes or a combination of electrodes. The usual carbon electrodes can be used with a damp sponge. In

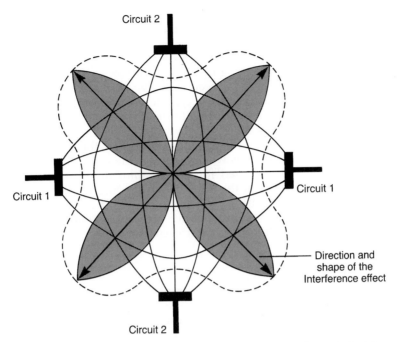

Figure 5–25. Current pathways and electrode placement for a static interferential field in a homogeneous medium. (From DeDomenico, G. [1988]: Interferential Stimulation: A Monograph. Chattanooga, TN, Chattanooga Corporation, p. 17.)

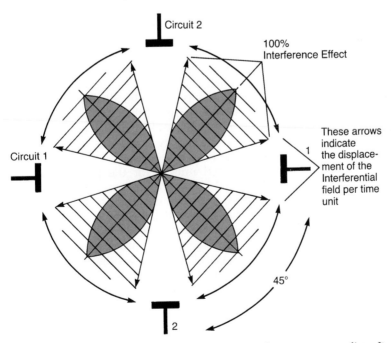

Figure 5–26. Movement of interference pattern in a homogeneous medium. It must be stressed that in the heterogeneous human tissue the position of the interference pattern is not as predictable. (From DeDomenico, G. [1988]: Interferential Stimulation: A Monograph. Chattanooga, TN, Chattanooga Corporation, p. 19.)

the past, IFC was commonly delivered using vacuum electrodes containing a damp sponge, which applied suction to the skin. The suction units added significant cost to the unit and could also be quite noisy. The use of suction electrodes has significantly decreased because of the advent of good multiuse self-adhesive electrodes. When using the suction system, it is recommended that the suction in the electrodes not exceed 0.25 atmosphere.[24] If the area being treated has significant edema, suction electrodes should not be used, as they may have a tendency to pull more fluid into the area.

IFC generators are primarily used for pain control, even though their effectiveness remains to be demonstrated.[121] Proponents suggest that they can be used for swelling and wound healing as well, but any evidence for these two uses is, at best, anecdotal. IFC can be used for motor stimulation, but two problems related to the common design of the units hamper its use for this purpose. The first problem is that many units do not have an on/off cycle adjustment; the second is that most units produce a maximum current of 40 mA, which may not be adequate to produce contractions of sufficient intensity for strengthening.

DIRECT CURRENT

DC electrical stimulation involves the uninterrupted, unidirectional flow of electrons. The flow of current is usually of long duration, lasting from about 1 second to the entire treatment time, depending on the application.[103] With the development and improved comfort of electrical stimulators using pulsed current characteristics, DC stimulators are used primarily to stimulate denervated muscle and in iontophoresis.

Stimulation of Denervated Muscle

Because of the extremely long duration of stimulus, application current intensities are relatively low, about 0.5 to 1.0 mA/cm^2.[90] Even with these low levels of current flow, considerable charge accumulates in the skin and superficial tissues directly under the electrodes. The pH of the skin under the cathode (the negative electrode) gradually becomes more alkaline as positive ions are attracted to it, whereas the skin under the anode (the positive electrode) undergoes the opposite reaction. These chemical changes elicit a reflex vasodilation, presumably for the purpose of maintaining homeostatic pH. Because the alkaline reaction occurring under the cathode is considerably more harmful than the acidic reaction under the anode, it is recommended that the electrode that serves as the cathode be increased in size.[90] This reduces current density under the cathode, thus diluting the ensuing chemical changes in the tissues.

Electrical stimulation of denervated muscle for the purpose of preventing disuse atrophy has been a traditional practice. As is true for the use of many of the electrical modalities, however, research on the use of this technique is contradictory. What is clear is that electrical stimulation cannot accelerate or enhance the reinnervation process, nor can its use ensure that reinnervation will occur. At best, it may slow down the degenerative process the muscle undergoes when denervated, but it cannot prevent it from occurring. It is possible to make a case for its use with axonotmesis lesions, but there is little evidence to substantiate its use with neuropraxic or neurotmesis lesions.

Iontophoresis

Iontophoresis is the other primary clinical use of direct current. In iontophoresis, charged molecules of medication are driven into the tissues by being placed under an electrode of the same polarity. When a direct current is applied, these molecules move away from the electrode into the skin and toward the target tissues. Neither pulsed current nor AC can be used because uniform forward movement of the molecules does not occur. Both animal and human studies on the efficacy of iontophoresis are inconclusive, with a slight edge to those studies substantiating its effectiveness.[46] Clinically, the advantages to using iontophoresis instead of more traditional drug delivery systems are that the clinician can introduce various medications into specific areas of the body, significantly reducing the systemic side effects of drugs delivered orally, and that damage to tissue from the introduction of a needle and a bolus of medication through or into delicate structures is avoided. Disadvantages include the risk of burns, the possibility of a less than therapeutic concentration of medication reaching the target tissue, the inability to use this method to treat deep structures, and finally, the lack of guidelines on frequency and dosage of medication for safe use.

Application. The amount of medication introduced into the tissues is determined by various factors: the intensity and duration of the current, skin resistance to ion movement, pH of the skin, ionization potential of the medication or its solvent, and electrode size (Fig. 5–27).[46]

Because patient tolerance to DC varies, instead of describing treatment protocols in terms of intensity and duration, many protocols are described in terms of current dosage. Current dosage is defined by multiplying the current intensity (in milliamperes) by the total treatment time (in minutes). For example, if the recommended current dosage of a medication is 80 mA · minute, it can be achieved with an intensity of 4 mA applied for a 20-minute duration or with any other combination that when multiplied is equal to 80 mA/minute. For safety reasons, the maximum current intensity allowed by commercial units is commonly 4 to 5 mA.

Electrodes can be made by the clinician by interposing a medication-soaked gauze pad between the athlete's skin and a conducting electrode attached to a DC generator. Commercially prepared electrodes are available and, in most instances, are more convenient to use. Commercial electrodes are constructed with a gel matrix or fiber pad that is then filled with the desired medication.[20]

It is highly recommended that iontophoresis be performed on DC stimulators designed specifically for this purpose. Stimulators designed for iontophoresis

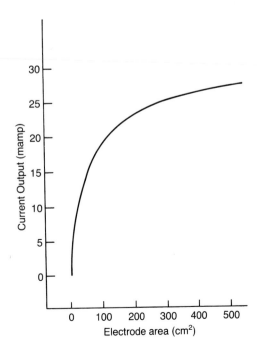

Figure 5–27. Recommended currents for electrodes of various sizes. (From Glick, E., and Snyder-Mackler, L. [1989]: *In:* Snyder-Mackler, L., and Robinson, A.J. [eds.]: Clinical Electrophysiology. Baltimore, Williams & Wilkins, p. 257.)

have several safety features to reduce the risk of burns, features not commonly found on regular DC stimulators. The primary safety feature is that the units automatically shut off if tissue impedance becomes too high or if the contact area becomes disconnected.[46] Another feature is simply the limitation of maximum current to 4 or 5 mA.

Depending on the drug used, iontophoresis is indicated for a wide variety of conditions, including bursitis, tendinitis, adhesive capsulitis, open wounds, scar tissue, calcium deposits, and hyperhidrosis.[46] Table 5–8 was developed by Kahn[59] and lists medications and their uses. Iontophoresis is contraindicated for patients with anesthetic skin or a known drug allergy. Initial sessions should be conducted with caution because allergic reactions are always possible and can be serious medical emergencies.

MICROAMPERAGE PULSATILE STIMULATION

Microamperage pulsatile stimulators, referred to clinically as MENS (microcurrent electrical neuromuscular stimulators), are the most recent class of stimulators to become commercially available. This class of stimulators produces pulsed current with maximum amplitudes of 1000 μA. This maximum amplitude is equivalent to 1 mA. Most units produce a monophasic waveform and can be set to automatically reverse the polarity of the electrodes periodically. The frequency choices on clinical units commonly range from 0.1 Hz to 1000 Hz.

One rationale for using microamperage intensities stems from the finding of Cheng and associates[19] that suggests that intensities greater than 1000 μA (macroamp) inhibit cellular respiration. This was an in vitro study, and the results have yet to be demonstrated in vivo. In addition, the stimulator used in this study was a microamperage DC unit and not the pulsatile unit that is sold commercially as MENS.

Application. Proponents of this form of stimulation suggest that it can be used for pain control, wound healing, and edema control.[98] To date there are no studies to support the clinical effectiveness of MENS for pain control.[114] If indeed this form of stimulation does have an impact on pain, it does not do so under the previously described mechanisms, because the intensity is typically set at a subsensory level, and this is not enough to produce action potentials. With regard to efficacy for edema control, these claims have not been substantiated with clinical research studies.

Research results for MENS as a modality to facilitate wound healing have been mixed. Neither Byl and associates[17] nor Leffman et al[65] found any treatment effect using MENS for surgically induced wounds in animal models. Results from a multicenter study using a blinded experimental protocol suggest that MENS increased the rate of recovery for patients with chronic stage II and stage III ulcers.[131]

Few guidelines as to the appropriate frequency, phase duration, or treatment time exist. Picker has suggested some guidelines for these parameters, but they are not based on experimental findings.[98] It is suggested that the intensity be maintained at a subsensory level.[98] Units commonly offer a variety of electrode choices for attended treatment options, as well as the standard electrodes for unattended treatment.

OTHER MODALITIES

Biofeedback

Biofeedback units are designed to monitor a physiologic process, objectively measure that process, and convert the measurement of the process into meaning-

Table 5–8. Nonsteroidal Ions and Radicals

ION OR RADICAL (CHARGE)	FEATURES*
Magnesium (+)	From magnesium sulfate (Epsom salts), 2% aqueous solution; excellent muscle relaxant, good vasodilator, mild analgesic
Mecholyl (+)	Familiar derivative of acetylcholine, 0.25% ointment; powerful vasodilator, good muscle relaxant and analgesic; used with discogenic low back radiculopathies and sympathetic reflex dystrophy
Iodine (−)	From Iodex ointment, 4.7%; bactericidal, fair vasodilator, excellent sclerolytic agent; used successfully with adhesive capsulitis ("frozen shoulder"), scars
Salicylate (−)	From Iodex with methyl salicylate, 4.8% ointment (if desired without the iodine, can be obtained from Myoflex ointment—trolamine salicylate, 10%—or from a 2% aqueous solution of sodium salicylate powder); a general decongestant, sclerolytic, and anti-inflammatory agent; used successfully with frozen shoulders, scar tissue, warts, and other adhesive or edematous conditions
Calcium (+)	From calcium chloride, 2% aqueous solution; believed to stabilize the irritability threshold in either direction, as dictated by the physiologic needs of the tissues; effective with spasmodic conditions, tics, "snapping joints"
Chlorine (−)	From sodium chloride, 2% aqueous solution; good sclerolytic agent; useful with scar tissue, keloids, burns
Zinc (+)	From zinc oxide ointment, 20%; trace element necessary for healing; especially effective with open lesions and ulcerations
Copper (+)	Form 2% aqueous solution of copper sulfate crystals; fungicide, astringent, useful with intranasal conditions (e.g., allergic rhinitis—hay fever), sinusitis, and dermatophytosis (athlete's foot)
Lidocaine (+)	From Xylocaine, 5% ointment; anesthetic and analgesic, especially with acute inflammatory conditions (e.g., bursitis, tendinitis, tic douloureux, and temporomandibular joint pain
Lithium (−)	From lithium chloride or carbonate, 2% aqueous solution; effective as an exchange ion with gouty tophi and hyperuricemia†
Acetate (−)	From acetic acid, 2% aqueous solution; dramatically effective as a sclerolytic exchange ion with calcific deposits‡
Hyaluronidase (+)	From Wydase crystals in aqueous solution, as directed; for localized edema
Tap water (+/−)	Usually administered with alternating polarity, sometimes with glycopyrronium bromide in hyperhidrosis
Ringer's solution (+/−)	With alternating polarity; used for open decubitus lesions
Citrate (+)	From potassium citrate, 2% aqueous solution; reported effective in rheumatoid arthritis
Priscoline (+)	From benzazoline hydrochloride, 2% aqueous solution; reported effective with indolent ulcers
Antibiotics Gentamycin sulfate (+)	8 mg/ml; for suppurative ear chondritis

From Kahn, J. (1987): Non-steroid iontophoresis. Clin. Management, 7:15. Reprinted from CLINICAL MANAGEMENT with the permission of the American Physical Therapy Association.

*All solutions are 2%; ointments are also low-percentage compounds. The literature and clinical reports agree that the lower the percentage, the more effective the ionic exchange and transfer. Whether this is purely a physical chemistry phenomenon or an example of the Arndt-Schultz law, which states that "the smaller the stimulant, the greater the physiological response," remains to be proven.

†The lithium ion replaces the weaker sodium ion in the insoluble sodium urate tophus, converting it to soluble lithium urate.

‡The acetate radical replaces the carbonate radical in the insoluble calcium carbonate calcific deposit, converting it to soluble calcium acetate.

ful information.[97] Biofeedback units used in rehabilitation typically do not measure physiologic events directly; rather, they record some aspect that is highly correlated with the physiologic event.[97] There are several types of biofeedback units. Electromyographic (EMG) units are most commonly used in the rehabilitation process because they measure the amount of electrical activity in skeletal muscle through the use of either implanted or surface-mounted electrodes (Fig.

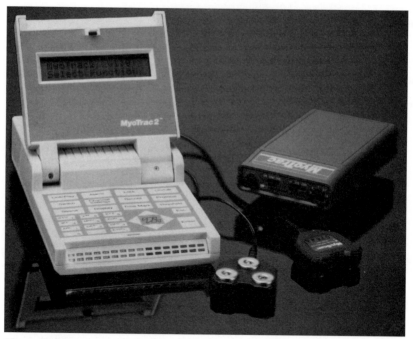

Figure 5–28. MyoTrac2 dual-channel, portable electromyographic biofeedback unit and a "clip-on" model are shown. (Photo courtesy of Thought Technology, Montreal, Quebec, Canada.)

5–28). EMG biofeedback has gained popularity in the past few years and is being used more often to help athletes develop greater voluntary control during neuromuscular relaxation or muscle re-education after injury.

Although few studies have evaluated the clinical efficacy of EMG biofeedback, those on the use of EMG biofeedback to facilitate muscle re-education demonstrate positive effects.[9, 31, 32, 51, 77] A greater peak torque and EMG output for the quadriceps muscle were found in healthy subjects who used biofeedback-facilitated quadriceps exercises versus those who used exercise alone.[51, 77] Additionally, Draper[31] reported increased isometric peak torque at 12 weeks after anterior cruciate ligament surgery in those subjects in whom EMG biofeedback was used to monitor performance on quad sets and straight leg raises versus a control group. Electrical stimulation has for a long time been the modality of choice for muscle re-education. Proponents of EMG biofeedback believe that biofeedback-assisted exercise requires the person to formulate a motor strategy, initiate the muscle contraction, and voluntarily maintain the contraction during the hold time.[32] By contrast, electrical stimulation provides an artificial stimulus for contraction, and it will maintain the contraction independent of patient effort.[32]

Both electrical stimulation and EMG biofeedback have been shown to be more effective than voluntary isometric exercise alone in the recovery of the quadriceps muscle force after anterior cruciate ligament reconstruction.[27, 31, 32, 38, 109] Only one study, by Draper and Ballard,[32] has compared EMG biofeedback with electrical muscle stimulation. Their results indicate that there was a greater recovery of isometric peak torque after anterior cruciate ligament reconstruction at 6 weeks with EMG biofeedback than with electrical stimulation. However, the clinical efficacy of this study is in question because of the experimental design, electrical stimulator type, and current intensity. Thus, at this time more clinical trials need to be performed to determine whether electrical stimulation or EMG biofeedback is better than exercise alone.

Application. The athlete receives visual or auditory feedback from the EMG unit as it monitors the physiologic state of the muscle or muscles over which the electrodes are placed. Visual feedback may be in the form of a numeric scale, and it can quantify the muscle activity. However, there is no universally accepted standardized measurement scale, and thus different brands of biofeedback units cannot be compared with each other. Auditory feedback can occur by the unit's converting the signals it is monitoring into sound. The pitch of the sound will increase or decrease depending on the amount of neuromuscular activity.

Clinically, surface electrodes are generally used for EMG biofeedback versus indwelling electrodes. Because indwelling electrodes must be inserted percutaneously, they are not practical clinically. Surface electrodes may be disposable or nondisposable and come in various types and sizes. In order to ensure an adequate connection for the surface electrode, the skin should be cleaned with an alcohol-prep pad and excess hair should be removed. The following guidelines should be used for placing the electrodes[99]:

- Electrodes should be placed as close to the muscle being monitored as possible.
- Electrodes should be secured to the body part in the position in which it will be monitored so that movement of the skin will not alter the positioning of the electrodes over a particular muscle.
- Electrodes should be applied parallel to the direction of the muscle fibers to ensure that a better sample of muscle activity is monitored while extraneous electrical activity is reduced (Fig. 5–29A).

EMG electrodes consist of two active electrodes that should be placed in proximity to one another and a reference electrode that may be placed anywhere on the body. Typically, in biofeedback, the reference electrode is placed between the two active electrodes. Most EMG biofeedback units today use commercially available electrodes that have an electrode that resembles the illustration in Figure 5–29B.

The sensitivity setting is used to set the threshold necessary to acquire feedback. High sensitivity levels should be used for relaxation training, and low sensitivity levels are used for muscle re-education. When using EMG biofeedback for muscle re-education, the sensitivity may be set at a high level, with gradual reduction to lower levels as the athlete learns to voluntarily recruit the particular muscle or muscles. This will require the athlete to produce a stronger muscle contraction to receive feedback from the unit.

When using EMG biofeedback to facilitate neuromuscular re-education, the following guidelines should be used when applying the unit[99, 120]:

- The body part should be as relaxed as possible.
- The body part should be placed in the desired position for the exercise.
- The sensitivity range should be set to the lowest value that elicits feedback when the athlete performs a maximal isometric muscle contraction. The sensitivity level may need to be adjusted during the treatment as the athlete is able to perform a more powerful muscle contraction.
- The athlete should be instructed to perform a maximum isometric contraction of the target muscle,

keeping the visual or audio feedback at maximum for 6 to 10 seconds, and then to relax completely.

- Treatments should be given daily if used for early muscle re-education and should consist of 10 to 15 contractions or 5 to 10 minutes, depending upon muscle fatigue. The authors also suggest that the treatment be incorporated in the entire exercise program to facilitate proper muscle recruitment with functional activities.

If the athlete is unable to contract the muscle, the clinician may (1) have the athlete contract the muscle on the opposite extremity, then attempt to contract the involved muscle; (2) have the athlete look at the involved muscle; (3) stroke or tap the target muscle; or (4) place the unit on the contralateral limb, have the athlete practice the muscle contraction on this limb, and then place the unit back on the involved limb and have the athlete try the muscle contraction again.[99, 120] Another alternative is to use electrical stimulation to initially elicit a muscle contraction if none is present; once a visible contraction is established, biofeedback can be used for proper muscle recruitment.

Indications and Contraindications. EMG biofeedback is indicated for neuromuscular re-education, muscle relaxation, and pain reduction. With this modality, pain reduction is a by-product of muscle re-education and relaxation. In

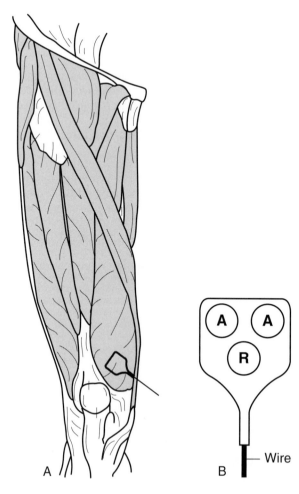

Figure 5–29. *A,* Example of electromyographic biofeedback electrode placement for the vastus medialis. *B,* Example of a typical electromyographic biofeedback electrode. A, active; R, reference.

general, EMG biofeedback is contraindicated for conditions in which muscular contractions would result in further damage to the tissues.[120]

Compression

The formation of edema after an injury is a common problem. Typically, edema forms from a blockage or overflow of the lymphatic drainage system or by frank bleeding within the tissues. Edema collects primarily in joints of soft tissues.[99] Frank bleeding, the result of ruptured capillaries, is associated with a hematoma, whose appearance is usually delayed by several hours to days after the original trauma. Edema formation not occurring because of actual bleeding is usually caused by leakage of plasma proteins out of the capillaries into the interstitial spaces. This can happen because of actual trauma to the capillaries themselves, allowing proteins to escape, or as a response to histamine or kinin action in the inflammatory process.[44]

As the serous or lymphatic edema accumulates in tissues, the normal contour of the body part is obliterated. This condition, known as pitting edema, is graded by the length of time required for a cavity, made by pressing a finger or thumb into the tissue, to fill. Although edema is a common response to injury, this makes it no less harmful to the athlete. Increased internal pressure caused by excess fluid can slow or even stop nutrient exchange, thus delaying the healing process. The pooling of fluid because of stasis results in a toxic environment, which promotes cell death, with consequent tissue necrosis. Additionally, the excess fluid can actually stretch or tear small structures in the edematous area, initiating the inflammatory response and worsening the situation.

Several tools are available to limit edema and thus to minimize the damage it can cause. The optimal technique for dealing with edema is to prevent its formation. Thus, after an injury in which edema is a likely consequence, many clinicians actively forestall edema formation, for example, by elevating the extremity and allowing gravity to assist lymphatic drainage. The application of a compression bandage, which increases external hydrostatic pressure and prevents fluid from moving into the interstitial spaces, is an almost universal practice and typically accompanies elevation of the limb. The bandage can be applied in a spiral wrap or in a figure-eight fashion. When these two methods were compared, the figure-eight method was found to be more effective than the spiral wrap technique.[130]

Once edema has formed it can be reduced or controlled in several different ways. These methods act to increase external hydrostatic pressure temporarily by compressing the limb, which prevents more fluid from leaking out of the capillaries and pushes fluid out of the extracellular space into the lymphatic-venous drainage system. If the edema is not too severe or is located in the hand, wrist, foot, or ankle, centripetal massage followed by application of a compression bandage can be sufficient to reduce edema. The hands of the operator are held in a pétrissage position and stroked repetitively in a centripetal direction along the limb. The goal is to stroke or milk the fluid into a more proximal location, into a muscle mass capable of pumping the fluid back into the lymphatics. Alternating contractions of major muscle groups (e.g., a muscle pump) in the area of the edema is another method that moves the excess fluid along and out of the tissues.

If the edema is widespread or severe, the clinician can apply intermittent compression using a mechanical pump and sleeve that covers the entire length of the upper or lower extremity (Fig. 5–30). Pressure is applied intermittently to force fluid into the lymph vessels, with periods of relaxation to allow fluid movement within the system. There is no consensus concerning the length or ratio of on-times to off-times between the compression and relaxation periods. Some have recommended that the time of compression should exceed the

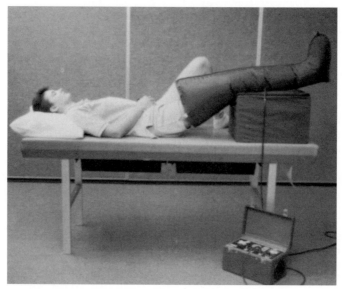

Figure 5–30. Intermittent compression, in which pressure is applied intermittently, alternating with periods of relaxation, is indicated for edema reduction.

time of relaxation by a factor of 2, 3, or even 4, whereas others have reversed this.[99, 108] The length of treatment varies and is determined by the athlete's tolerance of the procedure. In treating athletic injuries, 10- to 30-minute sessions are commonly used and seem to be effective for the types of conditions treated.[99]

Application. Prior to applying intermittent compression, both the involved and the uninvolved limbs should be measured either circumferentially or volumetrically to determine the amount of edema present. If circumferential measurements are taken, the location of the measurement should be the same at each session and should include the joint (if one is affected). Usually the length of the involved limb is divided into thirds, with measurements taken at these points.[108] Volumetric measurements are more precise and are determined by the amount of water displaced by the limb; however, they are also more time-consuming to perform and require special equipment.

For reasons of hygiene, a tubular stockinette covering is placed over the skin before the compression sleeve is placed on the extremity. The athlete's limb is placed in an elevated position so that the effects of gravity can be added to those of the compression pump. The time of treatment is set according to severity and expected tolerance. In the initial treatment session, it is recommended that the pressure be set at 80 mm Hg.[108] Successive settings can be either at this generic setting or 20 mm Hg below the athlete's systolic pressure.

At the end of a treatment session the involved extremity should be remeasured to determine the amount of edema removed from the limb, with care taken to use the same location if circumferential measurements are being taken. Optimally, the same person should perform the measurements. A compression bandage should be applied to the limb before upright or limb-dependent activities are resumed.

Portable units have been developed that use chemical coolants or ice water. The coolant or ice water circulates through a hand or foot sleeve, providing a cold modality in combination with compression. Although these units are convenient and provide an excellent tool for field treatment of injured athletes, they are not an adequate substitute for mechanical compression units because they do not provide as much pressure.

Indications and Contraindications. Mechanical compression is usually confined to the treatment of edema. It is contraindicated in patients with congestive heart failure, pulmonary edema, thrombophlebitis, and active inflammatory or infectious processes.[108]

Friction Massage

Friction massage is a specialized form of massage that uses subcutaneous friction of tissues for various purposes. It was popularized in the late 1970s by Dr. James Cyriax and is also known as deep transverse massage or cross-fiber massage. It is not a method of massage designed to promote relaxation, and it can be somewhat painful for the athlete, even if properly applied.

PHYSIOLOGIC EFFECTS

Friction massage has a number of effects on human tissues. Perhaps its most significant effect is on collagen fiber orientation. It is thought that friction massage causes healing collagen fibers to be laid down parallel to each other. This increases the strength of the involved tendon or ligament, allowing it to withstand greater levels of longitudinal stress. Generally, after an injury, these tissues are "rested" while adequate healing occurs. After this period the athlete is allowed to gradually resume a normal activity level. Without any stimulus to increase cross-sectional area, the ligament or tendon is usually weak when activities are resumed or the rehabilitation period is prolonged. Too much early stress to the tissue can result in reinjury. Use of friction massage during the interim healing period and rehabilitation process is believed to stimulate the ligament or tendon to orient its fibers longitudinally without actually stressing the tissue.[54] Friction massage also improves the extensibility of tissues.

Friction massage is believed to be useful in destroying adhesions. Adhesions, both those that bind the target tissue to structures around it and those between the fibers of the target tissue itself, are broken up and discouraged from re-forming.[54] This is the rationale for applying friction massage to surface scar tissue—to break down skin and subcutaneous tissue adhesions that would prevent full range of motion.

Friction massage produces a significant hyperemia in the target tissues.[54] This is especially important in the treatment of structures experiencing tissue breakdown caused by overuse or poor vascular perfusion. The combination of proper collagen fiber orientation and strengthening with improved circulation may be sufficient to allow an athlete to maintain a high level of activity that would have been impossible without treatment.

Application. The athlete is positioned comfortably, with the limb supported. If the purpose of the massage is to break up adhesions between the target tissue and adjacent structures, the target tissue is placed on slight stretch. To break up adhesions between a surface scar and subcutaneous tissues, a light to moderate pressure (sufficient to stretch the scar without damaging or blistering the skin) is applied along the length of the scar. The scar is stretched along its length with one finger or thumb, with tension being maintained until the second finger or thumb can be drawn up the scar. This process is repeated for several minutes. Greater pressure can be applied as some of the tenderness diminishes. Athletes should be instructed in the performance of this procedure at home on a daily to twice-daily basis. Pressure is never applied across or perpendicular to the scar because this can widen it, a cosmetically undesirable outcome.

If the purpose is to treat an underlying structure, the athlete is again positioned comfortably, this time with the target tissue slack (Fig. 5–31). The therapist or trainer is positioned in such a way that his or her fingers are perpendicular to the target structure and in a comfortable position. It is recommended that the therapist be seated.[54] Only one or two fingertips are used, and the others

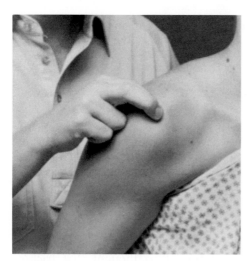

Figure 5–31. Deep friction massage to the supraspinatus tendon.

maintain positioning of the athlete. No oil or lotion is applied to the skin. The clinician applies enough pressure to the skin so that it moves with the fingers. The clinician rubs across the structure slowly in a controlled fashion. Only light pressure is applied initially, and the pressure is deepened as treatment progresses. Excursion of the movement should be small, no massage should be applied to any of the surrounding tissues, and there should be no tension on the skin, which might cause a blister.

The athlete generally reports some tenderness in the first 1 to 2 minutes of treatment, which should disappear. Pressure of the massage can then be increased. Greater pressure should not be applied, however, if tenderness has not diminished significantly or disappeared altogether. This may indicate that the initial pressure was too great. If the tenderness has not disappeared after 4 minutes or has actually increased, treatment should be discontinued.[54]

The length of treatment is 5 to 6 minutes for the initial session and is gradually increased in 3-minute increments to 12 to 15 minutes per session.[54] Treatment sessions are usually scheduled two to three times weekly, with most problems resolving within 2 to 3 weeks.

The stress that this technique may place on the joints of the therapist's or trainer's treatment fingers may be a problem. This can be reduced by stabilizing the affected joint with the opposite hand.[54]

Indications and Contraindications. Friction massage is ideal for overuse conditions of tissues that are poorly perfused or that have diminished energy-attenuating properties. Thus, conditions such as rotator cuff tendinitis, tennis and golfer's elbows, DeQuervain's tendinitis, plantar fasciitis, and mild or chronic sprains of the wrist, ankle, and surface ligaments of the knee are ideal for treatment with friction massage. Additionally, any surface scar that might prevent full range of motion can also benefit from treatment by friction massage. This technique is contraindicated in individuals with anesthetic skin who cannot report tenderness accurately and in acute inflammatory or infectious conditions.

A wide variety of tools are available to the therapist or trainer treating an injured athlete. Most of these are effective, if applied appropriately, and can be even more useful if combined with other modalities that reinforce their actions. For example, an athlete with a sprained ankle is expected to develop pain, edema, possible joint instability, and loss of function. These symptoms can be treated with ice packs and an assistive ambulatory device but would probably respond better if the ice treatment is combined with elevation, compression bandaging, and possibly electrical stimulation and if the joint is protected from hypermobility by a removable brace. Home treatment might include ice packs and the use of a TENS unit at night.

Although it seems reasonable to use these modalities in combination with other therapeutic techniques, the problem of overtreatment can develop from this strategy. The experienced clinician must determine, in each individual case, where the proper use of techniques and modalities ends and overtreatment begins. A worse problem is the unfortunate practice of treating the athlete with a combination of modalities that may actually counteract each other. This so-called shotgun strategy, used when the clinician does not know where to start treatment, at best provides no benefits to the athlete or clinician and may even retard healing.

The judicious, timely, and thoughtful use of various modalities requires time and energy on the part of the clinician, two factors frequently in short supply in busy training rooms and clinics. However, using a logical strategy in developing each athlete's treatment program, with frequent reappraisal, cannot fail to reward the clinician willing to make this effort.

References

1. Abramson, D.I., Bell, Y., and Tuck, S. (1961): Changes in blood flow, oxygen uptake and tissue temperatures produced by therapeutic physical agents. Am. J. Phys. Med., 40:5–13.
2. Abramson, D.I., Burnett, C., Bell, G., et al. (1960): Changes in blood flow, oxygen uptake, and tissue temperature produced by therapeutic physical agents. Am. J. Phys. Med., 39:51–62.
3. Alon, G. (1984): High Voltage Stimulation: A Monograph. Chattanooga, TN, Chattanooga Corporation.
4. Alon, G. (1987): Principles of electrical stimulation. In: Nelson, R.M., and Currier, D.P. (eds.): Clinical Electrotherapy. Norwalk, Appleton & Lange, pp. 29–80.
5. Baker, R.J., and Bell, G.W. (1991): The effect of therapeutic modalities on blood flow in the human calf. J. Orthop. Sports Phys. Ther., 13:23–27.
6. Balmaseda, M.T., Fatehi, M.T., Koozekanani, S.H., and Lee, A.L. (1986): Ultrasound therapy: A comparative study of different coupling media. Arch. Phys. Med. Rehabil., 67:147–150.
7. Balogun, J.A., Onilari, O.O., Akeju, O.A., and Marzouk, D.K. (1993): High voltage electrical stimulation in the augmentation of muscle strength: Effects of pulse frequency. Arch. Phys. Med. Rehabil., 74:910–916.
8. Bare, A.C., McAnaw, M.B., Pritchard, A.E., et al. (1996): Phonophoretic delivery of 10% hydrocortisone through the epidermis of humans as determined by serum cortisol concentrations. Phys. Ther., 76:738–747.
9. Beall, M.S., Diefenbach, G., and Allen, A. (1987): Electromyographic biofeedback in the treatment of voluntary posterior instability of the shoulder. Am. J. Sports Med., 15:175–178.
10. Benson, H.A., McElany, J.C., and Harland, R. (1989): Use of ultrasound to enhance percutaneous absorption of benzydamine. Phys. Ther., 69:113–118.
11. Bickford, R.H., and Duff, R.S. (1953): Influence of ultrasonic irradiation on temperature and blood flow in human skeletal muscle. Circ. Res., 1:534–538.
12. Bierman, W.S., and Friedlander, M. (1940): The penetrative effect of cold. Arch. Phys. Ther., 21:585–592.
13. Binder-Macleod, S.A., and McDermond, L.R. (1992): Changes in the force-frequency relationship of the human quadriceps femoris muscle following electrically and voluntarily induced fatigue. Phys. Ther., 72:95–104.
14. Brooks, M.E., Smith, E.M., and Currier, D.P. (1990): Effect of longitudinal versus transverse electrode placement on torque production by the quadriceps femoris muscle during neuromuscular electrical stimulation. J. Orthop. Sports Phys. Ther., 11:530–534.
15. Brown, S.A. (1987): Transdermal delivery of drugs. 1. Relationship between drug agents and carriers in skin preparation. Dermatol. Rep., 6:1–8.
16. Byl, N.N., McKenzie, A., Halliday, B., et al. (1993): The effects of phonophoresis with corticosteroids: A controlled pilot study. J. Orthop. Sports Phys. Ther., 18:590–600.
17. Byl, N.N., McKenzie, A.L., West, J.M., et al. (1994): pulsed microamperage stimulation: A controlled study of healing of surgically induced wounds in Yucatan pigs. Phys. Ther., 74:201–215.
18. Cameron, M.H., and Monroe, L.G. (1992): Relative transmission of ultrasound by media customarily used for phonophoresis. Phys. Ther., 72:142–148.
19. Cheng, N., Van Hoof, H., Bockx, E., et al. (1982): The effects of electrical currents on ATP generation, protein synthesis, and membrane transport in rat skin. Clin. Orthop., 171:264–272.
20. Ciccone, C.D. (1995): Iontophoresis. In: Robinson, A.J., and Snyder-Mackler, L. (eds.): Clinical Electrophysiology: Electrotherapy and Electrophysiological Testing. Baltimore, Williams & Wilkins, pp. 335–358.
21. Cline, P.D. (1963): Radiographic follow-up of ultrasound therapy in calcific bursitis. Phys. Ther., 43:16–17.

22. Cross, K.M., Wilson, R.W., and Perrin, D.H. (1996): Functional performance following an ice immersion to the lower extremity. Athl. Train., 31:113–116.
23. Davick, J.P., Martin, A.K., and Albright, J.P. (1988): Distribution and deposition of tritiated cortisol using phonophoresis. Phys. Ther., 68:1672–1675.
24. DeDomenico, G. (1988): Interferential Stimulation: A Monograph. Chattanooga, TN, Chattanooga Corporation.
25. Delitto, A., and Rose, S.J. (1986): Comparative comfort of three waveforms used in electrically eliciting quadriceps femoris contractions. Phys. Ther., 66:1704–1707.
26. Delitto, A., and Snyder-Mackler, L. (1990): Two theories of muscle strength augmentation using percutaneous electrical stimulation. Phys. Ther., 70:158–164.
27. Delitto, A., Rose, S.J., McKowen, J.M., et al.. (1988): Electrical stimulation versus voluntary exercise in strengthening thigh musculature after anterior cruciate ligament surgery. Phys. Ther., 68:660–663.
28. Delitto, A., Strube, M.J., Shulman, A.D., and Minor, S.D. (1992): A study of discomfort with electrical stimulation. Phys. Ther., 72:410–421.
29. Dowling, J.C. (1987): Shortwave diathermy. Sports Med. Update, 3:7–8.
30. Downing, D.S., and Weinstein, A. (1986): Ultrasound therapy for subacromial bursitis. Phys. Ther., 66:194–199.
31. Draper, V. (1990): Electromyographic biofeedback and recovery of quadriceps femoris muscle function following anterior cruciate ligament reconstruction. Phys. Ther., 70:11–17.
32. Draper, V., and Ballard, L. (1991): Electrical stimulation versus electromyographic biofeedback in the recovery of quadriceps femoris muscle function following anterior cruciate ligament surgery. Phys. Ther., 71:455–461.
33. Draper, D.O., and Ricard, M.D. (1995): Rate of temperature decay in human muscle following 3 MHz ultrasound: The stretching window revealed. Athl. Train., 30:304–307.
34. Draper, D.O., and Sunderland, S. (1993): Examination of the Law of Grotthus-Draper: Does ultrasound penetrate subcutaneous fat in humans? Athl. Train., 28:246–250.
35. Draper, D.O., Castel, J.C., and Castel, D. (1995): Rate of temperature increase in human muscle during 1 MHz and 3 MHz continuous ultrasound. J. Orthop. Sports Phys. Ther., 22:142–150.
36. Draper, D.O., Sunderland, S., Kirkendall, D.T., and Ricard, M. (1993): A comparison of temperature rise in human calf muscles following applications of underwater and topical gel ultrasound. J. Orthop. Sports Phys. Ther., 17:247–215.
37. Drez, D., Faust, D.C., and Evans, J.P. (1981): Cryotherapy and nerve palsy. Am. J. Sports Med., 9:256–257.
38. Eriksson, E., and Haggmark, T. (1979): Comparison of isometric muscle training and electrical stimulaton supplementing isometric muscle training in the recovery after major knee ligament surgery. Am. J. Sports Med., 7:168–171.
39. Evans, T.A., Faust, D.C., and Evans, J.P. (1981): Cryotherapy and nerve palsy. Am. J. Sports Med., 9:256–257.
40. Forrest, G., and Rosen, K. (1989): Ultrasound: Effectiveness of treatments given under water. Arch. Phys. Med. Rehabil., 70:28–29.
41. Forrest, G., and Rosen, K. (1992): Ultrasound treatments in degassed water. J. Sports Rehabil., 1:284–289.
42. Fox, R.H. (1961): Local cooling in man. Br. Med. Bull., 17:14–18.
43. Gann, N. (1991): Ultrasound: Current concepts. Clin. Management, 11:64–69.
44. Ganong, W. (1977): Review of Medical Physiology. Los Altos, CA, Appleton & Lange.
45. Gersh, M.R., and Wolf, S.L. (1986): Applications of transcutaneous electrical nerve stimulation in the management of patients with pain. Phys. Ther., 65:314–336.
46. Glick, E., and Snyder Mackler, L. (1989): Iontophoresis. In: Snyder Mackler, L., and Robinson, A.J. (eds.): Clinical Electrophysiology. Baltimore, Williams & Wilkins, pp. 247–259.
47. Griffin, J.E., and Touchstone, J.C. (1963): Ultrasonic movement of cortisol into pig tissues. I. Movement into skeletal muscle. Am. J. Phys. Med., 42:77–85.
48. Griffin, J.E., and Touchstone, J.C. (1968): Low-intensity phonophoresis of cortisol in swine. Phys. Ther., 48:1336–1344.
49. Griffin, J.E., Echternach, J.L., Price, R.E., and Touchstone, J.C. (1967): Patients treated with ultrasonic-driven hydrocortisone and with ultrasound alone. Phys. Ther., 47:594–601.
50. Griffin, J.E., Touchstone, J.C., and Liu, A.C.Y. (1965): Ultrasonic movement of cortisol into pig tissues. II. Movement into paravertebral nerve. Am. J. Phys. Med., 44:20–25.
51. Hald, R.D., and Bottjen, E.J. (1987): Effect of visual feedback on maximal and submaximal isokinetic test measurements of normal quadriceps and hamstrings. J. Orthop. Sports Phys. Ther., 9:86–93.
52. Hayes, K.W. (1992): The use of ultrasound to decrease pain and improve mobility. Crit. Rev. Phys. Med. Rehabil. Med., 3:271–287.
53. Henley, E.J. (1982): Fluidotherapy: Clinical Applications and Techniques. Sugarland, TX, Henley International.
54. Hertling, D., and Kessler, R.M. (1990): Management of Common Musculoskeletal Disorders, 2nd ed. Philadelphia, J.B. Lippincott.
55. Hocutt, J.E., Jaffe, R., Rylander, C.R., and Beebe, J.K. (1982): Cryotherapy in ankle sprains. Am. J. Sports Med., 10:316–319.

56. Jette, D.U. (1986): Effect of different forms of transcutaneous electrical nerve stimulation on experimental pain. Phys. Ther., 66:187–193.
57. Johnson, D.J., and Leider, F.E. (1977): Influence of cold bath on maximal handgrip strength. Percept. Mot. Skills, 44:323–326.
58. Johnson, M.I., Ashton, C.H., Bousfield, D.R., and Thompson, J.W. (1989): Analgesic effects of different frequencies of transcutaneous electrical stimulation on cold-induced pain in normal subjects. Pain, 39:231–236.
59. Kahn, J. (1987): Non-steroid iontophoresis. Clin. Management, 7:14–15.
60. Kessler, R.M, and Hertling, D. (1983): Management of Common Musculoskeletal Disorders. Philadelphia, Harper & Row.
61. Kleinkort, J.A., and Wood, F. (1975): Phonophoresis with 1 percent versus 10 percent hydrocortisone. Phys. Ther., 55:1320–1324.
62. Kloth, L.C. (1995): Electrical stimulation in tissue repair. In: McCulloch, J.M., Kloth, L.C., and Feeder, J.A. (eds.): Wound Healing Alternatives in Management. Philadelphia, F.A. Davis, pp. 275–314.
63. Knight, K.L. (1995): Cryotherapy in Sport Injury Management. Champaign, IL, Human Kinetics Publishers.
64. Kramer, J.F. (1985): Effect of therapeutic ultrasound intensity on subcutaneous tissue temperature and ulnar nerve conduction velocity. Am. J. Phys. Med., 64:1–9.
65. Leffman, D.J., Arnall, D.A., Holmgren, P.R., and Cornwall, M.W. (1994): Effect of microamperage stimulation on rate of wound healing in rats: A histological study. Phys. Ther., 74:195–200.
66. Lehmann, J.F. (1982): Therapeutic Heat and Cold, 3rd ed. Baltimore, Williams & Wilkins.
67. Lehmann, J.F., DeLateur, B.J., and Silverman, D.R. (1966): Selective heating effects of ultrasound in human beings. Arch. Phys. Med. Rehabil., 66:331–339.
68. Lehmann, J.F., DeLateur, B.J., and Stonebridge, J.B. (1969): Selective muscle heating by short-wave diathermy with a helical coil. Arch. Phys. Med. Rehabil., 50:117–123.
69. Lehmann, J.F., DeLateur, B.J., Stonebridge, J.B., and Warren, C.G. (1967): Therapeutic temperature distribution produced by ultrasound as modified by dosage and volume of tissue exposed. Arch. Phys. Med. Rehabil., 48:662–666.
70. Lehmann, J.F., Masock, A.J., Warren, C.G., and Koblanski, J.N. (1970): Effect of temperature on tendon extensibility. Arch. Phys. Med. Rehabil., 51:481–487.
71. Lehman, J.F., Stonebridge, J.B., DeLateur, B.J., et al. (1978): Temperatures in human thighs after hot pack treatment followed by ultrasound. Arch. Phys. Med. Rehabil., 59:472–475.
72. Levy, D., Kost, J., Meshulam, Y., and Langer, R. (1989): Effect of ultrasound on transdermal drug delivery to rats and guinea pigs. J. Clin. Invest., 83:2074–2078.
73. Lewis, T. (1930): Observations upon the reactions of the vessels of the human skin to cold. Heart, 15:177–208.
74. Licht, S. (1965): Therapeutic Heat and Cold, 2nd ed. Baltimore, Waverly Press.
75. Lota, M.J. (1965): Electronic plethysmography and tissue temperature studies of effect of ultrasound on blood flow. Arch. Phys. Med. Rehabil., 46:315–322.
76. Lowdon, B.J., and Moore, R.J. (1975): Determinants and nature of intramuscular temperature changes during cold therapy. Am. J. Phys. Med., 54:223–233.
77. Lucca, J.A., and Recchiuti, S.J. (1983): Effect of elecromyographic biofeedback on an isometric strengthening program. Phys. Ther., 63:200–203.
78. Maxwell, L. (1995): Therapeutic ultrasound and the metastasis of a solid tumor. J. Sports Rehabil., 4:273–281.
79. Mayer, D.J., and Price, D.D. (1989): Neurobiology of pain. In: Snyder Mackler, L., and Robinson, A.J. (eds.): Clinical Electrophysiology. Baltimore, Williams & Wilkins, pp. 141–201.
80. McDiarmind, T., and Burns, P.N. (1987): Clinical application of therapeutic ultrasound. Physiotherapy, 73:155–169.
81. McElany, J.C., Matthews, M.P., Harland, R., and McCafferty, D.F. (1985): The effect of ultrasound on the percutaneous absorption of lignocaine. Br. J. Clin. Pharmacol., 20:421–424.
82. McMaster, W.C., Liddle, S., and Waugh, T.R. (1978): Laboratory evaluation of various cold therapy modalities. Am. J. Sports Med., 6:291–294.
83. McNeal, D.R., and Baker, L.L. (1988): Effects of joint angle, electrodes and waveform on electrical stimulation of the quadriceps and hamstrings. Ann. Biomed. Eng., 16:299–310.
84. Mendel, F.C., and Fish, D.R. (1993): New perspectives in edema control via electrical stimulation. J. Athl. Train., 28:63–74.
85. Merrick, M.A., Knight, K.L., Ingersoll, C.D., and Potteiger, J.A. (1993): The effects of ice and compression wraps on intramuscular temperatures at various depths. Athl. Train., 28:236–245.
86. Michlovitz, S. (1986): Thermal Agents in Rehabilitation. Philadelphia, F.A. Davis.
87. Michlovitz, S., Smith, W., and Watkins, M. (1988): Ice and high voltage pulsed stimulation in treatment of acute lateral ankle sprains. J. Orthop. Sports Phys. Ther., 9:301–304.
88. Misasi, S., Morin, G., Kemler, D., et al. (1995): The effect of a toe cap and bias on perceived pain during cold water immersion. Athl. Train., 30:49–52.
89. Mohr, T., Carlson, B., Sulentic, C., and Landry, R. (1985): Comparison of isometric exercise and high volt galvanic stimulation on quadriceps femoris muscle strength. Phys. Ther., 65:606–612.
90. Nelson, R.M., and Currier, D.P. (1987): Clinical Electrotherapy. Los Altos, CA, Appleton & Lange.

91. Newton, R.A., and Karselis, T.C. (1983): Skin pH following high voltage pulsed galvanic stimulation. Phys. Ther., 63:1593–1596.
92. Nolan, M.F. (1991): Conductive differences in electrodes used with transcutaneous electrical nerve stimulation devices. Phys. Ther., 71:746–751.
93. Oakley, E.M. (1978):Dangers and contraindications of therapeutic ultrasound. Physiotherapy, 64:173–174.
94. Oliver, R.A., Johnson, D.J., Wheelhouse, W.W., and Griffin, P.P. (1979): Isometric muscle contraction response during recovery from reduced intramuscular temperature. Arch. Phys. Med. Rehabil., 60:126–129.
95. Oziomek, R.S., Perrin, D.H., Herold, D.A., and Denegar, C.R. (1991): Effect of phonophoresis on serum salicylate levels. Med. Sci. Sports. Exerc., 23:397–401.
96. Paul, W.D., and Imig, C.J. (1955): Temperature and blood flow studies after ultrasonic irradiaton. Am. J. Phys. Med., 34:370–375.
97. Peek, C.J. (1987): A primer of biofeedback instrumentation. In: Schwartz, M.S. (ed.): Biofeedback: A Practitioner's Guide. New York, Guilford Press.
98. Picker, R.I. (1989): Current trends: Low-volt pulsed microamp stimulation. Part II. Clin. Management Phys. Ther., 9:28–33.
99. Prentice, W.E. (1994): Therapeutic Modalities in Sports Medicine, 2nd ed. St. Louis, Times Mirror/Mosby.
100. Reid, D.C., and Cummings, G.E. (1973): Factors in selecting the dosage of ultrasound. Physiother. Can., 25:5–9.
101. Rimington, S.J., Draper, D.O., Durrant, E., and Fellingham, G. (1994): Temperature changes during therapeutic ultrasound in the precooled human gastrocnemius muscle. Athl. Train., 29:325–327.
102. Robinson, A.J. (1989): Basic concepts and terminology in electricity and physiology of muscle and nerve. In: Snyder-Mackler, L., and Robinson, A.J. (eds.): Clinical Electrophysiology. Baltimore, Williams & Wilkins, pp. 3–19, 61–94.
103. Robinson, A.J. (1989): Basic concepts in electricity and contempory terminology in electrotherapy. In: Snyder-Mackler, L., and Robinson, A.J. (eds.): Clinical Electrophysiology. Baltimore, Williams & Wilkins, pp. 1–31.
104. Robinson, A.J. (1989): Instrumentation for electrotherapy. In: Snyder-Mackler, L., and Robinson, A.J. (eds.): Clinical Electrophysiology. Baltimore, Williams & Wilkins, pp. 33–80.
105. Rose, S., Draper, D.O., Schulthies, S.S., and Durrant, E. (1996): The stretching window part two: Rate of thermal decay in deep muscle following 1-MHz ultrasound. Athl. Train., 31:139–143.
106. Ruiz, D.H., Myrer, J.W., Durrant, E., and Fellingham, G.W. (1993): Cryotherapy and sequential exercise bouts following cryotherapy on concentric and eccentric strength in the quadriceps. Athl. Train., 28:320–323.
107. Schmidt, K.L., Ott, V.R., Rocher, G., and Schaller, H. (1979): Heat, cold and inflammation: A review. Z. Rheumatol., 38:391–404.
108. Sculley, R.M., and Barnes, M.R. (1989): Physical Therapy. Philadelphia, J.B. Lippincott.
109. Selkowitz, D.M. (1985): Improvement in isometric strength of the quadriceps femoris muscle after training with electrical stimulation. Phys. Ther., 65:186–196.
110. Shelbourne, N.A., and Nitz, P. (1990): Accelerated rehabilitation after anterior cruciate ligament reconstruction. Am. J. Sports Med., 18:292–299.
111. Sisk, T.D., Stralka, S.W., Deering, M.B., and Griffin, J.W. (1987): Effects of electrical stimulation on quadriceps strength after reconstructive surgery of the anterior cruciate ligament. Am. J. Sports Med., 15:215–220.
112. Snyder-Mackler, L. (1989): Electrical stimulation for pain modulation. In: Snyder-Mackler, L., and Robinson, A.J. (eds.): Clinical Electrophysiology. Baltimore, Williams & Wilkins, pp. 205–227.
113. Snyder-Mackler, L. (1989): Electrical stimulation for tissue repair. In: Snyder-Mackler, L., and Robinson, A.J. (eds.): Clinical Electrophysiology. Baltimore, Williams & Wilkins, pp. 231–244.
114. Snyder-Mackler, L. (1995): Electrical stimulation for pain modulation. In: Robinson, A.J., and Snyder-Mackler, L. (eds.): Clinical Electrophysiology: Electrotherapy and Electrophysiological Testing. Baltimore, Williams & Wilkins, p. 285.
115. Snyder-Mackler, L. (1995): Electrical stimulation for tissue repair. In: Robinson, A.J., and Snyder-Mackler, L. (eds.): Clinical Electrophysiology: Electrotherapy and Electrophysiological Testing. Baltimore, Williams & Wilkins, pp. 319–322.
116. Snyder-Mackler, L., Delitto, A., Bailey, S.L., and Stralka, S.W. (1995): Strength of the quadriceps femoris muscle and functional recovery after reconstruction of the anterior cruciate ligament. J. Bone Joint Surg. [Am.], 77:1166–1173.
117. Snyder-Mackler, L., De Luca, P.F., Williams, P.R., et al. (1994): Reflex inhibition of the quadriceps femoris muscle after injury or reconstruction of the anterior cruciate ligament. J. Bone Joint Surg. [Am.], 76:555–560.
118. Snyder-Mackler, L., Ladin, Z., Schepsis, A.A., and Young, J.C. (1991): Electrical stimulation of the thigh muscles after reconstruction of the anterior cruciate ligament. J. Bone Joint Surg. [Am.], 73:1025–1036.
119. Synder-Mackler, L., Delitto, A., Stralka, S.W., and Bailey, S.L. (1994): Use of electrical stimulation to enhance recovery of quadriceps femoris muscle force production in patients following anterior cruciate ligament reconstruction. Phys. Ther., 74:901–907.
120. Starkey, C. (1993): Therapeutic Modalities for Athletic Trainers. Philadelphia, F.A. Davis.

121. Taylor, K., Newton, R.A., Personius, W.J., and Bush, F.M. (1987): Effects of interferential current stimulation for treatment of subjects with recurrent jaw pain. Phys. Ther., 67:346–350.

122. Thieme, H.A., Ingersoll, C.D., Knight, K.L., and Ozmun, J.C. (1996): Cooling does not affect knee proprioception. Athl. Train., 31:8–11.

123. Vaughn, D.T. (1973): Direct method versus underwater method in the treatment of plantar warts with ultrasound. Phys. Ther., 53:396–397.

124. Ward, A.R., and Robertson, V.J. (1996): Dosage factors for the subaqueous application of 1 MHz ultrasound. Arch. Phys. Med. Rehabil., 77:1167–1172.

125. Warren, C.G., Koblanski, J.N., and Sigelmann, R.A. (1976): Ultrasound coupling media: Their relative transmissivity. Arch. Phys. Med. Rehabil., 57:218–222.

126. Warren, C.G., Lehmann, J.F., and Koblanski, J.N. (1976): Heat and stretch procedures: An evaluation using rat tail tendon. Arch. Phys. Med. Rehabil., 57:122–126.

127. Weber, M.D., and Woodall, W.R. (1993): The effect of polarity on maximally tolerated stimulation contractions of the quadriceps. Phys. Ther., 73 (Suppl):RO63.

128. Wessling, K.C., DeVane, D.A., and Hylton, C.R. (1987): Effects of static stretch versus static stretch and ultrasound combined on triceps surae muscle extensibility in healthy women. Phys. Ther., 67:674–679.

129. Wessman, H.C., and Kottke, F.J. (1967): The effect of indirect heating on peripheral blood flow, pulse rate, blood pressure, and temperature. Arch. Phys. Med. Rehabil., 48:567–576.

130. Whitmore, J.J., Burt, M.M., and Fowler, R.S. (1972): Bandaging the lower extremity to control swelling: Figure 8 versus spiral technique. Arch. Phys. Med. Rehabil., 53:487–490.

131. Wood, J.M., Jacobson, W.E., Schallreuter, K.U., et al. (1992): Pulsed low-intensity direct current (PLIDC) is effective in healing chronic decubitus ulcers in stages II and III. J. Invest. Dermatol., 92:574S.

132. Woodall, W.R., and Weber, M.D. (1993): The effect of polarity in a bipolar electrode technique on stimulated contractions of the quadriceps femoris. Phys. Ther., 73 (Suppl):RO62.

133. Wright, V., and Johns, R.J. (1960): Physical factors concerned with the stiffness of normal and diseased joints. Bull. Johns Hopkins Hosp., 106:215–231.

134. Zankel, H.T. (1966): Effect of physical agents on motor conduction velocity of the ulnar nerve. Arch. Phys. Med. Rehabil., 47:787–792.

Chapter 6

Range of Motion and Flexibility

Gary L. Harrelson, Ed.D., A.T.,C., and
Deidre Leaver-Dunn, M.Ed., A.T.,C.

Range of motion is the available amount of movement of a joint, whereas flexibility is the ability of soft-tissue structures, such as muscle, tendon, and connective tissue, to elongate through the available range of joint motion. Whether it is undergoing therapeutic stretching during postinjury rehabilitation or during a routine flexibility program, connective tissue is the most important physical focus of range-of-motion exercises. Connective tissue involved in the body's reparative process after trauma or surgery often limits normal joint motion. Understanding the biophysical factors of connective tissue is important for determining optimal ways of increasing range of motion. Histologic evidence has shown that fibrosis can occur within 4 days of the onset of immobility.[46] Additional pathologic connective tissue conditions such as scarring, adhesions, and fibrotic contractures must also be addressed therapeutically.[21, 29] Similarly, soft tissues, including the muscle sheath and connective tissue framework, provide most of the resistance to the stretching of normal relaxed muscle.[46] Awareness of the structures and processes associated with limiting stretching to healthy tissue is crucial in the development and implementation of programs for improving and maintaining range of motion and flexibility.

STRETCHING

Biophysical Considerations

PROPERTIES OF CONNECTIVE TISSUE

Connective tissue is composed of collagen and other fibers within a ground substance, a protein-polysaccharide complex. A thorough discussion of connective tissue composition is found in Chapter 2. Connective tissue has viscoelastic properties, defined as two components of stretch, which allow elongation of the tissue.[15, 21, 44, 46] The viscous component permits a plastic stretch that results in permanent tissue elongation after the load is removed. Conversely, the elastic component allows for an elastic stretch, a temporary elongation, with the tissue returning to its previous length once the stress is removed. Range-of-motion exercise techniques should primarily be designed to produce plastic deformation.

NEUROPHYSIOLOGY

All stretching techniques are based on the premise of the stretch reflex, which involves two muscle receptors—the Golgi tendon organ (GTO) and the muscle spindle—that are sensitive to changes in muscle length.[53] The GTO is also affected by changes in muscle tension. These receptors must be considered in the process of selecting any stretching procedure. The intrafusal muscle spindle responds to rapid stretch by initiating a reflexive contraction of the muscle being stretched.[53] If a stretch is held long enough (at least 6 seconds),[38] this protective mechanism can be negated by the action of the GTO, which can override the impulses from the muscle spindle.[53] This reflexive relaxation that results is referred to as autogenic inhibition, and it allows effective stretching of the muscle tissue. Additionally, an isotonic contraction of an agonist muscle causes a reflex relaxation in the antagonist muscle, allowing it to stretch. This phenomenon is referred to as reciprocal inhibition. Conversely, a quick stretch of the antagonist muscle will cause a contraction of the agonist muscle. For example, when the quadriceps muscle contracts, a reflexive relaxation of the hamstring muscles occurs. In other words, once a tight muscle or muscles have been identified, an isotonic contraction of its antagonist will result in relaxation of the tight muscles and an improved range of motion. Autogenic inhibition and reciprocal inhibition are two components on which proprioceptive neuromuscular facilitation (PNF) stretching is based.

DURATION

The amount and duration of the applied force and the tissue temperature during performance of the stretch are the principal factors determining how much elastic or plastic stretch occurs with connective tissue stretching. Elastic stretch is enhanced by high-force, short-duration stretching, whereas plastic stretch results from low-force, long-duration stretching. Numerous studies have noted the effectiveness of prolonged stretching at low to moderate tension levels.[1, 11, 12, 15, 16, 21, 22, 27, 44, 47, 54, 55] A precise time frame for holding a static stretch has not been determined. Research has suggested that static stretches be held between 6 and 60 seconds,[38] with 15- to 30-second holds most commonly advocated.

TEMPERATURE OF CONNECTIVE TISSUE

Research has shown that temperature has a significant influence on the mechanical behavior of connective tissue under tensile stretch.[25, 44, 56] Because connective tissue is composed of collagen, which is resistant to stretch at normal body temperature, the effect of increased tissue temperature on stretch has been studied. It was concluded that higher therapeutic temperatures at low loads produce the greatest plastic tissue elongation with the least damage. Lentell and colleagues[26] reported greater increases in range of motion of healthy shoulders after heat application.

Increased connective tissue temperature decreases connective tissue resistance to stretch and promotes increased soft-tissue extensibility.[22, 25] It has been reported that collagen is very pliable when heated to a range between 102° and 110° F.[23, 44] The use of ultrasound prior to joint mobilization has proved effective in elevating deep tissue temperature and extensibility.[24] Draper and Ricard[9] have demonstrated the presence of a "stretching window" after a 3-MHz ultrasound application. This window indicates that for optimal tissue elongation, stretching should be performed during ultrasound treatment or within 3.3 minutes after termination of the treatment.[9] In a follow-up study, Rose and colleagues[42] reported that after application of 1-MHz ultrasound, the deeper tissues cooled at a slower rate than did superficial tissues; thus, the stretching window was open longer for deeper structures than for superficial ones. Although superior stretching results have been reported with the application of heat before and during stretching, other studies have reported greater increases in flexibility after the application of cold packs. Brodowicz and colleagues[3] reported improved hamstring flexibility in healthy subjects after 20 minutes of hamstring stretching with an ice pack applied to the posterior thigh compared with the group that received heat or that performed stretching without application of any therapeutic agent. Kottkeet and colleagues[21] have also shown that a greater plastic stretch results if the tissue is allowed to cool before tension is released, whereas others[26] have reported that the use of cold during the end stages of stretching diminished the cumulative gains in flexibility that occurred after application of heat. Moreover, it appears that the use of either a superficial heat or a cold modality in conjunction with stretching results in greater improvements in flexibility than stretching alone.[3, 26]

Types of Stretching Techniques

Limited joint range of motion caused by soft-tissue restriction often inhibits the initiation or completion of the rehabilitative process. Conservative treatment of contractures meets with only moderate success, and overly aggressive stretching may result in undesired adverse effects. Optimal stretching is achieved only when voluntary and reflex muscle resistance are overcome or eliminated. Contraindications of stretching are indicated in Table 6–1.

Three types of stretching techniques are generally recognized: ballistic, static, and PNF. Ballistic stretching consists of repetitive bouncing movements that stretch a muscle group. Ballistic stretching has not been advocated because forces could be applied to a muscle that exceed its extensibility or that activate the muscle spindles described previously, with resultant microtrauma to the muscle fibers. However, it has been reported that because many physical activities involve dynamic movement, ballistic stretching should follow a static stretching routine.[38] Static stretching involves stretching a muscle to a point of discomfort and holding the stretch for a length of time. PNF involves alternating muscle contractions and stretching.[20] The efficacy of all three techniques has been evaluated.[4–7, 10, 12, 14, 28, 30, 32–34, 36, 43, 48, 50, 53, 57] It appears that all three stretching techniques will increase flexibility, with static stretching being the safest of the three.[4, 32, 33] In some cases static stretching has been advocated over PNF because it is easier to teach and perform.[57] However, PNF stretching does allow for stretching in functional planes of movement.

PASSIVE AND ACTIVE-ASSISTED STRETCHING TECHNIQUES

Various mechanical passive and active-assisted techniques augment manual passive stretching. Methods of achieving the desired outcome are often limited only by creativity and improvisational skills. Once the soft-tissue restriction has been assessed, the clinician should analyze appropriate and effective ways of

---

Table 6–1. Contraindications for Stretching

Limitation of joint motion by a bony block
Recent fracture
Evidence of an acute inflammatory or infectious process (heat and swelling) in or around joints
Sharp, acute pain with joint movement or muscle elongation
Hematoma or other indications of tissue trauma
Contractures or shortened soft tissues providing increased joint stability in lieu of normal
    structural stability or muscle strength
Contractures or shortened soft tissues forming the basis for increased functional abilities,
    particularly in individuals with paralysis or severe muscle weakness.

Data from Kisner, C., and Colby, L. (1985): Therapeutic Exercise: Foundations and Techniques. Philadelphia, F.A. Davis.

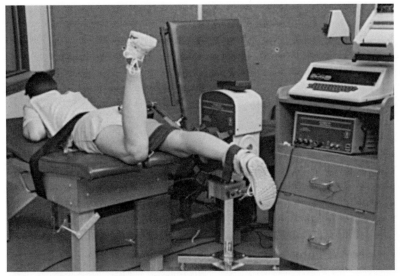

Figure 6–1. Prone weighted stretch of the knee.

carrying out the treatment and rehabilitation plan. Several methods of stretching can be used.

Spray and Stretch

This technique has been described in detail by Travell and Simons.[51] Spraying of Fluori-Methane* cools taut muscle fibers and desensitizes palpable myofascial trigger points, thereby facilitating stretching of the muscle to its full length. Passive stretch remains the central component within this technique.

Prolonged Weighted Stretch

The rationale for a prolonged-duration, low-load stretch has been discussed. Figure 6–1 illustrates a method of prolonged weighted stretching for the knee using the Cybex as a support and stabilizer. With the athlete in a prone position, a weight is attached to the ankle to help decrease any extension limitations present. Figure 6–2 shows a weighted stretch that can be used to help improve elbow range of motion. Also, Figure 14–9 illustrates a technique for providing a low-load, long-duration stretch for the elbow.

Assistive Devices

These appliances aid in gaining and maintaining end range of motion. Assistive devices include pulleys, extremity traction,[25, 44] T bars or wands, and continuous passive range-of-motion units. Pulleys are commonly used for joint restriction of the shoulder and knee (Figs. 6–3 and 6–4). Wands, T bars, towels, sport sticks, or other similar apparatus may be used for individual active-assisted stretching of the upper extremities.

Continuous passive range-of-motion units are often a valuable mechanical device that can benefit various joints. They can provide constant movement of the joint or joints after surgical repair. A passive mode can be used on other equipment, including isokinetic units, to allow a controlled passive range of motion with a pause to provide a stretch at the end range of motion (Fig. 6–5).

*Available from Gebauer Chemical Co., Cleveland, Ohio.

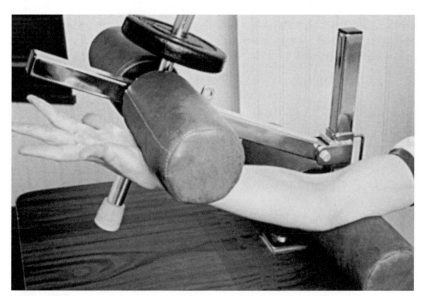

Figure 6–2. Weighted elbow stretch. (Courtesy of Sports Medicine Update. Birmingham, Alabama, HealthSouth Rehabilitation Corporation.)

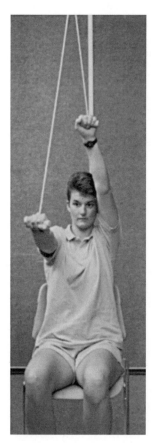

Figure 6–3. Active-assisted range of motion of the shoulder with the use of pulleys.

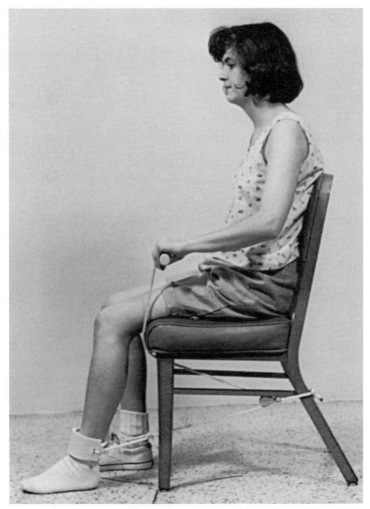

Figure 6–4. Active-assisted range of motion of the knee with the use of pulleys.

Dynamic Splints

Adjustable dynamic splints can produce low-intensity, prolonged-duration force. The construction of these devices offers a lower progressive load that can be self-adjusted and graduated as orthotic tolerance time increases (Figs. 6–6 to 6–8). Dynamic splints have been used successfully in the treatment of motion restrictions of the knee and elbow.[15, 16]

MYOFASCIAL RELEASE TECHNIQUES

Myofascial release techniques have been anecdotally reported as being effective for relieving restrictions and increasing range of motion. These claims have not been well investigated in controlled settings. Hanten and Chandler[14] have compared the effectiveness of the PNF contract-relax technique and the myofascial release leg pull technique in increasing hip flexion range of motion. Their results demonstrated significant gains in range of motion after use of both techniques, with significantly greater improvements with the contract-relax stretch as compared to the leg pull.

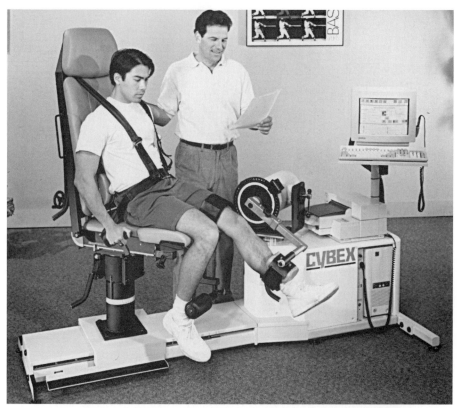

Figure 6–5. Isokinetic setup in a passive mode. (Photo courtesy of Cybex, Ronkonkoma, New York.)

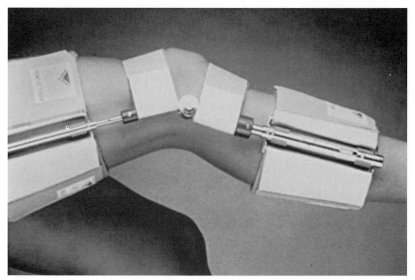

Figure 6–6. Knee Dynasplint. (Photo courtesy of Dynasplint Systems, Baltimore, Maryland.)

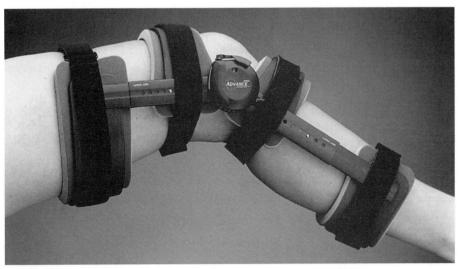

Figure 6–7. Advanced Dynamic ROM knee orthosis. (Photo courtesy of Empi, Inc., Minneapolis, Minnesota.)

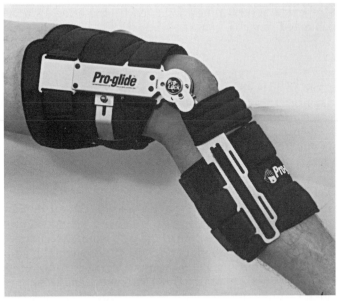

Figure 6–8. Pro-glide knee orthosis. (Photo courtesy of Thera-Kinetics, Inc., Mount Laurel, New Jersey.)

PROPRIOCEPTIVE NEUROMUSCULAR FACILITATION TECHNIQUES

PNF can be defined as a method of promoting or hastening the response of neuromuscular mechanisms through stimulation of the mechanoreceptors.[20, 52] PNF stretching techniques are based on the reduction of sensory activity through spinal reflexes in order to cause relaxation of the muscle to be stretched. Sherrington's principle of reciprocal inhibition demonstrates relaxation of the muscle being stretched (agonist) through voluntary concentric contraction of its opposite (antagonist) muscle.[20, 32, 50] Many studies[5–7, 10, 13, 14, 32–34, 36, 43, 50, 53] support the efficacy of PNF and show greater increases in flexibility when PNF is used, when compared with static or dynamic stretching techniques. Other investigations[4, 28, 30, 48, 57] have found PNF to be at least as effective as other types of stretching.

PNF patterns can be performed in a straight line, such as flexion-extension, or in rotational and diagonal patterns. PNF techniques generally comprise five trials of 5 seconds of passive stretching followed by a 5- to 10-second maximal voluntary contraction, as indicated by the technique used. The work of Cornelius and colleagues[7] showed that significant increases in systolic blood pressure occurred after three trials consisting of a protocol of 5 seconds of passive stretching, followed by a 6-second maximal voluntary antagonist contraction.

Contract-Relax

The contract-relax technique[7, 14, 33, 34, 49, 52] achieves increased range of motion in the agonist pattern by using consecutive isotonic contractions of the antagonist. The body part to be stretched is moved passively into the agonist pattern until range-of-motion limitation is felt. At this point, the athlete contracts isotonically into the antagonist pattern against strong manual resistance. When the clinician realizes that relaxation has occurred, the body part is again moved passively into as much range of motion as possible until limitation is again felt. The procedure is repeated several times, followed by the athlete's moving actively through the obtained range (Fig. 6–9).

Hold-Relax

Hold-relax[6, 7, 20, 49] is a PNF technique used to increase joint range of motion and is based on an isometric contraction of the antagonist performed against maximal resistance. This technique is performed in the same sequence as the contract-relax technique, but because no motion is allowed on isometric contraction, this is the method of choice when joint restriction is accompanied by muscle spasm and pain. The intensity of each contraction is gradually increased with each successive repetition (Fig. 6–10).

Slow Reversal Hold-Relax

The slow reversal hold-relax technique[20, 52] uses reciprocal inhibition, as does the hold-relax technique. The body part is moved actively into the agonist pattern to the point of pain-free limitation. An isometric contraction is then performed in the antagonist pattern for a 5- to 10-second hold, and the agonist muscle group actively brings the body part into a greater range of motion in the agonist pattern. The process is repeated several times. The technique is good for increasing range of motion when the primary limiting factor is the antagonist muscle group (Fig. 6–11).

JOINT MOBILIZATION

Techniques

Manual joint mobilization techniques are a form of passive range of motion used to improve joint arthrokinematics. The proper use of mobilization helps

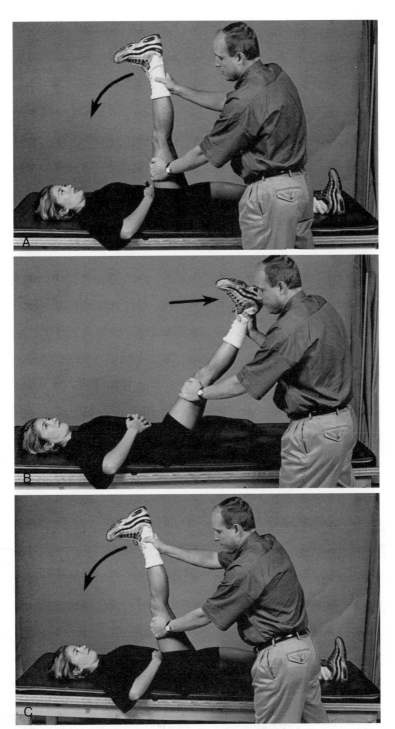

Figure 6–9. Contract-relax proprioceptive neuromuscular facilitation pattern for the hamstrings. *A,* The body part is moved passively by the clinician into the agonist pattern until limitation is felt. *B,* The athlete performs an isotonic contraction through the antagonist pattern. *C,* The clinician applies a passive stretch into the agonist pattern until limitation is felt. The procedure is repeated.

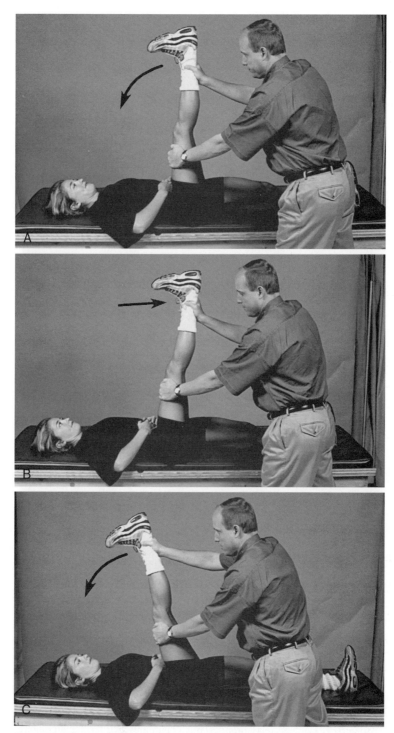

Figure 6–10. Hold-relax proprioceptive neuromuscular facilitation pattern for the hamstrings. *A,* The body part is moved passively by the clinician into the agonist pattern until limitation is felt. *B,* The athlete performs an isometric contraction into the antagonist pattern. *C,* The clinician applies a passive stretch into the agonist pattern until limitation is felt. The procedure is repeated.

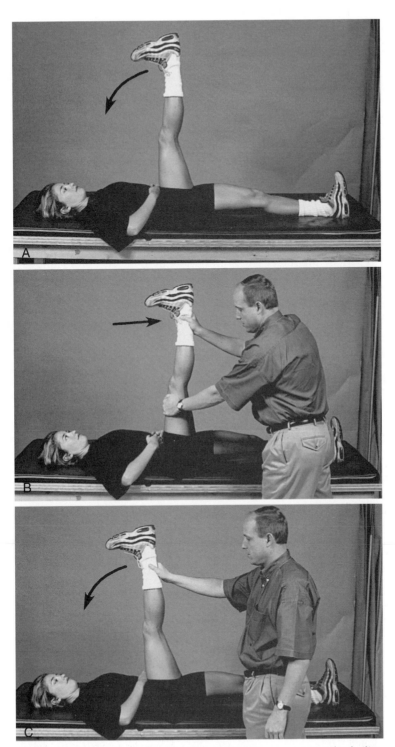

Figure 6–11. Slow reversal hold-relax proprioceptive neuromuscular facilitation pattern for the hamstrings. *A,* The athlete performs an active movement of the body part into the agonist pattern. *B,* The athlete performs an isometric contraction into the antagonist pattern. *C,* The athlete actively moves the body part further into the agonist pattern. The procedure is repeated.

Table 6–2. Stretching Versus Mobilization

STRETCHING	MOBILIZATION
Used when muscular resistance is encountered	Used when ligament or capsule resistance is encountered
Effective only at the end of the physiologic range of motion	Performed at any point in the range of motion
Limited to one direction	Can be done in any direction
Increased pain with increased range of motion	Decreased pain with increased range of motion
Used for tight muscular structures	Used for tight articular structures
Employs long lever arm techniques	Safer—employs short lever arm techniques

From Quillen, W.S., Halle, J.S., and Rouillier, L.H. (1992): Manual therapy: Mobilization of the motion-restricted shoulder. J. Sports Rehabil., 1:237–248.

facilitate healing, reduce disability, relieve pain, and restore full range of motion.[31] The traditional approach to restore loss of joint motion is to apply a passive sustained stretch without regard to a defined cause of motion limitation. This can result in an increased stimulation of pain receptors and a reflexive contraction of muscles, which may interfere with attempts at increasing motion.[40, 41] Table 6–2 compares physiologic (stretching) and accessory (mobilization) movement techniques.[41]

Joint motion is composed of both physiologic and accessory motions. Physiologic movement comprises the major portion of the range and can be measured with a goniometer (see Chap. 4). Physiologic joint movements occur in the cardinal movement planes and include flexion-extension, abduction-adduction, and rotation.[37] Accessory motion, also referred to as arthrokinematics, is necessary for normal physiologic range of motion; it occurs simultaneously with physiologic motion and cannot be measured precisely. Accessory motion occurs between the two articulating surfaces and is described by the terms spin, roll, and glide. Spin involves rotation about a stationary axis. Roll occurs when two joint surfaces that are not congruent move on one another. Glide occurs involuntarily when two surfaces slide with respect to one another. Both rolling and gliding motions occur simultaneously at some point in the range of motion.[37]

Because accessory motion is necessary for physiologic motion to occur, an assessment to determine the cause of the restricted motion is necessary. When restriction of a joint is assessed on passive movement, determination should be made as to whether the restriction is in a capsular or noncapsular pattern. A capsular pattern is found only in synovial joints that are controlled by muscles.[2] Capsular patterns or restrictions indicate loss of mobility of the entire joint

Table 6–3. Normal and Pathologic Endfeels

ENDFEEL	DESCRIPTION AND EXAMPLE
Normal	
Capsular	Firm; forcing the shoulder into full external rotation
Bony	Abrupt; moving the elbow into full extension
Soft-tissue approximation	Soft; flexing the normal knee or elbow
Muscular	Rubbery; tension of tight hamstrings
Pathologic	
Adhesions and scarring	Sudden; sharp arrest in one direction
Muscle spasm	Rebound; usually accompanies pain felt at the end of restriction
Loose	Ligamentous laxity; a hypermobile joint
Boggy	Soft, mushy; joint effusion
Internal derangement	Springy; mechanical block such as a torn meniscus
Empty	No resistance to motion

Data from Cyriax, J.H. (1975): Textbook of Orthopaedic Medicine, 6th ed, Vol. 1. Diagnosis of Soft-Tissue Lesions. Baltimore, Williams & Wilkins.

capsule from fibrosis, effusion, or inflammation. Differentiation can be made by noting the endfeel at the extremes of movement. The endfeels described in Table 6–3 may be normal or pathologic.[8] Joint restrictions from noncapsular patterns fall into three categories: ligament adhesions, internal derangement, and extra-articular limitation.[8]

- Ligament adhesions: These occur when adhesions form about a ligament after an injury and may cause pain or a restriction of mobility. Some movements will be painful, some are slightly limited, and some are pain free.
- Internal derangement: Restriction in joint mobility is the result of a loose fragment within the joint. The onset is sudden, pain is localized, and movements that engage against the block are limited, whereas all others are free.
- Extra-articular limitation: Loss in joint mobility results from adhesions in structures outside the joint. Movements that stress the adhesion will be limited and painful.

Physiologic Effects

Joint mobilization techniques serve to restore the accessory motions. Effects of joint mobilization include mitigating capsular restrictions and breaking adhesions, distracting impacted tissue, and providing movement and lubrication for normal articular cartilage. Pain reduction and decreased muscle tension are achieved through the stimulation of fast-conducting fibers to block small pain fibers and through activation of dynamic mechanoreceptors to produce reflexive relaxation. Joint mobilization is indicated for the treatment of capsular restrictions. Contraindications are described in Table 6–4.

Fundamentals

SYSTEMS OF GRADING MOBILIZATION

Systems of grading joint mobilization have been described by Maitland,[29] Kaltenborn,[17] and Paris.[35] Maitland[29] has described five grades of mobilization techniques (Table 6–5). Grade I and grade II mobilizations are used primarily for treatment of pain, and grades III and IV are used for treating stiffness. It is necessary to treat pain first and stiffness second.[29]

Traction is used to separate the joint surfaces to varying degrees into an open-packed position, thus increasing the mobility of the joint.[37, 39] Kaltenborn has

Table 6–4. Contraindications for Joint Mobilization

Premature stressing of surgical structures	Vascular disease
Hypermobility	Advanced osteoarthritis
Acute inflammation	Neurologic signs
Infection	Congenital bone deformities
Fractures	Osteoporosis
Malignancy	Rheumatoid arthritis

Data from Barak, T., Rosen, E.R., and Sofer, R. (1990): Basic concepts of orthopaedic manual therapy. *In:* Gould, J.A. (ed.): Orthopaedic and Sports Physical Therapy. St. Louis, C.V. Mosby, pp. 195–211; and Prentice, W.E. (1992): Techniques of manual therapy for the knee. J. Sports Rehabil., 1:249–257.

Table 6–5. Grades of Mobilization Techniques

GRADE	DESCRIPTION
I	This is a small-amplitude movement at the beginning of the range of motion, used when pain and spasm limit movement early in the range of motion.
II	This is a large-amplitude movement within the midrange of motion. It is used when spasm limits movement sooner with a quick oscillation than with a slow one or when slowly increasing pain restricts movement halfway into the range.
III	This is a large-amplitude movement up to the pathologic limit in the range of motion. It is used when pain and resistance from spasm, inert tissue tension, or tissue compression limit movement near the end of the range.
IV	This is a small-amplitude movement at the very end of the range of motion, used when resistance limits movement in the absence of pain and spasm.
V	This is a small-amplitude, quick thrust delivered at the end of the range of motion, usually accompanied by a popping sound called a manipulation.

Data from Maitland, G.D. (1977): Extremity Manipulation, 2nd ed. London, Butterworth Publishers.

proposed a system that uses traction combined with mobilization as a means of reducing pain or mobilizing hypomobile joints.[17] All joints have some looseness that is described by Kaltenborn as slack, and some degree of slack is necessary for normal joint motion. Kaltenborn's stages of traction are described in Table 6–6.[17] It has been recommended that 10-second intermittent stage I and stage II traction be used, distracting the joint surfaces up to stage III and then releasing distraction until the joint returns to its resting position.[39] Also, stage III traction should be used with mobilization glides to treat joint hypomobility.[17] Traction and translatoric gliding can be applied separately or together in various mobilization techniques (Fig. 6–12).[2]

JOINT POSITION AND FORCE APPLICATION

Successful joint mobilization depends upon position of the joint to be mobilized, direction of the force, and magnitude of the force applied. Correct positioning of a joint is critical when mobilizing a joint. A joint may be in either a close-packed or an open-packed position. A joint is in a close-packed position when the joint surfaces are most congruent. In a close-packed position the major ligaments are maximally taut, the intracapsular space is minimal, and the surfaces cannot be pulled apart by traction forces.[2] This position is used as a testing position but is never used for mobilization because there is no freedom of movement.[2] The maximal open-packed position is known as the resting position

Table 6–6. Kaltenborn's Stages of Traction

STAGE	DESCRIPTION
I (piccolo)	This is traction that neutralizes pressure in the joint without actual separation of the joint surfaces. The purpose is to relieve pain by reducing griding when performing mobilization techniques. This stage is analogous to a grade I mobilization.
II (take up the slack)	This is traction that effectively separates the articulating surfaces and takes up the slack or eliminates play in the joint capsule. Stage II is used to relieve pain and is the same as a grade IV mobilization.
III (stretch)	This is traction that involves actual stretching of the soft tissue surrounding the joint for the purpose of increasing mobility in a hypomobile joint.

Data from Kaltenborn, F.M. (1980): Mobilization of the Extremity Joints: Examination and Basic Treatment Techniques. Oslo, Olaf Noris Bokhandel; and Prentice, W.E. (1992): Techniques of manual therapy for the knee. J. Sports Rehabil., 1:249–257.

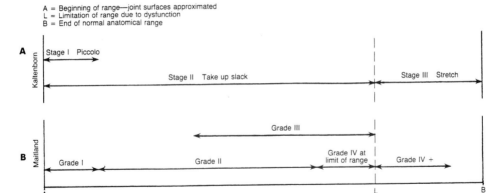

A = Beginning of range—joint surfaces approximated
L = Limitation of range due to dysfunction
B = End of normal anatomical range

Figure 6–12. Comparison of mobilization technique applications. *A,* Kaltenborn's technique. *B,* Maitland's technique. (From Barak, T., Rosen, E.R., and Sofer, R. [1990]. Basic concepts of orthopaedic manual therapy. *In:* Gould, J.A. [ed]: Orthopaedic and Sports Physical Therapy, 2nd ed. St. Louis, C.V. Mosby, pp. 195–211.)

and is characterized by the surrounding tissues being as lax as possible and the intracapsular space being its greatest.[2] The maximal open-packed position of a joint is the optimal position for joint mobilization.[2, 17–19, 29, 31] Kaltenborn[17] has described resting positions for all joints.

The direction of the mobilizing force is dependent on the contour of the joint surface of the structure to be mobilized. In most articulations, one joint surface is considered to be concave and the other convex. The concave-convex rule[29, 35] takes these joint surface configurations into account and states that when the concave surface is stationary and the convex surface is mobilized, a glide of the convex segment should be in the direction opposite to the restriction of joint movement.[19, 39] If the convex articular surface is stationary and the concave surface is mobilized, gliding of the concave segment should be in the same direction as the restriction of joint movement (Fig. 6–13). Typical treatment of a joint may involve a series of three to six mobilizations lasting up to 30 seconds, with one to three oscillations per second.[29, 37] General application principles for applying mobilizations are summarized in Table 6–7, and the contraindications for mobilization are listed in Table 6–4. The grades of mobilization and stages of traction have been previously described in this chapter. Traction should be used in conjunction with mobilization techniques to treat hypomobile joints. Prentice[39] reports that grade III traction stretches the joint capsule and increases the space between the articulating surfaces, placing the joint in an open-packed position. Applying grade III and grade IV oscillations within the athlete's pain limitations should maximally improve joint mobility.[39]

Table 6–7. Joint Mobilization Application Principles

Remove jewelry and rings.
Be relaxed (both athlete and clinician).
Always examine the contralateral side.
Use an open-packed joint position.
Avoid pain.
Perform smooth, regular oscillations.
Apply each technique for 20–60 sec.
Repeat each technique only 4–5 times per treatment session; it is easy to overmobilize.
Mobilize daily for pain and 2–3 times per week for restricted motion.
Follow mobilization with active range-of-motion exercises.

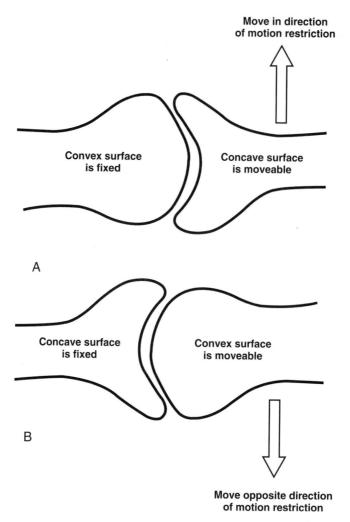

Figure 6–13. The concave-convex rule. If the joint surface of the limb to be moved is concave, move it in the direction of motion restriction. If the joint surface to be moved is convex, mobilize opposite the direction of motion restriction. (Modified from Quillen, W.S., and Gieck, J.H. [1988]. Manual therapy: Mobilization of the motion-restricted knee. Athl. Train., 23:123–130.)

APPLICATION TECHNIQUES

Upper Extremity

SHOULDER
Humeral Distraction with Anterior, Posterior, and Inferior Glides

Use:	This technique is effective for pain reduction.
Position:	The athlete is supine, with the arm resting at the side.
Stabilization:	The scapula may be stabilized with a small towel roll at the posterior aspect and with one of the

clinician's hands held at the inferior aspect of the glenoid.

Procedure: The mobilizing hand or hands grasp the humerus just above the elbow. A distraction force is then applied along the long axis of the humerus. The head of the humerus can be mobilized anteriorly, posteriorly, and inferiorly. As the athlete relaxes, the arm can be gradually moved into various degrees of abduction (Fig. 6–14).

Inferior Humeral Glide

Use: This technique is effective for increasing flexion.

Position: The athlete is supine, with the shoulder and elbow maximally flexed.

Stabilization: The scapula may be stabilized with a small towel roll at the posterior aspect.

Procedure: The mobilizing hands grasp the proximal humerus with the fingers interlaced. A posteriorly directed force is applied along the long axis of the humerus (Fig. 6–15).

Anterior and Posterior Acromioclavicular Glides

Use: This technique is effective for reducing pain and facilitating horizontal shoulder girdle movements that require gliding or rolling of the clavicle.

Position: The athlete is in the seated position.

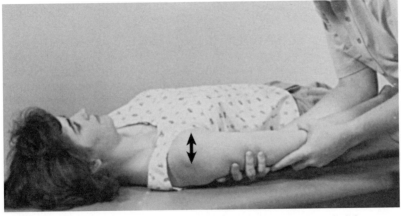

Figure 6–14. Humeral distraction with anterior, posterior, and lateral glides.

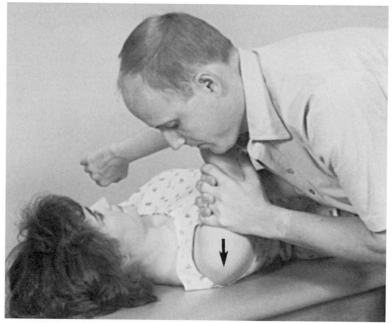

Figure 6–15. Inferior humeral glide.

Stabilization:	The distal clavicle or acromion process of the scapula is stabilized with one of the clinician's hands.
Procedure:	The clavicle is grasped between the clinician's thumb and forefinger and mobilized anteriorly or posteriorly (Fig. 6–16).
Note:	This procedure can also be applied to the sternoclavicular joint.

ELBOW

Radioulnar Distraction

Use:	This technique is effective for increasing extension.
Position:	The athlete is supine, with the arm by the side, elbow flexed, and forearm in neutral position.
Stabilization:	The distal humerus is stabilized with one of the clinician's hands.
Procedure:	The forearm is grasped by the clinician's hand and a distraction force is applied along the long axis of the forearm. A slight supination force can also be applied. The elbow may be gradually extended as movement increases (Fig. 6–17).

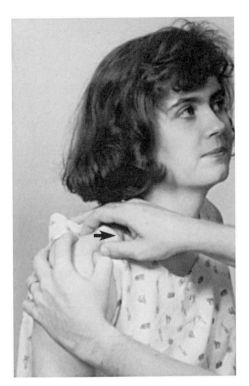

Figure 6-16. Anterior and posterior acromio-clavicular glides.

Anterior and Posterior Radioulnar Glides

Use: This technique is effective for increasing supination and pronation.

Position: The athlete is supine, sitting, or standing.

Stabilization: The ulna is stabilized proximally by one of the clinician's hands.

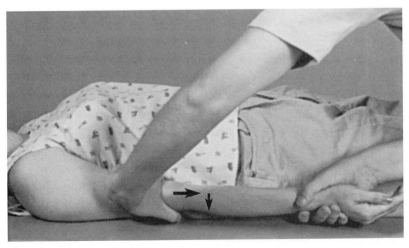

Figure 6-17. Radioulnar distraction.

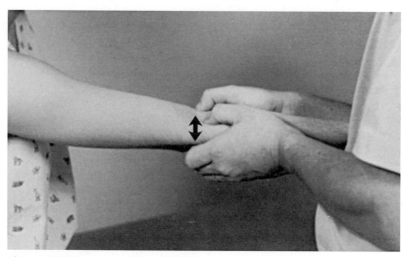

Figure 6–18. Anterior and posterior radioulnar glides.

Procedure: The radius is grasped proximally by the clinician's other hand. Posteriorly or anteriorly directed force is applied perpendicular to the long axis of the forearm (Fig. 6–18).

Note: This procedure can be repeated by moving distally along the forearm.

WRIST

Radiocarpal Distraction

Use: This technique is effective for reducing pain.

Position: The athlete is seated, with the hand hanging over the edge of the table. The forearm may be supported over a small towel roll.

Stabilization: The forearm is stabilized just proximal to the wrist by one of the clinician's hands.

Procedure: The proximal row of carpals is grasped by one

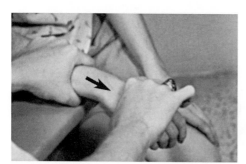

Figure 6–19. Radiocarpal distraction.

of the clinician's hands, and a distraction force is applied along the long axis of the forearm (Fig. 6–19).

Dorsal and Volar Radiocarpal Glides

Use:

This technique is effective for increasing flexion and extension.

Position:

The athlete is seated, with the hand hanging over the edge of the table. The forearm may be supported over a small towel roll.

Stabilization:

The forearm is stabilized just proximal to the wrist by one of the clinician's hands.

Procedure:

The clinician grasps the proximal carpals and applies dorsal and volar glides perpendicular to the long axis of the forearm (Fig. 6–20).

THUMB AND FINGERS

Interphalangeal Distraction with Volar, Dorsal, Medial, and Lateral Glides

Use:

This technique is effective for reducing pain and increasing flexion and extension at the interphalangeal joint.

Position:

The athlete is seated, with the forearm and hand in a resting position on the table.

Stabilization:

The distal aspect of proximal joint component is stabilized by the clinician's thumb and forefinger.

Procedure:

The dorsal and volar sides of the proximal end of the distal joint component are grasped between the clinician's thumb and forefinger. A long axis distraction force is applied. Volar and dorsal glides can be used to increase flexion and extension, respectively (Fig. 6–21).

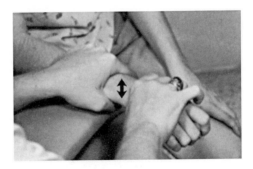

Figure 6–20. Dorsal and volar radiocarpal glides.

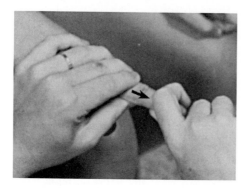

Figure 6–21. Interphalangeal distraction with volar, dorsal, medial, and lateral glides.

Note:

The position of the mobilizing fingers can be moved to the medial and lateral aspects of the phalanx, and medial and lateral glides can be used to increase abduction and adduction. These same procedures can be used at the metacarpophalangeal joint and, in the lower extremity, for the metatarsophalangeal joint and toe interphalangeal joints.

Lower Extremity

KNEE

Inferior and Superior Patellar Glides

Use:

This technique is effective for increasing patellar mobility and facilitating knee extension.

Position:

The athlete is supine with the knee slightly flexed.

Procedure:

The patella is grasped between the clinician's thumbs and forefingers. Alternating inferiorly and superiorly directed forces are applied (Figs. 6–22 and 6–23).

Medial and Lateral Patellar Glides

Use:

This technique is effective for increasing patellar mobility.

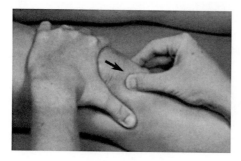

Figure 6–22. Inferior patellar glide.

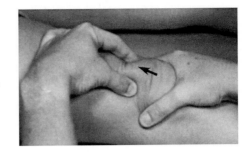

Figure 6–23. Superior patellar glide.

Position:	The athlete is supine, with the knee slightly flexed.
Procedure:	The clinician grasps the patella between the thumbs and forefingers of both hands. The patella is forced medially and laterally (Figs. 6–24 and 6–25).

Anterior and Posterior Tibial Glides

Use:	This technique is effective for increasing knee flexion and extension.
Position:	The athlete is supine, with the knee flexed to approximately 90° and the foot resting on the table.
Stabilization:	The athlete's foot is stabilized under the edge of the clinician's thigh as with the anterior and posterior drawer tests for knee laxity.
Procedure:	The clinician grasps the proximal tibia with fingers interlaced in the popliteal space and applies an anteriorly directed force to facilitate extension. For increasing flexion, the clinician's thumbs are placed over the proximal tibia, and a posteriorly directed force is applied to the tibia.

Posterior Tibial Glide in Extension

Use:	This technique is effective for increasing flexion.
Position:	The athlete is seated, with the knee flexed over the edge of the table.

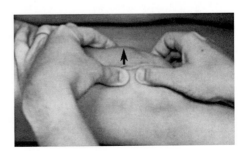

Figure 6–24. Medial patellar glide.

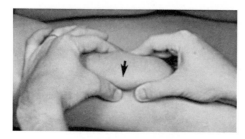

Figure 6–25. Lateral patellar glide.

Stabilization: Standing on the medial side of the athlete's leg, the clinician grasps the athlete's ankle and supports the leg in full extension.

Procedure: The clinician places the palm of the hand on the proximal aspect of the athlete's tibia and extends the elbow to provide a posteriorly directed force to the proximal tibia (Fig. 6–26).

ANKLE

Talocrural Joint Distraction

Use: This technique is effective for reducing pain.

Position: The athlete is supine, with the ankle resting in a neutral position.

Procedure: With both hands, the clinician grasps the rearfoot with fingers interlaced over the dorsum of the foot. A distraction force is applied parallel to the long axis of the leg.

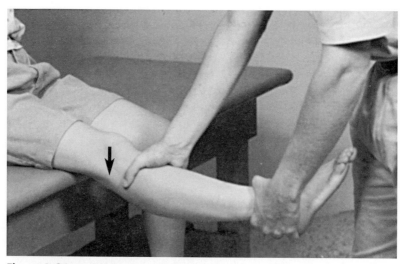

Figure 6–26. Posterior tibial glide in extension.

Talar Distraction with Posterior, Medial, and Lateral Glides

Use: This technique is effective for increasing dorsiflexion, inversion, and eversion.

Position: The athlete is supine, with the leg supported and the heel over the edge of the supporting surface.

Stabilization: The clinician stabilizes the leg by grasping the distal tibia and fibula with one hand.

Procedure: The clinician's hand grasps the athlete's rearfoot on the dorsal surface and applies a posteriorly directed glide to the talus in order to increase dorsiflexion. To increase eversion, the clinician grasps below the talus along the calcaneus and applies a medially directed force. Lateral glides in the same position will increase inversion (Fig. 6–27).

Anterior Talar Glide

Use: This technique is effective for increasing plantar flexion.

Position: The athlete is prone, with the foot hanging over the edge of table. A towel may be placed under the lower leg and ankle for comfort.

Stabilization: The clinician stabilizes the lower leg by grasping around the distal tibia and fibula.

Procedure: The web space of the clinician's other hand is placed on the posterior aspect of the talus and calcaneus. The calcaneus is distracted and an anteriorly directed force is applied to the calcaneus and talus (Fig. 6–28).

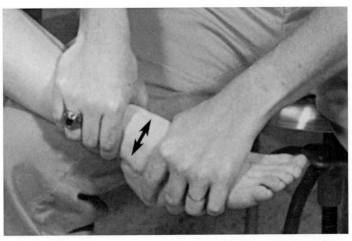

Figure 6–27. Talar distraction with posterior, medial, and lateral glides.

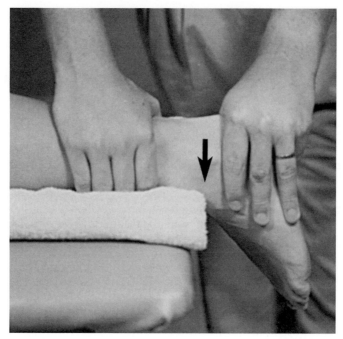

Figure 6–28. Anterior talar glide.

References

1. Bandy, W.D., and Irion, J.M. (1994): The effect of time on static stretch on the flexibility of the hamstring muscles. Phys. Ther., 74:845–852.
2. Barak, T., Rosen, E.R., and Sofer, R. (1990): Basic concepts of orthopaedic manual therapy. *In:* Gould, J.A. (ed.): Orthopaedic and Sports Physical Therapy. St. Louis., C.V. Mosby, pp. 195–211.
3. Brodowicz, G.R., Welsh, R., and Wallis, J. (1996): Comparison of stretching with ice, stretching with heat, or stretching alone on hamstring flexibility. J. Athl. Train., 31:324–327.
4. Condom, S.M., and Hutton, R.S. (1987): Soleus muscle electromyographic activity and ankle dorsiflexion range of motion during four stretching procedures. Phys. Ther., 67:24–30.
5. Cornelius, W.L., and Craft-Hamm, K. (1988): Proprioceptive neuromuscular facilitation flexibility techniques: Acute effects on arterial blood pressure. Physician Sportmed., 16:152–161.
6. Cornelius, W.L., Ebrahim, K., Watson, J., et al. (1992): The effects of cold application and modified PNF stretching techniques on hip joint flexibility in college males. Res. Q. Exerc. Sport, 63:311–314.
7. Cornelius, W.L., Jensen, R.L., and Odell, M.E. (1995): Effects of PNF stretching phases on acute arterial blood pressure. Can. J. Appl. Physiol., 20:222–229.
8. Cyriax, J.H. (1975): Textbook of Orthopaedic Medicine, 6th ed. Vol. I. Diagnosis of Soft Tissue Lesions. Baltimore, Williams & Wilkins.
9. Draper, D.O., and Ricard, M.D. (1995): Rate of temperature decay in human muscle following 3 MHz ultrasound: The stretching window revealed. J. Athl. Train., 30:304–307.
10. Etnyre, B.R., and Abraham, L.D. (1986): Gains in range of ankle dorsiflexion using three popular stretching techniques. Am. J. Phys. Med., 65:189–196.
11. Gillette, T.M., Holland, G.J., Vincent, W.J., et al. (1991): Relationship of body core temperature and warm-up to knee range of motion. J. Orthop. Sports Phys. Ther., 12:126–131.
12. Godges, J.J., MacRae, H., Longdon, C., et al. (1989): The effects of two stretching procedures on hip range of motion and gait economy. J. Orthop. Sports Phys. Ther., 11:350–357.
13. Godges, J.J., MacRae, P.G., and Engelke, K.A. (1993): Effects of exercise on hip range of motion, trunk muscle performance, and gait economy. Phys. Ther., 73:468–477.
14. Hanten, W.P., and Chandler, S.D. (1994): Effects of myofascial release leg pull and sagittal plane isometric contract-relax techniques on passive straight leg raise angle. J. Orthop. Sports Phys. Ther., 20:138–144.
15. Hepburn, G.R. (1987): Case studies: Contracture and stiff joint management with Dynasplint. J. Orthop. Sports Phys. Ther., 8:498–504.
16. Hepburn, G.R., and Crivelli, K.J. (1984): Use of elbow Dynasplint for reduction of elbow flexion contractures: A case study. J. Orthop. Sports Phys. Ther., 5:269–274.
17. Kaltenborn, F.M. (1980): Mobilization of the Extremity Joints: Examination and Basic Treatment Techniques. Oslo, Olaf Noris Bokhandel.

18. Kessler, R.N., and Hertling, D. (1983): Management of Common Musculoskeletal Disorders. Philadelphia, Harper & Row.
19. Kisner, C., and Colby, L. (1985): Therapeutic Exercise: Foundations and Techniques. Philadelphia, F.A. Davis.
20. Knott, M., and Voss, D.E. (1968): Proprioceptive Neuromuscular Facilitation, 2nd ed. New York, Harper & Row.
21. Kottke, F.J., Pauley, D.L., and Ptak, K.A. (1966): The rationale for prolonged stretching for correction of shortening of connective tissue. Arch. Phys. Med. Rehabil., 47:345–352.
22. Laban, N.M. (1962): Collagen tissue: Implications of its response to stress in vitro. Arch. Phys. Med. Rehabil., 43:461–466.
23. Lehman, J.F., and DeLateur, B.J. (1982): Therapeutic heat. In: Lehmann, J.F. (ed.): Therapeutic Heat and Cold. Baltimore, Williams & Wilkins, pp. 404–405, 428.
24. Lehmann, J.F., DeLateur, B.J., and Silverman, D.R. (1966): Selective heating effects of ultrasound in human beings. Arch. Phys. Med. Rehabil., 47:331–339.
25. Lehmann, J.F., Masock, A.J., Warren, C.G., et al. (1970): Effect of therapeutic temperatures on tendon extensibility. Arch. Phys. Med. Rehabil., 51:481–487.
26. Lentell, G., Hetherington, T., Eagan, J., et al. (1992): The use of thermal agents to influence the effectiveness of a low-load prolonged stretch. J. Orthop. Sports Phys. Ther., 16:200–207.
27. Light, K.E., Nuzik, S., Personius, W., et al. (1984): Low load prolonged stretch versus high load restretch treating knee contractures. Phys. Ther., 64:330–333.
28. Lucas, R.C., and Koslow, R. (1984): Comparative study of static, dynamic, and proprioceptive neuromuscular facilitation stretching techniques on flexibility. Perceptual Motor Skills, 58:615–618.
29. Maitland, G.D. (1977): Extremity Manipulation, 2nd ed. London, Butterworth Publishers.
30. Medeiros, J.M., Smidt, G.L., Burmeister, L.F., et al. (1977): The influence of isometric exercise and passive stretch on hip joint motion. Phys. Ther., 57:518–523.
31. Mennell, J. (1964): Joint Pain. Boston, Little, Brown & Co.
32. Moore, M.A., and Hutton, R.S. (1980): Electromyographic investigation of muscle stretching technique. Med. Sci. Sports Exerc., 12:322–329.
33. Osternig, L.R., Robertson, R., Troxel, R., et al. (1987): Muscle activation during Proprioceptive Neuromuscular Facilitation (PNF) stretching techniques. Am. J. Phys. Med., 66:298–307.
34. Osternig, L.R., Robertson, R.N., Troxel, R.K., et al. (1990): Differential responses to proprioceptive neuromuscular facilitation (PNF) stretch techniques. Med. Sci. Sports Exerc., 22:106–111.
35. Paris, S.V. (1979): Extremity Dysfunction and Mobilization. Atlanta, Institute Press.
36. Prentice, W.E. (1983): A comparison of static stretching and PNF stretching for improving hip joint flexibility. Athl. Train., 18:56–59.
37. Prentice, W.E. (1992): Techniques of manual therapy for the knee. J. Sports Rehabil., 1:249–257.
38. Prentice, W.E. (1994): Maintaining and improving flexibility. In: Prentice, W.E. (ed.): Rehabilitation Techniques in Sports Medicine. St. Louis, C.V. Mosby, pp. 42–45.
39. Prentice, W.E. (1994): Mobilization and traction techniques in rehabilitation. In: Prentice, W.E. (ed.): Rehabilitation Techniques in Sports Medicine. St. Louis, C.V. Mosby, pp. 138–163.
40. Quillen, W.S., and Gieck, J.H. (1988): Manual therapy: Mobilization of the motion-restricted knee. Athl. Train., 23 123–130.
41. Quillen, W.S., Halle, J.S., and Rouillier, L.H. (1992): Manual therapy: Mobilization of the motion-restricted shoulder. J. Sports Rehabil., 1:237–248.
42. Rose, S., Draper, D.O., Schulthies, S.S., et al. (1996): The stretching window part two: Rate of thermal decay in deep muscle following 1-MHz Ultrasound. J. Athl. Train., 31:139–143.
43. Sady, S.P., Wortman, M., and Blanke, D. (1982): Flexibility training: Ballistic, static, or proprioceptive neuromuscular facilitation? Arch. Phys. Med. Rehabil., 63:261–263.
44. Sapega, A., Quedenfeld, T.C., Moyer, R.A., et al. (1981): Biophysical factors in range of motion exercise. Physician Sportsmed., 9:57–65.
45. Reference deleted.
46. Stap, L.J., and Woodfin, P.M. (1986): Continuous passive motion in the treatment of knee flexion contracture. Phys. Ther., 66:1720–1722.
47. Stromberg, D., and Wiederhielm, C.A. (1969): Viscoelastic description of a collagenous tissue in simple elongation. J. Appl. Physiol., 26:857–862.
48. Sullivan, M., Dejulia, J.J., and Worrell, T.W. (1992): Effects of pelvic position and stretching method on hamstring muscle flexibility. Med. Sci. Sports Exerc., 24:1383–1389.
49. Sullivan, P.E., and Markos, P.D. (1987): Clinical Procedures in Therapeutic Exercise. Norwalk, CT, Appleton & Lange.
50. Tanijawa, M.D. (1972): Comparison of the hold relax procedure in passive immobilization on increasing muscle length. Phys. Ther., 52:725–735.
51. Travell, J.G., and Simons, D.G. (1983): Myofascial Pain and Dysfunction: The Trigger Point Manual. Baltimore, Williams & Wilkins.
52. Voss, D.E., Ionta, M.K., and Myers, B.J. (1985): Proprioceptive Neuromuscular Facilitation: Patterns and Techniques, 3rd ed. Philadelphia, Harper & Row.
53. Wallin, D., Ekblon, B., Grahn, R., et al. (1985): Improvement of muscle flexibility. Am. J. Sports Med., 13:263–268.
54. Warren, C.G., Lehmann, J.F., and Koblanski, J.N. (1971): Elongation of rat tail tendon: Effect of load and temperature. Arch. Phys. Med. Rehabil., 52:465–474.

55. Warren, C.G., Lehmann, J.F., and Koblanski, J.N. (1976): Heat and stress procedures: An evaluation using rat tail tendon. Arch. Phys. Med. Rehabil., 57:122–126.
56. Wiktorsson Moller, M., Oberg, B., Ekstrand, J., et al. (1988): Effects of warming up, massage, and stretching and range of motion for muscle strength in the lower extremity. Am. J. Sports Med., 11:249–252.
57. Worrell, T.W., Smith, T.L., and Winegardner, J. (1994): Effect of hamstring stretching on hamstring muscle performance. J. Orthop. Sports Phys. Ther., 20:154–159.

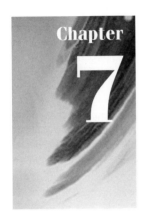

Chapter 7

Introduction to Rehabilitation

Gary L. Harrelson, Ed.D., A.T.,C., and
Deidre Leaver-Dunn, M.Ed., A.T.,C.

Rehabilitation, or reconditioning, is a dynamic program of prescribed exercise for preventing or reversing the deleterious effects of inactivity while returning an individual to his or her former level of competition.[86] Unlike conventional rehabilitation, in which complete return of function may not be possible, athletic rehabilitation combines exercise and therapeutic modalities to restore athletes to their supernormal level of activity. Athletic rehabilitation not only includes complete restoration of unrestricted performance but also strives for a level of conditioning greater than that which the athlete had prior to injury. It must take into account muscular strength, power, flexibility, and endurance, as well as balance, proprioception, timing, and cardiovascular performance.[86] Each rehabilitation program must be individualized to meet the special needs of each athlete.

Athletic rehabilitation primarily encompasses the restoration of traumatized musculoskeletal structures. Rarely is an injury so mild that some form of rehabilitation is not necessary, and as a rule, the more serious an injury, the more prolonged and necessary the rehabilitation.[5] The effectiveness of rehabilitation in the recovery period, either postinjury or postsurgery, usually determines the degree and success of future athletic competition.[5, 62] Moreover, injuries sustained during athletic participation are usually produced under circumstances inherent to the specific sport; therefore, the athlete can be exposed to identical recurrent trauma, making reinjury likely.[76] This potential for reinjury necessitates thorough and complete rehabilitation. Figure 7–1 illustrates the body's response to injury and the result of inadequate rehabilitation.

In any injury, specific physiologic events occur in response to trauma (see Chap. 2). It is the clinician's role to reduce the severity of these physiologic effects, optimize healing time, and return the athlete to competition as soon as possible without compromising the athlete's well-being. The goals of any rehabilitation program include the following:

1. Decrease in pain
2. Decrease in inflammatory response to trauma
3. Return of full, pain-free, active range of motion
4. Decrease in effusion
5. Return of full muscular strength, power, and endurance
6. Return to full asymptomatic functional activities at the preinjury level

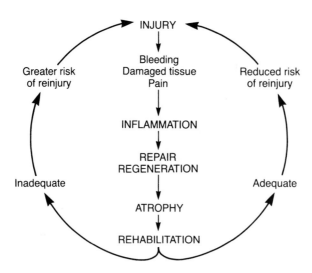

Figure 7–1. The body's response to injury and the role of rehabilitation. (From Welch, B. [1986]: The injury cycle. Sports Med. Update, 1:1.)

Swelling, pain, and spasm can inhibit early institution of a rehabilitation program. The use of various modalities can be instrumental in controlling and reducing these responses, allowing the athlete to begin early range-of-motion and strengthening exercises. The modality itself, however, is never considered the cure for most athletic injuries. Only through therapeutic exercise can the injured body part or parts be returned to the preinjury level. If a rehabilitation program is not instituted in conjunction with therapeutic modalities, the injury cycle may continue.

Early exercise is essential to rehabilitation. Athletes can improve their physical condition by about 1% daily, whereas they lose from 3% to 7% of their fitness daily if they remain totally inactive. Therefore, the longer an athlete is inactive, the longer it takes to complete the rehabilitation program.[20, 60] The proper use of exercise can expedite the healing process, and the lack of exercise during the early stages of rehabilitation may result in permanent disability. Caution must be observed, however, because exercise that is too vigorous also can result in permanent disability. Some limitations may be required to protect a surgical repair or allow an injury to heal properly. Optimal conditions for healing depend on a fine balance between protection from stress and return to normal function at the earliest possible time.

Each rehabilitation program must be individualized; there is no "cookbook" rehabilitation program for every injury that can be used for every athlete. A rehabilitation program should be designed to meet the athlete's needs, to address the specific deficiencies, and to take into account the athlete's specific functional demands for the sport, rather than to fit the athlete into a treatment plan.

The general goals of rehabilitation have already been mentioned. Before the rehabilitation program begins, the clinician and athlete should develop a set of short- and long-term goals based on the athlete's injury or surgical procedure. The use of pre-established rehabilitation protocols as guidelines for advancement of the athlete through the rehabilitation program can be valuable. Protocols should be grounded in principles derived from research on healing time and joint kinematics. Goals can be outlined in relationship to range of motion, weight bearing, and progressive-resistance exercise (PRE) weight progression. Rehabilitation protocols are only guidelines, however, and individuals tolerate pain differently and heal at varying rates. The athlete's rehabilitation advancement should be based on the clinician's daily assessment of subjective reports and objective findings. Advancement from one rehabilitation phase to another should not occur until the athlete has achieved the goals outlined in the current phase.

REHABILITATION CONCEPTS

Healing Constraints

The most important factors to consider in designing a rehabilitation program are the physiologic constraints to healing. Houglum, in her review[61] of the literature on tensile strength of various structures, reports the general agreement that immediately after an injury there is little or no loss of tensile strength, but within the first few days a significant loss of tensile strength can be observed. The length of time for this reduction in tensile strength is highly variable, depending on the extent of injury and the structures involved. This phase of reduction in tensile strength may last from day 1 to day 16 after injury.[61] Wounds in muscle and skin are usually closed securely within 5 to 8 days.[23] Tendons and ligaments recover much more slowly than muscle, which has been reported to reach near-normal tensile strength in 7 to 11 days.[44, 45] Tendons and ligaments may take 3 to 5 weeks to heal before progressing to a level of increased tensile strength.[23, 61] The reported times for tendons and ligaments to reach their near-normal strengths are varied, ranging from 4 months to 1 year, depending on the extent of injury and the duration of immobilization.[61] Animal investigations by Bosch and Kasperczyk[14] suggest that tendinous tissues used in the reconstruction of ligaments may never approach the strength of the original ligament. The rate of healing in bone is highly variable and may be estimated by considering the patient's age, the site and type of injury, and the blood supply to the area.[23] Because physiologic healing is affected by the age, health, and nutritional status of the athlete and the magnitude of the pathology, the rehabilitation program must be structured around these restraints.

Management of Pain and Swelling

Pain and swelling are major factors in the initiation of a therapeutic exercise program and are usually the first signs of injury. Pain varies according to the nature of the injury and the athlete's pain tolerance. In treating pain, it is first necessary to classify pain as acute or chronic. Pain is a symptom that helps in evaluating an injury and in determining the course of treatment. Acute pain is typically of short duration and is associated with an injury or surgery. It is often a protective response by the body, warning that something is wrong and inducing a cycle of muscle spasm and protective guarding. Chronic pain is present for a long period, frequently recurs, and often serves no purpose. It may exist long after the original injury has healed, as a result of such factors as altered biomechanics or learned habits of guarding. In the person with chronic pain, the pain may become a dysfunction in itself.[85]

It is important to know the underlying cause of pain because this has a direct bearing on the approach to pain management. Numerous therapeutic modalities can be used to control or manage pain. Continuous passive motion has also been shown to be effective in reducing pain associated with the acute stage of inflammation.[89] It is necessary for the clinician to understand the principles and applications of specific therapeutic choice or choices for pain management (see Chap. 5).

Control of existing swelling and prevention of further effusion are critical in the rehabilitation process. Swelling can compress sensory nerve endings and contribute to pain. In the acute injury state, ice, compression, and elevation should be used. Ice helps prevent secondary hypoxic injury and helps control hemorrhage and edema. Application of external pressure to the injury site helps control the amount of swelling. Compression wraps should be applied in a distal to proximal direction, with a decreasing pressure gradient. Tubi-Grip* or a stockinette is excellent for compression and can be applied and removed easily by the athlete. Elevation assists the lymphatic system in moving any extracellular tissue fluid away from the injury site.

Various modalities may be used in the management of swelling. The use of intermittent compression units in conjunction with elevation aids greatly in reducing edema. Electrical muscle stimulation can be used to create a muscle-pumping effect, facilitating removal of excess fluid. This can be further enhanced by voluntary isometric muscle contractions, as tolerated. Contrast hydrotherapy may be implemented after the acute phase of inflammation to facilitate removal and resorption of excess fluid. In addition, centripetal massage in conjunction with extremity elevation assists the lymphatic system in dissipating swelling.

Therapeutic exercise itself helps diminish swelling, which is an advantage of early motion. Pain and swelling can often cause transitory paralysis of a body part. This has been described in the knee as neural inhibition of the quadriceps muscle.[34] Along with the use of electrical muscle stimulation for muscle re-education, as the pain and effusion decrease, the athlete's ability to recruit and control the quadriceps muscle improves.[125]

Kinematic Chain

The term kinematic chain was introduced by Reuleaux[98] in 1875 to refer to a mechanical system of links in engineering. In engineering, a kinematic chain is usually a closed system of links joined together so that if any free link is moved on a fixed link, all the other links move in a predictable pattern. Steindler[108] first suggested the terms open kinetic chain (OKC) and closed kinetic chain (CKC) and defined a kinetic chain in the human body as a combination of successively arranged joints that constitutes a complex motor unit. The CKC is exemplified by the erect, weight-bearing standing position. With few exceptions, however, the system of skeletal links in the human body is generally composed not of closed chains but of open ones, because the peripheral extremities can move freely.[48, 92] The lower extremity is considered to be an OKC when the foot is off the ground and a CKC when the foot is in contact with a supporting surface. The kinetic chain concept allows the action of the entire lower or upper extremity to be viewed in a functional relationship.

Steindler[109] described an OKC as being characterized by the distal segment terminating freely in space, whereas in a CKC the distal segment of the joint is fixed and meets with considerable external resistance, which prohibits or restrains its free motion. Eventually the external resistance may be overcome, and the peripheral portion of the joint may move against this resistance.[109] Initially, closed kinetic chain exercise (CKCE) was characterized by the distal segment being fixed, the body weight being supported by the extremity, and considerable external resistance (Fig. 7–2); open kinetic chain exercise (OKCE) was characterized by the distal segment not being fixed, body weight not being supported, and negligible external resistance. As research has examined CKCE and OKCE, the basic characteristics have expanded (Table 7–1).

Although characterization of CKCE and OKCE has broadened, there is some debate regarding the application of lower extremity CKCE principles to the upper extremity. Because of the unique anatomic and biomechanical features of the shoulder, as well as the functional aspects,[130] applying the traditional definitions of OKCE and CKCE is difficult. Wilk and colleagues state the following[130]:

> The conditions that apply to the lower extremity such as weight-bearing forces, which create a closed kinetic chain effect, do not routinely occur in the upper extremity. However, due to the unique anatomical configuration of the glenohumeral

*Available from Sepro, Montgomeryville, Pennsylvania

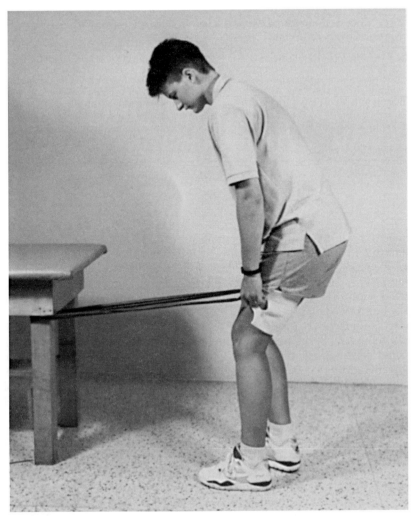

Figure 7-2. The closed-chain terminal knee extension represents the early definition of closed kinetic chain exercise. The distal segment is fixed and the body weight is supported by the extremity and an external resistance.

joint, whereas the stabilizing muscles contract producing a joint compression force that stabilizes the joint much to the same effect as closed kinetic chain exercise for the lower extremity. It is for this reason we believe that the principle of closed kinetic chain exercise is explained for the lower extremity may not apply for upper extremity exercises. Rather, we suggest specific terminology for the upper extremity exercise program under specific conditions, such as weight bearing or axial compression.

Because of incongruities between the lower and upper extremities, some authors[32, 79] have recommended different classification systems for describing OKCE and CKCE for the upper extremity. Dillman and colleagues[32] proposed three classifications for OKCE and CKCE for the upper extremity based on mechanics. The system takes into account the boundary condition and the external load encountered at the distal segment. The boundary condition of the distal segment may be either fixed or moveable, and an external load may or may not exist at the distal link. Thus, the categories include a fixed boundary with an external load (FEL), a moveable boundary with an external load (MEL), and a moveable boundary with no external load (MNL). The terms FEL and MNL correspond to the extremes of CKC and OKC exercises, respectively, and MEL refers to the "gray" region between these two extremes. The exercises

Table 7–1. Characteristics of Closed Kinetic Chain Exercise Versus Open Kinetic Chain Exercise

CLOSED KINETIC CHAIN EXERCISE	OPEN KINETIC CHAIN EXERCISE
Large resistance and low acceleration forces	Large acceleration and low resistance forces
Greater compressive forces	Distraction and rotatory forces
Joint congruency	Promotion of a stable base
Decreased shear	Joint mechanoreceptor deformation
Stimulation of proprioceptors	Concentric acceleration and eccentric deceleration
Enhanced dynamic stabilization	Assimilation of function

Data from Lephart, S.M., and Henry, T.J. (1995): Functional rehabilitation for the upper and lower extremity. Orthop. Clin. North Am., 26:579–592.

performed for each classification system appear in Table 7–2. Muscle function was determined by electromyography. This investigation found that once the external load became considerable, muscle activation was similar regardless of the boundary. These authors suggest that the confusing terms OKC and CKC be eliminated and that the biomechanics, load, and muscular response of the exercises be stressed.

Lephart and Henry[79] proposed a functional classification system (FCS) for upper extremity rehabilitation with the objective of restoring functional stability of the shoulder by re-establishing neuromuscular control for overhead activities. This system addresses three areas of the shoulder complex: scapulothoracic stabilization, glenohumeral stabilization, and humeral control. The FCS considers boundary and load and also the direction in which the load is applied. Table 7–3 summarizes the FCS.

There appears to be agreement that the traditional classification system for OKC and CKC exercises, which considers the fixation of the distal segment, the body weight, and the external resistance, is not adequate in describing exercises for the upper extremities. Both open- and closed-chain exercises have characteristics that are important in restoring strength and neuromuscular control to an injured upper extremity, and both should be incorporated into an upper extremity rehabilitation program.[79, 130]

The advantages of CKCE over OKCE have been well reported in the literature and include a decrease in shear forces, stimulation of proprioceptors, enhancement of joint stability, allowance for more functional patterns of movement, and greater specificity for athletic activities.[15, 49, 54, 130]

Most of the research regarding CKCE has targeted the lower extremity, specifically the knee joint. With regard to the effect of CKCE on the knee, most investigations have examined anterior tibial displacement and the resultant

Table 7–2. Examples of Exercises in the Closed Kinetic Chain Exercise Classification System for the Upper Extremity

CATEGORY	EXERCISES
Movable boundary, no external load	Bench press–type motions without weight
Movable boundary, external load	Bench press (135, 95, and 45 lb)
	Arm extension (25-lb dumbbell)
Fixed boundary, external load	Push-up from knees
	Push-up with a plus
	Two-handed wall press
	Axial wall press

From Dillman, C.J., Murray, T.A., and Hintermeister, R.A. (1994): Biomechanical differences of open and closed chain exercises with respect to the shoulder. J. Sports Rehabil., 3:228–238.

Table 7-3. Summary of Functional Classification System

CLASSIFICATION	CHARACTERISTICS	EXAMPLES
Fixed boundary: external, axial load	Considerable load, slow velocity NM reaction: active or reactive MM action: coactivation, acceleration, deceleration Coactivation of force couples Joint compression Minimal shear forces Promotion of dynamic stability	Axial loading in tripod position Slide board Unstable platform
Moveable boundary: external, axial load	Considerable load, variable velocity MM action: coactivation, acceleration, deceleration Coactivation of force couples Promotion of dynamic stability Activation of prime movers Minimal shear forces	Closed-chain protraction/retraction on an isokinetic dynamometer Traditional bench press Rhythmic stabilization activities
Movable boundary: external, rotatory load	Variable load, functional speeds NM reaction: active or reactive MM action: coactivation, acceleration, deceleration Stability of scapular and glenohumeral base Activation of prime movers Functional joint kinematics Functional motor patterns	Isokinetics in functional diagonal patterns Multiaxial machine Resistance tubing exercise Proprioceptive neuromuscular facilitation exercise
Movable boundary: no load	Negligible load, variable velocity NM reaction: active or passive MM action: acceleration, deceleration, or perceptual Activation of muscles, proximal to distal Low muscle activation without resistance Functional significance	Joint sensibility training: active and passive

From Lephart, S.M., and Henry, T.J. (1996): The physiological basis for open and closed kinetic chain rehabilitation for the upper extremity. J. Sports Rehabil., 5:77.
MM, Muscular; NM, neuromuscular.

stresses placed on the anterior cruciate ligament. The following conclusions may be drawn from these investigations:

- Joint compressive forces are increased as a result of the lower extremity being loaded by the body weight.[49, 87, 103]
- Anterior translation of the tibia on the femur is decreased.[33, 49, 58, 84, 87, 103, 127, 134, 135]
- Elongation force on the ACL is decreased.[33, 84, 87, 127, 135]
- Patellofemoral pain is less.[16, 103]
- The quadriceps and hamstrings cocontract.[134]
- Proprioceptors are stimulated.[15, 107]

On the other hand, the following results are obtained with use of OKCE in the lower extremity:

- Knee motions are isolated, and cocontractions are absent at the knee.[95]
- Patellofemoral compression is increased.[63]
- Anterior shear forces are increased.[33, 49, 58, 87, 135]
- The anterior cruciate ligament is elongated.[58, 87]

CKCEs involving locomotion have received additional attention. Flynn and Soutas-Little[37, 38] and others[58, 87] examined mechanical power, muscle action, and patellofemoral joint compressive forces during forward and backward running. Results from these studies show that backward running is associated with concentric and isometric quadriceps contractions[37] and with decreased patellofemoral compressive forces.[38] Similarly, Zimmerman and colleagues[136] examined muscle action during forward and retrograde stepping on a step ergometer. In this research, the forward condition was found to be more effective for general lower extremity muscle activation.[136]

Historically, criteria for returning an athlete to activity have been peak torque values and muscle girth. Unfortunately, these criteria do not relate to returning an athlete to previous functional levels.[81] OKCE assessment does allow for quantitative clinical assessment of muscle strength.[81] Unfortunately, a strong relationship between OKCE and functional activity has not been established,[15] nor does isokinetic testing appear to correlate with the efficacy of CKCE.[99] It has been suggested that CKCE be tested functionally.[134]

Types of Exercises

As defined previously, therapeutic exercise involves body movements prescribed to restore or favorably alter specific functions in an individual after injury. Figure 7–3 classifies the various therapeutic exercises that a clinician can incorporate into a therapeutic rehabilitation program.

STATIC EXERCISE

Static exercise incorporates isometric contractions in which force is generated without restricting movement or changing the joint angle (Fig. 7–4). The muscle being used maintains a fixed length, with the tension generated being equal to the resistance encountered. Isometric contractions are exertional where the velocity is zero.[86] Isometric exercise is the least effective method of building strength because, although circumference and strength increase, the strength gains are limited to the joint angle at which the contraction occurred. In the early phases of rehabilitation this may be the only type of exercise permitted, and it is preferable to no exercise at all.

PASSIVE EXERCISE

Passive exercise techniques attempt to restore physiologic and accessory joint motions. Restoration of physiologic motion is usually performed for the injured athlete by the clinician or by a mechanical appliance such as a continuous passive motion unit or isokinetic dynamometer set in the passive mode. Moreover, accessory motion can be restored through mobilization and manipulation techniques. Accessory motions (spins, rolls, and glides) are necessary for physiologic motion to occur (see Chap. 6).

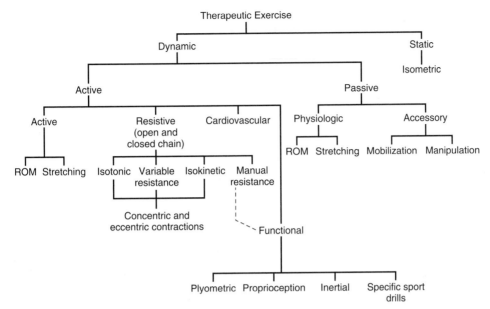

Figure 7–3. Classification of therapeutic exercise. ROM, range of motion. (Modified from Irrgang, J.J. [1995]: Rehabilitation. *In:* Fu, F.H., and Stone, D. [eds.]: Sports Injuries: Mechanisms, Prevention, Treatment. Baltimore, Williams & Wilkins.)

Passive exercise is carried out by the application of some external force, with minimal participation of muscle action by the injured athlete. It may be forced or nonforced. Nonforced exercises are those used to help maintain normal joint motion and are usually kept within a painless range of motion. Conversely, forced passive exercises generally produce movement beyond the limits of free range of motion and are associated with some discomfort to the individual.

ACTIVE EXERCISE

Exercise movements may be active or passive. Active exercise is purposeful voluntary motion that is performed by the injured athlete, with or without resistance and with or without the aid of gravity. Active exercise may be assisted, in which the clinician helps the athlete perform the movement, or resisted, in which there is some form of resistance to the movement. Resisted movements can be further categorized as dynamic or static. Dynamic training refers to moving the resistance through a range of motion. Static exercise refers to contraction against a fixed resistance.

Concentric and Eccentric Contractions

Two types of muscle contractions exist with dynamic training: concentric, in which a shortening of muscle fibers results in a decrease in the angle of the associated joint; and eccentric, in which the muscle resists its own lengthening so that the joint angle increases during the contraction.[86] Concentric and eccentric contractions may also be referred to as positive work and negative work, respectively. Concentric contractions function to accelerate a limb; for example, the shoulder internal rotators accelerate the arm during the acceleration phase of throwing. Conversely, eccentric contractions function to decelerate a limb and provide shock absorption; for example, the shoulder external rotators decelerate the shoulder during the follow-through phase of throwing.[71] The type of muscle contraction determines the amount of force generated. A maximum eccentric

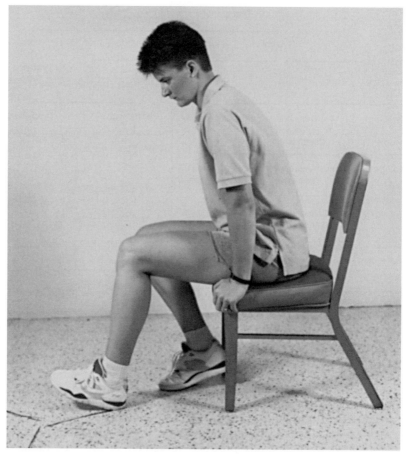

Figure 7–4. Isometric cocontractions of the quadriceps and hamstrings. This is an example of an isometric exercise in which the velocity is zero and the muscle maintains a fixed length.

contraction may generate forces 14% to 50% greater than a concentric contraction of the same group.[26]

Although considered to be more functional than concentric contractions, eccentric contractions are associated with the production of delayed-onset muscle soreness (DOMS).[19, 28, 123] DOMS has been defined as muscular pain or discomfort 1 to 5 days after unusual muscular exertion.[71] The syndrome of DOMS also includes joint swelling[19] and weakness.[19, 28, 123] Of clinical importance is the demonstration of continued weakness after the cessation of pain.[19] Additionally, the onset and degree of DOMS are inversely proportional to the intensity of eccentric exercise.[71] To help minimize the effects of DOMS, eccentric exercises should be progressed gradually.

Dynamic Exercise

Dynamic exercise can be of several types: isotonic, in which the fixed weight is moved through a range of motion; variable-resistance, in which resistance varies in a fixed ratio through a full range of motion; and isokinetic (accommodating variable-resistance), in which the speed of motion is fixed and the resistance varies to accommodate the force input. Additionally, functional exercises such as plyometric, proprioceptive, and inertial exercises and sport-specific drills are also a part of the dynamic exercise spectrum and are necessary for complete rehabilitation of the injured athlete.

Isotonic Exercise

With isotonic exercise, the actual muscle length changes as the muscle causes or resists a change in joint angle. In pure isotonic exercise, the resistance remains constant, whereas the velocity of movement is inversely proportional to the load. This type of exercise is readily available in the form of exercises performed with ankle weights, free weights, and weight machines (Fig. 7–5). Additionally, both eccentric and concentric contractions can be achieved with isotonic exercises. Some disadvantages are inherent, however, and include the fact that the weight is fixed and does not adjust to strength differences in various ranges of motion and the fact that with speed work, the weight is propelled so that the strength required diminishes at the extremes of motion.

In variable-resistance exercise, the resistance varies through the range of motion to match the difference in strength through that specific range. With these types of machines, the axis of rotation of the weight generates an isokinetic-like feel to the motion, but because angular velocity is not controlled, this equipment cannot provide isokinetic resistance (Fig. 7–6).

Manual PRE is a variation of accommodating variable-resistance exercise. The clinician provides the resistance with this mode of exercise and can modify the resistance and speed during the exercise as the athlete's fatigue is recognized. This exercise mode is applicable during early rehabilitation phases and, like proprioceptive neuromuscular facilitation techniques, can produce patterns that cannot be duplicated on machines.

Isokinetic Exercise

Isokinetic exercise, or accommodating variable-resistance exercise, is performed at a set speed, with resistance matching the input of force at that speed. As the force input changes, the resistance changes to match the input, but the speed remains constant. The application of one's own muscular resistance is met with a proportional amount of resistance through full agonist and antagonist ranges of motion (Fig. 7–7). Chapter 8 provides an in-depth discussion of isokinetics.

Inertial Exercise

Inertial loading is a recent addition to the exercise spectrum.[4] This mode of exercise simulates the momentum and velocity changes of functional activity through the reciprocal acceleration and deceleration of a variable mass.[116] Inertial exercise is performed with an Impulse* machine (Fig. 7–8). Albert[3] described the

---

*Available from EMA Inc., Newnan, Georgia

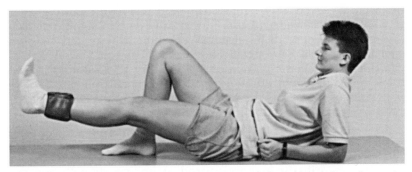

Figure 7–5. Traditional straight leg raises. This is an example of an isotonic exercise in which the resistance remains constant and the velocity is inversely proportional to the load.

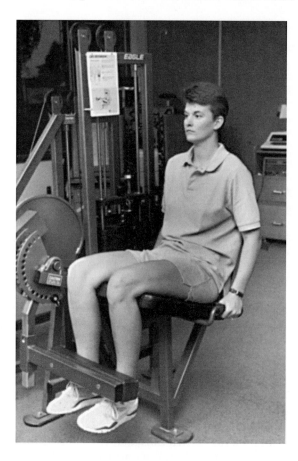

Figure 7–6. Variable-resistance exercise. This offers an isokinetic-like feel through a cam, but because the angular velocity is not controlled, it cannot provide isokinetic resistance.

type of loading that the impulse machine produces as "horizontal, sub-maximal, gravity eliminated plyometrics."

Several studies have examined the efficacy of inertial exercise. Albert and colleagues[4] examined the effectiveness of inertial exercise in producing muscle torque increases in the biceps brachii. In this study, 40 subjects showed significant increases in peak torque at 60° per second and 120° per second after a 5-week inertial exercise training program. Muscle activity during inertial exercise has been investigated by Tracy and colleagues.[116] The authors gathered electromyographic data from the biceps brachii and triceps brachii of 12 subjects during elbow flexion on an inertial exercise system with five random loads. Simultaneous measures of angular velocity and platform acceleration were gathered with a digital motion analysis system. Results of this work indicate that higher velocities were achieved with lighter loads and that significantly greater peak angular velocities occurred with the phasic exercise. No significant difference was seen in peak biceps brachii electromyographic activity between tonic and phasic techniques; however, significantly greater triceps brachii activity was identified during the phasic portion of the exercise. These studies indicate that inertial exercise may be an effective tool for functional muscle strengthening. However, when using inertial exercise, the clinician must consider the effects of load and phase on the desired outcome.

Plyometrics

Plyometrics are drills or exercises aimed at linking strength and speed of movement to produce an explosive-reactive type of muscle response.[126, 129] Plyometrics were initially used in off-season strength-training programs, and only

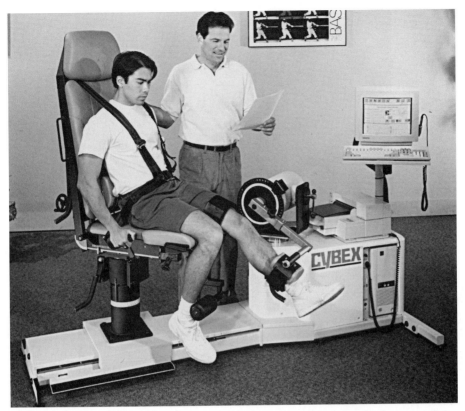

Figure 7–7. The Cybex Single Chair Extremity System (Norm) is an example of accommodating variable-resistance equipment. The resistance changes to match the input, but the speed remains constant. (Photo courtesy of Cybex, Medway, MA.)

recently have they become part of therapeutic rehabilitation. Plyometrics involve a prestretching of a muscle, thereby activating the stretch reflex. The purpose of plyometric training is to heighten the excitability of the neurologic receptors for improved reactivity of the neuromuscular system.[121, 131] By means of an eccentric contraction, the muscle is fully stretched immediately preceding the concentric contraction. The greater the stretch placed on the muscle from its resting length immediately before the concentric contraction, the greater the load the muscle can lift or overcome. Thus, plyometrics have been referred to as "stretch-shortening" drills or "reactive neuromuscular" training.[131] Wilk and colleagues[131] describe three phases of a plyometric exercise:

1. Eccentric phase: this is the preloading period in which the muscle spindle is prestretched prior to activation.
2. Amortization phase: this is the time between the eccentric contraction and initiation of a concentric force. The rate of the stretch is more critical than the duration of the stretch. Therefore, the more quickly an athlete can overcome the yielding eccentric force and produce a concentric force, the more powerful the response.
3. Concentric phase: this is a summation of the eccentric and amortization phases, with the product being an enhanced concentric contraction.

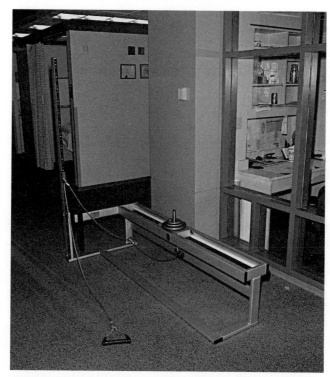

Figure 7–8. Impulse machine for inertial exercise.

Originally used to describe box jumps or depth jumps for the lower extremity, plyometrics have evolved to include hops and bounds that can be used to increase the athlete's speed, power, and skill of movement (Figs. 7–9 and 7–10). Plyometric exercise for the lower extremity has been described in the literature.[17, 18] In addition, the inclusion of plyometrics in a rehabilitation program for upper extremity pathologies has been advocated[128, 129] and described in the literature.[40, 121, 128, 129, 131] These upper extremity plyometric drills are usually insti-

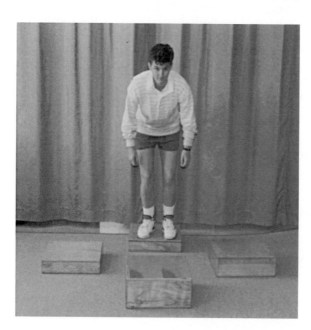

Figure 7–9. Plyometric jumps using small boxes and directional changes.

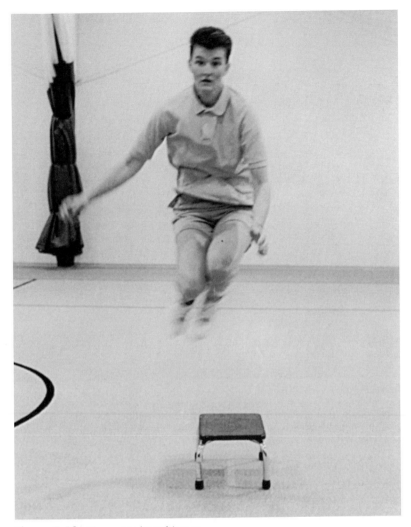

Figure 7-10. Plyometric lateral jumps.

tuted with the use of items such as a medicine ball, surgical tubing, plyoback, and boxes (Figs. 7–11 to 7–13). Plyometrics should be implemented in the late stages of rehabilitation and should mimic a sport-specific skill.

Plyometrics should be used judiciously, however, because they can cause overuse injuries. In order to reduce the chance of injury, plyometric exercises should be progressed from low intensity to high intensity, the athlete should be instructed in the correct technique for performing the exercises, the exercises should be terminated when the athlete can no longer perform them correctly, and an appropriate period for recovery should be allowed. The clinician should remember that postexercise soreness and delayed-onset muscle soreness are by-products of this type of exercise.

Plyometric exercises can be manipulated through intensity, volume, frequency, and recovery.[120] Intensity refers to the amount of effort exerted. In traditional weight-lifting programs, this variable can be manipulated by the amount of weight used. In plyometrics, effort can be increased by raising the height of a step or box, increasing the amount of external weight used, or progressing from a simple to a more complex activity. Volume is the total amount of work performed in a single exercise session. Volume correlates to repetitions in the traditional weight-lifting program. For plyometrics, repetitions may be the num-

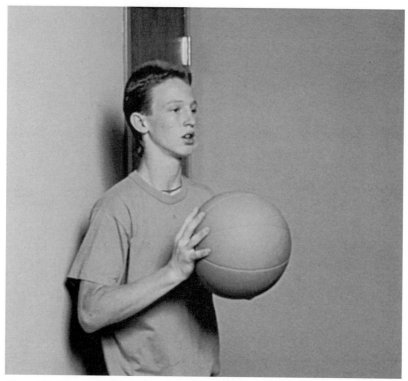

Figure 7–11. The medicine ball can be used by the athlete in various upper extremity plyometric exercises, such as the chest pass demonstrated here. The athlete catches the ball out in front of the body and decelerates the force of the ball before it hits the chest, initiating the stretch reflex. The athlete then explodes forward with the arms to pass the ball back.

ber of foot contacts, jumps, passes, or rotations. Volume should be inversely proportional to intensity. As intensity increases, volume should decrease and vice versa. Frequency is the number of times an exercise session is performed. Although the optimum frequency has not been determined, it is generally regarded that two to three sessions weekly, in conjunction with functional activities, is a reasonable plyometrics schedule. The intensity of the plyometrics

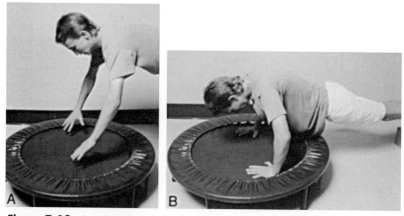

Figure 7–12. *A* and *B*, Plyometric push-ups bounding from the minitrampoline. (Photo courtesy of Sports Medicine Update. Birmingham, Alabama, HealthSouth Rehabilitation Corporation.)

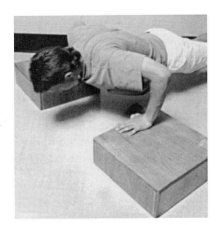

Figure 7–13. Box push-up. (Photo courtesy of Sports Medicine Update. Birmingham, Alabama, HealthSouth Rehabilitation Corporation.)

schedule should determine the recovery time; the higher the intensity, the longer the recovery period should be (48 to 72 hours). Finally, recovery is the rest time between exercise sets. If the goal is power training, a work-to-rest ratio of 1:3 or 1:4 is recommended. If endurance training is the desired outcome, the work-to-rest ratio should be shortened to 1:1 or 1:2.[120]

Absolute contraindications for plyometrics include acute surgery, gross instability, pain, and an athlete not being in a weight program previously. A variety of plyometric exercises are outlined in Appendix A.

Proprioception

A comprehensive rehabilitation program must not overlook the component of neuromuscular control that is necessary for joint stability. The repair of static or dynamic restraints and the strengthening of the appropriate muscles does not prepare a joint for the sudden changes in position that it is exposed to in the athletic arena. To adequately address this phenomenon, the clinician must appreciate the structures contributing to proprioception, as well as the process by which articular sensations contribute to functional stability.

When describing joint sensation, the terms proprioception and kinesthesia are often erroneously interchanged. Proprioception describes the awareness of posture, movement, and changes in equilibrium and the knowledge of position, weight, and resistance of objects in relation to the body.[1] Kinesthesia, however refers to the ability to perceive the extent, direction, or weight of movement.[1] These two definitions are combined into a comprehensive, operational definition: "Proprioception is considered a specialized variation of the sensory modality of touch and encompasses the sensations of joint movement (kinesthesia) and joint position (joint position sense)."[80] As Lephart describes, conscious and unconscious proprioception, respectively, are essential for proper joint function in sports and other daily tasks as well as for reflex stabilization.[78] These articular sensations are the direct focus of proprioceptive rehabilitation and are crucial for efficient, noninjurious movement.

PHYSIOLOGY OF PROPRIOCEPTION

The determinants of proprioceptive sense have been investigated since the mid-1800s. In 1863, Hilton described the innervation of joints by articular branches arising from nerves supplying the muscles of each articulation.[59] Sherrington[104] was the first to note the presence of receptors in the pericapsular structures. He coined the term proprioception to include all neural input originating from the joints, muscles, tendons, and associated deep tissues.[104] Abbott and colleagues[2] later proposed that knee articular sensations were one component of a dynamic stabilization system. This suggestion was supported by subsequent work identifying receptors in various articular structures.[70, 101, 102] Recent research has addressed the alteration of proprioception following injury to the ankle,[43, 47, 50, 75] knee,[6, 8, 55, 80, 82] and shoulder.[53, 106]

The extrinsic innervation of articular structures occurs via afferent stimulation of periarticular receptors (Hilton's law).[59] This stimulation results in the initiation of protective reflexes designed to oppose injurious movement. Hilton's law has been substantiated in animal experiments, with the consensus that maximal firing of the articular receptors occurs when the joint is stressed in the positions of maximal flexion and extension.[25]

The receptors identified by Sherrington[104] have been categorized by location into three separate groups: articular, deep (muscle-tendon related), and superficial (cutaneous). The functions of these receptors are summarized in Table 7–4. Articular receptors are located within the joint capsule, ligaments, and any intra-articular structures within the body.[66] The human joint capsule has been studied extensively and has been found to contain four very distinct types of nerve endings[42, 52, 102]: Ruffini's corpuscles, Golgi receptors, pacinian corpuscles, and free nerve endings. Ruffini's corpuscles are sensitive to stretching of the joint capsule, whereas, Golgi receptors are intraligamentous and have been shown to become active when the ligaments are stressed in the extremes of joint movement. Pacinian corpuscles are sensitive to high-frequency vibration, and the free nerve endings are sensitive to mechanical stress.

Table 7–4. Summary of Mechanoreceptor Function

RECEPTORS	LOCATION	CHARACTERISTICS
Ruffini's corpuscle	Joint capsule	Sensitive to changes in intra-articular pressure Monitors the direction and speed of capsular stretch and amplitude and velocity of joint position change Slowly adapting receptor
Pacinian corpuscle	Joint capsule	Silent in the immobile joint but is activated by the onset or cessation of joint movement; this enables it to signal joint acceleration and deceleration. Thus, it appear to be a rate of motion detector. Rapidly adapting receptor
Golgi-Mazzoni corpuscle	Joint capsule	Responds to perpendicular compression of the capsule but not to stretching of the capsule Slowly adapting receptor
Golgi ligament ending	Joint capsule	Sensitive to tension and stretch on ligaments Monitors position of the bony segments that contribute to a joint Inactive when the joint is immobile Similar to Golgi tendon organ Slowly adpating receptor
Free nerve ending	Joint capsule	Basically a pain receptor Slowly adapting receptor
Golgi tendon organ	Muscle/tendon	Respnds to both contraction and stretch of the musculotendinous junction Provides central nervous system with information concerning the contractile state of muscles Located in the tendon, near the musculotendinous junction Slowly adapting receptor
Muscle spindle	Muscle belly	Responds to muscle length (stretch) as well as to the rate of change of muscle length Appreciates joint position Slowly adapting receptor Contains both motor and sensory nerves

The importance of ligamentous structures in the perception of joint position sense has been documented by various authors.[70, 101, 102] Stimulation of these Golgi receptors causes them to act as mechanical stabilizers as they initiate reflexive muscular contraction in situations of abnormal stress.

Recently the belief that articular receptors alone provide the information necessary to signal joint position sense has shifted. The most conclusive evidence spurring this shift was derived from the study of surgically replaced knees by Skinner and colleagues.[105] This study demonstrated a remarkable maintenance of proprioception in knees after arthroplasty, suggesting a diminished role of articular receptors in the maintenance of proprioception. From these results, the list of structures deemed responsible for joint position sense was expanded to include deep receptors such as muscle spindles, Golgi tendon organs, and receptors of pressure and pain.

The muscle spindle is considered to be the third most complex sensory organ, after the eye and ear. Arranged in parallel with muscle fibers, the muscle spindle is innervated by both afferent and efferent fibers.[132] It detects muscle length and, more importantly, the rate of change in muscle length. Muscle tension is measured by the Golgi tendon organs that are located in the tendon as well as in the fascia.[132]

The final group of receptors that has been postulated to determine proprioceptive sense is the cutaneous receptors. Cutaneous receptors have been classified as mechanoreceptors, thermoreceptors, and nociceptors.[132] Mechanoreceptors include Meissner's, pacinian, and Ruffini's corpuscles, as well as receptors associated with the hair follicles. The thermoreceptors and nociceptors are primarily free nerve endings. Impetus for the suggestion that cutaneous receptors contribute to joint position sense comes from the work of Barrett and colleagues.[8] These investigators studied proprioceptive sense in the knees of patients with osteoarthritis and after total joint replacement. Proprioception and subjective reports of joint position sense were assessed under three conditions: with an elastic bandage, with a neoprene sleeve, and with no support. Objective and subjective measures indicated that the elastic and neoprene sleeves enhanced proprioception. The results of this study support the role of cutaneous receptors as mediators of proprioception.

ASSESSMENT OF PROPRIOCEPTION

Proprioception is assessed by measuring the characteristics that make up the proprioceptive mechanism. This includes kinesthetic sensibility, which is the perception of joint motion, and joint position sensibility, which is the perception of joint position.[13] When peripheral mechanoreceptors are deformed from joint motion, the proprioceptive mechanism is initiated.

Two primary methods have been used to objectively assess kinesthetic sensibility and joint position sensibility: threshold to detection of passive movement (TTDPM) and active or passive repositioning of joint movements. TTDPM is used as a functional indicator of kinesthesia and is used most often to assess afferent activity after ligament injury. Lephart and colleagues[80] have described a device for assessing TTDPM in the knee (Fig. 7–14). The testing mechanism uses a rotational transducer interfaced with a digital microprocessor to provide passive movement of the knee at a constant velocity of 0.5° per second in the frontal plane. A hand-held disengagement switch is activated by the subject when motion is first detected. Cutaneous, auditory, and visual inputs are eliminated through the use of a pneumatic boot, headphones, and a blindfold, respectively. An excellent test-retest reliability ($r = 0.92$) has been established for this device. A similar apparatus has been developed by Borsa and colleagues[13] for assessing TTDPM in the shoulder. This device assesses the subject's ability to detect passive movement in the transverse plane with the shoulder in 90° of abduction

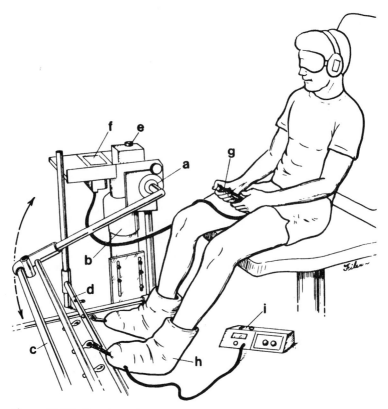

Figure 7–14. Proprioceptive testing device. a, Rotational transducer; b, motor; c, moving arm; d, stationary arm; e, control panel; f, digital microprocessor; g, hand-held disengage switch; h, pneumatic compression boot; and i, pneumatic compression device. Threshold to detection of passive movement is assessed by measuring the angular displacement until the subject senses motion in the knee. (From Lephart, S.M., Kocher, M.S., Fu, F.H., et al. [1992]: Proprioception following anterior cruciate ligament reconstruction. J Sports Rehabil., 1:188–196.)

and elbow in 90° of flexion. External and cutaneous stimuli are eliminated as with the knee-testing device.

Whereas the detection of passive movement is the hallmark of kinesthesia assessment, the ability to actively or passively reproduce a joint angle is the standard for functional measurement of joint position sense. Isokinetic dynamometers with internal goniometers are used in repositioning studies, with the subject situated as for joint testing.[55, 77, 113] As with TTDPM measurement, external stimuli are eliminated by blindfold and pneumatic devices. After the subject is positioned, the extremity is passively moved by the clinician to a predetermined joint angle and held at that angle for several seconds before being passively returned to a starting position. The subject is then instructed to actively move the extremity through an arc of motion to reposition the joint at the first angle. The electrogoniometer within the dynamometer records the subject's repositioning angle; the difference between the passive and the repositioned angle is taken as the score for that trial.

Studies using TTDPM and reproduction of active or passive position sense have predominantly been performed on the knee joint. The results of these investigations have shown decreased kinesthesia with increasing age,[7] with osteoarthritis,[8] and following anterior cruciate ligament disruption,[6, 80] which continues after reconstruction.[80, 82] The inability to actively and passively reproduce the joint angle in dorsiflexion and plantar flexion planes of sprained ankles showed decreased kinesthetic awareness in the involved ankle.[43, 47] Shoulder proprioception studies have shown deficits in TTDPM and repositioning of passive position in unstable shoulders.[13, 106]

Although active joint repositioning has been the basis for several studies of joint position sense,[55, 77, 96, 113] its reliability has been questioned.[111] Szczerba and colleagues assessed active and passive repositioning of ankle inversion-eversion angles in 20 healthy subjects. An isokinetic dynamometer with an internal electrogoniometer was used with a testing speed of 5° per second. Active repositioning was performed as described previously. The protocol for assessment of passive repositioning was similar in that the ankle was passively moved to a preselected angle and then passively returned to a resting position. As the investigator moved the subject's ankle back through the initial arc of motion, the subject was instructed to contract the ankle maximally in the opposite direction when it was perceived that the testing angle had been reached. The difference between the test angle and the subject's repositioned angle was recorded as the error score for each trial in each condition. Analysis of the data revealed significantly smaller error scores for passive repositioning at one testing angle. The results of this study indicate the need for further research to develop standardized, reliable protocols for the assessment of joint position sense.

PROPRIOCEPTION TESTING AND TRAINING

Balance exercises have been used for lower extremity proprioception testing and training. Thus, the ability to quantify balance would help the clinician in objectively determining proprioception deficits. Unfortunately, measurement of balance is difficult because of the many variables that compose it. Attempting to control for all of these variables in a research design is difficult. Currently, research on balance and its correlation to proprioception is in its infancy with respect to published studies. As additional investigations are performed and published, more will become known regarding this rehabilitation parameter. It is hypothesized that injury to the mechanoreceptors results in altered peripheral sensation that affects motor control. These deficits in motor control are thought to result in altered balance.[65] It has been documented that proprioceptors are damaged as a result of injury and must be rehabilitated. The optimal method, mode, duration, and frequency have not been scientifically determined. Additionally, no normative data on proprioception exist for purposes of comparison; typically, proprioception data have been compared to the uninvolved side.

However, some subjective and objective techniques are available. Guiskiewicz and Perrin[51] have described many of the common balance assessment techniques. Subjective clinical measurement of proprioception has included static balance tests, such as Romberg's test, in which the athlete stands with feet together, arms at the sides, and eyes closed. The clinician looks for a tendency to sway or fall to one side. The single-leg stance test requires the athlete to balance on one leg for a specified amount of time with eyes open or closed. Finally, the tandem Romberg's test[35] requires placement of one foot in front of the other (heel to toe). All of these are classified as static assessment techniques and are criticized because of their lack of sensitivity and objectivity.

More recently, high-technology methods of objectively assessing static and dynamic balance have been introduced (Figs. 7–15 and 7–16). Most of these systems attempt to quantify functional balance through analysis of postural sway.[51] Very little data have been published on the reliability of these instruments. Two studies, one by Irrgang and Lephart[64] and the other by Mattacola and colleagues,[88] have assessed the reliability of the Chattecx Balance System.* Irrgang and Lephart[64] reported reasonable reliability within and between days

---

*Available from Chattecx Corporation, Hixon, Tennessee

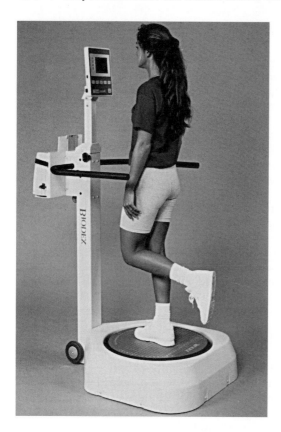

Figure 7-15. Biodex Stability System (Photo courtesy of Biodex Corp., Shirley, New York.)

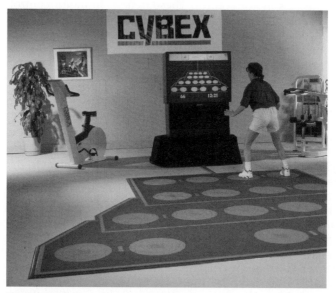

Figure 7-16. Reactor, which can be used to collect data not only on static balance but also on dynamic movements such as hopping, jumping, and pivoting. (Photo courtesy of Cybex, Medway, MA.)

for stable nonmoving measures of balance. Mattacola and colleagues,[88] who examined the intertester reliability values for static and dynamic balance reported a wide range of reliability values and concluded that variability exists for the measure of postural sway for static and dynamic testing conditions. The concept of balance is multifaceted, and assessment must account for vestibular, central nervous system, mechanoreceptor, and visual function, age, muscular strength and fatigue, as well as the environment in which the test is being performed and the subject's motor learning curve. At this time more investigations are needed to determine the efficacy of these instruments.

Proprioceptive exercises for the lower extremity[12, 114, 115] and upper extremity[13, 110, 114] have been described in the literature. Like other exercises, proprioceptive exercises should be specific to the type of activities that athletes will encounter in their sports. Static balancing activities can be used for those athletes who are required to maintain balance in a static position for a sustained period of time, or they may serve as preliminary training activities for those athletes who require balance and control during dynamic activities (Figs. 7–17 and 7–18).

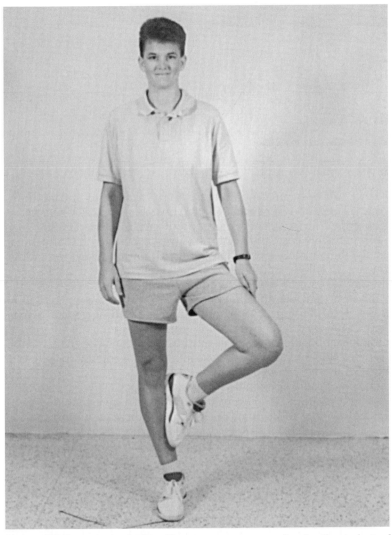

Figure 7–17. Stork stand. The athlete can progress to performing the stork stand with eyes open to eyes closed. Then, with eyes open, the athlete can further advance to playing catch with a ball.

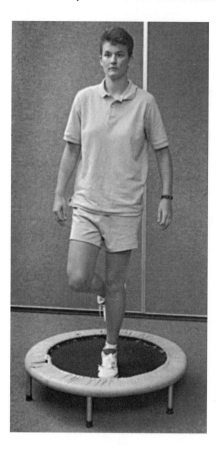

Figure 7–18. Stork stand on trampoline. The athlete can progress, while on the trampoline, to performing the stork stand with eyes open to eyes closed. Then, with eyes open, the athlete can further advance to playing catch with a ball.

Static balance exercises can be progressed from bilateral to unilateral, from eyes open to eyes closed, and from a stable to an unstable surface.[13] Dynamic activities such as running, jumping and landing, and cutting and pivoting require the athlete to repetitively lose and regain balance to perform the athletic activity.[13] Additionally, the athlete must be able to recruit muscles with the proper timing and sequence to allow smooth, coordinated movement (Figs. 7–19 to 7–22). Restoration of neurologic control to an injured area or extremity can be accomplished through exercises that include sudden alterations in joint positioning that necessitate reflex muscular stabilization (e.g., on a wobble board), open- and closed-chain exercises, proprioceptive neuromuscular facilitation patterns, and rhythmic stabilization exercises. Exercises to develop dynamic balance and control can be progressed from slow-speed to fast-speed, low-force to high-force, and controlled to uncontrolled activities.[13]

The effect of proprioception training on injured[27, 46, 119, 124] and uninjured[22] ankles has been studied. All the results from these investigations showed improved balance values following a training program and support the contention that proprioceptive deficits can be improved with training. Additionally, increased postural sway values have been correlated with increased risk of ankle injury.[118]

The effect of cold on proprioception has been investigated because cryotherapy is effective in decreasing nerve conduction velocity and altering cutaneous sensation. These changes suggest that proprioception would be negatively impacted by cold modalities. However, research on the ankle and knee has refuted this postulate. La Riviere and Osternig[77] assessed ankle joint position sense by measuring joint angle replication after ice immersion in 31 subjects with no history of ankle pathology. Their data showed no significant difference in reposi-

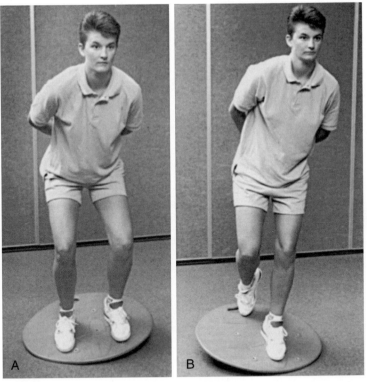

Figure 7–19. *A,* Bilateral Biomechanical Ankle Platform System board balancing. *B,* Progression to one-legged balancing.

tioning accuracy between either of the conditions, indicating that proprioception is not significantly altered by ice immersion.

The maintenance of proprioception following cryotherapy has also been demonstrated by Thieme and colleagues.[113] In this investigation, knee joint repositioning was measured in 37 subjects after 20 minutes of ice bag application and a control condition of 20 minutes of sitting. The repositioning measures showed no differences between the two conditions for each arc. In addition, the speeds with which subjects performed their repositioning trials were not different for the two conditions. These data further indicate that cooling does not inhibit proprioception.

Finally, the effect of taping or bracing on lower extremity proprioception has been addressed. Heit and colleagues[56] reported that ankle bracing and taping improved joint position sense in the stable ankle. Using a force plate, Friden and colleagues[39] reported decreased body sway in braced ankles. Tropp and colleagues,[117] using a force plate with a wobble board on top on which the subject stood, reported that ankle taping had no influence on balance values. The effect of knee bracing and wrapping on knee proprioception has also been examined. Lephart and colleagues[80] found that in subjects who had undergone anterior cruciate ligament reconstruction, kinesthesia (TTDPM) was improved while they were wearing neoprene sleeves. Barrett[8] reported similar results of enhanced proprioception when an elastic bandage or neoprene sleeve was applied to the injured knee in patients with osteoarthritic knees who had undergone total joint replacement. Perlau and colleagues[96] also reported that knee joint proprioception was improved in a group of uninjured subjects while they were wearing an elastic bandage. Other studies examining the effect of a func-

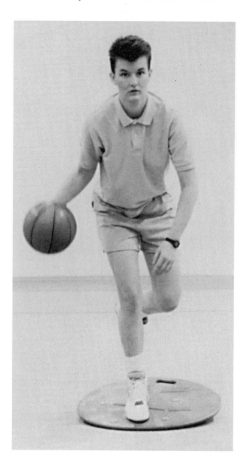

Figure 7-20. Biomechanical Ankle Platform System (BAPS) board dribbling on one leg, which can be a progression from bilateral BAPS board balancing while dribbling.

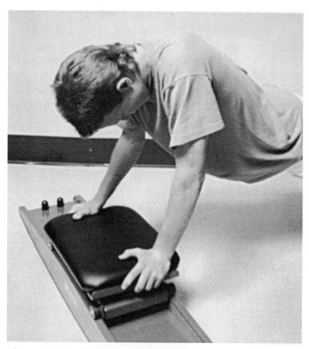

Figure 7-21. Upper extremity dynamic stabilization exercise using the Fitter. (Photo courtesy of Sports Medicine Update. Birmingham, Alabama, HealthSouth Rehabilitation Corporation.)

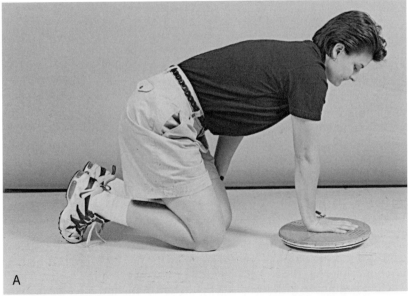

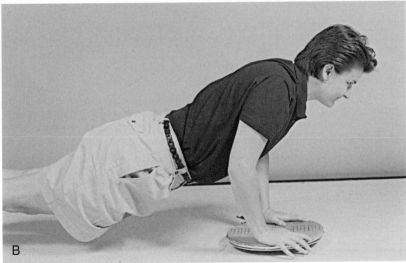

Figure 7-22. *A,* Proprioception training using a wobble board. *B,* Progression to a push-up on the wobble board.

tional knee brace[24] or a McDavid Knee Guard (M-202)[*67] showed that these braces have no effect on balance or joint position sense, respectively. These studies all have different experimental designs and instruments used for data collection, and therefore, comparison of these studies is not appropriate. More research needs to be conducted before the effects of taping or bracing on lower extremity proprioception can be determined.

Currently, it is generally agreed that kinesthetic deficits do occur as a result of injury and that these deficits can be overcome through training. The application of an elastic wrap or neoprene sleeve can heighten the kinesthetic sense, and cold appears to have little effect on proprioception. Data regarding the efficacy of high-technology balance machines that assess postural sway are still limited, and the validity and reliability of this equipment are still questionable. Answers

---

*Available from McDavid Knee Guard Inc., Chicago, Illinois

will come as more investigations are published, with the possible development of a predictive model for injury that is based on objective kinesthetic and proprioceptive data.

Progressive-Resistance Exercise

Before an athlete begins a PRE program, the athlete's range of motion must be assessed. If active range of motion is within normal limits when compared bilaterally, the athlete may begin active resistance exercise. It is not a prerequisite that full, pain-free active range of motion be attained before beginning active resistance exercise. As discussed previously, the athlete may begin isometric or manual-resistance exercise in a limited range of motion, provided that the healing process is not jeopardized. However, if an athlete lacks a significant amount of motion, remarkable strength gains will be impractical until functional motion is realized.[61]

Initiation of a PRE program is determined by the extent and nature of the injury. Athletes with chronic conditions may begin PRE on the first day of rehabilitation, whereas those with acute injuries may require several weeks or longer before beginning PRE because of pain, effusion, and biologic healing. The athlete may not be able to tolerate active movement or weight bearing in the early stages after injury or surgery. PRE is used to increase muscular strength and endurance in an orderly and progressive manner. This method permits an ever-increasing overload to be applied to the musculature and allows for the adaptation of bones, ligaments, tendons, and muscles so that the imposed overload is not applied too quickly, leading to further damage. This philosophy is based on the principle of specific adaptation to imposed demands.[122] This implies that the body responds to a given demand with a specific and predictable adaptation.[133] Stated another way, specific adaptation requires that a specific demand be imposed.[72] Therefore, if strength is to be developed in a particular muscle group, those muscles must be contracted to full capacity against resistance.

When using the PRE concept in therapeutic rehabilitation, the clinician must remember that it is an orderly progression, and the athlete should show improvement each day, whether this involves an increase in repetitions or an increase in weight. The theory behind therapeutic rehabilitation is to apply an overload to increase muscular strength and, at the same time, to maintain the integrity of the tissues of concern and not impede the healing process. Therapeutic rehabilitation should be based on the concept of low weight and high repetition. This not only builds muscular strength and endurance but helps retard and reverse the atrophy process, while negating some potential setbacks if the exercise is too aggressive.

THE DeLORME PROGRAM

DeLorme[29] first introduced the concept of PRE in 1945. The rationale for using PRE is that it creates a condition in which an individual muscle or muscles must work to full capacity against an ever-increasing resistance.[57] The ever-increasing intramuscular tension, caused by an ever-increasing resistance, produces an increase in muscle strength. Gardiner[41] has reported that it is essential for the resistance to be increased as the muscle strength improves. Furthermore, an increase in resistance that is too rapid results in overloading, preventing contraction and perhaps damaging the muscle; conversely, underloading will not increase strength.[41]

DeLorme's[29] initial concept of PRE was based on the amount of weight that could be carried through a full range of motion for 10 repetitions. This 10-repetition maximum (10 RM) was determined once a week, and a set of exercises of that 10-RM value was repeated 7 to 10 times during each exercise session.

This corresponds to 70 to 100 repetitions. On the last day of each exercise week, the maximum weight for only one repetition (1 RM) was determined, and the 10 RM for the following week was established from this 1 RM. DeLorme[29] has referred to this as heavy-resistance exercise because the weights used were great when compared with those used in previous strengthening methods and an all-out effort was necessary to lift them. This mode of PRE, however, is generally not applicable to athletes in the early postoperative stages. Subjects involved in DeLorme's research[29] were usually not diseased but had lost strength from disuse. The weight lifted in DeLorme's program does not take into account healing constraints in the early postoperative phases.

DeLorme and Williams[30] revised this original work in 1948. In their revised method, 20 to 30 repetitions were used. This permitted exercise with even heavier loads and thus resulted in a more rapid gain in strength and muscle volume. In the new regimen, the first one or two sets of repetitions were considered warm-ups for the 10-RM exercises. Their revised program can be outlined as follows:

1. First set of 10 repetitions: use one half of 10 RM
2. Second set of 10 repetitions: use three fourths of 10 RM
3. Third set of 10 repetitions: use full 10 RM

Still, DeLorme's PRE program was skewed toward the low-repetition, high-weight concept.

THE DAILY ADJUSTABLE PROGRESSIVE-RESISTANCE EXERCISE TECHNIQUE

There have been numerous modifications of the DeLorme PRE program.[60, 73, 100, 137] Knight's technique[73] of daily adjustable progressive-resistance exercise (DAPRE) uses the basic principle of PRE to a greater degree than did older programs. According to Knight,[73] the DAPRE technique allows for individual differences in the rate at which a person regains strength in the muscle and provides an objective method for increasing resistance in accordance with strength increases. The key to the program is that athletes perform as many full repetitions as they can in the third and fourth sets.[73] The number of repetitions performed in the third and fourth sets is then used to determine the amount of weight that is added to the working weight or sometimes removed from the working weight for the fourth set and the first set of the next session. The working weight is estimated for the initial reconditioning session. A good estimate would result in five to seven repetitions during the third set. More repetitions are performed if the estimate is low, and fewer are performed if it is too high.

During the first and second sets, the athlete performs 10 repetitions against half of the estimated working weight and six repetitions against three quarters of the working weight (Tables 7–5 and 7–6). These sets act to warm up and educate the muscles and neuromuscular structures involved.

Emphasis during the third and fourth sets is on performing the greatest number of full repetitions possible. The full working weight is used on the third set, and the athlete performs as many repetitions as possible. The number of full repetitions performed in the third set is used to determine the adjusted working weight for the fourth set, and the number performed is used to determine the working weight for the next day.

The DAPRE guidelines are based on the concept that if the working weight is ideal, the athlete can perform six repetitions when told to perform as many as

Table 7–5. Daily Adjustable Progressive Resistance Exercise

SET	PORTION OF WORKING WEIGHT USED	NUMBER OF REPETITIONS
1	Half	10
2	Three fourths	6
3*	Full	Maximum
4†	Adjusted	Maximum

From Knight, K.L. (1985): Guidelines for rehabilitation of sports injuries. Clin. Sports Med., 4:413.
*The number of repetitions performed during the third set is used to determine the adjusted working weight for the fourth set according to the guidelines in Table 7–6.
†The number of repetitions performed during the fourth set is used to determine the adjusted working weight for the next day according to the guidelines in Table 7–6.

possible.[9] If the athlete can perform more than six repetitions, the weight is too light. Conversely, if the athlete cannot perform six repetitions, the weight is too heavy. The number of repetitions also helps determine the amount of weight added during the adjustment.

Athletes exercise daily, except Sundays, until the working weight of the injured limb is equal to or within 5 pounds of that of the uninjured limb. Emphasis is then shifted from strength development to strength maintenance and to development of muscular endurance. The athlete should be in control of the weight at all times, performing the exercise slowly and deliberately, avoiding jerky or explosive contractions, and pausing at the extremes of motion.

THE HIGH-REPETITION, LOW-WEIGHT METHOD

For athletes with injuries of insidious onset and early postoperative rehabilitation, high-repetition, low-weight exercise has proved to be the best regimen.[11] Exercise involving high weight or intensity could potentially cause a breakdown of the supporting structures and only exacerbate the condition. Use of smaller weights and submaximal intensities provides a therapeutic effect that stimulates blood flow and diminishes tissue breakdown. To obtain the strengthening and endurance effect, higher repetitions must be used.[10, 11, 91]

The PRE program outlined here can be carried out early in rehabilitation using the low-weight, high-repetition concept (Table 7–7). Early rehabilitation begins with an active range of motion of two or three sets of 10 repetitions (or 20 to 30 repetitions), progressing to five sets of 10 repetitions (or 50 repetitions), as tolerated. The athlete should be able to do 20, 30, 40, or 50 of the prescribed exercises; it is not necessary for the number of repetitions to be divisible by 10

Table 7–6. General Guidelines for Adjustment of Working Weight

NUMBER OF REPETITIONS PERFORMED DURING SET	ADJUSTMENT OF WORKING WEIGHT FOR	
	FOURTH SET *	*NEXT DAY†*
0–2	Decrease by 5–10 lb and perform the set over	
3–4	Decrease by 0–5 lb	Keep the same
5–7	Keep the same	Increase by 5–10 lb
8–12	Increase by 5–10 lb	Increase by 5–15 lb
13+	Increase by 10–15 lb	Increase by 10–20 lb

From Knight, K.L. (1985): Guidelines for rehabilitation of sports injuries. Clin. Sports Med., 4:414.
*The number of repetitions performed during the third set is used to determine the adjusted working weight for the fourth set according to the guidelines in Table 7–5.
†The number of repetitions performed during the fourth set is used to determine the adjusted working weight for the next day according to the guidelines in Table 7–5.

Table 7-7. Preschedule for Initial Rehabilitation Stages

	DAY						
WEEK	*SUN*	*MON*	*TUES*	*WED*	*THUR*	*FRI*	*SAT*
1			Surgery	30 rep	40 rep	50 rep	30 rep@1 lb
2	40 rep@1 lb	50 rep@1 lb	30 rep@2 lb	40 rep@2 lb	50 rep@2 lb	30 rep@3 lb	40 rep@3 lb
3	50 rep@3 lb	30 rep@4 lb	40 rep@4 lb	50 rep@4 lb	30 rep@5 lb	40 rep@5 lb	50 rep@5 lb
	etc.						
•							
•							
•							
•							

rep, Repetitions.

before increasing the repetitions or weight. The repetitions can be split in half or can be performed consecutively, with no rest between repetitions. When the repetitions can be performed consecutively, the athlete's program should be upgraded by 10 repetitions the next day. The athlete should exercise two or three times per day, with the same exercises for a specific day performed in all sessions, even if the athlete fits the criteria for advancement. This technique allows the body and injured area to adjust to the demands placed on it.

When the athlete can perform 50 repetitions without stopping, 1 pound may be added, and the repetitions reduced to three sets of 10 repetitions, or 30 repetitions. At 50 repetitions, the cycle repeats, with the athlete adding another pound and reducing the repetitions to 30. Usually the athlete may progress along the PRE program as tolerable, with emphasis placed on proper lifting technique. All exercises should be performed smoothly, with a pause at the terminal position. The athlete must also concentrate on lowering the weight in a controlled fashion. In the later stages of rehabilitation, DeLorme's, Knight's, or any other type of PRE schedule may be used.

Some pain and discomfort are to be expected initially with the rehabilitation program. Moreover, the severity of the symptoms of many chronic injuries may slightly increase before it abates. Soreness after initiation of the rehabilitation program is common, and cryotherapy application postexercise may help with the soreness, pain, and inflammation. Postsurgically, cryotherapy is recommended for control of secondary hypoxic injury, pain, and edema.[74] Residual pain should be avoided as it generally indicates that the treatment is proceeding too quickly and should be reduced.

Prehab

Patient education plays an integral role in the rehabilitation program. If patients are educated about the surgical procedure and the methods and rationales for protecting a surgical repair, patient compliance with orthotic devices and treatment may be enhanced. Prehab is a term that refers to exercises and patient education before surgery. Ideally, particularly in the deconditioned athlete or individual, the initiation of a therapeutic exercise program 4 to 6 weeks prior to surgical intervention is preferable. This is thought to result in a decrease in morbidity and a reduction in loss of muscular strength and endurance postoperatively, because the individual is beginning at a higher level of conditioning. Generally, the program focuses on regaining range of motion and on therapeutic exercises that do not result in exacerbation of symptoms or further damage to the injured area. Usually the prehab concept can be used when a surgical procedure is not mandated immediately. If the injury proves to have progressed too far for conservative treatment, the conservative exercise program now becomes the preoperative exercise program.

Fortunately, a long period of prehab is usually not necessary for the conditioned athlete. In these individuals prehab may consist of only a short session to educate the athlete about the initial rehabilitation program and what is expected of the athlete in the early phases of rehabilitation; to perform gait training; to take baseline measurements, if indicated and tolerated by the athlete; and to fit any orthotic appliances that are to be used in the early postoperative phases. The athlete should also be informed about the surgical procedure to be performed, the prognosis after surgery, any potential complications, and precautions and limitations after surgery. Finally, the importance of rehabilitation, its function, and its approximate duration should also be discussed.

Following surgery, the exact findings and surgical procedure as well as the prognosis and any rehabilitation program changes should once again be discussed with the athlete. It is also recommended that at this time the topics that were discussed before surgery be reiterated so that the athlete has a clear understanding of them.

The preoperative and postoperative education of the athlete is often taken for granted, and the surgical procedure, extent of damage, prognosis, and rehabilitation course are often not discussed with the athlete. It is important that athletes become involved in goal setting, have input into their rehabilitation program, understand early rehabilitation restrictions, and realize the consequences of noncompliance with rehabilitation.

Crutch Training

The correct fitting of crutches and patient education in crutch use is often a neglected part of rehabilitation. Correct crutch fitting and instruction are imperative in preventing falls, reducing frustration, and increasing crutch compliance, when necessary. It is often assumed that the athlete knows how to ambulate on both flat surfaces and stairs using crutches, but usually this is not the case. Ideally, in patients with surgery of the lower extremity, in whom the potential for crutch use is the greatest, crutch training before surgery is encouraged. This results in a lower level of patient apprehension, less pain, and less risk of damage to repaired tissues or additional injury from a fall.

Improper crutch adjustment can cause early fatigue, axillary nerve injury, or a fall.[36] Moreover, properly adjusted crutches can help maintain good posture and can strengthen the trunk, shoulders, and arms. Athletes who have not been properly instructed in crutch use tend to rest their body weight on the axillary pads. This maneuver should be avoided because it can result in temporary or permanent numbness in the hands or arms resulting from pressure on the long thoracic nerve, a condition usually referred to as crutch palsy.

Crutch adjustment consists of the following[36]:

1. Adjustment with the athlete standing in good posture
2. Determination of crutch length by having the athlete stand with the feet close together and the rubber crutch tips 6 inches from the outer margin of each sole and 2 inches in front of the shoes
3. Adjustment of crutch height to allow a space of approximately two finger widths from the top of the crutch pad to the axillary skin fold
4. Adjustment of the hand grips to allow 25° to 30° of elbow flexion with the wrist straight (Figs. 7–23 and 7–24).

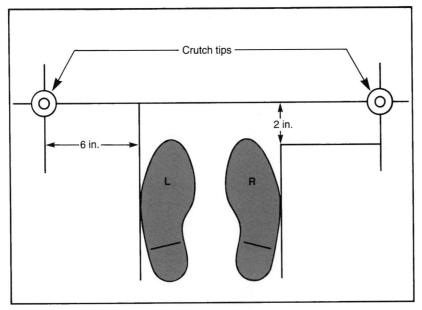

Figure 7-23. Schematic representation of properly adjusted axillary crutches. (From Flood, D.K. [1983]: Proper fitting and use of crutches. Phys. Sports Med., 11:75.)

Crutches are used to transfer body weight through the palms onto the hand grips. The arms may be almost fully extended at the elbow, and the axillary pads of the crutches are squeezed between the rib cage and upper arms while bearing weight.

There are five commonly used crutch gaits: two-point alternating gait, three-point gait, four-point alternating gait, swing-to gait, and swing-through gait.[36] In athletic arenas the three-point and swing-through gaits are used most often. The three-point gait is indicated when one extremity can support the body weight and the injured extremity is to be touched down or partially weight-bearing (Fig. 7–25). Just enough pressure is placed on the crutches to eliminate limping. The athlete can gradually increase the amount of weight bearing by decreasing the force transferred through the arms. The athlete should mimic a normal gait as closely as possible.

A swing-through gait is used when the athlete is to be non–weight-bearing, and weight is completely removed from the injured extremity. This technique should not be used longer than necessary because it can affect kinesthetic input to the lower extremity. It can also cause hip and knee tightness. In the swing-through gait, body weight is totally supported by the uninjured extremity while both crutches are placed 12 to 24 inches in front of the feet. Weight is then transferred to the crutches as the body is lifted and swung through to a point 12 to 24 inches in front of the crutches.

Negotiating stairs with crutches presents a different problem for the injured athlete. When instructing the athlete to maneuver on stairs it is a good idea to stand close to the athlete and hold on to the waist belt or to use an orthopedic safety belt. This allows the clinician to be in a better position to prevent or control a fall and helps the athlete maintain balance. In ascending stairs, the supportive limb is moved up to the first step while the body weight is supported on the crutch hand grips. The body weight is then transferred to the supportive limb, and the crutches in the affected limb are moved up the same step. This sequence is carefully repeated as the athlete ascends the stairs.

When the athlete is descending stairs on crutches, the affected limb is placed on a lower step while the unaffected extremity, supporting the body weight, is

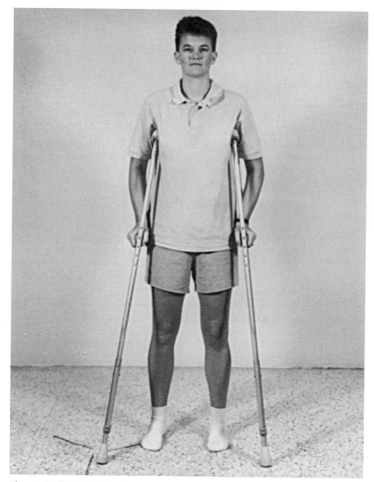

Figure 7–24. Correct posture for crutch adjustment.

on the upper step. Crutch placement on the lower step is critical for balance. The crutches must be placed toward the back of the step for greatest stability. After the body weight has been transferred from the unaffected extremity to the crutch hand grips, the unaffected limb is carefully brought down to the same step as the crutches and the affected extremity.

When a handrail is available, it should be used instead of one of the crutches because it is safer and more stable than crutches under both arms. The sequence of moving from one step to the next using the handrail is similar to the sequence followed when using crutches bilaterally. The athlete grips the handrail and applies a downward force with one hand while applying a downward force to the crutch grip with the other.[36] The extra crutch should be carried next to the crutch in use.

APPLICATION OF EXERCISE

Rehabilitation must prepare the athlete to return to competition as soon as possible without sacrificing healing time and predisposing the athlete to reinjury or to injury to another body part as a result of the initial trauma. Intensity, duration, frequency, specificity, rhythm, and progression of the program are all related to the functional capability that is developed.

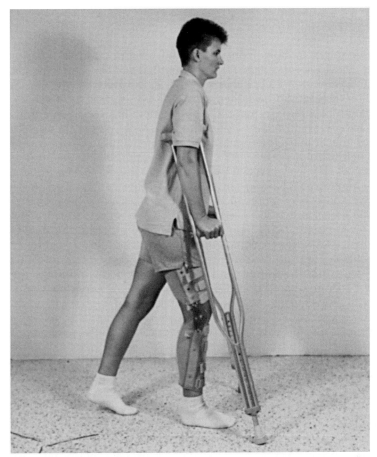

Figure 7–25. Partial weight bearing with two axillary crutches using a three-point gait.

Intensity

The goal of the rehabilitation program is to overload, not overwhelm.[31] Muscle and connective tissue must be subjected to a load greater than that of the usual stresses of daily activity if hypertrophy is to occur. Attempting to push too fast can result in reactive inflammatory changes.[31] After the program is underway, an increase in exercise intensity (higher weight, lower repetition) may increase the rate of strength gain. In the initial exercise regimen the high-weight, low-repetition concept is not applicable because of the greater stresses it places on the connective tissues, but it may be used later in the program. Exercise intensity varies according to injury.

Duration

The duration of the rehabilitation program is an estimate of how long it will take to return the athlete to full (100%) activity. It can vary from only a few days after a contusion to months after ligamentous injuries. Duration also encompasses the length of time the athlete is to be performing the rehabilitation program daily. This time shortens as pain, effusion, and soreness are alleviated.

Frequency

Frequency refers to how many times the rehabilitation program should be performed. Dickinson and Bennett[31] reported that exercise performed twice daily yields a greater improvement than exercise once daily in the early phases of rehabilitation. Houglum[60] described a natural rate of progress for individuals in a rehabilitation program. In the initial phase there is a relatively rapid improvement in strength, followed by a second phase, in which there is slowing or tapering of the improvement rate, and a third (final) phase, consisting of a progression toward a plateau state in which minimal or no improvement in strength occurs (Fig. 7–26). When the athlete is in the first phase of the rehabilitation development progression, an exercise routine can be implemented twice daily.[60] With the use of this concept, the athlete should be monitored, and a reduction in exercise may be needed periodically. As the athlete improves and comes closer to the final goal, a once-daily exercise program should be sufficient. This usually corresponds to a change in the PRE schedule toward higher weight, lower repetitions, and advancement toward functional activities. The reduction in routine should be instituted for two reasons: it helps minimize the athlete's chances of becoming bored and discontented with the program, and no reports have noted that exercising isotonically during the third phase more than once a day produces any significant physical benefits.[60] When the athlete returns to participation he or she can advance to a once- or twice-weekly program for maintenance. It is important that the athlete continue a rehabilitation maintenance program during the season, particularly if the regular weight-room regimen does not strengthen the appropriate muscles.

Specificity

There is a specific response to the type of exercise performed. An exercise program must be tailored to meet the specific needs of the individual. For example, exercises that mimic the throwing motion are ideal for the baseball pitcher but are not applicable for the football lineman. Activities or exercises that simulate part of the athlete's activity are ideal for this aspect of rehabilitation.[90]

Furthermore, the type of exercise is important. Athletes who are trained only with constant-resistance (isotonic) exercise perform better with this type of testing. Conversely, athletes trained with accommodating variable resistance show significant increases in strength when assessed by variable-resistance procedures, but these changes are less when assessed with constant-resistant proce-

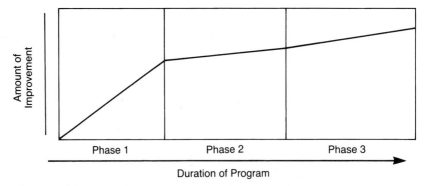

Figure 7–26. Typical progression rate during a rehabilitation program. (Adapted from Houghlum, P. [1977]: The modality of therapeutic exercise: Objectives and principles. Athl. Train., 12:43.)

dures.[90] Rhythm, or velocity, has also been shown to be specific, with greatest strength gains consistently occurring at training speeds.[90]

Speed

Speed refers to the rate at which the exercise is performed. The exercises should be performed in a slow and deliberate manner, with emphasis placed on concentric and eccentric contractions. The athlete should pause at the end of the exercise and should exercise through the full range of motion that is allowed, avoiding jerky movements. In addition, the larger muscle groups should be exercised first, proceeding to the smaller muscle groups. This is done because it is difficult to reach the required condition of momentary muscular exhaustion in a large muscle if a smaller muscle group that serves as a link between resistance and the large muscle group has been previously exhausted.

In the late stages of rehabilitation, the exercise speed should be varied. Traditional PRE exercises are performed at a rate of about 60 degrees per second, a speed that is not functional for attempts at returning athletes to their sports. For example, a pitcher's throwing arm travels at approximately 7000° per second. The continuation of a PRE program as the only tool in restoring this baseball pitcher to function does not prepare him or her for the great demands placed on the throwing arm on return to competition. As Costill and associates[21] have noted, it is important to vary the type and speed of the exercise. Surgical tubing can be used to implement a high-speed regimen to produce a concentric or eccentric synergist pattern, and isokinetic units at the highest speeds on the spectrum can also be used.

Progression

Progression within the rehabilitation program is of the utmost importance. There should be some type of objective improvement each day, whether this is an increase in repetitions or an increase in the amount of weight lifted. Only if the athlete has complaints of increased or residual pain should the program be maintained at the current level or possibly be decreased. Muscles must be continually overloaded for strength to develop. If the athlete continues to improve with repetitions or weights, he or she is getting stronger. As noted by Houglum,[60] progression is quicker at the beginning of the rehabilitation program and slows down as the athlete enters the second and third phases of rehabilitation.

In addition, there is an orderly progression from initial range-of-motion exercises to isometric, isotonic, isokinetic, and functional activities. Each phase proceeds from another, with some overlap in exercise types. Exercises should progress from a low-intensity to high-intensity level, with ever-increasing demands placed on the athlete as the healing process allows.

FUNCTIONAL REHABILITATION

Determining whether an athlete has been successfully rehabilitated or can safely return to competition can be difficult. Clinical techniques, however sophisticated, cannot predict the complex interaction of a rehabilitated joint in response to the demands of competition. As an aid to rehabilitation, functional progressions help the clinician and physician determine an athlete's status at any time throughout the rehabilitation process and can help the clinician prepare the athlete for competition.

Kegerreis[68] popularized the use of functional progressions in athletic rehabilitation. Several authors[79, 83, 97, 114] have further outlined and expanded its role. In a prospective follow-up study of 35 athletes with isolated medial collateral ligament injuries, Reider and colleagues[97] found that early functional rehabilitation was safe and effective. The subjects in this study subjectively rated their knees as good to excellent; all returned to full activity. They also achieved this return earlier than did athletes with similar injuries who were treated with surgery or a longer period of immobilization.

Additional support of the effectiveness of functional rehabilitation is found in the work of Mandelbaum and colleagues.[83] This prospective study followed 29 athletes who underwent functional rehabilitation after Achilles tendon repair. Twenty-seven of the patients returned to full activity within 6 months after surgery. Minimal strength deficits were seen on isokinetic testing at this time. At 1 year postsurgery, no deficits were seen in motion, strength, or endurance, and all of the athletes had returned to preinjury activity levels.

Implementation of functional progressions must be based on knowledge of the athlete's limitations, the inherent demands of the sport, and the provision of enough time for maturation of collagen-containing tissue, because there is a greater risk of injury during functional levels of activity.[68, 69] Taylor and colleagues[112] have demonstrated lower tensile strength and shorter lengths to complete rupture after experimental muscle strains in New Zealand White rabbits. From these results, the authors conclude that controlled functional activity is appropriate in the rehabilitation of muscle strain injuries.[112]

The basis of any rehabilitation effort is whether the athlete can perform effectively and safely. Noyes and colleagues[93] have labeled this concept "functional stability." Functional stability is provided by passive restraints of the ligaments, joint geometry, active restraints generated by the muscles, and joint compressive forces that occur with activity and that force the joint together. They concluded that laxity tests alone do not provide a reliable prediction of functional stability.[94] Rehabilitation should be directed toward improving strength and endurance and, perhaps primarily, increasing neuromuscular coordination,[79] proprioception,[79] and agility. The use of functional activities also helps the apprehensive athlete to acclimatize gradually to the inherent demands of the sport. Because each successive stage builds on the preceding stages, this ensures the return of physical prowess and instills confidence in the athlete with regard to ability to complete required tasks.[68, 69]

Initial considerations for implementation of a functional progression program revolve around the physical parameters of the athlete's intended activity. This involves an analysis of the demands of specific athletic endeavors, which are assessed for difficulty and complexity of response. The tasks are then placed on a continuum of difficulty with respect to the athlete's status. Overlaps occasionally occur as a particular task is accomplished but still remains in the athlete's program for solidification as the next task is begun. Care should be taken to ensure the blending of task progressions with specific restrictions concerning the nature of the pathology.

Just as in the PRE concept, functional progressions are based on the principle of specific adaptation to imposed demands. The intensity, duration, and frequency of the activity are related to the functional capability that is developed. Typical advancement follows a progression of half-speed to three-fourths–speed activity, increasing gradually until full-speed activity is reached. The athlete may be performing four or five tasks in a functional progression at one time. Conceivably, the athlete can be performing one task at half speed while performing a less demanding skill at full speed. Functional progressions and activities have been described in detail by Tippett and Voight.[114]

Functional activities may begin as soon as 2 to 3 days after injury or as late as 3 to 4 months after injury when a surgical procedure has been performed. Functional activities should be performed in conjunction with the rehabilitation program and not as a substitute for it. The athlete must ultimately be able to perform each activity asymptomatically. Functional tasks that result in apparent swelling or pain, particularly residual pain, immediate instability, or athlete anxiety should be curtailed in favor of a less aggressive activity. Prophylactic icing postexercise is controversial.[74] The clinician should recall the principal effects of cold and thermal agents when applying modalities postexercise.

It is common for the athlete to have occasional setbacks requiring regression to a former functional task. Tasks are considered completed when they are performed at competitive speeds with adequate repetitions without residual pain, edema, and loss of range-of-motion skills. Communication is important between the clinician and physician with regard to the current functional status of the athlete.

Clinical isokinetic data can be used to determine the athlete's strength, power, and endurance, but they do not predict performance when the athlete returns to competition. Functional activities progressed along an increasing continuum of difficulty can provide the clinician and physician with some idea of functional performance when an athlete returns to their respective sport.

SUMMARY

Rehabilitation or reconditioning is a dynamic method or program of prescribed exercise to prevent or reverse the deleterious effects of inactivity while returning an athlete to the former level of competition. Athletic rehabilitation requires the athlete to return to a performance level equal to or higher than that of the preinjury state. The goals of rehabilitation include decreasing pain, inflammation, and effusion; regaining full, pain-free, active range of motion; achieving full muscular strength, power, and endurance; and asymptomatically returning to full functional activities. Early exercise is essential to restoring the athlete to his or her former conditioning level as soon as possible, but a fine balance must be achieved between early mobilization and that which is too aggressive, which can set back the rehabilitation process.

In designing a rehabilitation program, the clinician must consider arthrokinematics and properties of the tissues that have been traumatized or surgically repaired. Ideally rehabilitation begins with a preoperative prehab phase. Later, initial phases of rehabilitation should primarily be concerned with reducing acute responses to injury. Once these reactions have been controlled, the athlete may proceed with early range-of-motion and active exercises. Strengthening exercises should include CKC activities in order to incorporate functional and proprioceptive training, as well as OKC exercises. The intensity of exercise should be progressed through a consistent PRE protocol. Duration, specificity, frequency, rhythm, and progression are additional important factors that must be addressed when designing a rehabilitation program. It is important to restore muscular strength, power, and endurance and to provide neuromuscular education and cardiovascular endurance during the reconditioning phases. A well-balanced rehabilitation program will provide for an orderly progression of exercises that include exercises that are both open and closed chain, train muscles across varying speeds of movement and varying functional contraction patterns (concentric and eccentric), and incorporate movements that mimic the athlete's sport-specific demands.

Finally, the athlete should be tested in regard to functional ability before returning to participation. The rehabilitation program should include functional progressions that athletes may encounter in their sport, advancing in difficulty from easy to challenging. Solid performance on objective measurements and full-speed functional activity tests with no pain or effusion indicate that the athlete is ready for return to full sport participation.

References

1. Taber's Cyclopedic Medical Dictionary (1977): 13th ed. Philadelphia, F.A. Davis.
2. Abbott, J.C., Saunders, J.B., and Dec, M. (1994): Injuries to the ligaments of the knee joint. J. Bone Joint Surg. [Am.], 26:503–521.
3. Albert, M. (1991): Inertial training concepts. *In:* Albert, M. (ed.): Eccentric Muscle Training in Sports and Orthopaedics. New York, Churchill Livingston, pp. 75–97.
4. Albert, M.S., Hillegas, E., and Spiegel, P. (1994): Muscle torque changes caused by inertial exercise training. J. Orthop. Sports Phys. Ther., 20:254–261.
5. Allman, F.L. (1985): Rehabilitative exercises in sports medicine. Instr. Course Lect., 34:389–392.
6. Barrack, R.L., Skinner, H.B., and Buckley, S.L. (1989): Proprioception of the anterior cruciate deficient knee. Am. J. Sports Med., 17:1–6.
7. Barrack, R.L., Skinner, H.B., Cook, S.D., et al. (1983): Effect of articular disease and total knee arthroplasty on knee joint-positioning sense. J. Neurophysiol., 50:684–687.
8. Barrett, D.S., Cobb, A.G., and Bentley, G. (1991): Joint proprioception in normal, osteoarthritic, and replaced knees. J. Bone Joint Surg. [Br.], 73:53–56.
9. Berger, R.A. (1962): Optimal repetitions for the development of strength. Res. Q. Exerc. Sport, 33:334–338.
10. Berger, R.A. (1982): Applied Exercise Physiology. Philadelphia, Lea & Febiger.
11. Blackburn, T.A. (1987): Rehabilitation of the shoulder and elbow after arthroscopy. Clin. Sports Med., 6:587–588.
12. Blair, D.F. (1990): Practical devices for proprioception. Athl. Train., 25:261–263.
13. Borsa, P.A., Lephart, S.M., Kocher, M.S., et al. (1994): Functional assessment and rehabilitation of shoulder proprioception for glenohumeral instability. J. Sports Rehabil., 3:84–104.
14. Bosch, U., and Kasperczyk, W.J. (1992): Healing of the patellar tendon autograft after posterior cruciate ligament reconstruction: A process of ligamentization? An experimental study in a sheep model. Am. J. Sports Med., 20:558–566.
15. Bunton, E.E., Pitney, W.A., Kane, A.W., et al. (1993): The role of limb torque, muscle action and proprioception during closed kinetic chain rehabilitation of the lower extremity. Athl. Train., 28:10–20.
16. Bynum, E.B., Barrack, R.L., and Alexander, A.H. (1995): Open versus closed chain kinetic exercise after anterior cruciate ligament reconstruction. Am. J. Sports Med., 23:401–406.
17. Chu, D. (1984): Plyometric exercise. Natl. Strength Condition. Assoc. J., 6:56–62.
18. Chu, D.A. (1992): Jumping into Plyometrics. Champaign, IL, Human Kinetics Publishers.
19. Cleak, M.J., and Eston, R.G. (1992): Muscle soreness, swelling, stiffness, and strength loss after intense eccentric exercise. Br. J. Sports Med., 26:267–272.
20. Cooper, D.L., and Fair, J. (1976): Reconditioning following athletic injuries. Phys. Sports Med., 4:125–128.
21. Costill, D.L., Fink, W.J., and Habansky, A.J. (1971): Muscle rehabilitation after knee surgery. Phys. Sports Med., 5:71–77.
22. Cox, E.D., Lephart, S.M., and Irrgang, J.J. (1993): Unilateral balance training in noninjured individuals and the effects on postural sway. J. Sports Rehabil., 2:87–96.
23. Cummings, G.S., Crutchfield, C.A., and Barnes, M.R. (1983): Soft tissue changes in contractures. *In:* Orthopedic Physical Therapy Series, Vol I. Atlanta, Stokesville Publishing.
24. Davies, G., Romeyn, R., and Shenton, D.W. (1992): Objective quantification of kinesthesia (balance) in 116 patients with knee ligament injuries while wearing or not wearing a functional knee brace. J. Orthop. Sports Phys. Ther., 15:54.
25. de Andrade, J.R., Grant, C., and Dixon, A.S. (1965): Joint distension and reflex inhibition in the knee. J. Bone Joint Surg. [Am.], 47:313–322.
26. Dean, E. (1988): Physiology and therapeutic implication of negative work. Phys. Ther., 68:233–237.
27. DeCarlo, M.S., and Talbot, R.W. (1986): Evaluation of ankle joint proprioception following injection of the anterior talofibular ligament. J. Orthop. Sports Phys. Ther., 8:70–76.
28. Dedrick, M.E., and Clarkson, P.M. (1990): The effects of eccentric exercise on motor performance in young and older women. Eur. J. Appl. Physiol., 60:183–186.
29. DeLorme, T.L. (1945): Restoration of muscle power by heavy resistance exercise. J. Bone Joint Surg., 27:645–667.
30. DeLorme, T.L., and Williams, A.L. (1948): Techniques of progressive resistance exercise. Arch. Phys. Med., 29:263–268.
31. Dickinson, A., and Bennett, K. (1985): Therapeutic exercise. Clin. Sports Med., 4:417–429.
32. Dillman, C.J., Murray, T.A., and Hintermeister, R.A. (1994): Biomechanical differences of open and closed chain exercises with respect to the shoulder. J. Sports Rehabil., 3:228–238.
33. Drez, D., Paine, R., and Neuschwander, D.C. (1992): In vivo testing of closed versus open kinetic chain exercises in patients with documented tears of the anterior cruciate ligament. Orthop. Trans., 16:43–47.
34. Fahere, H., Rentsch, H.U., and Gerber, N.J. (1988): Knee effusion and reflex inhibition of the quadriceps. J. Bone Joint Surg. [Br.], 70:635–638.
35. Fisher, A., Wietlisbach, S., and Wilberger, J. (1988): Adult performance on three tests of equilibrium. Am. J. Occup. Ther., 42:30–35.

36. Flood, D.K. (1983): Proper fitting and use of crutches. Physician Sportsmed., 11:75–78.
37. Flynn, T.W., and Soutas-Little, R.W. (1993): Mechanical power and muscle action during forward and backward running. J. Orthop. Sports Phys. Ther., 17:108–112.
38. Flynn, T.W., and Soutas-Little, R.W. (1995): Patellofemoral joint compressive forces in forward and backward running. J. Orthop. Sports Phys. Ther., 21:277–282.
39. Friden, T., Zatterstrom, R., Lindstrand, A., et al. (1989): A stabilometric technique for evaluation of lower limb instabilities. Am. J. Sports Med., 17:118–122.
40. Gambetta, V., and Odgers, S. (1991): The Complete Guide to Medicine Ball Training. Sarasota, FL, Optimum Sports Training.
41. Gardiner, M.D. (1975): The Principles of Exercise Therapy. London, G. Belt and Sons.
42. Gardner, E. (1948): The innervation of the knee joint. Anat. Rec., 101:109–130.
43. Garn, S.N., and Newton, R.A. (1988): Kinesthetic awareness in subjects with multiple ankle sprains. Phys. Ther., 68:1667–1671.
44. Garrett, W.E., and Lohnes, J. (1990): Cellular and matrix response to mechanical injury at the myotendinous junction. In: Leadbetter, W.B., Buckwalter, J.A., and Gordon, S.L. (eds.): Sports-Induced Inflammation. Park Ridge, IL, Amercian Academy of Orthopaedic Surgeons, pp. 215–224.
45. Garrett, W.E., and Tidball, J. (1988): Myotendinous junction: Structure, function, and failure. In: Woo, S.L.-Y., and Buckwalter, J.A. (eds.): Injury and Repair of the Musculoskeletal Soft Tissue. Park Ridge, IL, American Academy of Orthopaedic Surgeons, pp. 171–207.
46. Gauffin, H., Tropp, H., and Odenrick, P. (1988): Effect of ankle disk training of postural control in patients with functional instability of the ankle joint. Int. J. Sports Med. 9:141–144.
47. Glencross, D., and Throton, E. (1981): Position sense following joint injury. J. Sports Med., 21:23–27.
48. Gowitzke, B.A., and Morris, M. (1988): Scientific Basis of Human Movement, 3rd ed. Baltimore, Williams & Wilkins.
49. Graham, V.L., Gehlsen, G.M., and Edwards, J.A. (1993): Electromyographic evaluation of closed and open kinetic chain knee rehabilitation exercises. Athl. Train., 28:23–30.
50. Gross, M.T. (1987): Effects of recurrent lateral ankle sprains on active and passive judgements of joint position. Phys. Ther., 67:1505–1509.
51. Guskiewicz, K.M., and Perrin, D.H. (1996): Research and clinical applications of assessing balance. J. Sports Rehabil., 5:45–63.
52. Halata, F., Rettig, T., and Schulze, W. (1985): The ultrastructure of sensory nerve endings in the human knee joint capsule. Anat. Embryol., 172:265–275.
53. Hall, A.L., and McCloskey, D.I. (1983): Detection of movement imposed in finger, elbow and shoulder joints. J. Physiol., 335:519–533.
54. Harter, R.A. (1996): Clinical rationale for closed kinetic chain activities in functional testing and rehabilitation of ankle pathologies. J. Sports Rehabil., 5:13–24.
55. Harter, R.A., Osternig, L.O., and Singer, K.M. (1992): Knee joint proprioception following anterior cruciate ligament reconstruction. J. Sports Rehabil., 1:103–110.
56. Heit, E.J., Lephart, S.M., and Rozzi, S.L. (1996): The effect of ankle bracing and taping on joint position sense in the stable ankle. J. Sports Rehabil., 5:206–213.
57. Hellebrandt, F.A. (1951): Physiological bases of progressive resistance exercise. In: DeLorme, T.L., and Watkins, A.L. (eds.): Progressive Resistance Exercise. New York, Appleton-Century-Crofts.
58. Henning, C.E., Lynch, M.A., and Glick, K.R. (1985): An in vivo strain gage study of elongation of the anterior cruciate ligament. Am. J. Sports Med., 13:22–26.
59. Hilton, J. (1863): On the influence of mechanical and physiological rest in the treatment of accidents and surgical diseases, and the diagnostic value of pain: A course of lectures. London, Bell and Daldy.
60. Houglum, P. (1977): The modality of therapeutic exercise: Objectives and principles. Athl. Train., 12:42–45.
61. Houglum, P.A. (1992): Soft tissue healing and its impact on rehabilitation. J. Sports Rehabil., 1:19–39.
62. Hughston, J.C. (1980): Knee surgery: A philosophy. Am. Phys. Ther., 60:1611–1614.
63. Hungerford, D., and Barry, M. (1979): Biomechanics of the patellofemoral joint. Clin. Orthop., 144:9–15.
64. Irrgang, J.J., and Lephart, S. (1992): Reliability of measuring postural sway during unilateral stance in normal individuals using the Chattecx balance system. Phys. Ther., 72:566.
65. Irrgang, J.J., Whitney, S.L., and Cox, E.D. (1994): Balance and proprioceptive training for rehabilitation of the lower extremity. J. Sports Rehabil., 3:68–83.
66. Jimmy, M.L. (1988): Mechanoreceptors in articular tissues. Am. J. Anat., 182:16–32.
67. Kaminski, T.W., and Perrin, D.H. (1996): Effect of prophylactic knee bracing on balance and joint position sense. J. Athl. Train., 31:131–136.
68. Kegerreis, S. (1983): The construction and implementation of functional progressions as a component of athletic rehabilitation. J. Orthop. Sports Phys. Ther., 5:14–19.
69. Kegerreis, S., Malone, T., and McCaroll, J. (1984): Functional progressions: An aid to athletic rehabilitation. Physician Sportsmed., 12:67–71.
70. Kennedy, J.C., Alexander, I.J., and Hayes, K.C. (1982): Nerve supply of the human knee and its functional importance. Am. J. Sports Med., 10:329–335.

71. Keskula, D.R. (1996): Clinical implications of eccentric exercise in sports medicine. J. Sports Rehabil., 5:321–329.
72. Knight, K. (1985): Guidelines for rehabilitation of sports injuries. Clin. Sports Med., 4:405–416.
73. Knight, K.L. (1979): Rehabilitating chondromalacia patellae. Physician Sportsmed., 7:147–148.
74. Knight, K.L. (1995): Cryotherapy in Sports Injury Management. Champaign, IL, Human Kinetics Publishers, p. 11.
75. Konradsen, L., and Raven, J.B. (1990): Ankle instability caused by prolonged peroneal reaction time. Acta Orthop. Scand. (Suppl.), 61:388–390.
76. Kraus, H. (1959): Evaluation and treatment of muscle function in athletic injury. Am. J. Surg., 98:353–362.
77. La Riviere, J., and Osternig, L.R. (1994): The effect of ice immersion on joint position sense. J. Sports Rehabil., 3:58–67.
78. Lephart, S. (1994): Reestablishing proprioception, kinesthesia, joint position sense, and neuromuscular control in rehabilitation. In: Prentice, W.E. (ed.): Rehabilitation Techniques in Sports Medicine. St. Louis, C.V. Mosby.
79. Lephart, S.M., and Henry, T.J. (1995): Functional rehabilitation for the upper and lower extremity. Orthop. Clin. North Am., 26:579–592.
80. Lephart, S.M., Kocher, M.S., Fu, F.H., et al. (1992): Proprioception following anterior cruciate ligament reconstruction. J. Sports Rehabil., 1:188–196.
81. Lephart, S.M., Perrin, D.H., Fu, F.H., et al. (1992): Relationship between selected physical characteristics and functional capacity in the anterior cruciate-deficient athlete. J. Orthop. Sports Phys. Ther., 16:174–181.
82. MacDonald, P.B., Hedden, D., Pacin, O., et al. (1996): Proprioception in anterior cruciate ligament-deficient and reconstructed knees. Am. J. Sports Med., 24:774–778.
83. Mandelbaum, B.R., Myerson, M.S., and Forster, R. (1995): Achilles tendon rupture: A new method of repair, early range of motion, and functional rehabilitation. Am. J. Sports Med., 23:392–395.
84. Mangine, R.E., and Noyes, F.R. (1992): Rehabilitation of the allograft reconstruction. J. Orthop. Sports Phys. Ther., 15:294–302.
85. Mannheimer, J.S., and Lampe, G.N. (1984): Clinical Transcutaneous Electrical Nerve Stimulation. Philadelphia, F.A. Davis.
86. Marino, M. (1986): Current concepts of rehabilitation in sports medicine: Research and clinical interrelationship. In: Nicholas, J.A., and Hershman, E.D. (eds.): The Lower Extremity in Sports Medicine. St. Louis, C.V. Mosby, pp. 126–128.
87. Markolf, K.L., Gorek, J.F., and Kabo, J.M. (1990): Direct measurement of resultant forces in the anterior cruciate ligament. J. Bone Joint Surg. [Am.], 72:557–567.
88. Mattacola, C.G., Lebsack, D.A., and Perrin, D.H. (1995): Intertester reliability of assessing postural sway using the Chattecx balance system. J. Athl. Train., 30:237–241.
89. McCarthy, M.R., Yates, C.K., Anderson, M.A., et al. (1993): The effects of immediate continuous passive motion on pain during the inflammatory phase of soft tissue healing following anterior cruciate ligament reconstruction. J. Orthop. Sports Phys. Ther., 17:96–101.
90. Morrissey, M.C., Harman, E.A., and Johnson, M.J. (1995): Resistance training modes: Specificity and effectiveness. Med. Sci. Sports Exerc., 27:648–660.
91. Moss, C.L., and Grimmer, S. (1993): Strength and contractile adaptations in the human triceps surae after isotonic exercise. J. Sports Rehabil., 2:104–114.
92. Norkin, C., and Levangie, P. (1983): Joint Structure and Function: A Comprehensive Analysis. Philadelphia, F.A. Davis.
93. Noyes, F.R., Grood, E.S., and Butler, D.L. (1980): Knee ligament tests. Phys. Ther., 60:1578–1581.
94. Noyes, F.R., Grood, E.S., Butler, D.L., et al. (1980): Clinical laxity tests and functional stability of the knee: Biomechanical concepts. Clin. Orthop., 146:84–89.
95. Palmitier, R.A., An, K.-N., Scott, S.G., et al. (1991): Kinetic chain exercise in knee rehabilitation. Sports Med., 11:402–412.
96. Perlau, R., Frank, C., and Fick, G. (1995): The effect of elastic bandages on human knee proprioception in the uninjured population. Am. J. Sports Med., 23:251–255.
97. Reider, B., Sathy, M.R., Talkington, J., et al. (1993): Treatment of isolated medial collateral ligament injuries in athletes with early functional rehabilitation. Am. J. Sports Med., 22:470–477.
98. Reuleaux, F. (1875): Theoretische Kinematic: Grundigeiner Theorie des Maschinenwessens. Braunschweig, I.F. Vieweg und Sohn. In: The Kinematic Theory of Machinery: Outline of a Theory of Machines, A.B.W. Translated by Kennedy, Editor. Macmillan, London.
99. Reynolds, N.L., Worrell, T.W., and Perrin, D.H. (1992): Effect of lateral step-up exercise protocol on quadriceps isokinetic peak torque values and thigh girth. J. Orthop. Sports Phys. Ther., 15:151–155.
100. Schram, D.A. and Bennett, R.L. (1951): Underwater resistance exercise. Arch. Phys. Med., 32:222–226.
101. Schultz, R.A., Miller, D.C., and Kerr, C.S. (1984): Mechanoreceptors in human cruciate ligament: A histological study. J. Bone Joint Surg. [Am.], 69:1072–1076.
102. Schutte, M.J., Dabezies, E.J., and Zimny, M.L. (1987): Neural anatomy of the human anterior cruciate ligament. J. Bone Joint Surg. [Am.], 69:243–247.
103. Shelbourne, K., and Nitz, P. (1990): Accelerated rehabilitation after anterior cruciate ligament reconstruction. Am. J. Sports Med., 18:192–299.

104. Sherrington, C.S. (1906): On the proprioceptive system, especially in its reflex aspects. Brain, 29:467–479.
105. Skinner, H.B., Wyatt, M.P., and Hudgdon, J.A. (1986): Effect of fatigue on joint position of the knee. J. Orthop. Res., 4:112–118.
106. Smith, R.L., and Brunolli, J. (1989): Shoulder kinesthesia after anterior glenohumeral dislocation. Phys. Ther., 69:106–112.
107. Snyder-Mackler, L. (1996): Scientific rational and physiological basis for the use of closed kinetic chain exercise in the lower extremity. J. Sports Rehabil., 5:2–12.
108. Steindler, A. (1955): Kinesiology of the Human Body. Springfield, IL, Charles C Thomas.
109. Steindler, A. (1970): Kinesiology of the Human Body Under Normal and Pathological Conditions. Springfield, IL, Charles C Thomas.
110. Stone, J.A., Partin, N.B., Lueken, J.S., et al. (1994): Upper extremity proprioceptive training. J. Athl. Train., 29:15–18.
111. Szczerba, J.E., Bernier, J.N., and Perrin, D.H. (1995): Intertester reliability of active and passive ankle joint position sense testing. J. Sports Rehabil., 4:282–291.
112. Taylor, D.C., Dalton, J.D., Seaber, A.V., et al. (1993): Experimental muscle strain injury: Early functional and structural deficits and the increased risk for reinjury. Am. J. Sports Med., 21:190–194.
113. Thieme, H.A., Ingersoll, C.D., and Knight, K.L. (1996): Cooling does not affect knee proprioception. J. Athl. Train., 31:8–11.
114. Tippett, S.R., and Voight, M.L. (1995): Functional Progressions for Sports Rehabilitation. Champaign, IL, Human Kinetics Publishers, pp. 3–18.
115. Tomaszewski, D. (1991): "T-band kicks" ankle proprioception program. J. Athl. Train., 26:216–219.
116. Tracy, J.E., Obuchi, S., and Johnson, B. (1995): Kinematic and electromyographic analysis of elbow flexion during inertial exercise. J. Athl. Train., 30:254–258.
117. Tropp, H., Ekstrand, J., and Gillquist, J. (1984): Factors affecting stabilometry recordings of single limb stance. Am. J. Sports Med., 12:185–188.
118. Tropp, H., Eskstrand, J., and Gillquist, J. (1984): Stabilometry in functional instability of the ankle and its value in predicting injury. Med. Sci. Sports Exerc., 16:64–66.
119. Tropp, H., Odenrick, P., and Gillquist, J. (1985): Stabilometry recording in functional and mechanical instability of the ankle joint. Int. J. Sports Med., 6:180–182.
120. Voight, M., and Tippett, S., Plyometric exercise in rehabilitation. In: Prentice, W.E. (ed.): Rehabilitation Techniques in Sports Medicine. St. Louis, C.V. Mosby, pp. 88–97.
121. Voight, M.L., and Draovitch, P. (1991): Plyometrics. In: Albert, M. (ed.): Eccentric Muscle Training in Sports and Orthopaedics. New York, Churchill Livingstone, pp. 45–73.
122. Wallis, E.L., and Logan, G.A. (1964): Figure Improvement and Body Composition Through Exercise. Englewood Cliffs, NJ, Prentice-Hall.
123. Weber, M.D., Servedio, F.J., and Woodall, W.R. (1994): Effect of three modalities on delayed onset muscle soreness. J. Orthop. Sports Phys. Ther., 20:236–242.
124. Wester, J.U., Jespersen, S.M., Nielsen, K.D., et al. (1996): Wobble board training after partial sprains of the lateral ligaments of the ankle: A prospective randomized study. J. Orthop. Sports Phys. Ther., 23:332–336.
125. Wigerstad-Lossing, I., Grimby, G., and Jonsson, T. (1988): Effects of electrical muscle stimulation combined with voluntary contractions after knee ligament surgery. Med. Sci. Sports Exerc., 20:93–98.
126. Wilk, K.E. (1990): Plyometrics for the upper extremity. In: Advances on Shoulder and Knee Symposium. Cincinnati, OH, Cincinnati Sportsmedicine and Deaconess Hospital.
127. Wilk, K.E., and Andrews, J.R. (1993): Current concepts in the treatment of anterior cruciate ligament disruption. J. Orthop. Sports Phys. Ther., 15:279–293.
128. Wilk, K.E., and Arrigo, C. (1993): Current concepts in the rehabilitation of the athletic shoulder. J. Orthop. Sports Phys. Ther., 18:365–378.
129. Wilk, K.E., Arrigo, C., and Andrews, J.R. (1993): Rehabilitation of the elbow in the throwing athlete. J. Orthop. Sports Phys. Ther., 17:305–317.
130. Wilk, K.E., Arrigo, C.A., and Andrews, J.R. (1996): Closed and open kinetic chain exercise for the upper extremity. J. Sports Rehabil., 5:88–102.
131. Wilk, K.E., Voight, M.L., Keirns, M.A., et al. (1993): Stretch-shortening drills for the upper extremities: Theory and clinical application. J. Orthop. Sports Phys. Ther., 17:225–239.
132. Willis, W.D., and Grossman, R.G. (1981): Medical Neurobiology, 3rd ed. St. Louis, C.V. Mosby.
133. Wilmore, J.H. (1976): Athletic Training and Physical Fitness. Boston, Allyn & Bacon.
134. Worrell, T.W., Borchert, B., Erner, K., et al. (1993): Effect of lateral step-up exercise protocol on quadriceps and lower extremity performance. J. Orthop. Sports Phys. Ther., 18:646–653.
135. Yack, H.J., Collins, C.E., and Whieldon, T.J. (1993): Comparison of closed and open kinetic chain exercise in the anterior cruciate ligament-deficient knee. Am. J. Sports Med., 21:49–54.
136. Zimmerman, C.L., Cook, T.M., and Bravard, M.S. (1994): Effects of stair-stepping exercise direction and cadence on EMG activity of selected lower extremity muscle groups. J. Orthop. Sports Phys. Ther., 19:173–180.
137. Zinovieff, A.N. (1951): Heavy resistance exercise: The Oxford technique. Br. J. Phys. Med., 14:129–132.

Chapter 8

Application of Isokinetics in Testing and Rehabilitation

George J. Davies, M.Ed., P.T., S.C.S, A.T.,C., C.S.C.S., and Todd S. Ellenbecker, M.S., P.T., S.C.S, C.S.C.S.

Isokinetics plays a significant role in evaluation and rehabilitation of injured athletes. The utilization of isokinetics changed as the interest in isokinetics has varied over the past 25 years. Isokinetics was developed in the 1960s and was increasingly used during the 1970s. However, research on this subject was minimal and the potential uses and applications of isokinetics were not understood. In the 1980s isokinetics came into its own, with increasing popularity and, most importantly, with an increasing body of knowledge through numerous publications that supported the appropriate use of isokinetics in the testing and rehabilitation of athletes. During this period, isokinetics was increasingly used in many different areas and with many different applications. The first book dedicated solely to isokinetics was published in the early 1980s[25]; it provided an overview of the testing and application of isokinetics using a combination of published research and empirically based clinical experiences. However, in the 1990s, there has been a trend away from the utilization of isokinetics as part of the total evaluation and rehabilitation process. Despite extensive publications on isokinetics (over 2000 published articles regarding the utilization and efficacy of isokinetics, an entire journal dedicated to the art and science of isokinetics [*Isokinetics and Exercise Science*], and four books dedicated exclusively to isokinetics[18, 27, 43, 120]), many practicing clinicians have discontinued using isokinetics on the grounds that it is not functional. Although admittedly most athletes do not sit and flex and extend their knees as a functional activity, there is a high correlation between isokinetic testing of the knee and functional testing. Unfortunately, many clinicians are disregarding the extensive documentation of isokinetics in the evaluation and treatment of athletes and are embracing closed kinetic chain (CKC) exercises as a panacea without significant documentation of efficacy. We do not advocate that only isokinetics should be used or that CKC exercises should not be used; we would, however, like to emphasize the need for an integrated approach that uses many modes of testing and rehabilitation.

The purposes of this chapter will be to

- present an overview of the terminology used with isokinetics
- present the concept of a functional testing algorithm as an integrated approach to evaluate the athlete and to highlight the use of both CKC isokinetic testing and open kinetic chain (OKC) isokinetic testing

- present some general guidelines regarding the application of isokinetic testing
- present specific applications of isokinetic assessment of muscular power in the upper extremities
- present the application of isokinetics as part of rehabilitation programs
- present the scientific and clinical rationale for the use of isokinetics in evaluation and rehabilitation of sports injuries

OVERVIEW AND TERMINOLOGY

There are numerous modes of exercise that can be utilized in the evaluation and rehabilitation of athletes. These include isometrics, isotonics, plyometrics, isoacceleration, isodeceleration, and isokinetics.

The concept of isokinetic exercise was developed by James Perrine in the late 1960s, and it proved to be a revolution in exercise training and rehabilitation. Instead of the traditional exercises that were performed at variable speeds against a constant weight or resistance, Perrine developed the concept of isokinetics, which involves a dynamic preset fixed speed with resistance that is totally accommodating throughout the range of motion (ROM). Since the inception of isokinetics, this form of testing and exercise has become increasingly popular in clinical, athletic, and research settings, with the first article describing isokinetic exercise being published in 1967.[30] Since then, numerous articles and research presentations have documented the use of isokinetics for objective testing or for training.

Isokinetics means that exercise is performed at a fixed velocity (anywhere from 1° per second to approximately 1000° per second), with an accommodating resistance. Accommodating resistance means that isokinetic exercise is the only way to dynamically load a muscle to its maximum capability through every point throughout the ROM. Therefore, the resistance varies to exactly match the force applied by the athlete at every point in the ROM. This is important because, as the joint goes through the ROM, the amount of torque that can be produced varies because of the Blix curve (musculotendinous length-to-tension ratio) and because of the physiologic length-to-tension ratio changes that occur in the muscle-tendon unit and in biomechanical skeletal leverage.

Isokinetics offers several advantages[28]:

- Efficiency: It is the only way to load a dynamically contacting muscle to its maximum capability at all points throughout the ROM.
- Safety: An individual will never meet more resistance than he or she can handle, because the resistance is equal to the force applied.
- Accommodating resistance: Accommodating resistance occurs, which is predicated on changes in the musculotendinous length-to-tension ratio, changes in the skeletal leverage (biomechanics), fatigue, and pain.
- Decreased joint compressive forces at higher speeds: This is an empiric clinical observation that one of us (G.J.D.) has made in over 25 years of using isokinetics in testing and rehabilitation of athletes. This occurs because often an athlete exercises at a slow speed and pain develops; however, if the athlete

exercises at a faster velocity, pain does not develop. Furthermore, at faster speeds, there is less time to develop force, and the torque decreases with concentric isokinetics according to the force-velocity curve.

- Physiologic overflow through the velocity spectrum: When an athlete exercises at a particular speed, there is a specificity response, with the greatest power gains occurring at the speed of training; however, a concomitant increase in power gain occurs at other speeds as well. The majority of studies demonstrate that this phenomenon occurs at the slower speeds, although some research demonstrates an overflow in both directions from the training speed.[28]
- Velocity spectrum training[28]: Because of the various velocities at which functional and sporting activities are performed, the ability to train at various functional velocities is important, because of the specificity of training. It is important to train the muscles neurophysiologically to develop a normal motor recruitment pattern of neural contraction of the muscle.
- Minimal postexercise soreness with concentric isokinetic contractions
- Validity of the equipment
- Reliability of the equipment
- Reproducibility of physiologic testing (reliability)
- Development of muscle recruitment quickness (time rate of torque development)
- Objective documentation of testing
- Computer feedback provided so an athlete can train at submaximal or maximal levels

Admittedly, there are also certainly limitations of isokinetics, and these can be identified in *A Compendium of Isokinetics in Clinical Usage*,[28] as well as in the literature. These involve isolated joint/muscle testing, nonfunctional patterns of movement, limited velocities to replicate the actual speeds of sports performance, increased compressive forces at slower speeds, and increased tibial translation at slow speeds without proximal pad placement.

The previous definitions and terminology will be used in this chapter to describe the application of isokinetics to the evaluation and rehabilitation of the athlete.

Open Kinetic Chain

An OKC assessment or rehabilitation exercise is considered to be an activity in which the distal component of the extremity is not fixed but is free in space. It is questionable whether many exercises are pure OKC, CKC, or combinations of the two. Nevertheless, an operational definition of an OKC test or exercise, within the limitations of this chapter, is one in which the distal end of the extremity is free and not fixed to an object. One of the best examples of the OKC pattern is performing a knee flexion-to-extension pattern while sitting. This OKC pattern will serve as the model to describe OKC exercises.

Closed Kinetic Chain

A CKC assessment or rehabilitation exercise is considered to be an activity in which the distal component of the extremity is fixed. The fixed end may be either stationary or moveable. An example of a CKC exercise in which the distal end is stationary is a squat exercise in which the foot is fixed to the ground. An example of a CKC exercise in which the distal end is moveable is exercise on a leg press system in which the athlete's body is stationary and there is a moveable footplate.

The terms OKC and CKC will be used frequently throughout this chapter in describing both testing and rehabilitation applications of isokinetic exercise.

FUNCTIONAL TESTING ALGORITHM WITH EMPHASIS ON EVALUATION OF ISOKINETIC POWER

Evaluation of isokinetic power is one part of the comprehensive examination or serial reassessment of the injured athlete. Davies[29, 31, 36] has developed a progressive functional testing algorithm (FTA) that can be used as one method of evaluation of isokinetic power in the injured athlete (Table 8–1). The FTA is predicated on a systematic progressive testing sequence proceeding from controlled testing to more functional testing. The FTA for the lower extremity is described in Figure 8–1. A similar approach to testing can be applied to the upper extremity, with functional testing being utilized.[35]

A brief overview of the FTA is presented because the evaluation of isokinetic power of the athlete has to be performed within the context of various evaluation strategies and tools. Isokinetic power is only one of the many parameters that need to be assessed, whether it is for preseason screening, preoperative evaluation, serial reassessments during rehabilitation, or discharge and return to activity.

A summary of the process of using the FTA as a progressive examination strategy and the appropriate rehabilitation interventions is described in Figure 8–2.

The FTA has primary components consisting of basic measurements, strength testing, and functional testing.

Table 8–1. Criteria for Progression in the Functional Testing Algorithm

TESTS	EMPIRIC GUIDELINES
Sport-specific testing	
Lower extremity functional test	M: <1 min 30 sec; F: <2 min
Functional hop test	<15% difference with normative (height) data; <10% bilateral comparison
Functional jump test	<20% of normative (height) data
Standing CKC test	<25% difference with bilateral comparison
OKC test	<25% difference with bilateral comparison
Supine CKC test	<30% difference with bilateral comparison
Digital Balance Evaluator	<0.6
KT-1000 tests	<3 mm difference with bilateral comparison
Basic measurements	<10% difference with bilateral comparison
Subjective measurements (pain)	<3 (on an analog pain scale of 0–10)

CKC, Closed kinetic chain; F, females; M, males; OKC, open kinetic chain.

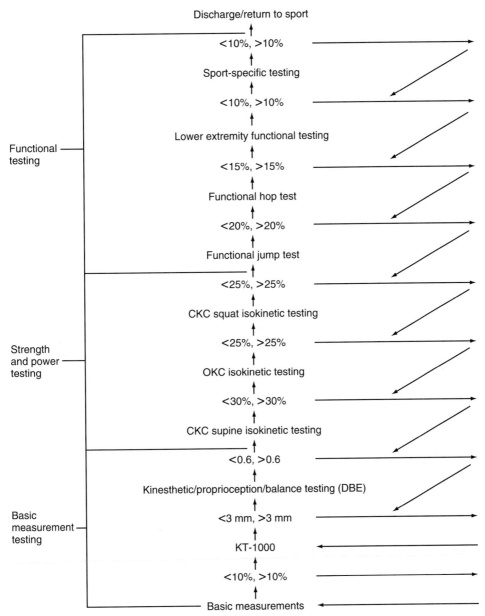

Figure 8-1. Functional testing algorithm. CKC, closed kinetic chain; OKC, open kinetic chain; DBE, Digital Balance Evaluator.

Basic Measurements

Basic measurements are the traditional measurements commonly used to evaluate athletes such as leg length, posture, special tests, and goniometric, flexibility, and anthropometric measurements.

If an athlete still has a 10% or greater deficit in these measurements, rehabilitation is continued to correct the problems. With a deficit less than 10%, the athlete is allowed to progress to the next level of the testing algorithm.

KT-1000 Tests

If the athlete has a cruciate ligament injury, KT-1000 tests are performed to evaluate the laxity of the knee or the integrity of an anterior cruciate ligament

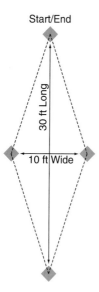

Start/End

30 ft Long

10 ft Wide

Figure 8–2. Functional testing algorithm (FTA) as the foundation for a progressive rehabilitation program. CKC, closed kinetic chain; OKC, open kinetic chain.

(ACL) reconstruction graft. If the athlete's manual maximum KT-1000 test measurements are 3 mm or less in the early stages of rehabilitation, the rehabilitation program can progress according to the clinic protocol. If the manual maximum KT-1000 tests are greater than 3 mm, the protocol is altered to protect the knee.

Kinesthesia/Proprioception/ Balance Testing

Different methods are used to assess proprioception. If deficits are present, the athlete is not allowed to progress in rehabilitation until the deficits are within normal limits of the test parameter. There is some controversy regarding the method of testing lower extremity function, because of the various studies that have researched the effects of CKC exercise in rehabilitation.[17, 37, 40, 41, 64, 102, 103, 124, 132, 139, 169] Therefore, the FTA acknowledges the advantages and disadvantages of testing both the OKC and the CKC and consequently incorporates both modes of testing for kinesthetic/proprioception/balance testing.

CKC Supine Isokinetic Testing

We begin the isokinetic power testing with CKC supine isokinetic testing.[29–32, 36] This is a safe starting position in which most of the variables, such as weight-bearing status, ROM, speed, varus, valgus, and rotational stresses, and translatory joint forces are controlled. The CKC position allows for axial loading in the joint, and consequently, the joint compressive forces help with joint stabilization.[83, 106, 140, 141] In the CKC position, there is also coactivation of the muscles around the knee, thereby creating a dynamic stabilization phenomenon as well.[45, 141] If the athlete has more than a 30% deficit, then various rehabilitation intervention strategies are implemented, with emphasis on bilateral CKC exercises. Once the athlete improves to less than a 30% bilateral deficit, he or she can progress to the next stage of the FTA strength testing for OKC.

Descriptive data for CKC computerized isokinetic data for female and male athletes' lower extremities are described in Table 8–2.[30, 31, 36]

Table 8–2. Descriptive Closed Kinetic Chain Computerized Isokinetic Data for Athletes' Lower Extremities (Linear Pattern)

	FORCE/BW	
SPEED	MALES	FEMALES
Slow (10 in./sec)	≈3 × BW	≈2.5 × BW
Medium (20 in./sec)	≈2.5 × BW	≈2 × BW
Fast (30 in./sec)	≈2 × BW	≈1.5 × BW

BW, Body weight.

OKC Isokinetic Testing

OKC isokinetic testing is performed because it allows for individual isolation of a muscle and, therefore, the ability to selectively isolate and evaluate portions of the kinetic chain. As with the CKC isokinetic testing, we feel this is a safe test, because all the following variables are controlled: weight-bearing status, ROM, speed, varus, valgus, rotational stresses, and translatory joint forces. With use of a proximally placed pad,[82, 90, 160] higher speeds,[160, 168] and limited ROM,[71, 90] OKC isokinetic testing is also safe for ACL reconstructions.[28,38]

Although muscles do not work in isolation functionally, the only way to determine whether a deficit exists within the kinetic chain is to perform power assessments in isolated muscle groups. Although some research indicates there is no correlation between OKC testing and functional performance,[3, 68] there are several studies that demonstrate that a correlation does exist. In other words, if an athlete tests well with OKC isokinetics, he or she will perform well in a variety of functional tests.[9, 74, 135, 148, 159, 167] Research by Davies[29–31, 36] demonstrates that just doing CKC isokinetic testing of several muscle groups in a functional lower extremity pattern does not identify existing weaknesses in major muscle groups. Therefore, there is a need to test isolated muscle groups.

Standardized isokinetic testing techniques to determine total leg strength (TLS), as described by Nicholas et al,[120] Gleim et al,[62] and Davies,[29, 30, 36] can be used for testing various lower extremity muscles.

The athlete must have a less than 25% deficit to progress to the next stage of the FTA. If a deficit exists, then specific OKC exercises or specific exercises targeted to isolate and strengthen the weak muscles are included in the rehabilitation program. Once the deficits are overcome, the athlete can progress to the weight-bearing testing position.

Descriptive data for OKC computerized isokinetic data for female and male athletes' quadriceps are included in Table 8–3.

CKC Squat Isokinetic Testing

The next step in the progression is to test the athlete in the CKC weight-bearing position and to perform squat isokinetic testing.[122, 123] In this position,

Table 8–3. Descriptive Open Kinetic Chain Computerized Isokinetic Quadriceps Torque Scores

	TORQUE/BW	
SPEED	MALE ATHLETES	FEMALE ATHLETES
Slow (60°/sec)	≈100%	≈90%
Medium (180°/sec)	≈66%	≈60%
Fast (300°/sec)	≈50%	≈45%

BW, Body weight.

most variables can still be controlled, but the athlete is now placed in the functional weight-bearing position. The variables of ROM, speed, and varus, valgus, and rotational forces are still well controlled and can be limited.

The fully weight-bearing CKC position allows for a controlled functional assessment. The athlete should have less than a 25% deficit before continuing on to the next stage of the FTA, which progresses to functional testing.

Functional Jump Test

The functional jump test (with both legs)[28, 34] is the next phase of testing, and it leads to the progressive series of functional tests.

Once functional testing begins, there is no longer control of most stresses to the extremity. Shock-type weight bearing (ground reaction force impact loading) occurs, ballistic concentric and eccentric muscle actions occur, ROM varies, control over speed is lost, and significant varus, valgus, and rotational stresses are imposed on the extremities. There is thus progress from the "controlled stress test" environment to an "uncontrolled stress test" situation.

In the functional jump test, the female athlete should jump within at least 20% of the descriptive normative data, which is based on the athlete's height. The male athlete should jump within 10% of the descriptive normative data (Table 8–4).[28]

If the athlete still has more than a 20% deficit, various exercises with emphasis on power activities and plyometrics are incorporated into the rehabilitation program, with bilateral emphasis. Once the athlete can jump to within 20% of the descriptive data in Table 8–4, the athlete progresses to the next stage of the FTA, which is to test each limb separately to compare the uninvolved with the involved extremity.

Functional Hop Test

A functional hop test (one-legged)[28, 39, 67, 84] is performed with all of the same considerations as for the jump test, except that the exercise is performed on one leg. Here, the athlete is expected to hop within 15% of the distance hopped with the uninvolved leg and to within 10% to 15% of the descriptive data in Table 8–4 for women and men. If the athlete cannot meet the these criteria, the rehabilitation is continued, with emphasis on single-leg power exercises and plyometrics. Once the athlete performs with less than a 15% deficit, the next stage of the FTA involves the lower extremity functional test (LEFT).

Lower Extremity Functional Test

In order to incorporate the various functional activities[61, 98, 99] that are inherent in many sports, an LEFT is performed.[28, 31] This is a test for agility and is also an anaerobic test.

Table 8–4. Descriptive Normative Data for Functional Jump Test and Functional Hop Test for Male and Female Athletes*

	MALE	FEMALE
Jump test (both legs)	90%–100%	80%–90%
Hop test (single leg)†		
Uninvolved extremity	80%–90%	70%–80%
Involved extremity	80%–90%	70%–80%

*Data are normalized to body height.
†Bilateral comparison should be within 10%–15%.

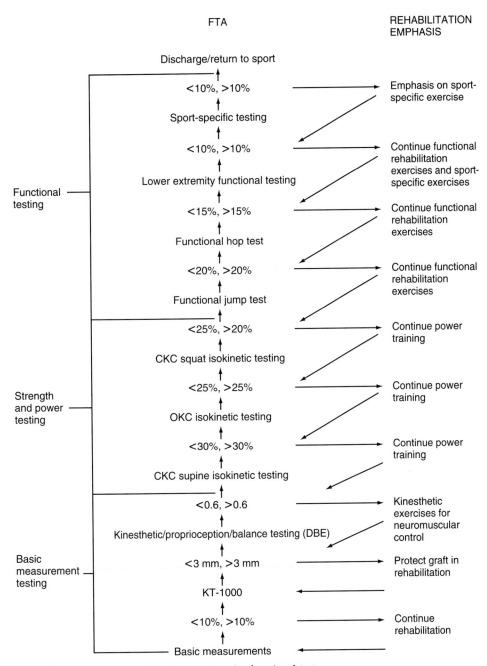

Figure 8–3. Components of the lower extremity functional test.

The test involves a series of different movements to functionally stress the lower extremity in order to replicate various sports performance movements. Figure 8–3 lists the components of the LEFT. Table 8–5 contains the descriptive normative data for the LEFT[28, 31] for women and men.

Sport-Specific Testing

Once an athlete has passed the hierarchy of tests designed to progressively stress the athlete from controlled to noncontrolled environments, sport-specific

Table 8–5. Descriptive Data in a Lower Extremity Functional Test

TIME	MALE	FEMALE
Average	1 min 30 sec	2 min
Range	1–2 min	1 min 30 sec–2 min 30 sec

testing should be performed to determine the athlete's readiness for return to specific sports activity.

ISOKINETIC TESTING

This section will briefly describe some general guidelines and principles of isokinetic testing. For more detailed information, the reader is referred to *A Compendium of Isokinetics in Clinical Usage and Rehabilitation Techniques.*[28]

The purposes for isokinetic testing are several: to obtain objective records, to screen athletes, to establish a database, to quantify objective information, to obtain objective serial reassessments, to develop normative data, to correlate isokinetic torque curves with pathologies, and to use the shape of the curve to individualize the rehabilitation program to a specific athlete's needs.

Isokinetic assessment allows the clinician to objectively assess muscular performance in a way that is both safe and reliable.[167] It affords the clinician objective criteria and provides reproducible data for assessing and monitoring an athlete's status. Isokinetic testing has been demonstrated to be reliable and valid.[8, 28, 57, 60, 70, 87, 89, 111, 113, 115, 116, 127, 131, 143, 149, 151, 158, 162]

Absolute and relative contraindications for testing and using isokinetics in rehabilitation must be established, as with any methodology in medicine. Examples of such contraindications are soft-tissue healing constraints, pain, limited ROM, effusion, joint instability, acute strains and sprains, and occasionally, subacute conditions.

A standard test protocol should be established, which will enhance the reliability of the testing. There are numerous considerations, which include the following: (1) educating the athlete regarding the particular requirements of the test, (2) testing the uninvolved side first to establish a baseline and to demonstrate the requirements so that the athlete's apprehension is decreased, (3) providing appropriate warm-ups at each speed, (4) having consistent verbal commands regarding instructions to the athlete, (5) having a consistent protocol for testing the different joints, (6) having properly calibrated equipment, and (7) providing proper stabilization.

A standard orthopedic testing protocol should be followed during isokinetic testing.[28]

- Educate the athlete: The athlete must be first informed and educated about the purpose, procedures, and requirements of the testing.
- Test the uninvolved side first: The uninvolved side is tested first to establish a baseline and to decrease the athlete's apprehension before testing the involved extremity.
- Perform warm-ups: The athlete should perform several submaximal gradient warm-ups and at least one maximal warm-up before each test. The submaximal warm-ups (25%, 50%, and 75%) prepare

the extremity for the test and allow the athlete to get a feel for the machine. The maximal effort is performed to create a positive learning transfer from a maximal warm-up to a maximal testing effort. This procedure improves the reliability of the testing sequence.[28, 111]

- Give consistent verbal commands: These should be standardized and remain the same throughout the testing sequence in order to improve test-retest reliability.

- Use standardized test protocols: The recommended testing protocols for each joint have been described in detail. The specific anatomic position and stabilization guidelines, ROM, speed, and other considerations have been described.[28]

- Test at different speeds: We recommend the use of a velocity spectrum testing protocol. Velocity spectrum testing refers to testing at slow (0° per second to 60° per second), intermediate (60° per second to 180° per second), fast (180° per second to 300° per second), and functional (300° per second to 1000° per second) contractile velocities. Performing three to five test repetitions at each speed and 20 to 30 repetitions at a fast speed (240° per second or 300° per second) for an endurance test is recommended.

Isokinetic testing allows for a variety of testing protocols ranging from power to endurance tests (see Davies[28] for a detailed description of the various isokinetic testing protocols). Our primary recommendation is to perform velocity spectrum testing so that the test will assess the muscle's capabilities at different speeds, thus simulating various activities. Often, deficits in a muscle's performance may show up at one speed and not at others. For example, athletes with a patellofemoral problem often have more power deficits at slow speeds, whereas after various surgical procedures of the knee, athletes will have fast-velocity deficits.

ISOKINETIC DATA AND ANALYSIS

One of the advantages of isokinetic testing is that it provides numerous objective parameters that can be used to evaluate and analyze an athlete's performance. Various isokinetic testing data that are frequently used to analyze an athlete's performance are peak torque, time rate of torque development, acceleration, deceleration, ROM, total work, average power, and shape of the torque curves.[28]

After these data are collected from the tests and analyzed regarding specific deficits and limitations of the athlete, the results need to be interpreted using some of the following criteria[28]:

- Bilateral comparison: Comparing the involved to the uninvolved extremity is probably the most common evaluation. Bilateral differences of 10% to 15% are considered to represent significant asymmetry. However, this single parameter by itself has limitations.

- Unilateral ratios: Comparing the relationship between the agonist and the antagonist muscles may identify particular weaknesses in certain muscle groups. This parameter is particularly important to assess with velocity spectrum testing, because the percentage relationships of the muscles change with changing speeds in many muscle groups. (Percentage relationship means that the unilateral ratio of antagonistic muscle torque is a certain percentage of agonist muscle torque. This percentage of torque production of the antagonist to the agonist muscle changes through the velocity spectrum.)
- Torque-to–body weight relationship: Comparing the torques to the body weight adds another dimension in interpreting test results. Often, even though bilateral symmetry and normal unilateral ratios are present, the torque-to-body weight relationship is altered.
- Total leg strength: Nicholas et al,[120] Gleim et al,[62] and Boltz and Davies[13] have published articles on the importance of considering the entire kinetic chain concept of total leg strength (TLS).
- Comparison to normative data: Although the use of normative data is controversial, if it is used properly relative to a specific population of athletes, it can be used to provide guidelines for testing or rehabilitation.

RATIONALE AND NEED FOR ISOKINETIC TESTING AND REHABILITATION

Although the purpose of this chapter is to describe the rationale and need for isokinetic rehabilitation, a few comments are necessary regarding why CKC exercises should be used instead of just OKC exercises. Many articles have described the rationale for using CKC exercises,[6, 14, 21, 23, 40, 45, 64, 72, 83, 122, 124, 133] particularly in rehabilitating athletes with ACL reconstructions.[2, 41, 44, 65, 74, 75, 78, 91, 102, 103, 105–110, 118, 122, 132, 135, 139–141] However, Crandall et al[25] performed a meta-analysis of 1167 articles on the treatment of athletes with ACL injuries published between 1966 and 1993 and found that only five articles (and three of these articles included data on the same athletes) met the criteria for meta-analysis of prospective, randomized, controlled, experimental clinical trials. Consequently, many of the articles that are commonly referred to as "definitive treatment articles" are simply descriptive studies. Therefore, although the benefits of using CKC exercises in rehabilitation have been described quite extensively, few scientifically based, prospective, randomized, controlled, experimental clinical trials[17, 37, 144] document the efficacy of CKC exercises.

The rationale for the use of only CKC is thus founded not on scientific studies that have documented its efficacy, but more on unverified empiric observations and descriptive studies.[24]

RATIONALE FOR OKC ISOKINETIC ASSESSMENT

Despite the many described disadvantages of OKC assessment, there are still several reasons why OKC exercises should be incorporated in both assessment and rehabilitation. These are as follows:

1. It is necessary to perform isolated testing of specific muscle groups usually affected by certain pathologic changes. If the component parts of the kinetic chain are not measured, the weak link will not be identified or adequately rehabilitated, which will affect the entire chain.[28, 30]

2. Muscle groups away from the specific site of injury must be assessed to determine other associated weaknesses (e.g., disuse, pre-existing problems).[62, 120]

3. CKC or total extremity testing may not demonstrate the true weakness that exists; often, proximal and distal muscles compensate for weak areas.[30, 36]

4. Performing OKC testing allows the clinician to have significant clinical control. The examiner can control ROM, speed, translational stresses (by shin pad placement), varus and valgus forces, and rotational forces. When CKC exercises are begun, control of these variables decreases, thereby increasing the potential risk of injury to the athlete.

5. Although most athletes do not sit flexing and extending their knees in an OKC pattern when they are performing, numerous studies (based on a variety of functional assessment tests) demonstrate a correlation between OKC testing and CKC functional performance.[9, 68, 137, 148, 150, 159, 167]

6. When an athlete has an injury or dysfunction related to pain, reflex inhibition, decreased ROM, or weakness, abnormal movement patterns often result and create abnormal motor learning. Isolated OKC training can work within the limitations to normalize the motor pattern.

7. Efficacy of rehabilitation with OKC exercises[29, 35-37, 91, 94, 95, 129, 142, 144, 150, 166, 167] has been demonstrated in numerous articles throughout the literature. The reader is encouraged to check the references for a more detailed description of the studies.

The primary purpose of performing OKC isokinetic assessment is the need to test specific muscle groups of a pathologic joint in isolation. Although the muscles do not work in an isolated fashion, a deficit, or "weak link," in a kinetic chain will never be identified unless specific isolated OKC isokinetic testing is performed. Furthermore, on serial retesting, one will not know how the athlete is progressing and if and when the athlete meets the parameters for discharge. Examples of the importance of performing isolated testing of the kinetic chain to identify specific dysfunctions have been offered by several authors including Nicholas et al[120] and Gleim et al.[62]

Nicholas et al[120] performed TLS isokinetic testing and developed a composite lower extremity score. They evaluated several groups of athletes with various pathologic conditions and determined that certain characteristic patterns of muscle weakness could be correlated with the specific pathologic syndromes. In ankle and foot problems, knee ligamentous instabilities, intra-articular defects, and patellofemoral dysfunctions, there was an irrefutable deficit in TLS ($p < 0.01$). For example, athletes with ankle and foot problems have statistically significant weaknesses of the ipsilateral hip abductors and adductors. Furthermore, there was a trend toward ipsilateral weakness of the quadriceps and hamstring muscles, although these trends are not statistically significant.

Gleim et al[62] also determined that the total percent deficit in the injured leg was the one value that was most informative. Typically, when a single muscle group is compared bilaterally, values that fall within 10% are empirically determined to be normal. Because the TLS composite score is more sensitive and minimizes the variability, Gleim et al suggested that even a 5% difference in bilateral comparison is significant.

It is important to note that the only way to document weaknesses in muscle groups distant to the site of injury is through performing isolated OKC testing. Furthermore, specific muscle weakness at the injury site can be identified only by isolated OKC testing.

Another example of the need for isolated testing was illustrated in the recent work by Davies,[30] who performed CKC computerized isokinetic tests on athletes with various knee injuries and also analyzed bilateral comparison data. Dynamic CKC isokinetic testing that required a linear motion with force production being measured in pounds at slow (10 inches per second), medium (20 inches per second), and fast (30 inches per second) velocities was done on a Linea computerized CKC isokinetic dynamometer system.* The same athletes were also tested on a Cybex OKC computerized isokinetic dynamometer,† and a bilateral analysis of the data was performed. Isolated joint testing was performed to provide rotational force and torque values, which were recorded at slow (60° per second), medium (180° per second), and fast (300° per second) angular velocities. The results of the testing demonstrate that more significant deficits were shown to exist in athletes after OKC isolated joint and muscle testing than after CKC multiple joint and muscle testing (Table 8–6).

Similar results were reported by Feiring and Ellenbecker[58] with isokinetic open- and closed-chain testing of 23 athletes 15 weeks after ACL reconstruction. Bilateral comparisons of open-chain knee extension isokinetic muscle function ranged from 74% to 77% of the uninjured extremity, whereas CKC isokinetic testing using a leg press extension-type movement pattern ranged between 91% and 93% of the uninjured extremity.

When testing multiple muscle groups and developing a summative composite score of their forces, the proximal and distal muscles apparently compensate for weak muscles and tend to demonstrate less of a deficit than actually exists in the area. We have made this empirically based observation for years, but now CKC isokinetic testing that objectively documents and quantifies performance has supported this observation. Again, if muscle's performance is not measured, a deficit cannot be identified. These research studies and examples provide justification for the need for OKC isokinetic testing.

Another major reason for performing OKC isokinetic testing is the clinical control afforded. When testing, the examiner controls ROM, speeds, translational stresses (by shin pad placement), varus and valgus stresses, and rotational forces. However, when one begins CKC testing, control of the these variables decreases, thereby increasing the potential risk to the athlete.

An often-cited example is that performing OKC isokinetic tests on an athlete who has had an ACL reconstruction can stretch or injure the graft. This is a situation of good science being applied to an inappropriate clinical setting. If the graft were actually to be stretched during OKC testing, the problem is more one of the clinician's performing an inappropriate test or testing at an inappropriate time rather than of the OKC test itself.[104]

When testing or rehabilitating an athlete after an ACL reconstruction, the following guidelines should be used to prevent injury:

---

*Available from Loredan Biomedical, West Sacramento, California
†Available from Cybex, Ronkonkoma, New York

Table 8–6. Comparisons Between Open Kinetic Chain and Closed Kinetic Chain Computerized Isokinetic Dynamometer Testing of 300 Patients with Various Pathologic Knee Conditions or After Surgery

CYBEX (OKC)			LINEA (CKC)		
PARAMETER	*VALUES*	*% DEFICIT*	*PARAMETER*	*VALUES*	*% DEFICIT*
Peak torque Force	60°/sec (quadriceps)	29%	Peak torque Force	10 in/sec	9%
U	142 ft lb		U	462 lb	
I	101 ft lb		I	420 lb	
Peak torque (BW) Force	60°/sec (quadriceps)	31%	Peak torque (%BW) Force	10 in/sec	11%
U	95%		U	298 lb	
I	66%		I	266 lb	
Peak torque Force	180°/sec	21%	Peak torque Force	20 in/sec	11%
U	99 ft lb		U	374 lbs	
I	78 ft lb		I	331 lbs	
Peak torque (BW) Force	180°/sec	25%	Peak torque (%BW) Force	20 in/sec	11%
U	64%		U	239 lb	
I	48%		I	253 lb	
Peak torque Force	300°/sec	20%	Peak torque Force	30 in/sec	16%
U	80 ft lb		U	302 lb	
I	64 ft lb		I	253 lb	
Peak torque (BW) Force	300°/sec	20%	Peak torque (%BW) Force	30 in/sec	11%
U	51%		U	193 lb	
I	41%		I	171 lb	

BW, Body weight; I, involved extremity; U, uninvolved extremity.

1. Know the type of surgery (e.g., whether autograft or allograft was used).
2. Know the fixation technique.
3. Determine the graft status (using KT-1000 testing).
4. Establish testing guidelines for particular pathologic conditions (exceptions always exist).
5. Respect soft-tissue healing times (based on clinical protocols).
6. Use a proximally placed pad.[90, 160]
7. Limit ROM (avoid 30° to 0° of knee flexion to extension).[71]
8. Use faster velocities.[160]

Correlation of OKC to CKC Functional Performance

In addition to obtaining clinical control, another reason to perform OKC isokinetic testing is because of the correlation of OKC isokinetic testing with CKC functional performance. Although athletes do not regularly function by sitting in a chair while flexing and extending their knees, and although some research indicates that there is no functional correlation,[3, 68] numerous studies do demonstrate a positive correlation between OKC testing and functional performance.[9, 74, 135, 137, 148, 150, 159, 167]

SPECIFIC APPLICATION OF ISOKINETIC ASSESSMENT OF MUSCULAR POWER IN THE UPPER EXTREMITY

Application of isokinetic exercise and testing for the upper extremity is imperative, because of the demanding muscular work required in sport-specific activities. The large unrestricted ROM of the glenohumeral joint and limited inherent bony stability necessitate dynamic muscular stabilization to ensure normal joint arthrokinematics.[112] Objective information regarding the intricate balance of agonist and antagonist muscular strength at the glenohumeral joint is a vital resource for rehabilitation and preventive evaluation of the shoulder. Utilization of therapeutic exercise and isolated joint testing for the entire upper extremity kinetic chain, including the scapulothoracic joint, is indicated for an overuse injury or postoperative rehabilitation of an isolated injury of the shoulder or elbow.[34]

Rationale for Utilization of Isokinetics in Upper Extremity Strength Assessment

Unlike the lower extremities, in which most functional and sport-specific movements occur in a CKC environment, the upper extremities function almost exclusively in an OKC format.[124] The throwing motion, tennis serve, and ground stroke all are examples of OKC activities for the upper extremity. OKC muscular strength assessment methodology allows for isolation of particular muscle groups, as opposed to closed-chain methods, which utilize multiple joint axes, planes, and joint and muscle segments. Traditional isokinetic upper extremity test patterns are open chain with respect to the shoulder, elbow, and wrist. The velocity spectrum (1° per second to approximately 1000° per second) currently available on commercial isokinetic dynamometers provides specificity with regard to testing the upper extremity by allowing the clinician to assess muscular strength at faster, more functional speeds. Table 8–7 lists the angular velocities of sport-specific upper extremity movements.

The dynamic nature of upper extremity movements is a critical factor in directing the clinician to optimal testing methodology for the upper extremity. Manual muscle testing (MMT) provides a static alternative for the assessment of muscular strength by using well-developed patient positions and stabilization.[25, 92] Despite the detailed description of manual assessment techniques,

Table 8–7. Upper Extremity Angular Velocities of Functional Activities

JOINT	MOVEMENT	SPORTS ACTIVITY	ANGULAR VELOCITY	SOURCE
Shoulder	Internal rotation	Baseball pitching	7000°/sec	Dillman et al[42]
Shoulder	Internal rotation	Tennis serve	1000–1500°/sec	Shapiro and Steine[138]
Shoulder	Internal rotation	Tennis serve	2300°/sec	Dillman et al[42]
Elbow	Extension	Baseball pitching	2500°/sec	Dillman et al[42]
Elbow	Extension	Tennis serve	1700°/sec	Dillman[43]
Wrist	Flexion	Tennis serve	315°/sec	Vangheluwe and Hebbelinck[152]

reliability of MMT is compromised because of differences in the size and strength of clinicians and patients and the subjective nature of the grading system.[119, 153]

Ellenbecker[49] compared isokinetic testing of the shoulder internal and external rotators to MMT in 54 subjects who exhibited symmetric normal grade (5/5) strength by manual assessment. Isokinetic testing found 13% to 15% bilateral differences in external rotation (ER) and 15% to 28% bilateral differences in internal rotation (IR). Of particular significance was the large variability in the size of this mean difference between extremities, despite the presence of bilateral symmetry on MMT. The use of MMT is an integral part of a musculoskeletal evaluation. MMT provides a time-efficient, gross screening of muscular strength of multiple muscles using a static, isometric muscular contraction, particularly in patients with neuromuscular disease or in athletes with large muscular strength deficits.[119, 153] The limitations of MMT appear to be most evident in instances in which there is only minor impairment of strength, as well as in the identification of subtle isolated strength deficits. Differentiation of agonist and antagonist muscular strength balance is also complicated when using manual techniques, as opposed to using isokinetic apparatus.[49]

Glenohumeral Joint Testing

Dynamic strength assessment of the rotator cuff musculature is of primary importance in rehabilitation and preventive screening of the glenohumeral joint. The rotator cuff forms an integral component of the force couple in the shoulder as described by Inman et al.[85] The approximating role of the supraspinatus muscle for the glenohumeral joint, as well as the inferior (caudal) glide component action provided by the infraspinatus, teres minor, and subscapularis muscles, must stabilize the humeral head within the glenoid cavity against the superiorly directed forces exerted by the deltoid muscle with humeral elevation.[96] Muscular imbalances, primarily in the posterior rotator cuff, have been objectively documented in athletes with glenohumeral joint instability and impingement.[157]

Shoulder Internal Rotation and External Rotation Strength Testing

Initial testing and training using isokinetics for rehabilitation of the shoulder typically involves the modified base position. The modified base position is obtained by tilting the dynamometer approximately 30° from the horizontal base position.[27, 28] This causes the shoulder to be placed in approximately 30° of abduction (Fig. 8–4). The modified base position places the shoulder in the scapular plane 30° anterior to the coronal plane.[136] The scapular plane is characterized by enhanced bony congruity and a neutral glenohumeral position that results in a midrange position for the capsular ligaments and scapulohumeral musculature.[136] This position does not place the suprahumeral structures in an impingement situation and is well tolerated by athletes.[27]

Isokinetic testing using the modified base position requires consistent testing of the athlete on the dynamometer. Studies have demonstrated significant differences in IR and ER strength with varying degrees of abduction, flexion, and horizontal abduction and adduction of the glenohumeral joint.[73, 145, 156] The modified base position uses a standing athlete position, which compromises both isolation and test-retest reliability. Despite these limitations, valuable data can be obtained early in the rehabilitative process using this neutral, modified base position.[26, 28, 50]

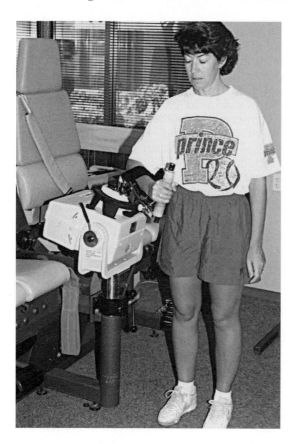

Figure 8–4. Modified neutral position for isokinetic testing of shoulder internal or external rotation.

Isokinetic assessment of IR and ER strength is also done with 90° of glenohumeral joint abduction. Specific advantages of this test position are greater stabilization in either a seated or supine test position on most dynamometers and placement of the shoulder in an abduction angle, corresponding to the overhead throwing position used in sports activities.[42, 56] As a precursor to using the 90°-abducted position, we require initial tolerance of the athlete to the modified base position. Ninety-degree abducted isokinetic testing can be performed in either the coronal or the scapular plane. The benefits of the scapular plane are similar to those discussed for the modified position and include protection of the anterior capsular glenohumeral ligaments and a theoretic length-tension enhancement of the posterior rotator cuff.[55, 69, 73] Changes in length-tension relationships and in the line of action of scapulohumeral and axiohumeral musculature are reported with 90° of glenohumeral joint abduction instead of a more neutral adducted glenohumeral joint position.[27] The 90°-abducted position for isokinetic strength assessment is more specific for assessing the muscular functions required for overhead activities.[12]

Heavy emphasis is placed on assessing IR and ER strength of the shoulder during rehabilitation. The rationale for this apparently narrow focus is provided by an isokinetic training study by Quincy et al.[129] Six weeks of isokinetic training of the internal and external rotators produced statistically significant improvements not only in IR and ER strength but also in flexion-extension and abduction-adduction strength. Isokinetic training for flexion-extension and for abduction-adduction produced improvements only in the position of training. The physiologic overflow of strength caused by training the internal and external rotators provides a rationale for the heavy emphasis on strength development and assessment in rehabilitation. Additional research has identified the IR and

ER movement pattern as the preferred testing pattern in athletes with rotator cuff tendinosis.[81]

INTERPRETATION OF SHOULDER INTERNAL AND EXTERNAL ROTATION TESTING
Bilateral Differences

As with isokinetic testing of the lower extremities, the assessment of the strength of an extremity relative to the contralateral side forms the basis for standard data interpretation. This practice is more complicated in the upper extremities because of limb dominance, particularly in unilaterally dominant sports athletes. In addition to the complexity caused by limb dominance, isokinetic descriptive studies demonstrate disparities in the degree of limb dominance, as well as in strength dominance only in specified muscle groups.[1, 20, 22, 47, 48, 51, 54, 79]

In general, a maximum limb dominance of the internal and external rotators of 5% to 10% is assumed in nonathletic persons and athletes engaging in recreational upper extremity sports.[123] Significantly greater IR strength has been identified in the dominant arm in professional,[16, 54] collegiate,[22] and high school[79] baseball players, as well as in elite junior[20, 48] and adult[47] tennis players. No difference between extremities has been demonstrated in concentric ER in professional[54, 163] and collegiate[22] baseball pitchers or in elite junior[20, 48] and adult[47] tennis players. This selective strength development in the internal rotators produces significant changes in agonist-antagonist muscular balance. The identification of this selectivity with isokinetic testing has implications for rehabilitation and prevention of injuries.

Normative Data Utilization

Normative or descriptive data can assist clinicians in further analyzing isokinetic test data. Care must be taken to use normative data that is both population- and apparatus-specific.[60] Tables 8–8 to 8–10 present data from large samples of specific athletic populations using two dynamometer systems. Data are presented using body weight as the normalizing factor.

Unilateral Strength Ratios (Agonist-to-Antagonist)

The assessment of muscular strength balance of the internal and external rotators is of vital importance when interpreting upper extremity strength tests. Alteration of this ER-to-IR ratio has been reported in athletes with glenohumeral joint instability and impingement.[157] The initial description of the ER-to-IR ratio on normal female subjects was published by Ivey[86] and confirmed by Davies[27] for both men and women. An ER-to-IR ratio of 66% is targeted in normal subjects. Biasing this ratio in favor of the external rotators has been advocated by clinicians,[25, 50, 161] both for preventing injury in throwing and racquet-sport athletes and for following injury or surgery to the glenohumeral joint.

Reports of alteration of the ER-to-IR ratio because of selective muscular development of the internal rotators without concomitant ER strength are widespread in the literature.[22, 47, 48, 54, 51, 79] This alteration has provided clinicians with an objective rationale for the global recommendation of preventive posterior rotator cuff ER-strengthening programs for athletes in high-level overhead activities.[50, 161] Examples of ER-to-IR ratios in specific athletic populations and with specific apparatus are presented in Tables 8–10 and 8–11.

Table 8–8. Isokinetic Peak Torque–to–Body Weight Ratios from 150 Professional Baseball Pitchers*

| SPEED | INTERNAL ROTATION | | EXTERNAL ROTATION | |
	DOMINANT ARM	NONDOMINANT ARM	DOMINANT ARM	NONDOMINANT ARM
180°/sec	27%	17%	18%	19%
300°/sec	25%	24%	15%	15%

From Wilk, K.E., Andrews, J.R., Arrigo, C.A., et al. (1993): The strength characteristics of internal and external rotator muscles in professional baseball pitchers. Am. J. Sports Med., 21:61–66.
*Data were obtained on a Biodex Isokinetic Dynamometer.

Table 8–9. Isokinetic Peak Torque–to–Body Weight and Work–to–Body Weight Ratios from 147 Professional Baseball Pitchers*

| SPEED | INTERNAL ROTATION | | EXTERNAL ROTATION | |
	DOMINANT ARM	NONDOMINANT ARM	DOMINANT ARM	NONDOMINANT ARM
210°/sec				
Torque	21%	19%	13%	14%
Work	41%	38%	25%	25%
300°/sec				
Torque	20%	18%	13%	13%
Work	37%	33%	23%	23%

Data from Ellenbecker, T.S., and Mattalino, A.J. (1997): Concentric isokinetic shoulder internal and external rotation strength in professional baseball pitchers. J. Orthop. Sports Phys. Ther., 25:323–328.
*Data were obtained on a Cybex 350 Isokinetic Dynamometer.

Table 8–10. Isokinetic Peak Torque–to–Body Weight Ratios, Single Repetition Work–to–Body Weight Ratios, and External Rotation–to–Internal Rotation Ratios in Elite Junior Tennis Players*

| | DOMINANT ARM | | NONDOMINANT ARM | |
	PEAK TORQUE (%)	WORK (%)	PEAK TORQUE (%)	WORK (%)
External rotation (ER)				
Male, 210°/sec	12	20	11	19
Male, 300°/sec	10	18	10	17
Female, 210°/sec	8	14	8	15
Female, 300°/sec	8	11	7	12
Internal rotation (IR)				
Male, 210°/sec	17	32	14	27
Male, 300°/sec	15	28	13	23
Female, 210°/sec	12	23	11	19
Female, 300°/sec	11	15	10	13
ER/IR ratio				
Male, 210°/sec	51	64	80	78
Male, 300°/sec	70	65	81	80
Female, 210°/sec	70	66	79	82
Female, 300°/sec	67	69	77	80

*A Cybex 300 series Isokinetic Dynamometer and 90° of glenohumeral joint abduction were used. Data are expressed in foot-pounds per unit of body weight.

Table 8–11. Unilateral External Rotation/Internal Rotation Ratios in Professional Baseball Pitchers

SPEED	DOMINANT ARM	NONDOMINANT ARM
180°/sec		
Torque	65	64
300°/sec		
Torque	61	70
210°/sec		
Torque	64	74
Work	61	66
300°/sec		
Torque	65	72
Work	62	70

Data from Wilk, K.E., Andrews, J.R., Arrigo, C.A., et al. (1993): The strength characteristics of internal and external rotator muscles in professional baseball pitchers. Am. J. Sports Med., 21:61–66, and Ellenbecker, T.S., and Mattalino, A.J. (1997): Concentric isokinetic shoulder internal and external rotation strength in professional baseball pitchers. J. Orthop. Sports Phys. Ther., 25:323–328.

Additional Glenohumeral Joint Testing Positions

SHOULDER ABDUCTION AND ADDUCTION

Isokinetic evaluation of shoulder abduction-adduction strength is an additional pattern frequently evaluated because of the key role of the abductors in the Inman force couple[85] and the functional relationship of the adductors to throwing velocity.[11, 91] Specific factors important in this testing pattern are the limitation of ROM to approximately 120° to avoid glenohumeral joint impingement and the consistent use of gravity correction.[76]

Interpretation of abduction-adduction isokinetic tests follows traditional bilateral comparison, normative data comparison, and unilateral strength ratios. Ivey,[86] testing normal adult women, reported ratios of 50% bilaterally. Similar findings were reported by Alderink and Kluck[1] in high school and collegiate baseball pitchers. Wilk[164, 165] reported dominant arm abduction-to-adduction ratios of 85% to 95% using a Biodex dynamometer. His data utilized a windowing technique that removed impact artifacts after free-limb acceleration and end-stop impact from the data. Upper extremity testing, using long input adapters and fast isokinetic testing velocities, can produce a torque artifact that significantly changes the isokinetic test result. Wilk recommended windowing the data by excluding all data obtained at velocities outside 95% of the present angular testing velocity.[165] (Because of free limb acceleration and deceleration, only a portion of the entire ROM is truly isokinetic. If the velocities differ from actual test speed by 5% or more, then the data are not valid isokinetic data and should not be used.)

SHOULDER FLEXION-EXTENSION AND HORIZONTAL ABDUCTION-ADDUCTION

Additional isokinetic patterns used to obtain a more detailed profile of shoulder function are flexion-extension and horizontal abduction-adduction. Both these motions are generally tested in a less-functional supine position to improve stabilization. Normative data on these testing positions are less prevalent in the literature. Flexion-to-extension ratios reported for normal subjects by Ivey[86] are 80% (4:5). Ratios for athletes with shoulder extension–dominant activities are reported at 50% for baseball pitchers[1] and 75% to 80% for highly skilled adult tennis players.[47] Normative data need to be developed further to define strength more clearly in these upper extremity patterns. Body position and gravity compensation are, again, key factors affecting proper interpretation of data.

SCAPULOTHORACIC TESTING
(PROTRACTION-RETRACTION)

In addition to the supraspinatus-deltoid force couple, the serratus anterior–trapezius force couple is of critical importance for a thorough evaluation of upper extremity strength. Gross manual muscle testing and screening attempting to identify scapular winging are commonly utilized in the clinical evaluation of the shoulder complex. Davies and Hoffman[35] have recently published normative data on 250 shoulders regarding isokinetic protraction-retraction testing. An approximately 1:1 relationship of protraction-retraction strength was reported. Testing and training the serratus anterior, trapezius, and rhomboid musculature enhances scapular stabilization and strengthens primary musculature involved in the scapulohumeral rhythm. Emphasis on the promotion of proximal stability to enhance distal mobility is a concept used and recognized by nearly all disciplines of rehabilitative medicine.[147]

Concentric versus Eccentric Considerations

The availability of eccentric dynamic strength assessment has made a significant impact, primarily in research investigations. The extrapolation of research-oriented isokinetic principles to patient populations has been a gradual process. Eccentric testing in the upper extremity is clearly indicated on the basis of the prevalence of functionally specific eccentric work. Maximal eccentric functional contractions of the posterior rotator cuff during the follow-through phase of the throwing motion and tennis serve provide a rationale for eccentric testing and training in rehabilitation and preventive conditioning.[88] Kennedy et al[93] found mode-specific differences between the concentric and eccentric strength characteristics of the rotator cuff. Further research regarding eccentric muscular training is necessary before widespread use of eccentric isokinetics can be applied to patient populations.

The basic characteristics of eccentric isokinetic testing, such as greater force production as compared to concentric contractions at the same velocity, have been reported for the internal and external rotators.[33, 53, 117] This enhanced force generation is generally explained by the contribution of the series elastic (non-contractile) elements of the muscle-tendon unit in eccentric conditions. An increase in postexercise muscle soreness, particularly of latent onset, is a common occurrence following periods of eccentric work. Therefore, eccentric testing would not be the mode of choice during early inflammatory stages of an overuse injury.[33] Many clinicians recommend the use of dynamic concentric testing before performing an eccentric test. Both concentric and eccentric isokinetic training of the rotator cuff have produced objective concentric and eccentric strength improvements in elite tennis players.[53, 117]

RELATIONSHIP OF ISOKINETIC TESTING TO FUNCTIONAL PERFORMANCE

Dynamic muscular strength assessment is used to evaluate the underlying strength and balance of strength in specific muscle groups. This information is used to determine the specific anatomic structure that requires strengthening, as well as to demonstrate the efficacy of treatment procedures. Isokinetic testing of the shoulder internal and external rotators has been used as one parameter for demonstrating the functional outcome after rotator cuff repair on select patient populations.[63, 130, 154, 155]

An additional purpose for isokinetic testing is to determine the relationship of muscular strength to functional performance. Several studies have tested upper extremity muscle groups and have correlated their respective levels of strength to sport-specific functional tests. Pedegana et al[126] found a statistical relationship between elbow extension, wrist flexion, shoulder extension-flexion, and ER strength measured isokinetically and throwing speed in professional pitchers. Bartlett et al,[11] in a similar study, found shoulder adduction to correlate with throwing speed. These studies are in contrast to those of Pawlowski and Perrin,[125] who did not find a significant relationship in throwing velocity.

Ellenbecker et al[53] determined that 6 weeks of concentric isokinetic training of the rotator cuff resulted in a statistically significant improvement in serving velocity in collegiate tennis players. Mont et al,[117] in a similar study, found serving velocity improvements following both concentric and eccentric IR and ER training. A direct statistical relationship between isokinetically measured upper extremity strength and tennis serve velocity was not obtained by Ellenbecker,[47] despite earlier studies showing increases in serving velocity after isokinetic training. The complex biomechanical sequence of segmental velocities and the interrelationship of the kinetic chain link with the lower extremities and trunk make delineation and identification of a direct relationship between an isolated structure and a complex functional activity difficult. Isokinetic testing can provide a reliable, dynamic measurement of isolated joint motions and muscular contributions to assist the clinician in the assessment of underlying muscular strength and strength balance. The integration of isokinetic testing with a thorough, objective clinical evaluation allows the clinician to provide optimal rehabilitation both in overuse injuries and in postsurgery cases.

APPLICATION OF ISOKINETICS IN DESIGNING REHABILITATION PROGRAMS

Many types of exercise programs are in widespread use for rehabilitating injured athletes. This section focuses on resistive rehabilitation programs, as well as on the specific progression of resistive exercise recommended during rehabilitation. The resistive rehabilitation programs vary from isometric, concentric, and eccentric isotonics to concentric and eccentric isokinetics to isoacceleration and isodeceleration programs. The scientific and clinical rationale for progression through a resistive exercise rehabilitation program is described, including the specific progression and inclusion of isokinetic exercise in the clinical rehabilitation of upper extremity overuse injuries.

Patient Progression Criteria

Several important concepts predicate the progression through the resistive exercise program. These include athlete status, signs and symptoms, time after surgery, and soft-tissue healing constraints. The athlete's progression up the various levels of the resistive exercise program is determined by continual charting and assessment of subjective and objective evaluative criteria (Table 8–12). This resistive exercise progression continuum[28] is based on the concept of a trial treatment. If any adverse changes occur, the rehabilitation program continues at the previous level of intensity of repetitions, sets, or duration without the athlete's progressing to the next level of the exercise progression continuum.

Table 8-12. Commonly Used Subjective and Objective Criteria for Patient Progress in a Rehabilitation Program

SUBJECTIVE CRITERIA (SYMPTOMS)	OBJECTIVE CRITERIA (SIGNS)
Pain	Anthropometric measurements
Stiffness	Goniometric measurements
Changes in function	Palpable cutaneous temperature changes
	Redness
	Manual muscle testing
	Isokinetic testing
	Kinesthetic testing
	Functional performance testing
	KT-1000 testing

From Davies, G.J. (1992): A Compendium of Isokinetics in Clinical Usage and Rehabilitation Techniques, 4th ed. Onalaska, WI, S & S Publishers.

If, however, an athlete performs the trial treatment without any negative effects, then the athlete progresses gradually to the next higher level in the exercise continuum. An athlete may enter the exercise rehabilitation continuum at any stage depending on the results of the initial evaluation. Furthermore, an athlete may also progress through several stages from one treatment session to the next depending primarily on the athlete's response. Before beginning the actual resistive exercise portion of the rehabilitation program, various warm-up exercises and mobilization-stretching exercises are appropriate.

Resistive Exercise Progression Continuum

The rehabilitation program is designed along a progression continuum. The program begins with the safest exercises and progresses to the more stressful exercises. These are illustrated in Figure 8–5 and Table 8–13.

MULTIPLE-ANGLE ISOMETRICS

The exercise rehabilitation program typically begins with multiple-angle isometrics that are performed at a submaximal intensity level. The isometrics are performed approximately every 20° through the ROM that is indicated, based on the athlete's safe and comfortable ROM demonstrated during examination. The rationale for using this particular exercise is the presence of a 20° physiologic overflow with the application of isometrics[28] (Fig. 8–6). Therefore, as an example (Fig. 8–7), if the athlete presents with a painful arc syndrome, which is common in a shoulder with rotator cuff pathology, the isometrics can be applied every 20° through the ROM, and the athlete will still obtain a concomitant strengthening effect throughout the entire ROM without increasing the symptomatic area. The painful arc that is typical in athletes with rotator cuff pathology occurs between 85° and 135° of elevation, at which point peak forces against the undersurface of the acromion occur.[101] Performing isometric exercise around the painful arc during the rehabilitation process is a prime example of applying isometrics early in rehabilitation of the shoulder after overuse injury or after surgery.

The next consideration with isometric exercise is that the athlete use the rule of tens: 10-second contractions, 10-second rest, 10 repetitions, and so on. The athlete is usually taught to perform the isometrics in the following sequence: (1) take 2 seconds to gradually build up the desired tension, whether working at a submaximal or maximal intensity level; (2) hold the desired tension of the

STAGES:

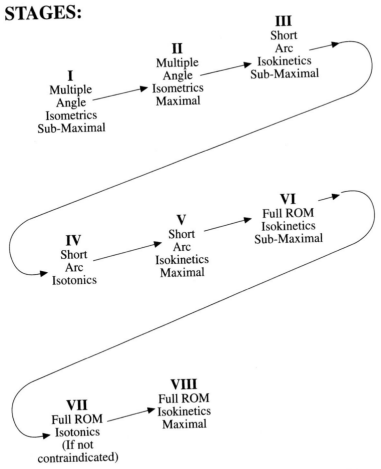

Figure 8–5. Stages of Davies' resistive exercise progression continuum. (From Davies, G.J. [1992]: A Compendium of Isokinetics in Clinical Usage and Rehabilitation Techniques, 4th ed. Onalaska, WI, S & S Publishers.)

isometric contraction for 6 seconds, which is the optimum duration for an isometric contraction[7]; and (3) gradually relax, releasing the tension in the muscle over the last 2 seconds (Fig. 8–8). This sequence allows for a controlled buildup and easing of the contraction with an optimum 6-second isometric contraction.

GRADIENT INCREASE AND DECREASE IN FORCE PRODUCTION

The concepts of a gradient increase and decrease in muscle force production are concepts that athletes have taught us over the years. As an example, if an athlete has effusion or pain in a joint and performs a muscle contraction, pain is often created. This is often the result of capsular distention from the internal pressure of the effusion. The submaximal muscle contraction places external pressure on the capsule, which is highly innervated,[134] and subsequently increases the pain. However, with a gradient increase in the muscle contraction to the desired intensity (submaximal or maximal), an accommodation is often created that either eliminates or minimizes pain. At the completion of the 6-second isometric contraction, the gradient decrease in the muscle contraction is performed. Again, when an effusion is present and the athlete suddenly releases the contraction, pain results. This is perhaps due to a rebound type of phenome-

Table 8-13. Davies' Resistive Exercise Progression Continuum

PERCENTAGE OF EXERCISE EFFORT	EXERCISE PROGRAM
100%	Submaximal multiple-angle isometrics
	Subjective/objective assessment and plan (SOAP)
	Trial treatment (TT) of maximal multiple-angle isometrics
50%/50%	Submaximal multiple-angle isometrics + maximal multiple-angle isometrics
	SOAP
100%	Maximal multiple-angle isometrics
	SOAP
	TT of submaximal short-arc isokinetics
50%/50%	Maximal multiple-angle isometrics + submaximal short-arc isokinetics
	SOAP
100%	Submaximal short-arc isokinetics
	SOAP
	TT of maximal short-arc isokinetics or short-arc isotonics
	SOAP
50%/50%	Submaximal short-arc isokinetics + maximal short-arc isokinetics
	SOAP
100%	Maximal short-arc isokinetics
	SOAP
	TT of submaximal full ROM isokinetics
	SOAP
50%/50%	Maximal short-arc isokinetics + submaximal full ROM isokinetics
	SOAP
100%	Submaximal full ROM isokinetics
	SOAP
	TT of maximal full ROM isokinetics
	SOAP
	(Full ROM isotonics here, if not contraindicated)
50%/50%	Submaximal full ROM isokinetics + maximal full ROM isokinetics
	SOAP
100%	Maximal full ROM isokinetics
	SOAP

From Davies, G.J. (1992): A Compendium of Isokinetics in Clinical Usage and Rehabilitation Techniques, 4th ed. Onalaska, WI, S & S Publishers.

non, because the effusion in the joint pushes the capsule out, and the muscular contraction that was pushing in against the capsule and compressing it causes an "equalizing" of the pressure. At the release of the muscular contraction, the external pressure is relieved; therefore, the internal pressure causes a rebound phenomenon, stretching the capsule and creating the discomfort. If the athlete gradually releases the muscle contraction, and some type of accommodation occurs, it either eliminates or minimizes the pain.

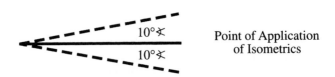

Point of Application
of Isometrics

20° ⪥ Physiologic Overflow

Figure 8-6. Isometric exercises and physiologic overflow through the range of motion. (From Davies, G.J. [1992]: A Compendium of Isokinetics in Clinical Usage and Rehabilitation Techniques, 4th ed. Onalaska, WI, S & S Publishers.)

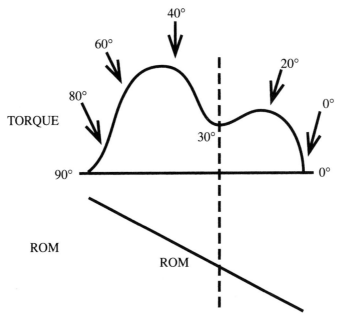

Figure 8–7. Application of isometric exercises through the range of motion with a "painful" deformation. Isometrics are applied every 20° through the range of motion. Note particularly the application of isometrics on each side of "painful" deformation. (From Davies, G.J. [1992]: A Compendium of Isokinetics in Clinical Usage and Rehabilitation Techniques, 4th ed. Onalaska, WI, S & S Publishers.)

DETERMINING SUBMAXIMAL EXERCISE INTENSITY

Submaximal exercise intensity can be distinguished from maximal exercise intensity in various ways. If a submaximal exercise is being applied, it can be determined by using the symptom-limited submaximal exercises (exercises performed at less than maximum efforts that do not cause pain) or a musculo-skeletal rating of perceived exertion for submaximal effort. Furthermore, the distinction must be made between "good" and "bad" pain after exercise. "Good" pain refers to the transient acute exercise-bout pain that is due to lactic acid accumulation, pH changes in the muscle, and an ischemic response. However, "bad" pain is pain that occurs at the site of the actual injury or at the muscle-

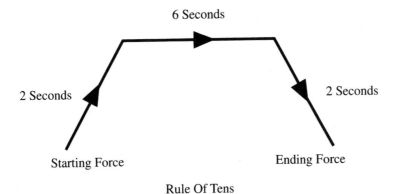

Figure 8–8. Isometric contraction applied by the rule of tens. (From Davies, G.J. [1992]: A Compendium of Isokinetics in Clinical Usage and Rehabilitation Techniques, 4th ed. Onalaska, WI, S & S Publishers.)

tendon unit of injury. An example of this pain classification used in shoulder rehabilitation would include a posteriorly oriented discomfort of pain over the infraspinous fossa after an external rotation exercise ("good" pain) versus anteriorly directed pain over the greater tuberosity or biceps long head tendon ("bad" pain).

GUIDELINES FOR PAIN DURING EXERCISE

The following are guidelines that we use during the rehabilitation program: (1) If no pain is present at the start of an exercise bout but it develops after the exercise, that particular exercise is stopped, and modifications to the exercise are made. (2) If pain is present at the start of the exercise and the pain increases, that exercise is terminated. (3) If pain is present at the start of an exercise and the pain plateaus, the athlete continues the exercise program.

TRIAL TREATMENT

When a rehabilitation program includes the progression of the athlete through a resistive exercise continuum, a key element is how to determine the progression from one stage to the next in the continuum. One of the keys to this progression is the use of a trial treatment. The trial treatment essentially consists of performing one set from the next stage in the exercise progression continuum that was illustrated in Figure 8–5. After the athlete completes the exercise program at one level of the exercise progression continuum, he or she performs a trial of the next stage of treatment. The athlete's signs and symptoms are then evaluated at the conclusion of that particular treatment session as well as at the next scheduled visit, at which time the athlete is re-evaluated and a decision is made on the basis of the athlete's signs and symptoms. If these have stayed the same or improved, the athlete can progress to the next level of exercise because the trial treatment has demonstrated that the athlete's muscle-tendon unit or joint is ready for the higher exercise intensity. Any negative sequels such as increased pain or effusion in the joint are an indication that the joint or muscle is not ready for progression, and consequently, the athlete continues to work at the same level of intensity. Further physical therapy is performed to decrease the irritability of the joint or muscle-tendon unit, and in the next visit, the trial treatment is once again attempted to determine whether the athlete's injury can tolerate the progression.

SUBMAXIMAL EXERCISE: FIBER RECRUITMENT

Several exercise modes can be performed at a submaximal level in order to enhance selective fiber recruitment. Preferential muscle fiber recruitment is predicated on the intensity of the muscle contraction to recruit either slow-twitch or fast-twitch A or fast-twitch B fibers. It is generally accepted that during voluntary contractions of human muscle there is orderly recruitment of motor units according to the size principle.[77] In mixed muscle containing both slow-twitch and fast-twitch fibers, this implies that the involvement of the slow-twitch fibers is obligatory, regardless of the power and velocity being generated with fast-twitch A and fast-twitch B muscle fibers that are recruited once higher intensities are generated.[66] Figure 8–9 summarizes this preferential muscular recruitment. The slow-twitch motor units have relatively low contraction velocities and long contraction times that require only low levels of stimulus to contract. In contrast, the fast-twitch motor units require a very high intensity stimulus to contract and have very short contraction times. The preferential recruitment of muscle fibers is an important concept for the clinician to understand relative to the manipulation of submaximal and maximal exercise intensi-

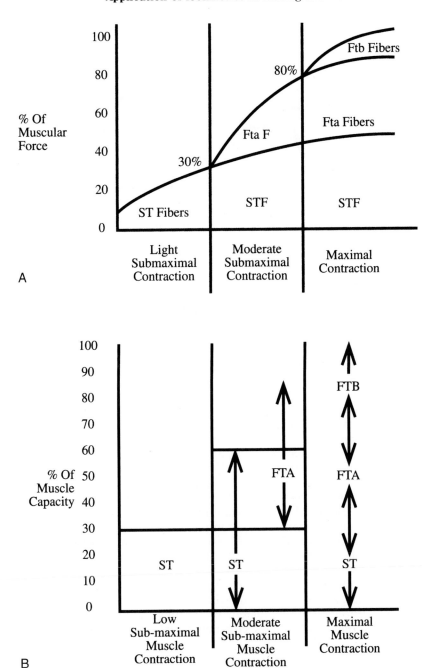

Figure 8–9. Preferential muscle fiber recruitment is predicated on the intensity of the muscle contraction. STF, slow-twitch fiber; FTA or Fta, fast-twitch A; FTB or Ftb, fast-twitch B. (From Davies, G.J. [1992]: A Compendium of Isokinetics in Clinical Usage and Rehabilitation Techniques, 4th ed. Onalaska, WI, S & S Publishers.)

ties with rehabilitative exercise. Submaximal exercise can stimulate the slow-twitch muscle fibers and allow athletes to exercise at lower, pain-free intensities early in the rehabilitation process, with a progression to higher exercise intensities later in rehabilitation, preferentially stimulating the fast-twitch fibers.

SHORT-ARC EXERCISES

The athlete next progresses from the static isometric exercises to more dynamic exercise. The dynamic exercises start with short-arc exercises and the ROM

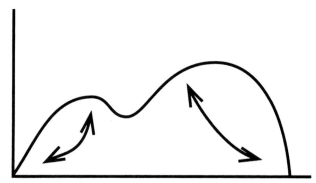

Figure 8–10. Short-arc isokinetic exercises being applied at different points in the range of motion. If an isokinetic torque curve has a deformity in the range of motion as illustrated, short arc isokinetic exercises can be applied to each side of the deformity. (From Davies, G.J. [1992]: A Compendium of Isokinetics in Clinical Usage and Rehabilitation Techniques, 4th ed. Onalaska, WI, S & S Publishers.)

within symptom and soft-tissue healing constraints. Short-arc exercises are often started using submaximal isokinetics (Fig. 8–10) because of the accommodating resistance inherent in submaximal isokinetic exercise that makes it safe for the athlete's healing tissues. With short-arc isokinetics, speeds ranging from 60° per second to 180° per second are utilized (Fig. 8–11). The athlete works with what is called a velocity spectrum rehabilitation protocol (VSRP). When the athlete is performing short-arc isokinetics, slower contractile velocities (60° per second to 180° per second) are chosen because of the acceleration and deceleration response (Fig. 8–12). Isokinetic exercise contains three major components, as identified in Figure 8–12: acceleration, deceleration, and load range. Acceleration is the portion of the ROM in which the athlete's limb is accelerating to "catch" the preset angular velocity; deceleration is the portion of the ROM in which the athlete's limb is slowing prior to cessation of that repetition; and the load range is the actual portion of the ROM in which the preset angular velocity is met by the athlete, and a true isokinetic load is imparted to the athlete. Load range is inversely related to isokinetic speed. A larger load range is found at slower contractile velocities, with a statistically shorter load range at faster contractile velocities.[15]

Consequently, the athlete's available ROM must be evaluated to determine the optimal ROM for exercise. With short-arc isokinetic exercise, there is a physiologic overflow of approximately 30° through the ROM (Fig. 8–13). Therefore, when an athlete with rotator cuff pathology is exercising, an abbreviated

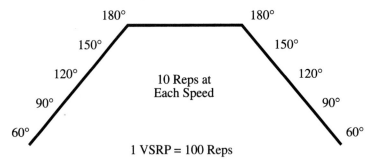

Figure 8–11. Short-arc isokinetic velocity spectrum rehabilitation protocol (VSRP) performed at intermediate contractile velocities. Reps, repetitions. (From Davies, G.J. [1992]: A Compendium of Isokinetics in Clinical Usage and Rehabilitation Techniques, 4th ed. Onalaska, WI, S & S Publishers.)

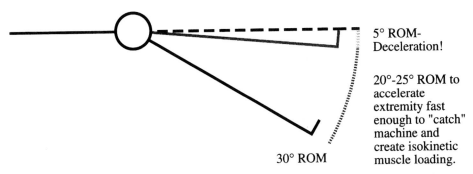

5° ROM-
Deceleration!

20°-25° ROM to
accelerate
extremity fast
enough to "catch"
machine and
create isokinetic
muscle loading.

30° ROM

Figure 8–12. Acceleration and deceleration range of motion (ROM) with short-arc isokinetic exercise. (From Davies, G.J. [1992]: A Compendium of Isokinetics in Clinical Usage and Rehabilitation Techniques, 4th ed. Onalaska, WI, S & S Publishers.)

ROM in internal-external rotation can be utilized in the pain-free range, with overflow into the painful ROM, without actually placing the injured structures into that movement range. Another example of isokinetic exercise for the upper extremities would be the limitation of external ROM to 90° during isokinetic training, even though the demands on the athletic shoulder in overhead activities exceed the 90° ER. Limiting the ER to 90° protects the anterior capsular structures of the shoulder, with physiologic overflow improving strength at ranges of ER exceeded during training.

In addition to ROM, the speed selected with isokinetic exercise is also of vital importance in a VSRP. The speeds in the protocol are designed so that the athlete will exercise 30° per second through the velocity spectrum. The reason for using an interval of 30° per second in the velocity spectrum is the physiologic overflow with respect to speed that has been identified with isokinetic research (Fig. 8–14).[18, 100, 114]

REST INTERVALS[4, 5]

When the athlete is performing either submaximal or maximal short-arc isokinetics using a VSRP, the rest interval between each set of 10 training repetitions may be as long as 90 seconds.[4] However, this is not a viable clinical rest time because it takes too much time to complete the exercise session. Consequently, rest intervals are often applied on a symptom-limited basis. If the athlete does complete a total VSRP, a rest period of 3 minutes after the completion of the VSRP has been shown to be an effective rest interval[5] (Fig. 8–15). Additional research provides guidance for rest interval selection with isotonic and isokinetic exercise in rehabilitation. According to Fleck,[59] 50% of the adenosine triphosphate and creatine phosphate is restored in 20 seconds after an acute bout of muscular

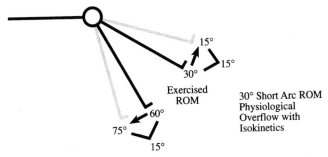

15°

15°

30°

Exercised
ROM

60°

75°

15°

30° Short Arc ROM
Physiological
Overflow with
Isokinetics

Figure 8–13. Thirty-degree short-arc range of motion (ROM) overflow with isokinetics. (From Davies, G.J. [1992]: A Compendium of Isokinetics in Clinical Usage and Rehabilitation Techniques, 4th ed. Onalaska, WI, S & S Publishers.)

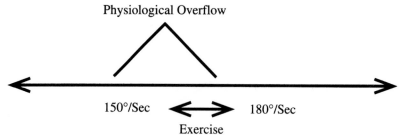

Figure 8–14. Thirty degrees per second physiologic overflow through the velocity spectrum. (From Davies, G.J. [1992]: A Compendium of Isokinetics in Clinical Usage and Rehabilitation Techniques, 4th ed. Onalaska, WI, S & S Publishers.)

work. Seventy-five percent and 87% of the intramuscular stores are replenished in 40 seconds and 60 seconds, respectively. Knowledge of the phosphagen replenishment schedule allows clinicians to make scientifically based decisions on the amount of rest needed or desired after periods of muscular work. Another factor in determining the optimum rest intervals with isotonic and isokinetic training is specificity. For example, during rehabilitation of the shoulder of a tennis player, a high-repetition format is used to improve local muscular endurance. Rest cycles are limited to 25 to 30 seconds because that is the time allotted during tennis play for rest between points. Applying activity or sport-specific muscular work rest cycles is an important consideration during rehabilitation.

When isotonic exercises are applied, they are implemented between isokinetic submaximal and maximal exercises (see Fig. 8–5). The reason is that isotonic muscle loading loads a muscle only at its weakest point in the ROM. Figure 8–16 demonstrates the effects of isotonic muscle loading through the ROM. Consequently, when isotonic muscle exercise is performed through the ROM, a combination of maximal and submaximal loading occurs, whereas with isokinetics, submaximal exercises can be performed throughout the ROM, or maximal intensity loading of the muscle is maximal throughout the ROM, because of the accommodating resistance phenomena inherent with isokinetic exercise.

FULL RANGE OF MOTION EXERCISES

The athlete next progresses to full ROM isokinetic exercise beginning with submaximal exercises and then progressing to maximal intensity (Fig. 8–17). Straight planar movements are used initially to protect the injured plane of movement. Faster contractile velocities are also used from 180° up to the maximum capabilities of the isokinetic dynamometer. There are numerous reasons for using the faster isokinetic speeds: physiologic overflow to slower speeds, specificity response, motor learning response, and decreased joint compressive forces.[28] Joint compressive forces are decreased, based on Bernoulli's principle

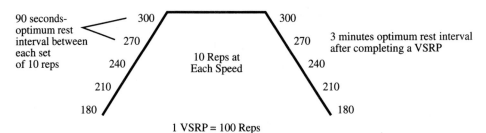

Figure 8–15. Optimum rest intervals. Reps, repetitions; VSRP, velocity spectrum rehabilitation protocol. (From Davies, G.J. [1992]: A Compendium of Isokinetics in Clinical Usage and Rehabilitation Techniques, 4th ed. Onalaska, WI, S & S Publishers.)

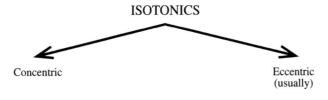

Figure 8-16. Concentric and eccentric isotonic muscle loading and submaximal and maximal loading through the range of motion (ROM). (From Davies, G.J. [1992]: A Compendium of Isokinetics in Clinical Usage and Rehabilitation Techniques, 4th ed. Onalaska, WI, S & S Publishers.)

that at faster speeds, there is a decreased surface pressure on the articular surface because of the synovial fluid interface.[10] This is probably due to the interfacing of the hydrodynamic pattern of the articular cartilage and the synovial fluid movement. Another consideration is the positioning of the athlete to use the length-tension curve of the muscle. With isokinetic exercise, the athlete's position is often modified to bias the respective muscles, for example, to stretch them to facilitate contraction or to place them in a shortened position if that is the functional position. Obviously, of greatest importance is to try to replicate the ultimate functional performance position of the individual.

CKC Rehabilitation

CKC exercises are implemented for the upper and lower extremities along with the traditional OKC positions. Because the upper extremity primarily functions in the OKC environment, many upper extremity OKC exercises are used, but there are many instances in which compression to the joint will facilitate stabilization of the joint through CKC exercises. A limited amount of upper extremity CKC research has been performed. Ellenbecker and Roetert[52] studied the closed-chain stance stability of elite junior tennis players and professional baseball pitchers. A unilateral stance similar to the starting position of a

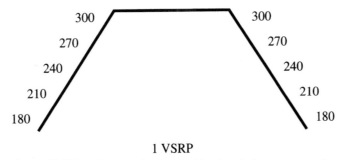

1 VSRP

Figure 8-17. Full range-of-motion isokinetic velocity spectrum rehabilitation protocol (VSRP) performed at fast contractile velocities. (From Davies, G.J. [1992]: A Compendium of Isokinetics in Clinical Usage and Rehabilitation Techniques, 4th ed. Onalaska, WI, S & S Publishers.)

one-arm push-up was used with a Fastex device* that measured the ability of the subject to stabilize over one upper extremity for 20 seconds. No significant differences were found between the dominant and the nondominant extremities in closed-chain stance stability. This is in contrast to previously published results on OKC isokinetic upper extremity testing on unilaterally dominant upper extremity athletes that indicated significantly greater IR, shoulder extension, forearm pronation, and wrist flexion-extension strength on the dominant extremity.[47, 48, 51] Clinical application of this research indicates that differences in muscular function and testing may occur between the OKC and the CKC states. This difference is further illustrated in the lower extremity in athletes after ACL reconstruction. Significant differences were found in bilateral comparisons of OKC knee extension strength and a closed-chain isokinetic leg press type of movement pattern.[58] With OKC knee extension testing at 15 weeks after ACL reconstruction, athletes showed approximately 70% quadriceps peak torque in single-repetition-work bilateral comparisons. In comparison, the CKC isokinetic leg press extension test showed 95% bilateral comparisons. Obviously, significant differences exist between 70% and 95% bilateral comparisons, and these indicate that caution be applied when comparing tests between the OKC and the CKC environments. Further research is necessary to clarify the important role of open- and closed-chain exercise and testing in rehabilitation and to determine the efficacy of applying open- and closed-chain exercise in rehabilitation.

Isoacceleration and Deceleration

Because functional activities are primarily accelerative and decelerative movement patterns, it is important to try to replicate these patterns when performing different types of rehabilitation activities. Also, because of the functional activities involved with various sports, such as the deceleration phase of tennis or baseball that is applied to the posterior rotator cuff or to the forearm or biceps muscles, the potential use of eccentric exercise may also be important. There are limited studies that demonstrate the efficacy of performing eccentric exercise or eccentric isokinetic rehabilitation programs at this time.[53] Ellenbecker et al[53] reported concentric strength improvement in internal and external rotation after 6 weeks of eccentric isokinetic training of the internal and external rotators in elite tennis players. Mont et al[117] found both concentric and eccentric strength improvements with eccentric isokinetic training of the rotator cuff in elite tennis players. Despite the lack of research on eccentric exercise training, particularly in athletes, specific application of eccentric exercise programs to the posterior rotator cuff, quadriceps, and other important muscle-tendon units that must perform extensive eccentric work may be indicated. Empirically, we support the integration and application of eccentric isokinetics as part of the whole rehabilitation program.

OUTCOMES RESEARCH

The evolution of rehabilitation modes over the past few decades can best be described as follows:

1970s: Functional rehabilitation
1980s: OKC assessment and rehabilitation (with emphasis on isokinetics)
1990s: CKC rehabilitation

---

*Available from Cybex, Ronkonkoma, New York

By 2000: Integrated assessment and rehabilitation that
  should include both OKC and CKC

Recently, Bynum et al[17] published the results of the first prospective randomized study comparing OKC and CKC exercises. With respect to the parameters
listed, their conclusions indicate the following about the CKC exercises:

1. Lower mean KT-1000 arthrometer side-to-side differences (KT-20, $p = 0.057$, not significant; KT-Max,
   $p = 0.018$, significant)
2. Less patellofemoral pain ($p = 0.48$, not significant)
3. Patients generally more satisfied with the end result
   ($p = 0.36$, not significant)
4. Patients returned to activities of daily living sooner
   than expected ($p = 0.007$, significant)
5. Patients returned to sports sooner than expected
   ($p = 0.118$, not significant)

The authors stated: "As a result of this study, we now use the CKC protocol
exclusively after anterior cruciate ligament reconstruction."[17] Surprisingly, Bynum
et al[17] came to several conclusions that were not statistically significant and
probably not clinically significant either. Yet they based their entire protocol
exclusively on these findings.

CKC exercises have almost replaced OKC exercises in the rehabilitation of
athletes after an ACL reconstruction. As indicated earlier, this change is not
founded on solid experimental or clinical studies, with limited published prospective randomized experimental studies to prove the efficacy of CKC exercises.[57] In contrast, the literature on OKC isokinetics and OKC isotonics is
extensive, but most clinicians have ignored past successes with OKC exercises
and have chosen to use CKC exercises without documentation.[102]

A recently published article by Snyder-Mackler et al[144] describes prospective
randomized clinical trials and the effects of intensive CKC rehabilitation programs and different types of electrical stimulation on athletes with ACL reconstructions. These researchers had previously demonstrated that the strength of
the quadriceps femoris muscle correlates well with the function of the knee
during the stance phase of gait. In the later study,[144] after an intensive CKC
rehabilitation program, they reported a residual weakness in the quadriceps that
produced alterations in the normal gait function of these athletes. The authors
concluded that CKC exercise alone does not provide an adequate stimulus to
the quadriceps femoris to permit more normal knee function in the stance phase
of gait in most athletes soon after ACL reconstruction. They suggested that the
judicious application of OKC exercises for the quadriceps femoris muscle (with
the knee in a position that does not stress the graft) improves the strength of
this muscle and the functional outcome after reconstruction of the ACL.

SUMMARY

Isokinetic assessment and treatment techniques are only one part of the evaluation and rehabilitation process. The diversity in assessment and rehabilitation is
tremendous, as illustrated by the fact that after ACL reconstruction, some athletes return to sports after 12 weeks, and others return after 12 months. Therefore,
we strongly encourage clinicians to use an integrated approach to assessment
and rehabilitation, to review the literature critically, and to contribute to the
advancement of the art and science of sports medicine by performing research
and sharing results through peer-reviewed publications.

References

1. Alderink, G.J., and Kluck, D.J. (1986): Isokinetic shoulder strength of high school and college aged pitchers. J. Orthop. Sports Phys. Ther., 7:163–172.
2. Anderson, A.F., and Lipscomb, A.B. (1989): Analysis of rehabilitation techniques after anterior cruciate reconstruction. Am. J. Sports Med., 17:154–160.
3. Anderson, M.A., Gieck, J.H., Perrin, D., et al. (1991): The relationship among isometric, isotonic and isokinetic concentric and eccentric quadriceps and hamstring force and three components of athletic performance. J. Orthop. Sports Phys. Ther., 14:114–120.
4. Ariki, P., Davies, G.J., Siewart, M., et al. (1985): Rest interval between isokinetic velocity spectrum rehabilitation speeds. Phys. Ther., 65:735–736.
5. Ariki, P., Davies, G.J., Siewart, M., et al. (1985): Rest interval between isokinetic velocity spectrum rehabilitation sets. Phys. Ther., 65:733–734.
6. Arms, S.W., Pope, M.H., Johnson, R.J., et al. (1984): The biomechanics of anterior cruciate ligament rehabilitation and reconstruction. Am. J. Sports Med., 12:8–18.
7. Astrand, P., and Rodahl, K. (1977): Textbook of Work Physiology. New York, McGraw-Hill Book Co.
8. Barbee, J., and Landis, D. (1984): Reliability of Cybex computer measures. Phys. Ther., 68:737.
9. Barber, S.D., Noyes, F.R., Mangine, R.E., et al. (1990): Quantitative assessment of functional limitations in normal and anterior cruciate ligament deficient knees. Clin. Orthop., 225:204–214.
10. Barnam, J.N. (1978): Mechanical Kinesiology. St. Louis, C.V. Mosby.
11. Bartlett, L.R., Storey, M.D., and Simons, B.D. (1989): Measurement of upper extremity torque production and its relationship to throwing speed in the competitive athlete. Am. J. Sports Med., 17:89–91.
12. Basset, R.W., Browne, A.O., Morrey, B.F., and An, K.N. (1994): Glenohumeral muscle force and moment mechanics in a position of shoulder instability. J. Biomech., 23:405–415.
13. Boltz, S., and Davies, G.J. (1984): Leg length differences and correlation with total leg strength. J. Orthop. Sports Phys. Ther., 6:23–129.
14. Brask, B., Lueke, R.H., and Soderberg, G.L. (1984): Electromyographical analysis of selected muscles during the lateral step-up exercise. Phys. Ther., 64:324–329.
15. Brown, L.E., Whitehurst, M., Findley, B.W., et al. (1995): Isokinetic load range during shoulder rotation exercise in elite male junior tennis players. J. Strength Conditioning Res., 9:160–164.
16. Brown, L.P., Neihues, S.L., Harrah, A., et al. (1988): Upper extremity range of motion and isokinetic strength of the internal and external shoulder rotators in major league baseball players. Am. J. Sports Med., 16:577–585.
17. Bynum, E.B., Barrack, R.L., and Alexander, A.H. (1995): Open versus closed chain kinetic exercises after anterior cruciate ligament reconstruction: A prospective randomized study. Am. J. Sports Med., 23:401–406.
18. Caizzo, V.J., et al. (1980): Alterations in the in-vivo force-velocity. Med. Sci. Sports Exerc. 12:134.
19. Chan, K.M., and Maffulli, N. (eds.) (1966): Principles and Practice of Isokinetics in Sports Medicine and Rehabilitation. Hong Kong, Williams & Wilkins.
20. Chandler, T.J., Kibler, W.B., Stracener, E.C., et al. (1992): Shoulder strength, power, and endurance in college tennis players. Am. J. Sports Med., 20: 455–458.
21. Chandler, T.J., Wilson, G.D., and Store, M.H. (1989): The effects of the squat exercise on knee stability. Med. Sci. Sports Exerc., 21:299–303.
22. Cook, E.E., Gray, V.L., Savinor-Nogue, E., et al. (1987): Shoulder antagonistic strength ratios: A comparison between college-level baseball pitchers, J. Orthop. Sports Phys. Ther., 8:451–461.
23. Cook, T.M., Zimmerman, C.L., Lux, K.M., et al. (1992): EMG comparison of lateral step-up and stepping machine exercise. J. Orthop. Sports Phys. Ther., 16:108–113.
24. Corwell, J.R. (1987): College football: To brace or not to brace (editorial). J. Bone Joint Surg. [Am.], 69:1.
25. Crandall, D., Richmond, J., Lau, J., et al. (1994): A meta-analysis of the treatment of the anterior cruciate ligament. Presented at American Orthopedic Society of Sports Medicine, Palm Desert, CA, June 1994.
26. Daniels, L., and Worthingham, C. (1986): Muscle Testing: Techniques of Manual Examination, 5th ed. Philadelphia, W.B. Saunders.
27. Davies, G.J. (1984): A Compendium of Isokinetics in Clinical Usage and Rehabilitation Techniques. La Crosse, WI, S & S Publishers.
28. Davies, G.J. (1992): A Compendium of Isokinetics in Clinical Usage and Rehabilitation Techniques, 4th ed. Onalaska, WI, S & S Publishers.
29. Davies, G.J. (1995): The need for critical thinking in rehabilitation. J. Sports Rehab., 4:1–22.
30. Davies, G.J. (1995): Descriptive study comparing OKC vs CKC isokinetic testing of the lower extremity in 200 patients with selected knee pathologies. Presented at World Confederation of Physical Therapy, June 1995.
31. Davies, G.J. (1995): Functional testing algorithm for patients with knee injuries. Presented at World Confederation of Physical Therapy, June 1995.
32. Davies, G.J., and Heiderschet, B. (1997): Reliability of the Lido Linea closed kinetic chain isokinetic dynamometer. J. Orthop. Sports Phys. Ther., 25:133–136.

33. Davies, G.J., and Ellenbecker T.S. (1992): Eccentric isokinetics. Orthop. Phys. Ther. Clin. North Am., 1(2): 297–336.

34. Davies, G.J., and Ellenbecker, T.S. (1993): Total arm strength rehabilitation for shoulder and elbow overuse injuries. Orthop. Phys. Ther., Home Study Course, Orthopaedic Section—American Physical Therapy Association.

35. Davies, G.J., and Hoffman, S.D. (1993): Neuromuscular testing and rehabilitation of the shoulder complex. J. Orthop. Sports Phys. Ther., 18:449–458.

36. Davies, G.J., and Malone, T. (1995): Proprioception, open and closed kinetic chain exercises and application to assessment and rehabilitation. Presented at American Orthopaedic Society of Sports Medicine, Toronto, July 1995.

37. Davies, G.J., and Romeyn, R.L.: Prospective, randomized single blind study comparing closed kinetic chain versus open and closed kinetic chain integrated rehabilitation programs of patients with ACL autograft infrapatellar tendon reconstructions. (Research in progress, August 1992 to present.)

38. Davies, G.J., Heiderscheit, B., and Clark, M.A. (1995): Open kinetic chain assessment and rehabilitation. Athletic training: Sports Health Care Perspect., 1:347–370.

39. DeCarlo, M., and Sell, K.E. (1994): Range of motion and single-leg hop values for normals and patients following anterior cruciate ligament reconstruction. J. Orthop. Sports Phys. Ther., 19:73.

40. DeCarlo, M., Porter, D.A., Gehlsen, G., et al. (1992): Electromyographic and cinematographic analysis of the lower extremity during closed and open kinetic chain exercise. Isokin. Exerc. Sci., 2:24–29.

41. DeCarlo, M., Shelbourne, K.D., McCarroll, J.R., et al. (1992): Traditional versus accelerated rehabilitation following ACL reconstruction: a one-year follow-up. J. Orthop. Sports Phys. Ther., 15:309–316.

42. Dillman, C.J., Fleisig, G.S., and Andrews, J.R. (1993): Biomechanics of pitching with emphasis upon shoulder kinematics. J. Orthop. Sports Phys. Ther., 18:402–408.

43. Dillman, C.J. (1991): Presentation on The Upper Extremity in Tennis and Throwing Athletes. United States Tennis Association Meeting, Tucson, AZ, March 1991.

44. Draganich, L.F., Jaeger, R.J., and Kralj, A.R. (1989): Coactivation of the hamstrings and quadriceps during extension of the knee. J. Bone Joint Surg. [Am.], 71:1075–1081.

45. Draganich, L.F., and Vahey, J.W. (1990): An in vitro study of anterior cruciate ligament strain induced by quadriceps and hamstring forces. J. Orthop. Res., 8:57–63.

46. Dvir, Z. (1993): Isokinetic Exercise and Assessment. Champaign, IL, Human Kinetics Publishers.

47. Ellenbecker, T.S. (1991): A total arm strength isokinetic profile of highly skilled tennis players. Isokin. Exerc. Sci., 1:9–21.

48. Ellenbecker, T.S. (1992): Shoulder internal and external rotation strength and range of motion of highly skilled junior tennis players. Isokin. Exerc. Sci., 2:1–8.

49. Ellenbecker, T.S. (1994): Muscular strength relationship between normal grade manual muscle testing and isokinetic measurement of the shoulder internal and external rotators. J. Orthop. Sports Phys. Ther., 1:72.

50. Ellenbecker, T.S., and Derscheid, G.L. (1988): Rehabilitation of overuse injuries in the shoulder. Clin. Sports Med., 8:583–604.

51. Ellenbecker, T.S., and Mattalino, A.J. (1997): Concentric isokinetic shoulder internal and external rotation strength in professional baseball pitchers. J. Orthop. Sports Phys. Ther., 25:323–328.

52. Ellenbecker, T.S., and Roetert, E.P. (1996): A bilateral comparison of upper extremity unilateral closed chain stance stability in elite tennis players and professional baseball players. Med. Sci. Sports Exerc., 8:S105.

53. Ellenbecker, T.S., Davies, G.J., and Rowinski, M.J. (1988): Concentric versus eccentric isokinetic strengthening of the rotator cuff: Objective data versus functional test. Am. J. Sports Med., 16:64–69.

54. Ellenbecker, T.S., Dehart, R.L., and Boeckmann, R. (1992): Isokinetic shoulder strength of the rotator cuff in professional baseball pitchers. Phys. Ther., 72:S81.

55. Ellenbecker, T.S., Feiring, D.C., Dehart, R.L., and Rich, M. (1992): Isokinetic shoulder strength: Coronal versus scapular plane testing in upper extremity unilaterally dominant athletes. Phys. Ther., 72:S80–S81.

56. Elliot, B., Marsh, T., and Blanksby, B. (1986): A three dimensional cinematographic analysis of the tennis serve. Int. J. Sport Biomech., 2: 260–271.

57. Farrell, M., and Richards, J.G. (1986): Analysis of the reliability and validity of the kinetic communicator exercise device. Med. Sci. Sports Exerc., 18:44, 1986.

58. Feiring, D.C., and Ellenbecker, T.S. (1995): Open versus closed chain isokinetic testing with ACL reconstructed patients. Med. Sci. Sports Exer., 27:S106.

59. Fleck, S. (1983): Interval training: Physiological basis. J. Strength Conditioning Res., 5:4–7.

60. Francis, K., and Hoobler, T. (1987): Comparison of peak torque values of the knee flexor and extensor msucle groups using the Cybex II and Lido 2.0 isokinetic dynamometers. J. Orthop. Sports Phys. Ther., 8:480–483.

61. Gauffin, H., Peterson Y., Tegner Y., and Tropp, H. (1990): Function testing in patients with old rupture of the anterior cruciate ligament. Int. J. Sports Med., 11:73–77.

62. Gleim, G.W., Nicholas, J.A., and Webb, J.N. (1978): Isokinetic evaluation following leg injuries. Physician Sportsmed., 6:74–82.

63. Gore, D.R., Murray, M.P., Sepic, S.B., and Gardner, G.M. (1986): Shoulder muscle strength and

range of motion following surgical repair of full thickness rotator cuff tears. J. Bone Joint Surg. [Am.], 68:266–272.

64. Graham, V.L., Gehlsen, G.M., and Edwards, J.A. (1993): Electromyographic evaluation of closed and open kinetic chain knee rehabilitation exercises. J. Athl. Train., 28:23–30.

65. Grana, W.A., and Muse, G. (1988): The effect of exercise on laxity in the anterior cruciate ligament deficient knee. Am. J. Sports Med., 16:586–588.

66. Green, H.J. (1986): Muscle power: fibre type, recruitment, metabolism and fatigue. In: Jones, N.L., McCartney, N., and McComas, A.J. (eds.): Human Muscle Power. Champaign, IL, Human Kinetics Publishers.

67. Greenberger, H.B., and Paterno, M.V. (1994): The test-retest reliability of a one-legged hop for distance in healthy young adults. J. Orthop. Sports Phys. Ther., 19:62.

68. Greenberger, H.B., and Paterno, M.V. (1994): Comparison of an isokinetic strength test and functional performance test in the assessment of lower extremity function. J. Orthop. Sports Phys. Ther., 19:61.

69. Greenfield, B.H., Donatelli, R., Wooden, M.J., and Wilkes J. (1990): Isokinetic evaluation of shoulder rotational strength between the plane of the scapula and the frontal plane. Am. J. Sports Med., 18:124–128.

70. Griffin, J.W. (1985): Differences in elbow flexion torque measured concentrically, eccentrically, and isometrically. Phys. Ther., 67:1205.

71. Grood, E.S., Suntay, W.J., Noyes, F.R., et al. (1984): Biomechanics of the knee-extension exercise. J. Bone Joint Surg. [Am.], 66:725–734.

72. Gryzlo, S.M., Patek, R.M., Pink, M., et al. (1994): Electromyographic analysis of knee rehabilitation exercises. J. Orthop. Sports Phys. Ther., 20:36–43.

73. Hageman, P.A., Mason, D.K., Rydlund, K.W., et al. (1989): Effects of position and speed on eccentric and concentric isokinetic testing of the shoulder rotators. J. Orthop. Sports Phys. Ther., 11:64–69.

74. Harter, R.A., Osternig, L.R., Singer, K.M., et al. (1988): Long-term evaluation of knee stability and function following surgical reconstruction for anterior cruciate ligament insufficiency. Am. J. Sports Med., 16:434–443.

75. Hefzy, M.S., Grood, E.S., and Noyes, F.R. (1989): Factors affecting the region of most isometric femoral attachments. Part II. The anterior cruciate ligament. Am. J. Sports Med., 17:208–216.

76. Hellwig, E.V., Perrin, D.H., Tis, L.L., and Shenk, B.S. (1991): Effect of gravity correction on shoulder external/internal rotator reciprocal muscle group ratios. J. Natl. Athl. Trainers Assoc., 26:154.

77. Henneman, E., Somjen, G., and Carpenter, D.O. (1965): Functional significance of cell size in spinal motorneurons. J. Neurophysiol., 28:560–580.

78. Henning, C.E., Lynch, M.A., and Glick, K.R. (1985): An in-vivo strain gauge study of elongation of the anterior cruciate ligament. Am. J. Sports Med., 13:22–26.

79. Hinton, R.Y. (1988): Isokinetic evaluation of shoulder rotational strength in high school baseball pitchers. Am. J. Sports Med., 16:274–279.

80. Hislop, H.J., and Perrine, J.J. (1967): The isokinetic concept of exercise. Phys. Ther., 47:114–117.

81. Holm, I., Brox, J.I., Ludvigsen, P., and Steen, H. (1996): External rotation-best isokinetic movement pattern for evaluation of muscle function in rotator tendonosis. A prospective study with a 2-year follow-up. Isokin. Exerc. Sci., 5:121–125.

82. Howell, S.M. (1990): Anterior tibial translation during a maximum quadriceps contraction: Is it clinically significant? Am. J. Sports Med., 18:573–578.

83. Hsieh, H., and Walker, P.S. (1976): Stabilizing mechanisms of the loaded and unloaded knee joint. J. Bone Joint Surg. [Am.], 58:87–93.

84. Hu, H.S., Whitney, S.L., Irrgang, J., and Janosky, J. (1992): Test-retest reliability of the one-legged vertical jump test and the one-legged standing hop test. J. Orthop. Sports Phys. Ther., 15:51.

85. Inman, V.T., Saunders, J.B. de C.M., and Abbot, L.C. (1944): Observations on the function of the shoulder joint. J. Bone Joint Surg. [Am.], 26:1–30.

86. Ivey, F.M., Calhoun, J.H., Rusche, K., et al. (1984): Normal values for isokinetic testing of shoulder strength. Med. Sci. Sports Exerc., 16:127.

87. Jackson, A.L., Highgenboten, C., Meske, N., et al. (1987): Univariate and multivariate analysis of the reliability of the kinetic communicator. Med. Sci. Sports Exerc., 19 (Suppl):23.

88. Jobe, F.W., Tibone, J.E., Perry, J., et al. (1983): An EMG analysis of the shoulder in throwing and pitching. A preliminary report. Am. J. Sports Med., 11:3–5.

89. Johnson, J., and Siegel, D. (1978): Reliability of an isokinetic movement of the knee extensors. Res. Q., 49:88.

90. Jurist, K.A., and Otis, J.C. (1985): Anteroposterior tibiofemoral displacements during isometric extension efforts. Am. J. Sports Med., 13:254–258.

91. Kannus, P.M., Jarvinen, M., Johnson, R., et al. (1992): Function of the quadriceps and hamstring muscles in knees with chronic partial deficiency of the ACL. Am. J. Sports Med., 20:162–168.

92. Kendall, F.D., and McCreary, E.K. (1983): Muscle Testing and Function, 3rd ed. Baltimore, Williams & Wilkins.

93. Kennedy, K., Altchek, D.W., and Glick, I.V. (1993): Concentric and eccentric isokinetic rotator cuff ratios in skilled tennis players. Isokin. Exerc. Sci., 3:155–159.

94. Knight, K.L. (1979): Knee rehabilitation by the daily adjustable progressive resistive exercise technique. Am. J. Sports Med., 7:336.

95. Knight, K.L. (1985): Quadriceps strengthening with DAPRE technique: Case studies with neurological implications. Med. Sci. Sports Exerc., 17:636.

96. Kronberg, M., Nemeth, F., and Brostrom, L.A. (1990): Muscle activity and coordination in the normal shoulder: An electromyographic study. Clin. Orthop., 257:76–85.

97. Lace, J.E. (1989): An isokinetic shoulder profile of collegiate baseball pitchers and its relation to throwing velocity (unpublished master's thesis). Arizona State University.

98. Lephart, S.M., et al. (1988): Functional assessment of the anterior cruciate insufficient knee. Med. Sci. Sports Exerc., 20:2.

99. Lephart, S.M., Perrin, D.H., Fu, F.H., and Minger, K. (1991): Functional performance tests for the anterior cruciate ligament insufficient athlete. J. Athl. Train., 26:44–50.

100. Lesmes, G.R., Costill, D.L., Coycle, E.F., and Fine, W.J. (1978): Muscle strengthening and power changes during maximal isokinetic training. Med. Sci. Sports Exerc., 10:266–269.

101. Lucas, D.B. (1973): Biomechanics of the shoulder joint. Arch. Surg., 107:425.

102. Lutz, G.E., Palmitier, R.A., An, K.N., et al. (1991): Closed kinetic chain exercises for athletes after reconstruction of the anterior cruciate ligament. Med. Sci. Sports Exerc., 23:413.

103. Lutz, G.E., Palmitier, R.A., An, K.N., et al. (1993): Comparison of tibiofemoral joint forces during open kinetic chain and closed kinetic chain exercises. J. Bone Joint Surg. [Am.], 75:732–739.

104. Maitland, M.E., Lowe, R., and Stewart, S. (1993): Does Cybex testing increase knee laxity after anterior cruciate ligament reconstructions? Am. J. Sports Med., 21:690–695.

105. Maltry, J.A., Noble, P.C., Woods, G.W., et al. (1989): External stabilization of the anterior cruciate ligament deficient knee during rehabilitation. Am. J. Sports Med., 17:550–554.

106. Markolf, K.L., Bargar, W.L., Shoemaker, S.C., et al. (1981): Role of joint load in knee stability. J. Bone Joint Surg. [Am.], 63: 579–585.

107. Markolf, K.L., Gorek, J.F., Kabo, J.M., et al. (1990): Direct measurement of resultant forces in the anterior cruciate ligament. J. Bone Joint Surg. [Am.], 72:557–567.

108. Markolf, K.L., Graff-Radford, A., and Amstutz, H.C. (1978): In-vivo knee stability. J. Bone Joint Surg. [Am.], 60:664–674.

109. Markolf, K.L., Kochan, A., and Amstutz, H.C. (1984): Measurement of knee stiffness and laxity in patients with documented absence of anterior cruciate ligament. J. Bone Joint Surg. [Am.], 66:242–253.

110. Markolf, K.L., Mensch, J.S., and Amstutz, H.C. (1976): Stiffness and laxity of the knee. The contributions of the supporting structures. J. Bone Joint Surg. [Am.], 58:583–594.

111. Mawdsley, R.H., and Knapik, J.J. (1982): Comparison of isokinetic measurements with test repetitions. Phys. Ther., 62:169.

112. Meister, K., and Andrews, J.R. (1993): Classification and treatment of rotator cuff injuries in the overhand athlete. J. Orthop. Sports Phys. Ther., 18:413–421.

113. Moffroid, M., Whipple, R., Hofkosh, J., et al. (1969): A study of isokinetic exercise. Phys. Ther., 49:735.

114. Moffroid, M.T., et al. (1970): Specificity of speed of exercise. Phys. Ther., 50:1693–1699.

115. Molnar, G.E., and Alexander, J. (1973): Objective, quantitative muscle testing in children: A pilot study. Arch. Phys. Med. Rehab., 54:225–228.

116. Molnar, G.E., Alexander, J., and Gudfeld, N. (1979): Reliability of quantitative strength measurements in children. Arch. Phys. Med. Rehab., 60:218.

117. Mont, M.A., Cohen, D.B., Campbell, K.R., et al. (1994): Isokinetic concentric versus eccentric training of the shoulder rotators with functional evaluation of performance enhancement in elite tennis players. Am. J. Sports Med., 22:513–517.

118. More, R.C., Karras, B.T., Neiman, R., et al. (1993): Hamstrings: An anterior cruciate ligament protagonist. An in vitro study. Am. J. Sports Med., 21:231–237.

119. Nicholas, J.A., Sapega, A., Kraus, H., and Webb, J.N. (1978): Factors influencing manual muscle tests in physical therapy. J. Bone Joint Surg. [Am.], 60:186.

120. Nicholas, J.A., Strizak, A.M., and Veras, G. (1976): A study of thigh muscle weakness in different pathological states of the lower extremity. Am. J. Sports Med., 4:241–248.

121. Nirschl, R.P., and Sobel, J. (1981): Conservative treatment of tennis elbow. Physician Sportsmed., 9:43–54.

122. Ohkoshi, Y., and Yasada, K. (1989): Biomechanical analysis of shear force exerted to anterior cruciate ligament during half squat exercise. Orthop. Trans., 13:310.

123. Ohkoshi, Y., Yasuda, K., Kaneda, K., et al. (1991): Biomechanical analysis of rehabilitation in the standing position. Am. J. Sports Med., 19:605–610.

124. Palmitier, R.A., An, K.N., Scott, S.G., et al. (1991): Kinetic chain exercise in knee rehabilitation. Sports Med., 11:402–413.

125. Pawlowski, D., and Perrin, D.H. (1989): Relationship between shoulder and elbow isokinetic peak torque, torque acceleration energy, average power, and total work and throwing velocity in intercollegiate pitchers. Athl. Train., 24:129–132.

126. Pedegana, L.R., Elsner, R.C., Roberts, D., et al. (1982): The relationship of upper extremity strength to throwing speed. Am. J. Sports Med., 10:352–354.

127. Perrin, D.H. (1986): Reliability of isokinetic measures. Athl. Train., 23:319.

128. Perrin, D.H. (1993): Isokinetic Exercise and Assessment. Champaign, IL, Human Kinetics Publishers.

129. Quincy, R., Davies, G.J., Kolbeck, K., et al.: Isokinetic exercise: The effects of training specificity on shoulder power. J. Sport Rehab., (submitted for publication).

130. Rabin, S.J., and Post, M.P. (1990): A comparative study of clinical muscle testing and Cybex evaluation after shoulder operations. Clin. Orthop., 258:147–156.
131. Reitz, C.L., Rowinski, M., and Davies, G.J. (1988): Comparison of Cybex II and Kin-Com reliability of the measures of peak torque, work, and power at three speeds. Phys. Ther., 69:782.
132. Renstrom, P., Arms, S.W., Stanwyck, T.S., et al. (1986): Strain within the anterior cruciate ligament during hamstring and quadriceps activity. Am. J. Sports Med., 14:83–87.
133. Reynolds, N.L., Worrell, T.W., and Perrin, D.H. (1992): Effect of a lateral step-up exercise protocol on quadriceps isokinetic peak torque values and thigh girth. J. Orthop. Sports Phys. Ther., 15: 151–155.
134. Rowinski, M.J. (1985): Afferent neurobiology of the joint. In: Davies, G.J., and Gould, J.A. (eds.): Orthopaedic and Sports Physical Therapy. St. Louis, C.V. Mosby.
135. Sachs, R.A., Daniel, D.M., Stone, M.L., et al. (1989): Patellofemoral problems after anterior cruciate ligament reconstruction. Am. J. Sports Med., 17:760–764.
136. Saha, A.K. (1971): Dynamic stability of the glenohumeral joint. Acta Orthop. Scand., 42:491–505.
137. Shaffer, S.W., Payne, E.D., Gabbard, L.R., et al. (1994): Relationship between isokinetic and functional tests of the quadriceps. J. Orthop. Sports Phys. Ther., 19:55.
138. Shapiro R., and Steine, R.L. (1992): Shoulder rotation velocities. Technical report submitted to the Lexington Clinic, Lexington, KY.
139. Shelbourne, K.D., and Nitz, P. (1990): Accelerated rehabilitation after anterior cruciate ligament rehabilitation. Am. J. Sports Med., 18:292–299.
140. Shoemaker, S.C., and Markolf, K.L. (1982): In-vivo rotatory knee stability. J. Bone Joint Surg. [Am.], 64:208–216.
141. Shoemaker, S.C., and Markolf, K.L. (1985): Effects of joint load on the stiffness and laxity of ligament-deficient knees. J. Bone Joint Surg. [Am.], 67:136–146.
142. Smith, M.J., and Melton, P. (1981): Isokinetic versus isotonic variable-resistance training. Am. J. Sports Med., 9:275–279.
143. Snow, D.J., and Johnson, K. (1988): Reliability of two velocity controlled tests for the measurement of peak torque of the knee flexors during resisted muscle shortening and resisted muscle lengthening. Phys. Ther., 68:781.
144. Synder-Mackler, L., Delitto, A., Bailey, S.L., et al. (1995): Strength of the quadriceps femoris muscle and functional recovery after reconstruction of the anterior cruciate ligament. J. Bone Joint Surg. [Am.], 77:1166–1173.
145. Soderberg, G.J., and Blaschak, M.J. (1987): Shoulder internal and external rotation peak torque production through a velocity spectrum in differing positions. J. Orthop. Sports Phys. Ther., 8:518–524.
146. Solomonow, M., Baratta, R., Zhov, B.H., et al. (1987): The synergistic action of the anterior cruciate ligament and thigh muscles in maintaining joint stability. Am. J. Sports Med., 15:207–213.
147. Sullivan, E.P., Markos, P.D., and Minor, M.D. (1982): An Integrated Approach to Therapeutic Exercise: Theory and Clinical Application. Reston, VA, Reston Publishing Co.
148. Tegner, Y., Lysholm, J., Lysholm, M., et al. (1986): A performance test to monitor rehabilitation and evaluate anterior cruciate ligament injuries. Am. J. Sports Med., 14:156–159.
149. Thorstensson, A., Grimby, G., and Karlsson, J. (1976): Force-velocity relations and fiber composition in human knee extensor muscles. J. Appl. Physiol., 40:12, 1976.
150. Timm, K.E. (1988): Post-surgical knee rehabilitation: A five year study of four methods and 5,381 patients. Am. J. Sports Med., 16:463–468.
151. Timm, K.E. (1988): Reliability of Cybex 340 and MERAC isokinetic measures of peak torque, total work, and average power at five test speeds. Phys. Ther., 69:782.
152. Vangheluwe, B., and Hebbelinck, K.M. (1986): Muscle actions and ground reaction forces in tennis. Int. J. Sports Biomech., 2:88–99.
153. Wakin, K.G., Clarke, H.H., Elkins, E.C., and Martin, G.M. (1950): Relationship betwen body position and application of muscle power to movements of joints. Arch. Phys. Med. Rehab., 31:81–89.
154. Walker, S.W., Couch, W.H., Boester, G.A., and Sprowl, D.W. (1987): Isokinetic strength of the shoulder after repair of a torn rotator cuff. J. Bone Joint Surg. [Am.], 69:1041–1044.
155. Walmsley, R.P., and Hartsell, H. (1992): Shoulder strength following surgical rotator cuff repair: a comparative analysis using isokinetic testing. J. Orthop. Sports Phys. Ther., 15:215–222.
156. Walmsley, R.P., and Szybbo, C. (1987): A comparative study of the torque generated by the shoulder internal and external rotator muscles in different positions and at varying speeds. J. Orthop. Sports Phys. Ther., 9:217–222.
157. Warner, J.P., Micheli, L.J., Arslanian, L.E., et al. (1990): Patterns of flexibility, laxity, and strength in normal shoulders and shoulders with instability and impingement. Am. J. Sports Med., 18:366–375.
158. Wessel, J., Mattison, G., Luongo, F., et al. (1988): Reliability of eccentric and concentric measurements. Phys. Ther., 68:782.
159. Wiklander, J., and Lysholm, J. (1987): Simple tests for surveying muscle strength and muscle stiffness in sportsmen. Int. J. Sports Med., 8:50–54.
160. Wilk, K.E., and Andrews, J.R. (1993): The effects of pad placement and angular velocity on tibial displacement during isokinetic exercise. J. Orthop. Sports Phys. Ther., 17:23–30.

161. Wilk, K.E., and Arrigo, C.A. (1993): Current concepts in the rehabilitation of the athletic shoulder. J. Orthop. Sports Phys. Ther., 18:365–378.

162. Wilk, K.E., and Johnson, R.E. (1988): The reliability of the Biodex B-200. Phys. Ther., 68:792.

163. Wilk, K.E., Andrews, J.R., Arrigo, et al. (1993): The strength characteristics of internal and external rotator muscles in professional baseball pitchers. Am. J. Sports Med., 61–66.

164. Wilk, K.E., Arrigo, C.A., and Andrews, J.R. (1991): Standardized isokinetic testing protocol for the throwing shoulder: The throwers series. Isokin. Exerc. Sci., 1:63–71.

165. Wilk, K.E., Arrigo, C.A., and Andrews, J.R. (1992): Isokinetic testing of the shoulder abductors and adductors: windowed vs nonwindowed data collection. J. Orthop. Sports Phys. Ther., 15:107–112.

166. Wilk, K.E., Voight, M.L., Keirns, M.A., et al. (1993): Stretch-shortening drills for the upper extremities: theory and clinical application. J. Orthop. Sports Phys. Ther., 17:225–239.

167. Wilk, K.E., Romaniello, W.T., Soscia, S.M., et al. (1994): The relationship between subjective knee scores, isokinetic (OKC) testing and functional testing in the ACL reconstructed knee. J. Orthop. Sports Phys. Ther., 20:60–73.

168. Wyatt, M.P., and Edwards, A.M. (1981): Comparison of quadriceps and hamstring torque values during isokinetic exercise. J. Orthop. Sports Phys. Ther., 3:48–56.

169. Yack, H.J., Collins, C.E., and Whieldon, T.J. (1993): Comparison of closed and open kinetic chain exercise in the anterior cruciate ligament-deficient knee. Am. J. Sports Med., 21:49–54.

Chapter 9

Lower Leg, Ankle, and Foot Rehabilitation

Edward P. Mulligan, M.S., P.T., S.C.S., A.T.,C.

The lower leg, ankle, and foot consist of 26 bones, all working as one unit to propel the body. The foot has three components: rearfoot, midfoot, and forefoot. The rearfoot and midfoot are composed of the tarsal bones. The rearfoot contains the subtalar joint, with the talus resting on top of the calcaneus. The midfoot is composed of the navicular and cuboid as they articulate with the talus and calcaneus to form the transverse tarsal joint. The three cuneiform bones are located within the midfoot. Five tarsal and 14 phalangeal bones make up the forefoot structure. The shape of the joint, orientation of its axis, supporting ligaments, and subtle accessory motions at the joint surface are important determinants of normal biomechanical behavior. The treatment of pathologic hypomobility or hypermobility is predicated on a thorough understanding of these principles and their functional intimacy.

ARTHROKINEMATICS

Tibiofibular Joint

The tibiofibular joint provides accessory motion to allow greater freedom of movement in the ankle. Fusion or hypomobility of this joint can restrict or impair ankle function. During ankle plantar flexion, the fibula slides caudad at the superior and inferior tibiofibular joint, while the lateral malleolus rotates mediad to cause an approximation of the two malleoli. With dorsiflexion, the opposite accessory motions provide a slight spread of the malleoli and accommodate the wider portion of the anterior talus. Accessory motion of the tibiofibular joint also occurs with supination (calcaneal inversion) and pronation (calcaneal eversion). The head of the fibula slides distally and posteriorly with supination and proximally and anteriorly during pronation.[25]

Talocrural Joint

The talocrural articulation is a synovial joint with a structurally strong mortice and supporting collateral ligaments. The concave surface of the mortice is made up of the distal tibial plafond and the tibial (medial) and fibular (lateral) malleoli. Within the mortice sits the convex surface of the talar dome. The joint derives ligamentous support from the deltoid ligament medially and the anterior talofibular, calcaneofibular, and posterior talofibular ligaments laterally.

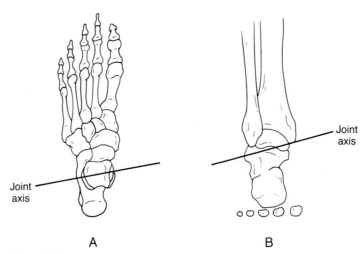

Figure 9–1. Joint axis for talocrural joint. *A,* Dorsal view. *B,* Posterior view. Axis of orientation runs from posterolateral inferior to anteromedial superior.

The lateral malleolus is positioned distally and posteriorly relative to the medial malleolus, causing the axis of motion for the ankle joint to run from posterolateral inferior to anteromedial superior (Fig. 9–1). This oblique orientation allows triplanar motion. Sagittal plane plantar flexion and dorsiflexion make up the primary movements of the joint and are coupled with adduction and abduction, respectively. Because the axis is nearly parallel to the transverse plane, inversion and eversion are negligible components of motion. Available range of motion is typically defined as approximately 20° of dorsiflexion and 50° of plantar flexion.[1]

A small amount of talocrural physiologic accessory motion also accompanies plantar flexion and dorsiflexion.[27] As the foot plantar flexes, the body of the talus slides anteriorly. Conversely, as the foot dorsiflexes, the direction of talar slide is posterior. Maximal stability to angular and torsional stresses occurs in the close-packed position of maximal dorsiflexion, in which the talus slides posteriorly and wedges within the mortice. The resting position of the ankle joint is 10° of plantar flexion (Table 9–1).

Subtalar Joint

The talocalcaneal articulation provides the triplanar motions of pronation and supination. The joint is supported by the medial and lateral collateral, interosseous talocalcaneal, and posterior and lateral talocalcaneal ligaments.

Table 9–1. Joint Positional Treatment Considerations

JOINT	CLOSE-PACKED POSITION	RESTING POSITION	CAPSULAR PATTERN
Talocrural	Maximal dorsiflexion	10° plantar flexion	Plantar flexion restricted greater than dorsiflexion
Subtalar	Maximal supination	Neutral	Increasing loss of varus until fixed in valgus
Midtarsal	Maximal supination	STJ neutral	Limitations in adduction and inversion
First MTP	Maximal dorsiflexion	Slight plantar flexion	Gross limitation of extension; slight limitation of flexion

MTP, Metatarsophalangeal; STJ, subtalar joint.

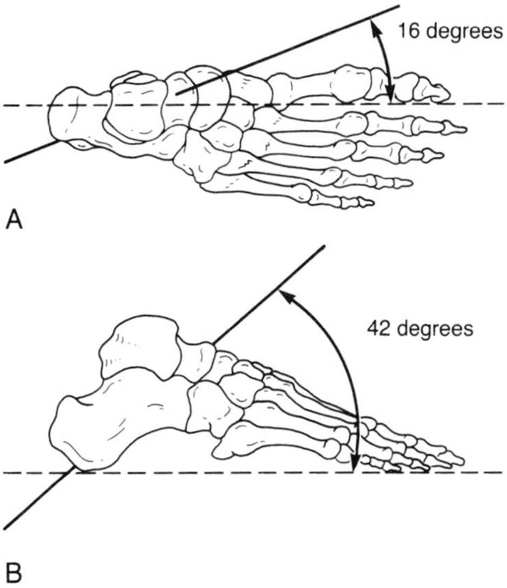

Figure 9–2. Subtalar joint axis lies approximately 16° from the sagittal plane *(A)* and 42° from the transverse plane *(B)*. (Reproduced by permission from Mann, Roger A.: Biomechanics of running. *In:* American Academy of Orthopaedic Surgeons: Symposium on the Foot and Leg in Running Sports. St. Louis, 1982, The C.V. Mosby Co.)

The joint axis runs from dorsal, medial, and distal to plantar, lateral, and proximal. It is oriented approximately 16° from the sagittal plane and 42° from the transverse plane (Fig. 9–2). Because of this axis of orientation, the joint provides the triplanar motions of pronation and supination. The pronation components of motion in an open kinetic chain are calcaneal dorsiflexion, abduction, and eversion. Conversely, open kinetic chain supination consists of calcaneal plantar flexion, adduction, and inversion. Functionally, however, the subtalar joint operates like a closed kinetic chain. Closed kinetic chain motion occurs when the distal segment is fixed and the proximal segment becomes mobile, as when the foot is in contact with the ground. The distal or terminal joints meet with considerable resistance, which prohibits or restrains free motion. During the weight-bearing portion of the stance phase of gait, friction and ground reaction forces prevent the abduction-adduction and plantar flexion–dorsiflexion elements of open kinetic chain subtalar motion. To counteract these forces, the talus functions to maintain the transverse and sagittal plane motions of supination and pronation.[31] Thus, in closed kinetic chain motion, subtalar joint pronation consists of talar plantar flexion–adduction and calcaneal eversion, whereas subtalar joint supination consists of talar dorsiflexion-abduction and calcaneal inversion (Fig. 9–3).[48] Note that calcaneal direction of movement is unaffected by the open-chain versus the closed-chain type of motion (Table 9–2).

The subtalar joint couples the function of the foot with the rest of the proximal kinetic chain. The prime function of the subtalar joint is to permit rotation of the leg in the transverse plane during gait. The rotation of the talus on the calcaneus allows the foot to become a directional transmitter and torque con-

Table 9–2. Calcaneal and Talar Motion in Open and Closed Kinetic Chain

MOTION OF FOOT	OPEN-CHAIN COMPONENT	CLOSED-CHAIN COMPONENT
Pronation	Calcaneal eversion Calcaneal abduction Calcaneal dorsiflexion	Calcaneal eversion Talar adduction Talar plantar flexion
Supination	Calcaneal inversion Calcaneal adduction Calcaneal plantar flexion	Calcaneal inversion Talar abduction Talar dorsiflexion

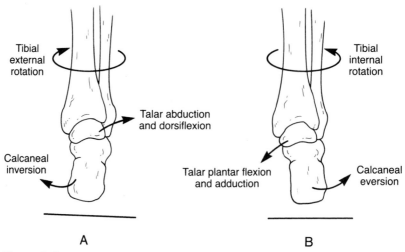

Figure 9–3. Closed-chain subtalar motion. *A,* Supination. *B,* Pronation.

verter to the kinetic chain.[37] These characteristics allow the foot to be a loose adaptor to the terrain in midstance and a rigid lever for propulsion.

Because the subtalar joint is angulated approximately 45° from the transverse plane, there is 1° of inversion or eversion for every 1° of tibial internal or external rotation. This relationship can be observed in gait. As the subtalar joint pronates, the tibial tuberosity is seen to be rotating internally (Fig. 9–4). High angles of inclination (greater than 45°) of the subtalar joint axis cause a relative decrease in calcaneal inversion-eversion motion and an increased tibial rotation motion,

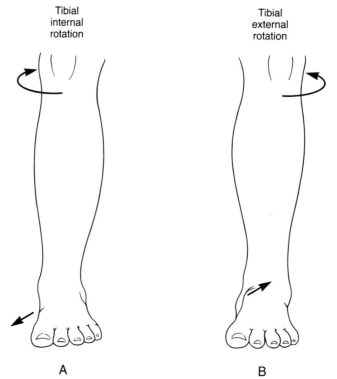

Figure 9–4. Relationship of the subtalar joint to the lower leg during gait. *A,* Subtalar pronation. *B,* Subtalar supination.

leading to posture-related pathologies secondary to poor absorption of ground reaction forces. Conversely, the athlete with a low angle of inclination (less than 45°) of the subtalar joint demonstrates a relative increase in calcaneal mobility, resulting in more foot-related overuse and fatigue problems secondary to the calcaneal hypermobility.[48]

The physiologic accessory motions of the subtalar joint occur in the frontal plane. The convex portion of the posterior calcaneus slides laterally during inversion (supination) and medially with eversion (pronation). The close-packed position of the subtalar joint is maximal supination, whereas the resting position is the subtalar neutral position. From its neutral position the subtalar joint can supinate approximately two times as much as it can pronate. This motion is measured in the frontal plane of calcaneal inversion and eversion. The normal subtalar range of motion is approximately 30°, with two thirds of that motion being represented as calcaneal inversion and one third as calcaneal eversion. Gait requires 8° to 12° of supination and 4° to 6° of pronation.[43]

Midtarsal Joint

The midtarsal joint consists of the talonavicular and calcaneocuboid articulations. They derive their ligamentous support from the calcaneonavicular (spring), deltoid, dorsal talonavicular, and calcaneocuboid (long and short plantar) ligaments.

The midtarsal joint has two separate axes. Functionally, these two axes work together to result in triplanar motion. The two axes of the midtarsal joint are the longitudinal and the oblique. The longitudinal axis is essentially parallel to the sagittal and transverse planes, allowing only frontal plane motions of inversion and eversion, whereas the oblique axis is parallel with the frontal plane, allowing motion in the sagittal (plantar flexion–dorsiflexion) and transverse (adduction-abduction) planes (Fig. 9–5). Because the oblique axis is angulated about equally[55] for the sagittal and transverse planes, plantar flexion–adduction and dorsiflexion-abduction are coupled equally.

From a clinical standpoint, there is no reliable method of quantifying motion in the midtarsal joint. Midtarsal joint motion is dictated by the position of the subtalar joint. When the subtalar joint is pronated, the axes of the talocalcaneal and calcaneocuboid joints are parallel, allowing the midtarsal joint to unlock

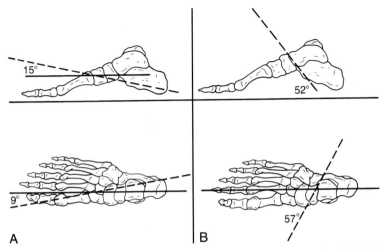

Figure 9–5. Axes of motion for the midtarsal joints. *A*, Longitudinal axis. *B*, Oblique axis.

and become an adaptor with increased mobility. As the subtalar joint supinates, the midtarsal joint's motion decreases as the two axes diverge and "lock" the forefoot on the rearfoot in preparation for its rigid lever function during the propulsive phase of gait (Fig. 9–6).

The position of the midtarsal joint is dictated by ground reaction forces during the contact and midstance phases of gait and by muscular activity on the joint during the propulsive phase of gait.[39] The standard clinical index for determining midtarsal joint position is to compare the plantar plane position of the five metatarsal heads to the plantar plane position of the neutral rearfoot when the midtarsal joint is maximally pronated about both its axes.

Physiologic accessory motions of the midtarsal joint that can be evaluated manually include dorsal and plantar glides of the navicular on the talus and of the cuboid on the calcaneus. Plantar glide accompanies supination, and dorsal glide accompanies pronation.

Tarsometatarsal, Metatarsophalangeal, and Interphalangeal Joints

The first ray represents a functional articulation consisting of the bones of the medial column. The joint axis runs from the distolateral to the proximomedial direction, almost parallel to the transverse plane. Motion occurs primarily in the sagittal (plantar flexion–dorsiflexion) and frontal (inversion-eversion) planes. The axis is angulated 45° from both these planes, so for every 1° of plantar flexion there is 1° of eversion (Fig. 9–7).

First-ray motion begins in the late-stance phase of gait and continues late into propulsion. As with the midtarsal joint, first-ray motion is controlled by the position of the subtalar joint. With the subtalar joint in pronation, the amount of first-ray motion is increased. As the subtalar joint supinates, the first-ray motion decreases. The normal extent of movement is 0.5 to 1 cm (a thumb width) in the plantar and dorsal directions.[39]

The clinical standard for determining the neutral position of the first metatarsal is to evaluate the position of the first ray relative to the three central metatarsal heads. It should lie in the same transverse plane, neither plantar flexed nor dorsiflexed.

The fifth ray operates about an independent axis with the same directional orientation as the subtalar joint. The central three rays have an axis orientation parallel to the frontal and transverse planes. Consequently, there is only plantar flexion–dorsiflexion motion in the sagittal plane. The metatarsophalangeal (MTP)

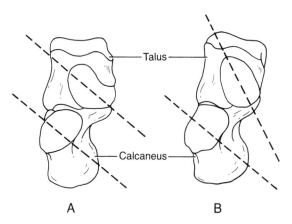

A   B

Figure 9–6. Axis of transverse tarsal joint. *A,* When calcaneus is in eversion, the conjoint axes between the talonavicular and calcaneocuboid joints are parallel to one another, so that increased motion occurs in the transverse tarsal joint. *B,* When the calcaneus is in inversion, the axes are no longer parallel, and there is decreased motion with increased stability of the transverse tarsal joint. (Reproduced by permission from Mann, Roger A.: Biomechanics of running. *In:* American Academy of Orthopaedic Surgeons: Symposium of the Foot and Leg in Running Sports. St. Louis, 1982, The C.V. Mosby Co.)

Talus

Calcaneus

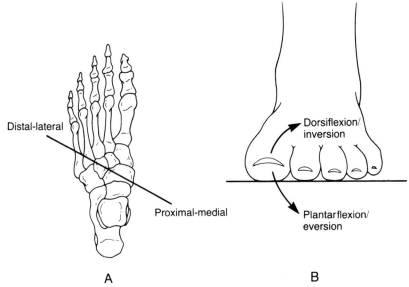

Figure 9–7. First ray axis and motion. *A,* First ray axis of motion, dorsal view. *B,* First ray motion.

joints also have an additional vertical axis, which is parallel to the frontal and sagittal planes to allow abduction and adduction of the joints.

The first MTP joint represents the articulation between the first metatarsal and the proximal phalanx of the big toe. Minimal normal first MTP range of motion with the first ray stabilized is about 20° to 30° of hyperextension. Without stabilization, the first MTP joint should hyperextend to at least 60° to 70°.[30] The MTP joints also have an additional vertical axis, which is parallel to the frontal and sagittal planes to allow abduction and adduction of the joints.

Physiologic accessory motions of the MTP joints include plantar and dorsal glides. Plantar glide of the convex first metatarsal accompanies extension, whereas dorsal glide accompanies toe flexion.

MUSCULAR FUNCTION OF THE LOWER LEG, ANKLE, AND FOOT

The phasic action of the muscles of the lower leg and foot can be determined by examining the musculotendinous unit's excursion from origin to insertion relative to the axis on which it acts (Fig. 9–8). Each muscle group has specific functions that control or provide the necessary forces to create movement. The muscles of the leg and foot can be divided into subgroups or compartments (Table 9–3; Fig. 9–9).

Posterior Superficial Muscle Group

The posterior superficial muscle group is composed of the gastrocnemius, soleus, and plantaris muscles. These muscles originate from above and below the knee joint and have a common insertion by way of the Achilles tendon on the posterior aspect of the calcaneus. In the open kinetic chain, the triceps surae provide flexion of the knee, plantar flexion of the ankle, and supination of the subtalar joint. With closed kinetic chain function, the gastrocnemius and soleus

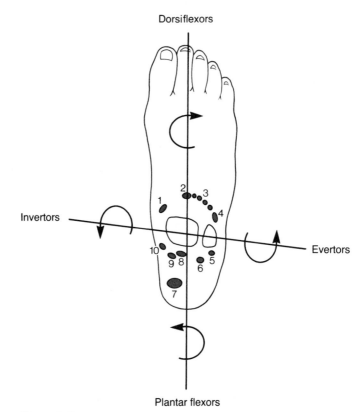

Figure 9–8. Motion diagram of the ankle. Tibialis anterior *(1)*, extensor hallucis longus *(2)*, extensor digitorum longus *(3)*, peroneus tertius *(4)*, peroneus brevis *(5)*, peroneus longus *(6)*, Achilles tendon *(7)*, flexor hallucis longus *(8)*, flexor digitorum longus *(9)*, and tibialis posterior *(10)*. (From Magee, D.J. [1987]: Orthopedic Physical Assessment. Philadelphia, W.B. Saunders.)

are active throughout the stance phase of gait. Initially, at heel strike, the gastrocnemius and soleus contract eccentrically to decelerate tibial internal rotation and forward progression of the tibia over the foot. Later, during midstance and heel-off, they provide subtalar joint supination (externally rotating the tibia) and ankle plantar flexion.

Posterior Deep Muscle Group

The posterior deep muscles of the lower leg include the posterior tibialis, flexor digitorum longus, and flexor hallucis longus. The posterior tibialis is a

Table 9–3. Lower Leg Muscle Groups

GROUP	MUSCLES
Posterior superficial	Gastrocnemius, soleus, plantaris
Lateral	Peroneals
Dorsal intrinsics	Extensor hallucis brevis, extensor digitorum brevis
Deep posterior	Posterior tibialis, flexor digitorum longus, flexor hallucis longus
Anterior pretibial	Anterior tibialis, extensor hallucis longus, extensor digitorum, peroneus tertius
Plantar intrinsics	Flexor digitorum brevis, flexor hallucis brevis, adductor and abductor hallucis, lumbricales

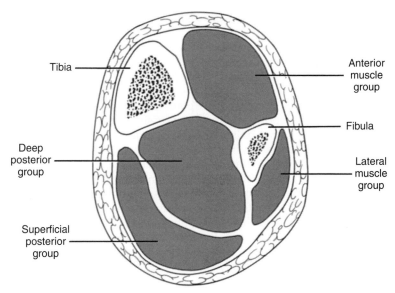

Figure 9–9. Cross section of the lower leg muscle groups.

strong supinator and invertor of the subtalar joint and functions to control and reverse pronation during gait. It decelerates subtalar joint pronation and tibial internal rotation at heel strike and then reverses its function to accelerate subtalar joint supination and tibial external rotation during stance. The posterior tibialis also maintains the stability of the midtarsal joint in the direction of supination around its oblique axis during the stance phase of gait.

The flexor digitorum longus functions as a supinator of the subtalar joint and flexor of the second through fifth MTP joints in the open kinetic chain. When the foot is in contact with the ground and the digits are stable, the flexor digitorum longus actively stabilizes the foot as a weight-bearing platform for propulsion. If the flexor digitorum longus works unopposed by the action of the intrinsic muscles, clawing of the toes results.[21]

The flexor hallucis longus has a function similar to that of the flexor digitorum longus in that it flexes the first MTP joint in the open kinetic chain. Both these long flexors help support the medial arch.

Lateral Muscle Group

The lateral muscle group includes the peroneus longus and brevis. The peroneus longus, because of its attachment to the first metatarsal and medial cuneiform on the plantar surface, functions to pronate the subtalar joint and to plantar flex and evert the first ray in the open kinetic chain. In the closed kinetic chain, the peroneus longus has many important functions. It provides support to the transverse and lateral longitudinal arches. During the latter portion of midstance and early heel-off, it actively stabilizes the first ray and everts the foot to transfer body weight from the lateral to the medial side of the foot.

The peroneus brevis is primarily an evertor in open kinetic chain motion. During gait it functions in concert with the peroneus longus. Its primary role is to stabilize the calcaneocuboid joint, allowing the peroneus longus to work efficiently over the cuboid pulley.

Anterior Muscle Group

The pretibial muscles include the anterior tibialis, extensor digitorum longus, extensor hallucis longus, and peroneus tertius. As a group they are active during the swing phase and the heel-strike to foot-flat phases of gait.

The anterior tibialis is primarily a dorsiflexor of the talocrural joint in open kinetic chain function. In gait, the anterior tibialis basically operates concentrically in the swing phase and eccentrically in the stance phase. At the end of toe-off, the anterior tibialis begins to contract concentrically to initiate dorsiflexion of the ankle and first ray, to assist in ground clearance at midswing, and then to supinate the foot slightly during late swing in preparation for heel strike. When the foot hits the ground, the anterior tibialis reverses its role to decelerate or control plantar flexion to foot-flat, prevent excessive pronation, and supinate the midtarsal joint's longitudinal axis. A weak anterior tibialis can lead to "foot-slap," or uncontrolled pronation in gait.

In non–weight-bearing function, the long extensors (extensor digitorum and hallucis longus) provide dorsiflexion of the ankle and extension of the toes. Because, unlike the anterior tibialis, these tendons pass laterally to the subtalar joint axis, they provide a pronatory force at the joint. In fact, a prime responsibility of the long extensors is to hold the oblique axis of the midtarsal joint in a pronated position at heel strike and then to assist the controlled deceleration of plantar flexion to foot-flat.

Intrinsic Muscle Group

Generally, the intrinsic muscles of the foot act together during most of the stance phase of gait. Their function is to stabilize the midtarsal joint and digits while keeping the toes flat on the ground until lift-off. An unstable, pronated midtarsal joint during midstance necessitates that the intrinsic muscles work harder and longer. This phenomenon explains the common complaint of foot fatigue in the athlete with a hypermobile foot.

ANTHROPOMETRIC ASSESSMENT

Anthropometric measurements of the leg, foot, and ankle provide objective evidence of effusion. Many techniques can be reliable. Volumetric displacement methods with submersion of the foot into a calibrated tank are highly reliable and easily performed. Other methods include girth assessments at selected sites using heel-lock and figure-eight tape measurement techniques (Fig. 9–10). Tatro-Adams demonstrated excellent intratester and intertester reliability with the figure-eight method of measurement.[45] Comparison with the uninvolved side is always appropriate.

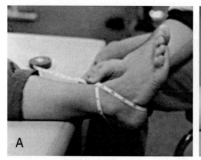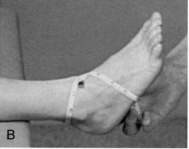

Figure 9–10. Ankle girth assessment. *A,* Heel-lock method. *B,* Figure-eight method.

Determination of Subtalar Joint Neutral Position

To assess inversion-eversion motion of the ankle, the clinician must first identify the subtalar neutral position. This can be found through palpation of the head of the talus as it articulates with the navicular. When the subtalar joint is pronated or supinated, the head of the talus is palpable medially or laterally. When the fourth and fifth metatarsal heads are loaded to pronate the forefoot to tissue resistance, the calcaneus is inverted and everted. When the subtalar joint is supinated, the medial side of the talus disappears, and the lateral aspect of the talus becomes prominent. The reverse is true when the subtalar is pronated. The neutral position is defined as that point at which there is talonavicular congruency and either the medial and lateral aspects of the talus are palpable or their protrusion is symmetric. This technique can be used in a closed-chain or open-chain assessment (Fig. 9–11). In a weight-bearing position, an easy visual assessment is to observe for equal concavities above and below the lateral malleolus.[39] A shallow curve superiorly and an accentuated curve inferiorly would suggest a pronated subtalar joint (Fig. 9–12).

Subtalar Range of Motion

Once the subtalar joint's neutral position has been established, assessment of calcaneal inversion-eversion range of motion can take place. Initially, the subtalar joint's neutral position is objectively quantified through goniometric measurement. Normal is considered 2° to 3° of varus. The goniometer's arms are aligned with the longitudinal midline of the posterior calcaneus and the posterior bisection of the tibia (Fig. 9–13). Care must be taken to disregard the Achilles tendon and calcaneal fat pads, because they may produce unreliable measurements. Readings are recorded following maximal passive calcaneal inversion and eversion (Fig. 9–14). Inversion and eversion amounts of motion are then determined based on the initial neutral position. Differences may be noted, depending on whether this assessment was performed in a weight-bearing or

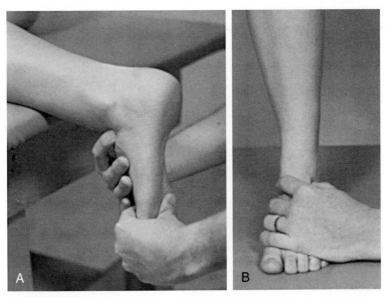

Figure 9–11. Subtalar neutral position. *A,* Non–weight-bearing palpation. *B,* Closed-chain palpation.

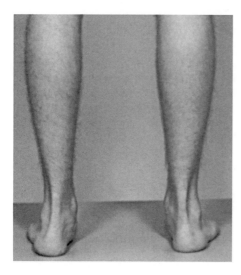

Figure 9-12. Pronated subtalar position with accentuated inferior curve.

non–weight-bearing posture. Lattanza and colleagues[29] have found an average increase of 37% in subtalar eversion as a component of pronation when measured in the closed-chain weight-bearing posture as compared to the traditional non–weight-bearing position. The intratester and intertester reliability of these measurement techniques have been investigated by a number of authors.[8, 35, 40, 42] Generally, the intratester reliability is considered to be fair and the intertester reliability poor. Measurement repeatability may be enhanced with experienced examiners using inclinometers in a weight-bearing assessment.

Plantar Flexion–Dorsiflexion Range of Motion

Ankle dorsiflexion range of motion must be assessed while maintaining the subtalar joint in a neutral position. If the subtalar joint is not monitored, pronator substitution may provide an inaccurate portrayal of gastrocnemius-soleus flexibility. When the subtalar joint is pronated, midtarsal mobility is increased, and dorsiflexion of the foot can occur around the oblique axis of the midtarsal joint.

A minimum of 10° dorsiflexion is needed at heel-off to allow for normal

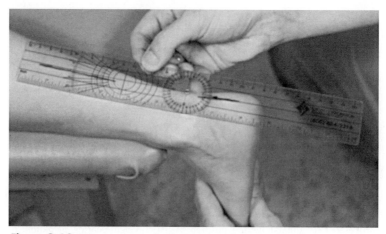

Figure 9-13. Measurement of subtalar neutral position.

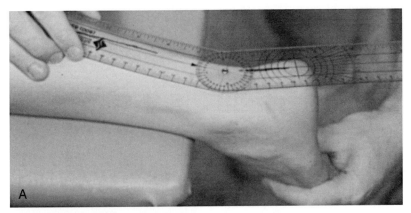

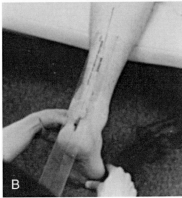

Figure 9-14. Measurement of subtalar range of motion. *A*, Inversion. *B*, Eversion.

ambulation.[4] Because the knee joint is fully extended at this point in the gait cycle, the two-joint gastrocnemius muscle is fully stretched over both joints. Consequently, the knee should be placed in full extension when evaluating the range of dorsiflexion excursion available in gait. To differentiate soleus extensibility, dorsiflexion range of motion is assessed in a knee-flexed posture so that the gastrocnemius is slack. An increase of 10° dorsiflexion to a total of 20° is anticipated.

To measure ankle dorsiflexion range of motion, the athlete is placed prone with the ankle extended off the end of the table. The clinician then palpates and establishes the subtalar neutral position. The distal arm of the goniometer is placed parallel to the lateral aspect of the calcaneus and the fifth metatarsal head, while the proximal arm is aligned with the bisection of the lateral aspect of the lower leg and the head of the fibula. The clinician then passively forces dorsiflexion while the athlete is actively assisting (Fig. 9–15). This active assistance provides reciprocal inhibition of the passive tension stored in the triceps surae group. Pronator substitution tendencies are manifested by calcaneal eversion. Calcaneal stabilization may have to be provided manually. This procedure should be performed with the knee extended and flexed. If the dorsiflexion range is equal in the flexed and extended postures, ankle equinus (bony block caused by osseous lipping in the anterior ankle joint) or soleus equinus should be suspected.[4]

Plantar flexion range of motion is expected to be 50° to 60° and is assessed with similar goniometric placement techniques.

Subtalar Joint Position

Subtalar joint position is determined by comparing the orientation of the calcaneus relative to the distal third of the leg when the calcaneus is in its neutral

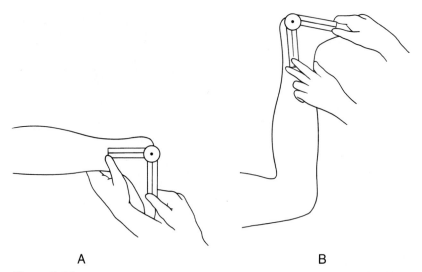

Figure 9–15. Goniometric assessment of ankle dorsiflexion range of motion. *A*, Knee extended. *B*, Knee flexed.

position. Rearfoot varus is defined as an inverted calcaneus when compared to the posterior bisection of the tibia in the non–weight-bearing position (Fig. 9–16*A*). Rearfoot valgus is the opposite situation, in which the calcaneus is everted relative to the tibia (Fig. 9–16*B*). Calcaneal varus and valgus are terms used to describe calcaneal position relative to the supporting surface. This position may represent a compensated position dependent upon the range of motion available at the subtalar joint.

In identifying an athlete's foot type it is important to evaluate the feet in their position of function. The neutral and resting calcaneal stance positions are accurate reflections of the way the lower extremity's kinetic chain interfaces with the supporting surfaces. The neutral calcaneal stance position is the angular relationship of the calcaneus and the ground with the subtalar joint in the neutral position. As described previously, this may be called a rearfoot varus or

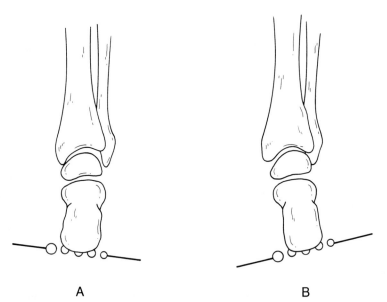

Figure 9–16. *A*, Rearfoot varus. *B*, Rearfoot valgus.

valgus posture. Resting calcaneal stance position is this same angular relationship in natural stance, in which compensation for deviations is allowed.

Assessment is made by placing the athlete in his or her angle and base of gait and measuring this relationship by placing one arm of a goniometer parallel to the ground and the other aligned with the posterior calcaneal bisection. Measurements are made in subtalar neutral and natural relaxed stances. Ideally, these values should be the same. The diagnostic hallmark of a rearfoot varus is an inverted neutral calcaneal stance position.[39] Compensation for these deformities depends on the availability of the subtalar range of motion. Rearfoot varus is considered fully compensated if the subtalar joint allows enough calcaneal eversion to reach a perpendicular position to the floor, where forces across the heel and forefoot are equilibrated (Fig. 9–17). Uncompensated rearfoot varus is indicated by having an inverted calcaneus in the neutral calcaneal stance position and less inversion in the resting or relaxed calcaneal stance position.

Midtarsal Joint Position

Midtarsal structure and foot type are determined by comparison of the forefoot position relative to the rearfoot. Forefoot varus is a structural abnormality in which the plantar plane of the forefoot is inverted relative to the plantar plane of the rearfoot, with the subtalar joint in its neutral position and the forefoot maximally pronated around both its midtarsal joint axes (Fig. 9–18A). Forefoot valgus is the opposite of forefoot varus in that the forefoot is everted relative to the rearfoot (Fig. 9–18B). An additional requirement for defining forefoot valgus is that the foot has a first ray that has normal range of motion. This differentiates forefoot valgus from a plantar-flexed first ray. Often, a plantar-flexed first ray gives the appearance of a forefoot valgus but can be differentiated by decreased range of motion associated with this deformity. A plantar-flexed first ray shows more plantar flexion than dorsiflexion range of motion (Fig. 9–18C).

Forefoot supinatus is a relatively fixed acquired soft-tissue deformity that typically occurs in athletes whose calcaneus is maintained in an everted position. The forefoot is supinated in relation to the rearfoot because of soft-tissue adapta-

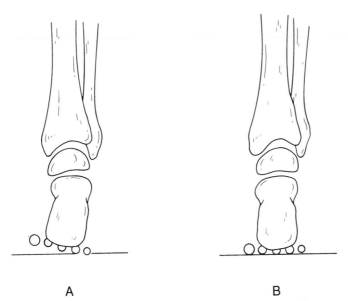

A   B

Figure 9–17. Rearfoot varus. *A,* Inverted calcaneus. *B,* Compensation accomplished by calcaneal eversion in natural resting stance.

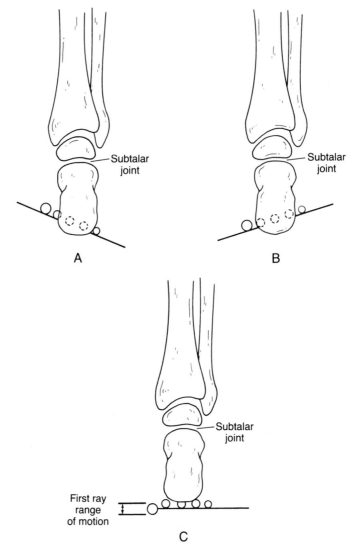

Figure 9–18. *A,* Forefoot varus, inverted forefoot. *B,* Forefoot valgus, everted forefoot. *C,* Plantar-flexed first ray.

tion, and the total midtarsal range of motion is reduced. The compensatory mechanism is the plantar-flexed attitude of the first ray to bring the medial forefoot in contact with the ground (Fig. 9–19).

When assessing midtarsal foot type it is important to assess the quality and quantity of midtarsal motion subjectively. Passive manual assessment techniques can identify the relative amounts of plantar flexion–dorsiflexion and abduction-adduction around the oblique axis and inversion-eversion of the longitudinal axis. Motion should be maximal with the subtalar joint held in pronation and should decrease as the subtalar joint is placed in a supinated position.

Postural Considerations

TIBIAL VARUM

Tibial varum is a structural deformity in which the distal tibia is closer to the midline than the proximal tibia. Its determination quantifies the amount of

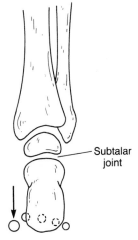

Figure 9-19. Forefoot supinatus: supinated forefoot with plantar-flexed first ray.

frontal plane deviation of the tibia. Assessment is made with the athlete bearing weight on the measured extremity in its angle and base of gait. The goniometer is placed with one arm parallel to the ground and the other parallel to the posterior bisection of the distal tibia (Fig. 9–20). The presence of tibial varum contributes to the total varus attitude of the lower extremity.

TIBIAL TORSION

To evaluate for tibial torsion, the clinician aligns the patient's legs straight so that the femoral condyles are in the transverse plane and the patellae face straight up. The clinician then assesses the amount of torsion by measuring the angle of the malleoli relative to the shaft of the tibia. The normal value is considered to be approximately 13° to 18° of external tibial torsion (Fig. 9–21).

FUNCTIONAL RELATIONSHIPS

The entire kinetic chain is intimately linked with every movement in sport. Each segment of the body depends on the role and function of adjoining and

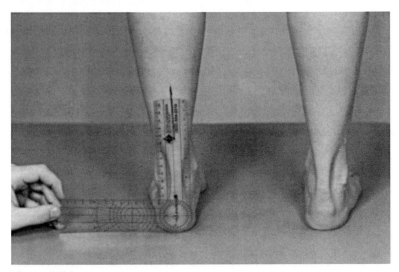

Figure 9-20. Measurement of tibial varum.

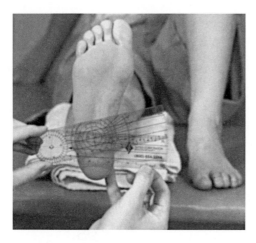

Figure 9–21. Measurement of tibial torsion.

distant structures. A prime example of this interdependence is displayed in overground ambulation. The following is a description of "normal" gait. Normal gait is a difficult entity to quantify, but this description can serve as a basis by which to evaluate a potentially pathologic type of movement.

Normal Gait

At heel strike, the ankle is in a neutral position and then plantar flexes to foot-flat under the eccentric control of the pretibial muscles. The subtalar and midtarsal joints are supinated at heel contact and begin the process of pronation to unlock the midtarsal joint, which allows foot adaptation to the terrain. At the knee joint, the tibia follows the directional input of the subtalar joint by internally rotating and flexing. Normal subtalar pronation during this phase of gait is a passive activity in the closed kinetic chain that directs movement and attenuates ground reaction forces.[15]

During midstance, from foot-flat to heel-off, the subtalar joint undergoes supination as the body weight shifts anterior to the weight-bearing extremity. The ankle joint is moving into its extreme of dorsiflexion. The supination movement of the subtalar joint dictates that the tibia rotate externally and allow the knee to reach full extension at the end of midstance. The posterior calf muscles eccentrically control the early pronation and concentrically shorten as the foot moves into supination. During this phase the foot reverses function, from that of a mobile adaptor to that of a rigid lever.

Propulsion from heel-off to toe-off shows the ankle joint plantar flexing while the midtarsal joint is locking on the supinating subtalar joint. This process prepares the foot for its role as a stable platform from which to push off. The MTP joints extend while the knee joint flexes in preparation for the swing phase of gait.

Swing-phase motion requires flexion of the knee and dorsiflexion of the ankle to provide ground clearance. The subtalar joint initially pronates in early swing to shorten the limb and assist in ground clearance. It then supinates in terminal swing to prepare for heel contact on the next step (Table 9–4; Fig. 9–22).

Dynamic Gait Assessment

Whereas assessment of lower quarter injuries with the athlete in a static posture is the benchmark for evaluation, dynamic assessment of movement patterns offers the most valid means for determining the athlete's functional

Table 9-4. Normal Gait Cycle

Joint		STANCE PHASE				SWING PHASE		
		HEEL CONTACT	**FOOT-FLAT**		**HEEL-OFF**	**TOE-OFF**		
		Forefoot Loading		*Midstance*	*Propulsion*	*Early Swing*	*Midswing*	*Terminal Swing*
		0%	15%	30%	45%	60%		100%
Tibiofemoral	position	Extended ——→ Mildly flexed		——→ Extended		——→ Maximally flexed		
	Motion	Flexion, tibial internal rotation		Extension, tibial external rotation	Flexion		Extension	
Talocrural	position	Neutral ——→ Maximally plantar flexed		——→ Maximally dorsiflexed	——→ Plantar flexed →Neutral → Dorsiflexed			
	Motion	Plantar flexion	Dorsiflexion		Very rapid plantar flexion	Dorsiflexion		
Subtalar	position	Mildly supinated ——→ Fully pronated		Supination ——→ Mildly supinated	——→ Fully supinated	Pronation		Supination
	Motion	Pronation		Supination	Mildly supinated	Pronation		Supination
Midtarsal	position	Everted ——→ Inverted		Inverted				
	Motion	Unlocking to adapt		Locking as rigid lever				

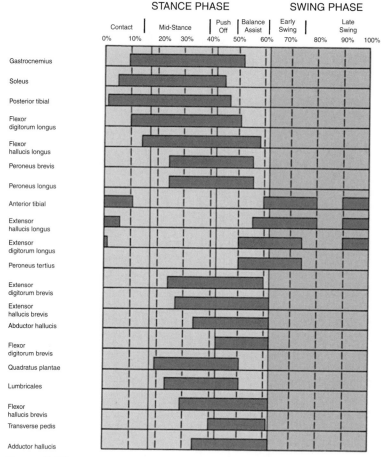

Figure 9–22. Muscular function in normal gait. (From McGlamry, E.D. [1987]: Fundamentals of Foot Surgery. © Williams & Wilkins, Baltimore.)

ability. Assessment of gait should be incorporated into all evaluations of the lower extremity. This can be performed in any setting, but a treadmill greatly enhances the convenience of analysis.

Brandel and Williams[3] have demonstrated a statistically insignificant difference in stride length, velocity, and cadence with treadmill analysis of gait versus normal walking at 2.5 to 3.2 miles per hour. A treadmill also allows easy control of gait speeds and inclination. With recently developed videotape-recording technology, an objective documentation of function is obtained, and the tape can be slowed down for careful analysis. A simple clinical setup requires only single positioning of the camera to allow anterior, posterior, and lateral views to be videotaped with the assistance of postural mirrors (Fig. 9–23).

General observations of gait should include head placement, shoulder height and position, arm swing and carry, cadence, step-stride length, weight acceptance, and single-limb stance stability. With a knowledge of normal gait mechanics, joint position and motion in the different phases of the gait cycle can be compared with expected norms. Hypotheses are then generated concerning the source of deviations and correlated with static evaluation findings. Some subtle weaknesses, inflexibilities, and postural asymmetries can be detected with this method of evaluation. Points of observation for recognizing subtalar joint position during videotape analysis of gait are presented in Table 9–5.

When evaluating gait it is important to recognize some of the general trends that differentiate walking, jogging, and running. As movement speed increases,

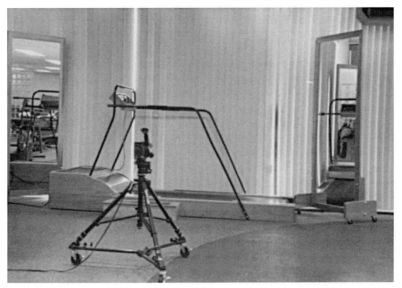

Figure 9–23. Video setup for gait analysis.

the total range of motion that each joint undergoes must increase. This increased range of motion takes place during a shorter period of time because the gait cycle is occurring at a more rapid pace. As a result, velocity of joint motion must be increased. During the stance phase of gait these higher velocities of motion cause high eccentric tensile contractions that must be dissipated and tolerated by the musculoskeletal system. Table 9–6 contrasts the parameters that define and differentiate walking, jogging, and running.

Pathologic Gait

COMMON PRONATORY DISORDERS

By having the foot function as a rigid lever during propulsion, the weight of the body is propelled off that limb with maximum efficiency. If the subtalar joint cannot reach the neutral position, heading toward a supinated position just prior to heel-off, an unstable base of support is used for propulsion. If a condition does not allow the forefoot to lock on the rearfoot, a situation exists that is analogous to walking in sand, in which the base of support gives way under push-off forces. It takes significantly more muscle energy to push off such unstable platforms, resulting in foot and leg fatigue secondary to overuse.

It must be appreciated that pronation is a normal and necessary component of gait. Only when the amount, timing, or sequence of the pronation-supination cycle is altered is it considered abnormal.[22] An athlete with rearfoot varus demonstrates this during midstance and, as a result, can have abnormal hyper-

Table 9–5. Recognition of Subtalar Joint Position

VIEW	PRONATION	SUPINATION
Posterior	Calcaneal inversion; calcaneal indentation concave to midline	Calcaneal eversion; calcaneal indentation convex to midline
Anterior	Internal rotation of tibia	External rotation of tibia
Lateral	Talar head adducts and plantar flexes; talar head bulges and medial arch flattens	Medial longitudinal arch heightens

Table 9–6. Contrast of Walking, Jogging, and Running

PARAMETER	WALKING	JOGGING	RUNNING
Speed	2–4 mph	5–10 mph	10+ mph
Stance time duration	0.6 second	0.3 second	0.2 second
Stance:swing time ratio	3:2	3:4	1:2
Vertical forces	Body weight	2–3 × body weight	2–3 × body weight
Support phase	Double-limb support	Single-limb support	Single-limb support
Base of gait	2–3 cm	1 cm	None or crossover

mobility and shearing forces within the foot. As can be seen in Figure 9–24, the athlete with rearfoot varus does obtain some supination in propulsion, but the subtalar joint is still in a pronated posture at the initiation of heel-off.

Forefoot varus is another condition that is compensated for by abnormal pronation of the subtalar joint. The subtalar joint remains pronated throughout the stance phase of gait to allow ground contact on the medial forefoot and creates a propulsive method of ambulation (Fig. 9–25).

Abnormal pronation can also be caused by factors and forces extrinsic to the foot. Flexibility deficiencies, postural deviations, and muscular weaknesses can alter the normal pronation-supination sequence extrinsically.[49] Equinus deformities caused by a tight gastrocnemius or soleus tend to cause a massive subtalar joint pronation just before propulsion begins.[39] A tight Achilles complex causes either early heel-off or prolonged subtalar joint pronation to compensate for the lack of adequate talocrural dorsiflexion range of motion. In both cases the subtalar joint has not supinated to neutral prior to heel-off.

Proximal inflexibilities, such as tight medial hamstrings, which shorten stride length or affect lower extremity external rotation during swing phase, are other examples of extrinsically induced abnormal pronation.[49] These inflexibilities do not allow enough time for full resupination of the subtalar joint during the late swing phase in its preparation for heel strike.

Postural deviations such as leg length discrepancies are a final example of abnormal pronation brought on by external causes. Subtalar pronation is a method by which leg length can be shortened in the closed kinetic chain.[28] Although this chapter deals with lower leg and foot pathology, it is important to note that dysfunction may originate proximal to the structure in which it is manifested.

SUPINATORY DISORDERS

Abnormal supination in gait is a less common occurrence than abnormal pronation but is seen in athletes who have forefoot valgus or a rigid, plantar-

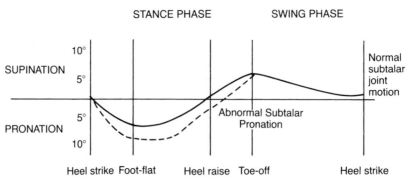

Figure 9–24. Graphic representation of subtalar joint motion in rearfoot varus.

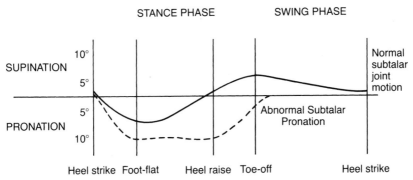

Figure 9–25. Graphic representation of subtalar joint motion in forefoot varus.

flexed first ray. Supinatory compensation is found first at the longitudinal axis of the midtarsal joint and then at the subtalar joint.[39] Rapid supination in midstance to bring the lateral side of the foot to the floor creates lateral instability of the ankle, making the athlete prone to inversion injuries. As can be seen in Figure 9–26, rapid supination alters the timing sequence of normal subtalar motion, and the joint pronates late in propulsion.

LOWER LEG, ANKLE, AND FOOT INJURIES AND THEIR MANAGEMENT

Lower Leg Injuries

TIBIOFIBULAR SYNOSTOSIS

Tibiofibular synostosis is a condition in which there is ossification of the interosseous membrane between the tibia and fibula at the inferior tibiofibular syndesmosis. The injury can occur because of a single inversion–internal rotation trauma or from recurrent, less severe episodes in which the anterior and posterior inferior tibiofibular ligaments and the interosseous membrane are damaged. Resultant spreading of the tibia and fibula allows bone formation from the periosteal insertions in the form of a flat exostosis or a synostosis that occurs proximally along the interosseous membrane.[20]

The athlete's chief complaint is difficulty in performing movements that require pivoting or cutting, and there is a sense of spasm and instability at the

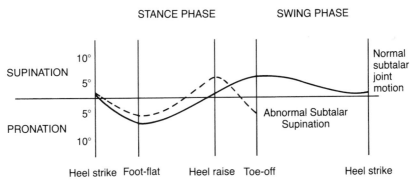

Figure 9–26. Graphic representation of subtalar joint motion in forefoot valgus or rigid plantar-flexed first ray.

ankle joint. This injury should be suspected whenever an athlete cannot recover from an "ankle sprain" and remains symptomatic longer than usual.

Conservative management includes treatment of the initial injury with ice, compression, and rest. Rehabilitation is aimed at restoring normal joint stability. If there are continued complaints of pain and instability, a surgical synovectomy is indicated, when the bone is mature, to reduce risk of recurrence.

ACHILLES TENDON RUPTURE

The Achilles tendon complex is prone to injury if there is a sudden and powerful eccentric contraction of the gastrocnemius-soleus muscles (considered together as the triceps surae). This mechanism is best demonstrated during jumping and landing activities, in which the knee is extending while the ankle is dorsiflexing eccentrically. The tendon usually ruptures at a point just proximal to the calcaneus (Fig. 9–27). Vascular impairment, nonspecific degeneration leading to tissue necrosis, and use of injectable corticosteroids may weaken this area and predispose it to injury.

The athlete reports an audible snap and the sensation of being kicked in the leg. Immediate plantar flexion weakness and pain, swelling, and a palpable defect are usually present. The diagnosis is confirmed with a positive Thompson test, in which the athlete is prone, with the knee flexed and the foot relaxed. A firm squeeze to the calf should produce calcaneal plantar flexion. The test is positive when there is no movement of the foot.

Acute care consists of ice application, with the ankle immobilized in slight

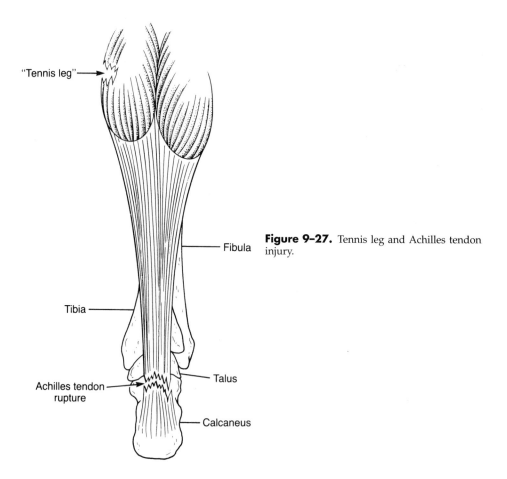

Figure 9–27. Tennis leg and Achilles tendon injury.

"Tennis leg"

Fibula

Tibia

Talus

Achilles tendon rupture

Calcaneus

plantar flexion. A non–weight-bearing crutch gait should be used until the severity of injury has been determined. Table 9–7 provides a treatment rationale for lesions of the triceps surae mechanism. Postsurgical or closed, nonsurgical care of complete ruptures traditionally required 4 to 8 weeks of cast immobilization. However, recent trends have shown that protected (early and controlled) motion and functional orthoses are as safe and effective as less aggressive and more strict immobilization methods.[8] Protected-arc, active plantar flexion range-of-motion activities may be started as early as 2 to 4 weeks postinjury. This allows collagen fibers to be laid down along the line of stress. A 1-inch heel lift is used when weight bearing is allowed and the height of the lift gradually decreased as the dorsiflexion range of motion improves. Surgical versus nonsurgical management decisions are based on the site and thickness of the tear in conjunction with the goals and ambitions of the patient. Both methods of management have shown acceptable results.[9]

TENNIS LEG

Previously thought to be a tear of the plantaris muscle, "tennis leg" has now been proved through surgical exploration to be a musculotendinous lesion of the medial gastrocnemius head (see Fig. 9–27).[33] The usual mechanism of injury is sudden extension of the knee with the foot in a dorsiflexed position. This places a tremendous tensile stress on the two-joint expansion of the gastrocnemius. Middle-aged athletes or those with previous degenerative changes in this anatomic area may be predisposed to this type of trauma.

The athlete feels a sudden, sharp twinge in the upper medial calf and immediately has difficulty in full weight bearing. Typically, there is rapid swelling and ecchymosis, with point tenderness or a palpable defect at the site of the lesion.

Acute care consists of immediate first-aid measures, including ice, compression, and elevation to the injured area. The ankle is placed in mild plantar flexion to alleviate stress on the area of injury. A non–weight-bearing crutch gait may be necessary, depending on the severity of the injury.

Gradual, gentle static stretching is initiated early in the subacute phase to align the healing scar tissue. Friction massage to the area also prevents random alignment of collagen fibers. As the athlete progresses to full weight bearing, heel lifts can be used in the shoe to protect against weight-bearing stresses. As Achilles tendon flexibility improves, the height of the lifts can be gradually reduced. Table 9–7 presents further details about the rehabilitation progression of Achilles tendon–related pathology.

TENDINOPATHIES

Tendinous lesions of the muscles of the lower leg frequently occur in athletes involved in activities of a repetitious nature. Microtraumatic damage caused by overuse, fatigue, or biomechanical abnormalities may be manifested by an inflammatory reaction of these tendons.

Achilles Tendinitis

The Achilles tendon is the common tendon of the gastrocnemius and soleus muscles. It inserts into the posterosuperior aspect of the calcaneus and is a frequent site of pathology in competitive and recreational athletes.[10, 24] It is surrounded by the paratenon, which functions as an elastic sleeve that envelops the tendon and allows free movement against surrounding tissues. In areas in which the tendon passes over zones of potential pressure and friction, the paratenon is replaced by a synovial sheath or bursa.[11]

The major blood supply to the Achilles tendon is provided through the paratenon. An area of reduced vascularity is found 2 to 6 cm proximal to the

Table 9–7. Gastrocnemius-Soleus Rehabilitation and Treatment

PARAMETER	IMMEDIATE (ACUTE PHASE)	INTERMEDIATE (SUBACUTE PHASE)	TERMINAL (CHRONIC PHASE)	RETURN TO ACTIVITY (FUNCTIONAL PHASE)
Goal	Rest Control inflammation and pain Promote healing Create "flexible" scar	Increase pain-free ROM Restore contractile capability	Increase musculotendinous tensile strength Modify, correct, or control abnormal biomechanics	Prepare and train for specific sport or activity
Modalities	Ice massage NSAIDs Gentle transverse friction massage to prevent adhesion formation HVGS in shortened position	Heat prior to rehabilitation Ice post rehabilitation Ultrasonography (pulsed vs continuous) Myofascial–soft-tissue mobilization techniques	Heat prior to rehabilitation Ice postrehabilitation Iontophoresis/phonophoresis Deep transverse friction massage to improve gliding between tissue planes	Modality sequence: 1. passive-active tissue and systemic warm-up 2. static stretching 3. activity or exercise 4. stretch again—mildly ballistic motion 5. cooldown 6. cryotherapy
ROM/flexibility	Immobilization or pain-free ROM dependent upon type and severity of pathology	Temperature-assisted, prolonged-duration, low-intensity, static stretching of antagonist Non-weight-bearing knee bent and straight towel stretches	Low-intensity, static stretching of involved musculotendinous unit Weight-bearing knee bent or straight wall leans Slant board stretching	Assess capability, tolerance, and response to ballistic motion of involved tissue
Exercise rationale	Isometrics progressing from submaximal to maximal intensity in protected ROM (knee flexed or ankle in plantar flexion). These exercises may have to be delayed 2–6 weeks in the case of surgically repaired ruptures.	Non-weight bearing submaximal to maximal effort isokinetics in progressively larger arcs of motion; concentric contractions at highest attainable speeds in a velocity spectrum to minimize tensile stress in this early phase	Weight-bearing concentric and eccentric isotonic exercise at increasing speeds of contraction as tolerated by tissue symptomatic response	Functional rehabilitation activities—toe walking Plyometric progressions—hopping, bounding, depth jumps, and box drills Sport-specific training

Proprioceptive rehabilitation	BAPS board training in non–weight-bearing positions if not immobilized	BAPS board training in partial to full weight-bearing position with increasing levels of ROM difficulty	BAPS board training in full weight-bearing position with posterior peg overload	Balance board training
Alternative conditioning	UBE	Gravity-reduced running with assistance of unloading device or flotation device in water	Gravity-reduced running; stationary cycling	Stairclimbers Stationary cross-country skier
Complementary exercise	Hip-knee-trunk strengthening and conditioning activities	Dorsiflexion, inversion, and eversion strengthening Exercise of foot intrinsic musculature	Lower extremity stretching and continuation of activities from previous phase	Ensure normal plantar-to-dorsiflexion strength ratios and muscle balance 3–4:1 ratio at slow speeds of contraction
Activity education modification	Controlled immobilization and rest prn Examine athletic shoes, training surface, and training regimens	Trial of low-amplitude rebounder running	Flat training surfaces only; avoid hilly and cambered terrain or muddy surfaces	Careful increases in training regimens; limit increase in program by more than 5%/week in intensity, duration, or frequency
Orthotic care	Crutches as necessary; weight-bearing status dictated by severity of pathology	Viscoelastic heel lift inserts to reduce stress on Achilles tendon and decrease ground reaction forces	Custom orthotic insert to control excessive or abnormal compensatory subtalar joint motion	Orthotic or taping techniques

BAPS, Biomechanical Ankle Platform System; HVGS, high-voltage galvanic stimulation; NSAIDs, nonsteroidal anti–inflammatory drugs; ROM, range of motion; UBE, upper body ergometer.

insertion.[41] This region of relative avascularity may play an etiologic role in the frequent onset of symptoms at this level.[41]

Although an Achilles tendon overuse injury is a common problem, the nomenclature used to identify this injury is often confusing. Classification is based on whether the Achilles tendon itself or the peritendinous tissue that surrounds it is involved. Achilles tendinitis is defined as disruptive lesions within the substance of the tendon itself, whereas peritendinitis involves inflammation in the paratenon.[11] These conditions could occur simultaneously or in isolation.

The onset of Achilles tendinitis or peritendinitis is usually gradual and insidious, although some precipitating factor may be identified. The athlete complains of a dull, aching pain during or after activity. On physical examination, slight edema or tendon thickening may be present. Point tenderness is usually elicited 2 to 3 cm proximal to the calcaneal attachment. Because this is a contractile lesion, pain usually increases with passive dorsiflexion and resisted plantar flexion.[13] Crepitation may be noted in plantar flexion movements in the subacute and chronic stages.[26]

Table 9–8 presents a suggested rationale for the conservative management and treatment of tendinitis and peritendinitis. The four stages of injury define potential entry points into the treatment system. An athlete could initially be seen at any one of these stages. Progression from one stage to the next is variable and is dictated by time, symptoms, and athlete response.

As is usually true, the best treatment for microtraumatic injuries such as Achilles tendinitis is prevention of onset. The frequency or severity of inflammatory Achilles injuries may be reduced if some suggested guidelines are followed:

1. Select appropriate footwear. The athletic shoe should have a firm, notched heel counter to decrease tendon irritation and control rearfoot motion. The midsole should have a moderate heel flare, provide adequate wedging, and allow flexibility in the forefoot. It is also important to maintain a relatively consistent heel height in all shoes worn during the day.

2. Avoid training errors. Achilles tendon microtrauma can be induced extrinsically because of training errors. Steady, gradual increases of no more than 5% to 10% per week in training mileage and speed on appropriate terrain should be emphasized. Use of cross-training principles may also reduce cumulative stresses on the Achilles tendon.

3. Ensure gastrocnemius-soleus flexibility. The talocrural joint should have 10° of dorsiflexion with the knee joint extended and 20° with the knee flexed. Normal gait requires 10° of dorsiflexion just prior to heel-off, during which the subtalar joint is in neutral position and the knee is extending in stance phase.[4]

4. Control pronation forces. Abnormal compensatory pronation forces can cause a whipping or bowstring effect on the medial edge of the Achilles tendon. Orthotic correction may be indicated if this abnormal pronation is of structural origin.[11]

5. Ensure adequate strength. The triceps surae musculotendinous unit must have adequate concentric and eccentric contractile capabilities. This includes dynamic symmetry in bilateral comparisons and

appropriate balance with its ipsilateral antagonist. A plantar flexion–to-dorsiflexion ratio of 3:1 or 4:1 has been suggested for slow isokinetic speeds of contraction.[16]

6. Perform postural screening for biomechanical malalignments. This may detect any abnormalities that could adversely affect the kinetic chain and increase stress on the Achilles tendon. Such conditions include leg length discrepancies, cavus foot resulting from metatarsal forefoot equinus, ankle equinus, tibial varum, and rotational influences of the femur or tibia.[4]

Anterior Tibialis Tendinitis

An inflammatory response of the anterior tibialis tendon occurs when it cannot absorb deceleration forces in the heel-strike phase to the foot-flat phase of gait. Uncontrolled or excessive pronation following heel strike stretches the anterior tibialis as it attempts to control the speed of forefoot loading.

Conditions that predispose the anterior tibialis to overuse usually include training errors and physical abnormalities. Frequently, the combination of excessive extrinsic forces placed on intrinsic abnormalities produces stresses that cannot be dissipated or tolerated by the athlete. Extrinsic factors include dramatic increases in mileage, overstriding, and excessive hill running, all of which can cause fatigue and injury. The athlete with a tight Achilles complex requires increased muscular output of the anterior tibialis to overcome the inherent posterior tautness. This condition is then magnified with uphill running, which necessitates full dorsiflexion range of motion. In downhill running, increased eccentric forces are necessary to control forefoot loading over an increased range of motion. If the anterior tibialis has undergone adaptive shortening in response to chronic hyperpronation, the musculotendinous unit cannot provide the necessary range of motion and absorption of tensile forces needed during the early stance phase.

This injury is characterized by pain and swelling over the dorsum of the foot. There may be crepitation along the tendon or at its point of insertion onto the navicular. Examination reveals pain with stretching into the extremes of plantar flexion and pronation and pain-inhibited weakness with manual muscle testing of anterior tibialis function.

Table 9–8 summarizes the treatment rationale for lower leg tendinopathies. Prime consideration should be given to correcting soft-tissue imbalances, improving eccentric muscular capabilities, and selecting appropriate footwear. Shoe selection should focus on midsole materials that attenuate shock and accommodate orthotic additions. A heel lift may be used for the athlete with structural equinus, or varus posting may be indicated if a forefoot varus or supinatus is prolonging the pronation process.

Peroneal Tendinitis

Inflammatory lesions of the peroneal muscle tendons or of their protective sheaths are common in athletes who, for compensatory reasons, overuse this musculature. The pathology is seen secondary to chronic lateral ankle sprains or in athletes with hypermobile first rays. In both situations, the peroneal muscle tendons are worked excessively in an attempt to provide stability. Any mechanical stress caused by abnormal forefoot structures that force the foot into a valgus position can also amplify this inflammatory response.

Pain and swelling typically occur in the area just posterior to the lateral malleolus. Occasionally, symptoms are manifested at the musculotendinous

Table 9–8. Lower Leg Tendinopathy Rehabilitation and Treatment

PARAMETER	IMMEDIATE (ACUTE PHASE)	INTERMEDIATE (SUBACUTE PHASE)	TERMINAL (CHRONIC PHASE)	RETURN TO ACTIVITY (FUNCTIONAL PHASE)
Goal	Rest Control inflammation and pain Promote healing Create "flexible" scar	Rehabilitation of musculotendinous unit Increase ROM Increase muscle contractile capability	Increase musculotendinous tensile strength Modify, correct, or control abnormal biomechanics	Prepare and train for specific sport or activity
Modalities	Ice massage NSAIDs Gentle transverse friction massage to prevent adhesion formation	Heat prior to rehabilitation Ice postrehabilitation Ultrasound (pulsed vs continuous) Myofascial–soft-tissue mobilization techniques	Heat prior to rehabilitation Ice postrehabilitation Iontophoresis/phonophoresis Deep transverse friction massage to improve gliding between tissue planes	Modality sequence: 1. passive-active tissue and systemic warm-up 2. static stretching 3. activity or exercise 4. stretch again—mildly ballistic motion 5. cooldown 6. cryotherapy
ROM/flexibility	Pain-free ROM exercises	Temperature-assisted, prolonged-duration, low-intensity, static stretching of antagonist	Low-intensity, static stretching of involved musculotendinous unit	Assess capability, tolerance, and response to ballistic motion of involved tissue
Exercise rationale	Isometrics	Submaximal to maximal effort isokinetics in progressively larger arcs of motion; concentric contractions at highest attainable speeds in a velocity spectrum to minimize tensile stress in this early phase	Eccentric exercise at increasing speeds of contraction as tolerated by tissue symptomatic response	Functional rehabilitation activities and plyometric progressions Sport-specific training

Proprioceptive rehabilitation	BAPS board training in non–weight-bearing positions	BAPS board training in partial to full weight-bearing position with increasing levels of ROM difficulty	BAPS board training in full weight-bearing position with resistance overload to appropriate muscle groups	Balance board training
Alternative conditioning	UBE	Gravity-reduced running with assistance of unloading device or flotation device in water	Gravity-reduced running; stationary cycling	Stairclimbers Stationary cross-country skier
Complementary exercise	Hip-knee-trunk strengthening and conditioning activities	Exercise of foot intrinsic musculature	Lower extremity stretching and continuance of activities from previous phase	Ensure normal agonist-to-antagonist strength ratios and muscle balance
Activity education modification	Controlled immobilization and rest prn Examine athletic shoes, training surface, and training regimens	Trial of low-amplitude rebounder running	Flat training surfaces only; avoid hilly and cambered terrain or muddy surfaces	Careful increases in training regimens; limit increase in program by more than 5%/week in intensity, duration, or frequency
Orthotic care	Heel lift if appropriate	Viscoelastic inserts to decrease ground reaction forces (especially in rigid cavus feet)	Custom orthotic insert to control excessive or abnormal compensatory subtalar joint motion	Orthotic or taping techniques

BAPS, Biomechanical Ankle Platform System; NSAIDs, nonsteroidal anti-inflammatory drugs; ROM, range of motion; UBE, upper body ergometer.

junction.[13] Tendon crepitus may be present in more chronic conditions. Pain and weakness are evident with passive overstretching of these contractile structures and when resistance is provided to plantar flexion and eversion of the first ray. Compared with peroneal longus tendinitis, peroneal brevis tendinitis is more affected by resistance to calcaneal eversion and ankle plantar flexion. The differential diagnosis must be made among peroneal subluxation, inversion ankle sprain, sural nerve entrapment, and subacute lateral compartmental syndrome, because subsequent management differs for each of these conditions.

Rehabilitation is aimed at providing symptomatic relief and identifying the causative factors. Muscular imbalances between the anterior or posterior tibialis and peroneals should be explored. Orthotic relief of structural abnormalities can be provided by a metatarsal pad with a first ray cutout. Transverse friction massage can be used to reduce symptoms and promote healing.[13] Table 9–8 presents further treatment considerations.

Posterior Tibialis Tendinitis

Posteromedial shin pain secondary to athletic overuse can indicate inflammatory microtrauma to the tendon of the posterior tibialis. Periosteal irritation and tibial stress reactions may also be suspected.

Medial tibial stress, whether tendinitis or periostitis, is generally the result of abnormal hyperpronation biomechanics (Fig. 9–28). The muscles in the superficial posterior compartment contract in a stretched position and are overworked in an attempt to stabilize the foot during propulsion. Common predisposing factors include improper training on crowned or banked surfaces, inappropriate footwear, and any structural condition that increases the varus attitude of the lower extremity.

Pain and swelling are present over the posteromedial crest of the tibia along the origin of the posterior tibialis. Tenderness and crepitation may be found anywhere along the course of the tendon as it passes behind the medial malleolus and inserts distally on the navicular and first cuneiform. Manual resistance to plantar flexion and inversion localizes the complaint. In subacute phases, repeated unilateral heel raises, which require plantar flexion and supination of the calcaneus, can be a source of symptom aggravation.

Differential diagnosis is important to rule out a tibial stress reaction, in which there is pain at the junction of the lower and middle thirds of the posteromedial tibia. Tibial stress fractures can occur in this area if the bony osteoblastic activity cannot keep pace with the osteoclastic stress placed on it. At approximately 2 weeks postsymptom awareness, a fracture through the tibial cortex may become evident on radiographs. Prior to this finding, a bone scan reveals increased calcium uptake in the area of injury. Clinical differentiation is accomplished by detection of tenderness in areas devoid of muscle on the tibial shaft or with percussion and tuning fork vibration techniques.

Treatment is aimed at alleviating abnormal pronation using a semirigid orthosis with a medial heel wedge. Attention should also be given to the training regimen and to finding shoes with a stable, firm, and snug heel counter.

Flexor Hallucis Longus Tendinitis

The athlete who must perform repetitive push-off maneuvers is especially prone to developing tendinitis in the long flexor of the great toe. Hyperpronation during propulsion also places excessive stress on the tendon as it contracts from a lengthened position. This condition is similar to posterior tibial tendinitis and can be differentiated through selected manual muscle testing. Pain with passive extension of the first MTP joint while the ankle is dorsiflexed confirms the diagnosis. The condition is managed with appropriate varus posting and tape restriction for excessive dorsiflexion of the first MTP joint.

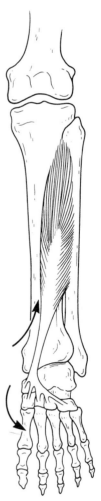

Figure 9–28. Etiology of posterior tibialis tendinitis: excessive traction stress placed on the posterior tibialis tendon with hyperpronation.

Flexor Digitorum Longus Tendinitis

The flexor digitorum longus is another musculotendinous unit in the superficial posterior compartment that is susceptible to overuse microtrauma. Pain is usually present in the posteromedial third of the leg as a result of overuse from forced, resistive dorsiflexion of the toes during propulsion.[21] The resultant cramping sensation in the forefoot and toes can be relieved with a viscoelastic metatarsal pad, which dorsally displaces the metatarsal heads and reduces the extension angle of the lesser four MTP joints. A more rigid sole in the athletic shoe may also help prevent excessive forced hyperextension of the digits in propulsion. Exercise rehabilitation focuses on correcting any intrinsic muscular imbalances that allow toe-clawing deformities and that require the flexor digitorum longus to work harder.[21] The intrinsic muscles of the foot can be isolated for emphasis during toe-curling exercises. This is accomplished by contracting the extensor hallucis longus to inhibit the long toe flexor's ability to contract (Fig. 9–29).

COMPARTMENTAL COMPRESSION SYNDROMES

There are four osseofascial compartments in the lower leg—the anterior, lateral, superficial posterior, and deep posterior compartments. The anterior com-

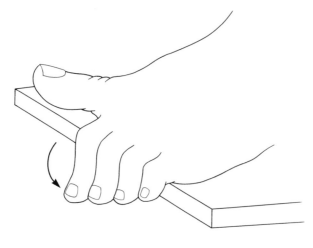

Figure 9–29. Isolation of intrinsic toe flexors to inhibit long toe flexor contribution.

partment is the most common site for compression ischemia. It is bordered by the interosseous membrane posteriorly, the tibia and fibula medially and laterally, and a tough, nonexpansive fascial covering anteriorly. If pressure increases within the compartment there is no space for expansion or accommodation. With increasing pressure, circulation and tissue function can be quickly compromised. There are two types of anterior compartmental compression syndrome: acute and recurrent.

Acute Anterior Compartmental Compression Syndrome

This condition is usually traumatic in onset. Contusions, crush injuries, fractures, or severe overexertion can cause a rapid increase in compartmental volume from bleeding or muscular swelling. Increased intercompartmental pressure leads to venous collapse and increased resistance to arterial circulation. These physiologic changes produce an ischemic pain and, ultimately, tissue necrosis if the process is left uninterrupted.

The athlete's chief complaint is intense pain that is disproportionate to the injury and not relieved by rest. Palpation reveals a "woody tension" over the muscles of the anterior compartment, and passive plantar flexion evokes pain. In the advanced stages, neurologic changes may be evident, and the dorsalis pedis and anterior tibial pulses may be diminished. Table 9–9 presents the neurologic changes manifested in the later stages of lower leg compartmental syndrome.

This condition is considered a medical emergency, because early muscle damage occurs in the first 4 to 6 hours, and irreversible tissue damage occurs within 18 hours after injury. Acute care consists of ice application without compression and monitoring of the neurovascular status. If pain and swelling do not respond to conservative treatment, an emergency surgical fasciotomy must be performed.

Table 9–9. Late Neurologic Changes in Compression Syndromes

COMPARTMENT	AREA OF PARESTHESIA	AREA OF WEAKNESS
Anterior	First dorsal web space	Dorsiflexion (drop foot)
Lateral	Anterior lateral leg	Eversion (peroneals)
Deep posterior	Medial arch	Inversion
Superficial posterior	Sural nerve distribution	Plantar flexion

Recurrent Compartmental Syndrome

Chronic, exertional compartmental syndrome has the same pathophysiology as acute compartmental syndrome, but its presentation and care are different (Table 9–10). The athlete complains of lower leg pain and tightness that occur at a constant interval after the initiation of physical activity. The symptoms subside with rest but return on resumption of the activity. Most patients have bilateral involvement with mild edema, tenderness, and occasional paresthesia. The diagnosis is confirmed with wick catheter measurement of intercompartmental pressure at rest and during activity.

Conservative management includes ice application before and after exercise, lower leg stretching, and balancing plantar flexion–dorsiflexion strength. Any alterations in the training program that decrease muscular workloads may also be helpful. Bevel-heeled shoes, softer training surfaces, and energy-absorbing orthoses may accomplish this goal. If conservative measures fail, a surgical fasciotomy is indicated. Postoperative rehabilitation consists of gentle stretching and stationary cycling beginning 7 to 10 days postsurgery, with expected return to activity after 2 to 3 months.

Ankle Injuries

Pathologic trauma to the ligamentous structures of the ankle is a common athletic injury. The majority of these injuries occur to the lateral side of the joint with an inversion component of motion. In the neutral position of 0° dorsiflexion, the calcaneofibular ligament is taut, but as the foot plantar flexes, the anterior talofibular ligament tightens as its fibers become parallel to the axis. Eighty percent to 90% of ankle sprains occur as the result of this plantar flexion–inversion mechanism. Initial damage is to the anterior talofibular ligament because of the direction of force, and further stress affects the calcaneofibular and posterior talofibular ligaments. The posterior talofibular ligament is not involved or injured until the other two ligaments have ruptured and some degree of lower extremity rotation has occurred. Injuries to the medial side of the joint and the deltoid ligament are less frequent and typically involve a hyperpronation force, such as when an athlete plants the foot and then cuts in the opposite direction. Table 9–11 outlines the common mechanisms of injury for bony and ligamentous structures of the ankle.

INVERSION SPRAINS

The signs and symptoms of ankle ligamentous injuries vary according to the severity of injury, the tissues involved, and the extent of their involvement. Varying degrees of pain, swelling, point tenderness, and functional disability are usually evident. Following inversion trauma, radiographic studies of the joint and bone structure are of paramount importance. Bony lesions must be ruled out before decisions about appropriate management of the injury can be made. Unstable bimalleolar fractures, proximal fibular fractures, and avulsion-type fractures all are possible and may require surgical fixation or longer periods of immobilization.

Table 9–10. Symptom Presentation of Acute versus Recurrent Compartmental Syndromes

	RECURRENT	ACUTE
Pathology	Reversible changes	Irreversible tissue damage possible
Effect of rest	Symptoms decrease	No change in symptoms
Nature of complaint	Cramping, aching	Intense pain
Involvement	Often bilateral	Usually unilateral

Table 9–11. Mechanism of Ankle Injuries

MECHANISM OF INJURY	COMMENTS	LIGAMENTOUS INJURY (PROGRESSION OF INCREASING SEVERITY OF PATHOLOGY)	POTENTIAL BONY LESIONS
Plantar flexion–inversion	Typical ankle sprain	ATF→ATF and CF→ATF, CF, and PTF	Transverse fracture of lateral malleolus; Avulsion fracture of base of fifth metatarsal
Supinated position–adduction force			Medial malleolus fracture
Plantar flexion–inversion and rotation	Crossover cut on a plantar flexed and inverted foot	ATF and tibfib→ATF, tibfib, and CF	
Supinated position–eversion force			Spiral fracture of lateral malleolus or fracture of neck of fibula
Pure inversion	Rare; landing on another's foot	CF→CF and ATF→CF, ATF, and PTF	
Pronation: Abduction-eversion-dorsiflexion	Open cut	Deltoid→deltoid, tibfib, and interosseus membrane	Avulsion fracture of medial malleolus
Pronated position–eversion force			Fibular fracture above the mortice line

ATF, Anterior talofibular ligament; CF, calcaneofibular ligament; PTF, posterior talofibular ligament; tibfib, anterior and posterior tibiofibular ligaments.

Table 9–12 outlines some criteria for assessing the severity of injury in lateral ankle sprains. This grading process provides a basis for logically estimating the rate and intensity at which the athlete can progress through the phases of treatment and rehabilitation, as well as for estimating the length of time before the athlete can return to full participation.

Treatment and Rehabilitation

The functional or chronic disability associated with ankle sprains can be the result of various abnormalities. These include anterior, posterior, or varus instability of the talus in the ankle mortice, instability of or adhesion formation in the subtalar joint, inferior tibiofibular diastasis, peroneal muscle weakness, and motor incoordination secondary to articular deafferentation.[5, 16, 19, 22, 27, 36]

Each potential problem must be addressed in the treatment and rehabilitation program. The damaged ligaments must be allowed to heal as a "flexible" restraint, the contractile elements must regain dynamic stabilization capabilities, and the proprioceptive system must be completely restored. Table 9–13 suggests a treatment plan for the conservative management of inversion ankle sprains. Each athlete's injury is unique, and progression through the various stages of rehabilitation may have to be altered, depending on the severity of tissue trauma, history, and goals of rehabilitation. Figures 9–30 to 9–42 illustrate some of the rehabilitation procedures used in the restoration of normal ankle joint function after ligamentous injury.

The goal of management is to provide dynamic stability to a potentially unstable joint. During the acute immobilization phase, emphasis is placed on controlling symptoms and on maintaining general conditioning and neuromuscular continuity. Various modalities are used to minimize effusion and decrease pain. Edema within the ankle joint distorts the capsule's normal configuration and adversely affects mechanoreceptor function. Ice, focal compression around the periphery of the fibular malleolus, electrotherapy, and gentle effleurage with the ankle elevated all facilitate anesthesia and reduction of edema and reverse

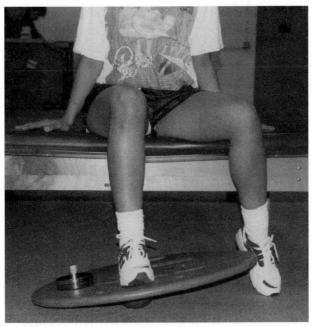

Figure 9–30. Biomechanical Ankle Platform System (BAPS): BAPS board with posterolateral overload.

Table 9–12. Signs and Symptoms of Lateral Ankle Sprains

GRADE	SEVERITY	INVOLVEMENT	FUNCTIONAL STATUS	SWELLING	PAIN/TENDERNESS	LIGAMENT LAXITY
I	Mild	Usually only ATF	Maintenance of joint integrity produces minimal functional disability	Variable, but usually slight	Mild, localized pain over ATF	Negative anterior drawer and talar tilt
II	Moderate	ATF and CF	Moderate disability, with difficulty in heel and toe walking	Variable, but more than in grade I, and resultant ecchymosis	Moderate pain and tenderness over involved ligaments	Laxity evident but distinct end points to stress
III	Severe	ATF and CF; possibly PTF	Functional disability, with loss of ROM and complete inability to bear weight	Anterolateral and spreading diffusely around the joint	Marked tenderness to palpation	Positive anterior drawer or talar tilt

ATF, Anterior talofibular ligament; CF, calcaneofibular ligament; PTF, posterior talofibular ligament; ROM, range of motion.

the neural inhibition of the dynamic stabilizers surrounding the joint. Support to the injured ligaments is provided by a neutral orthosis, Gibney's strapping (open basket-weave taping with a horseshoe pad to compress extracellular fluids back into circulation), and a posterior splint to maintain Achilles tendon flexibility. Because strict immobilization is no longer recommended, cautious and gentle motion in protected arcs can be initiated through Biomechanical Ankle Platform System* (BAPS) board activity (see Fig. 9–30).

Early mobilization allows earlier return to function without increase in pain, residual symptoms, or rate of reinjury.[17] Isometric exercises are also started during this phase to minimize or retard atrophy.

The weight-bearing status of the athlete is allowed to progress as symptoms and healing allow. Emphasis should be placed on maintaining a normal heel-to-toe gait and on keeping weight-bearing forces to below the pain symptom level. Early, pain-free weight bearing will maintain proprioceptive input, prevent stiffness, and provide a means for an active muscle pump to mobilize effusion.

In the intermediate or postimmobilization phase, attention is focused on the healing ligaments. Subpathologic stress through joint mobilization is placed on the injured ligaments to stimulate organized collagen formation along the direction of normal fibers. Care must be taken not to place traction forces on the joint with ankle-weight resistance on the foot. Closed-chain rehabilitation in a weight-bearing position is preferred because it can provide compressive forces that augment stability.

Weight bearing should progress in this stage to full weight bearing without ambulation assistance. The use of stirrup-type splints with heel-lock protection to limit excessive calcaneal inversion is indicated. Exercise rehabilitation may include Achilles tendon stretching; open-chain, cryotherapy-assisted active range of motion progressing toward submaximal effort isokinetics in limited arcs; and closed-chain functional activities such as soleus pumps, stork stands, stationary cycling, and body-weight transfers over stable or unstable surfaces (Figs. 9–31 to 9–34).

In the terminal phase of rehabilitation, progressive closed-chain activities with emphasis on restoring kinesthetic awareness and proximal hip strength are given

---

*Available from Camp International, Jackson, Michigan

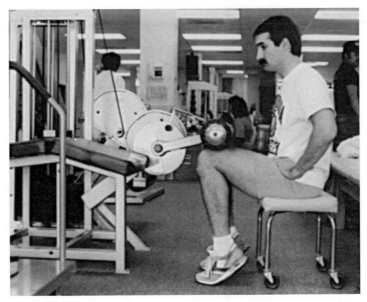

Figure 9–31. Soleus pumps.

Table 9–13. Conservative Management of Ankle Sprains

PHASE	IMMEDIATE (ACUTE)	INTERMEDIATE (SUBACUTE) (POSTIMMOBILIZATION)	TERMINAL (CHRONIC)	RETURN TO ACTIVITY (FUNCTIONAL)
Goals	Protect joint integrity Control inflammatory response Control pain, edema, and spasm	Optimal stimulation for tissue regeneration	Functional progression of CKC activities Proprioceptive retraining Correct/control biomechanics	Preparation for return to sport or activity
Weight-bearing status	Non–to touch-down weight-bearing	Crutch partial weight bearing progressing toward full weight bearing	Full weight bearing	Full weight bearing
Modalities	Ice Intermittent/constant compression Elevation TENS or HVGS Effleurage in elevated position	Cryotherapy (ice-ROM-ice) Contrast baths Friction massage at site of lesion	Cryokinetics (Ice-CKC activities-ice)	Ice postparticipation
External support	Neutral orthosis Gibney open basket-weave taping Posterior splint	Stirrup splint with heel-lock support	Stirrup splint with heel-lock support	Taping Aircast or lace-up Active ankle orthosis Orthosis
ROM/flexibility		Grade I or II joint mobilizations Achilles stretching in sitting and standing positions	Achilles stretching in supinated positions	

Open kinetic chain exercise	Isometrics	Alphabet ROM Toe curls and marble pickups Four-plane surgical tubing exercises Submaximal isokinetics in short arcs		Full-arc isokinetics
Closed kinetic chain exercise		CKC ROM trunk twists and squats Shuttle squats/heel raises/toe raises Soleus pumps Tubing lunge steps, TKEs, SKFI	Heel-raise progression Shuttle hops and bounds	Marching, running, sidesteps, backpedaling, cariocas, etc. Plyometric drills
Proprioception/agility/balance drills		BAPS in non- or partial weight-bearing position overload Stork stands Single plane tilt boards	BAPS in full weight bearing c/s overload Profitter or slide board Multiaxial tilt or balance boards Tubing walkaways/runaways Tubing contrakicks	Jump rope/jump platform Four-square hopping drills Functional running patterns Running in place tubing drills
Complementary alternative exercises	Gluteus medius strengthening	Pool therapy Stationary cycling	Rebounder minitrampoline drills Treadmill Stairmaster	Stationary cross-country skiing Lateral step-ups

BAPS, Biomechanical Ankle Platform System; CKC, closed kinetic chain; HVGS, high-voltage galvanic stimulation; ROM, range of motion; SKFI, single knee flexion initiation; TENS, transcutaneous electrical nerve stimulation; TKE, terminal knee extension.

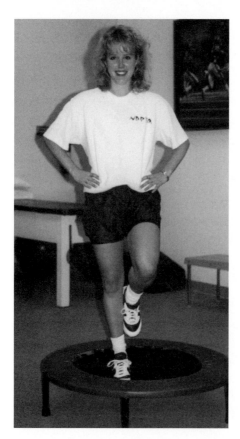

Figure 9–32. Stork stands.

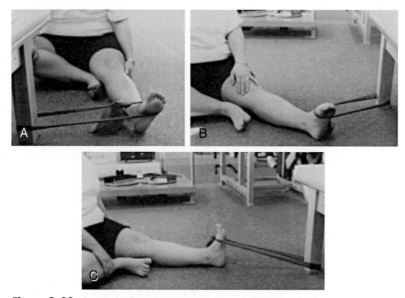

Figure 9–33. Surgical tubing resisted exercises. *A*, Eversion. *B*, Inversion. *C*, Dorsi-flexion.

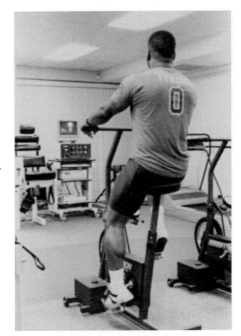

Figure 9–34. Ankle rehabilitation on stationary bike.

priority. Bullock-Saxton[6] showed that hip muscle function is compromised with severe ankle sprains. Gluteus maximus muscle recruitment may be delayed during hip extension in gait, and gluteus medius weakness may increase frontal plane inversion stress on the ankle secondary to a Trendelenburg gait. Tubing-resisted sidesteps are an excellent exercise to redevelop this strength deficit (Fig. 9–35). Physical agents at this point are used only as needed, but after rehabilitation, ice is usually necessary. Exercise rehabilitation becomes aggressive and

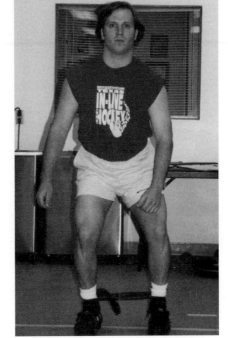

Figure 9–35. Tubing-resisted side steps.

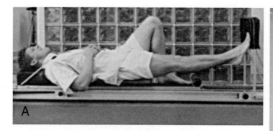

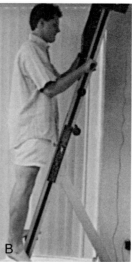

Figure 9–36. Closed-chain plantar flexion strengthening. *A,* Supine with gravity eliminated on Shuttle 2000. *B,* Standing on Versa-Climber.

includes slant board Achilles tendon stretching without allowing subtalar joint substitution, full-arc isokinetics, and heel-raise progression (Fig. 9–36). Balance and motor coordination are enhanced by the use of a ProFitter,* balance board, and rebounder minitrampoline (Figs. 9–37 to 9–39).

As the athlete prepares to return to high-level activities, a functional progression should be used to simulate those stresses, forces, and motions inherent to the activity that caused the original injury. Elastic tubing resistance to weight-bearing activities improves ankle strength and coordination and stimulates pro-

---

*Available from ProFitter, Calgary, Alberta, Canada

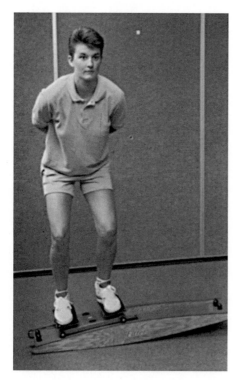

Figure 9–37. Ankle rehabilitation on ProFitter.

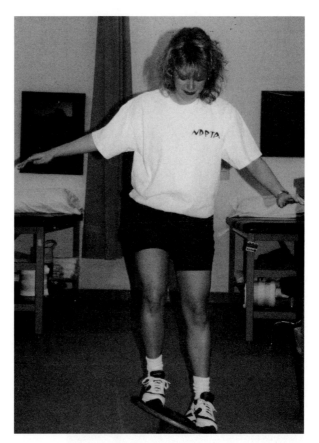

Figure 9–38. Balancing on multiaxial wobble board.

prioception for the entire lower extremity (Fig. 9–40). Progression from resistance in marching to running to motion on inclines can be employed (Fig. 9–41). Tubing resistance can come from all directions, and progression is based on pain-free exercise without effusion or tendency for the ankle to roll over.[36] Tape or external support should not be used during these controlled activities to allow full rehabilitative benefit. Clinical plyometrics on the Shuttle 2000 or with four-square hopping also represents an excellent means of re-creating athletic activity (Fig. 9–42). Finally, a functional movement progression that includes backpedaling, sidestepping, cariocas, pivoting, and cutting should be used in assessing readiness for return to athletic activities.

Orthotic and external support should be used to prevent recurrence of trauma. Athletes with an uncompensated rearfoot varus, compensated forefoot valgus, or rigidly plantar-flexed first ray alter their gait pattern with prolonged or excessive supination in midstance and are extremely susceptible to reinjury. Because it takes at least 20 weeks for a ligament to regain its normal histologic characteristics, ankle taping or ankle support should be provided for at least 5 to 6 months postinjury during participation in athletics.

SYNDESMOTIC ANKLE SPRAINS

The syndesmotic ankle sprain is often referred to as a "high" ankle sprain because of the anatomic location of the injury. Commonly, the athlete has tenderness and mild swelling over the anterior inferior tibiofibular ligament. The mechanism of injury is usually a combination of foot external rotation with lower leg internal rotation as pictured in Figure 9–43. External rotation stress to the foot and ankle with the knee held in 90° of flexion will reproduce pain over

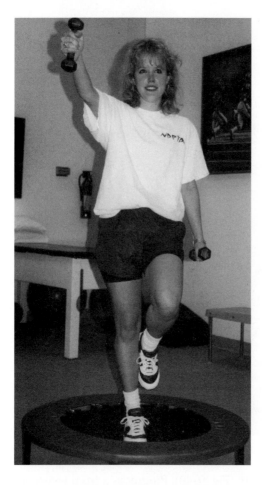

Figure 9–39. Balance training on mini-trampoline's unstable surface.

the ligament and syndesmosis. This type of injury is very slow to respond to conservative care. Boytin and colleagues[7] showed that players with syndesmotic ankle sprains missed significantly more games and required more treatment than did players who sustained lateral ankle sprains.

Postsurgical Management of Lateral Ankle Reconstructions

Sometimes surgical repair or reconstruction after lateral ligamentous injury is necessary to provide joint stability. Table 9–14 outlines common reconstructive

Table 9–14. Surgical Procedures for Lateral Ankle Instability

Nonanatomic reconstructions	
Watson-Jones procedure	Peroneus brevis tendon used to reconstruct the anterior talofibular ligament
Evans procedure	Peroneus brevis tendon rerouted to limit inversion at the ankle and subtalar joints
Chrisman-Snook procedure	Anterior talofibular and calcaneofibular ligaments reconstructed using half of the peroneus tendon
Anatomic repairs	
Modified Brostrom procedure	Direct repair of the anterior talofibular and calcaneofibular ligaments with reinforcement of the extensor retinaculum and lateral talocalcaneal ligament

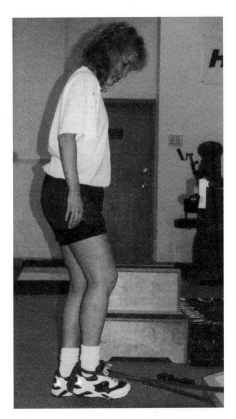

Figure 9–40. Contralateral kicks to simulate closed-chain pronation-supination.

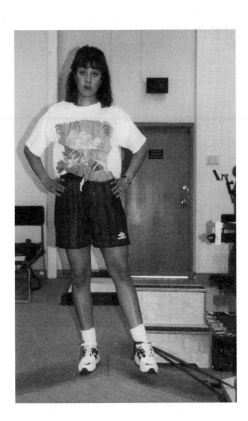

Figure 9–41. Proprioceptive training on inclined surface.

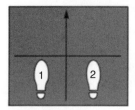

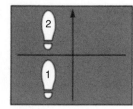

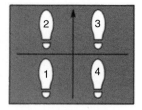

Side to side: Hop laterally between two quadrants.

Front to back: Hop forward and backward between two quadrants.

Four square: Hop from square to square in a circular pattern. Sets are performed clockwise and counterclockwise.

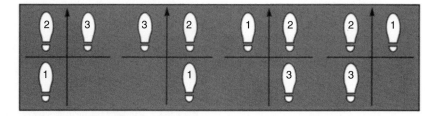

Triangles: Hop within three different quadrants. There are four triangles, each requiring a different diagonal hop.

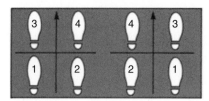

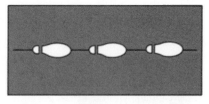

Crisscross: Hop in an X pattern.

Straight-line hop: Hop forward and then backward along a 15 to 20 ft. line.

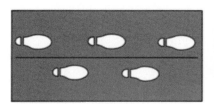

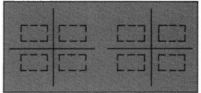

Line zigzag: Hop from side to side across a 15- to 20-ft. line while moving forward and then backward.

Disconnected squares: While performing the first five patterns, hop into squares marked in the quadrants.

Figure 9–42. Four-square hopping ankle rehabilitation. The eight basic hopping patterns in the four-square ankle rehabilitation program are arranged in order of increasing difficulty. The arrows denote the direction the athlete is facing. Number 1 is the starting point. (From Toomey, S.J. [1986]: Four-square ankle rehabilitation exercises. Physician Sportsmed., 14:281.)

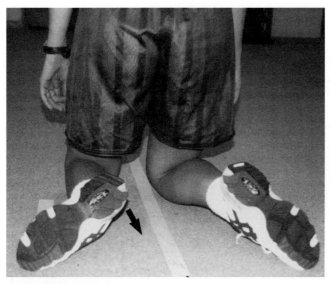

Figure 9–43. Mechanism of injury for syndesmotic ankle sprain.

or reparative surgical procedures used in the management of chronic lateral ankle instability. Recent research has indicated that direct anatomic repair procedures that reproduce anterior talofibular and calcaneofibular orientation are superior mechanical restraints to anterior talar displacement and tilt without compromising subtalar joint range of motion. The postoperative therapeutic management of these procedures involves principles similar to those used in the conservative care of grade III ankle injuries. Typically, a short-leg cast or brace is applied for 6 weeks with the ankle in 0° dorsiflexion and mild eversion. During the first 2 weeks the athlete uses a non–weight-bearing crutch gait. In the final 4 weeks of immobilization partial weight bearing on crutches is allowed. Strict immobilization is discontinued at 6 weeks, and active-assisted range-of-motion exercises in the sagittal plane are begun. At 8 weeks, active range-of-motion exercises for calcaneal inversion and eversion are begun, along with resistive exercises for the plantar flexors and dorsiflexors. When the athlete can walk without a detectable limp, functional rehabilitation progression may commence. Return to activity is expected after 4 to 6 months.

Rehabilitation of Postimmobilization Fractures

Rehabilitation following cast removal after ankle fractures is focused on restoring joint mobility. The immobilization time necessary for ensuring union of fractures causes capsular restrictions, muscular atrophy, and proprioceptive deficits. Emphasis is then placed on joint mobilization and on appropriate exercises to strengthen and mobilize the soft tissues. The mechanics of the fracture and its surgical fixation must be understood and appreciated to avoid excessive force or stress on the initial injury. Figures 9–44 to 9–53 demonstrate joint mobilization techniques that may be used carefully and rationally to restore accessory joint motion and normal joint arthrokinematics.

PERONEAL TENDON SUBLUXATION

The peroneal tendons lie in a deep groove posterior to the lateral malleolus. They are subject to subluxation out of this groove if the peroneal retinaculum is ruptured by sudden and violent dorsiflexion and eversion forces. This is com-

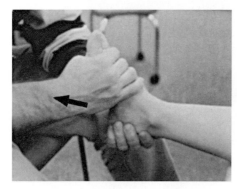

Figure 9–44. Talocrural joint traction to increase general mobility of ankle.

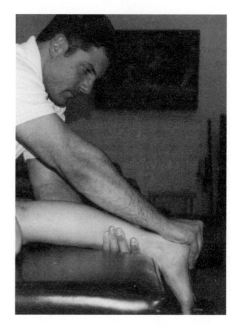

Figure 9–45. Subtalar joint traction to increase general mobility of subtalar joint.

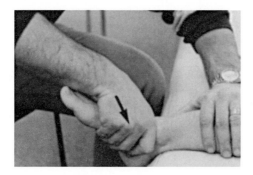

Figure 9–46. Talocrural joint: posterior glide of the talus to increase dorsiflexion range of motion.

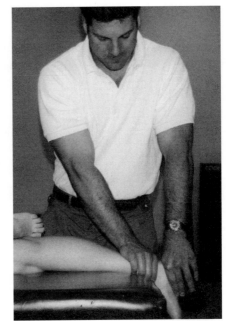

Figure 9–47. Talocrural joint: anterior glide of talus to increase plantar flexion range of motion.

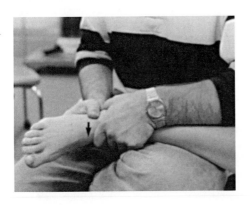

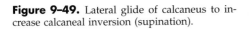

Figure 9–48. Medial glide of calcaneus to increase calcaneal eversion (pronation).

Figure 9–49. Lateral glide of calcaneus to increase calcaneal inversion (supination).

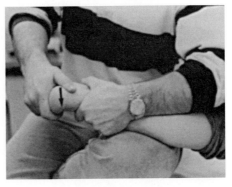

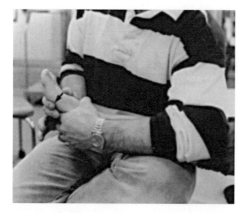

Figure 9–50. Plantar glide of midtarsal joint.

Figure 9–51. Dorsal glide of midtarsal joint.

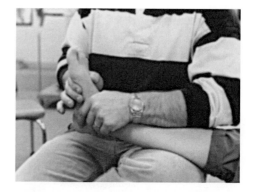

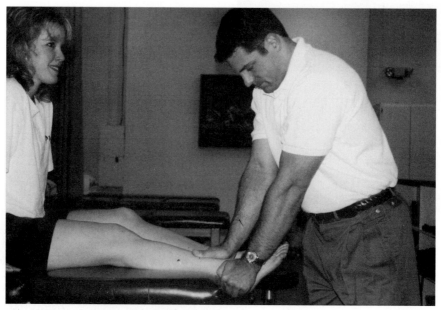

Figure 9–52. Tibiofibular joint: anterior glide of tibia.

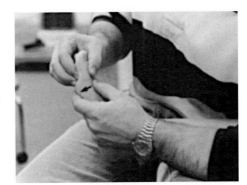

Figure 9–53. Plantar glide of first metatarsal at first metatarsophalangeal joint.

monly seen when a novice skier falls forward while loading the inner edge of the skis.

This injury is commonly confused with inversion ankle sprains because of the similarity in symptoms. The athlete relates a feeling of tenderness, instability, and swelling in an area around the lateral malleolus. Differential diagnosis can be determined if there is complaint of intense retromalleolar pain with resistive dorsiflexion and eversion or, in patients with a chronic condition, marked instability and audible snapping of the tendon in and out of its groove.

Conservative management involves reducing the inflammatory response with ice, compression, and elevation. Peroneal stabilization can be attempted with taping techniques that limit excessive motion and that incorporate a J-shaped pad that compresses the tendons as they pass around the lateral malleolus (Fig. 9–54). If conservative management fails to control the symptoms, surgical intervention may be elected. Surgical procedures generally attempt to reconstruct or reinforce the damaged peroneal retinaculum or use bony procedures to deepen the groove behind the lateral malleolus.

Calcaneal Injuries

HEEL BRUISES

Contusion injuries to the heel and calcaneal fat pad are among the most disabling in sports. Athletic activities that require frequent jumping or changes of direction seem to be especially likely to produce this type of injury. Runners with leg length discrepancy who overstride on the side of the short leg and who, as a result, have increased impact forces at the heel-strike area are also especially vulnerable to this type of trauma. Contusion injuries that cause subperiosteal bleeding and tender scar formation are sensitive to tissue compression monitored by pressure nerve endings in the area.

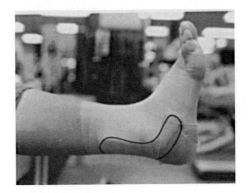

Figure 9–54. J-pad stabilization of peroneal tendons.

The athlete will complain of severe pain in the plantar aspect of the calcaneus, which is greatly aggravated by weight bearing. Treatment must include some element of rest to minimize continued, repetitive trauma. As the athlete returns to play, the heel should be taped and placed in a heel cup. It is also helpful if a shoe with a firm, well-fitting heel counter is selected for participation. The tape and heel cup strengthen and support the columnar septa and lobules, which provide the calcaneal fat pad with its impact-absorbing qualities.

OS TRIGONUM INJURY

Injury to the os trigonum is common in athletes who function on their toes (e.g., ballet dancers) or who encounter resistance to dorsiflexion while in the extreme of plantar flexion (e.g., soccer players who have a kick blocked). Accessory bone fracture or soft-tissue pinching produces severe local pain in the posterolateral portion of the ankle. Conservative treatment involves taping techniques to limit end-range plantar flexion. If this motion is necessary for performance, surgical excision may be necessary.

CALCANEAL APOPHYSITIS

Traction epiphyseal injuries in active adolescents are common when they wear cleated shoes or when they rapidly alter the heel height of their athletic shoes. The tight Achilles tendon pulls on the calcaneal epiphyseal attachment, producing a disruption of circulation and possible fragmentation (also known as Sever's disease). The young athlete complains of pain on the posterior heel at the insertion point of the Achilles tendon, which is aggravated by activity and relieved by rest. This condition ends at skeletal maturity, when the epiphysis closes. Until then, judicious rest and the insertion of bilateral heel lifts can help alleviate injurious stresses.

RETROCALCANEAL BURSITIS

Long-distance running and repetitive jumping can create a bursal inflammation between the Achilles tendon and calcaneus. This condition is aggravated by excessive compensatory pronation, which results in cumulative trauma and pressure to the posterolateral aspect of the heel. A structural predisposition to bursal inflammation may exist in the cavus foot if there is spurring on the posterosuperior aspect of the calcaneus.

This condition is characterized by pain, swelling, and discoloration on the posterolateral and posterosuperior aspects of the heel. Tenderness is elicited anterior to the Achilles tendon but posterior to the talus.

Ice, anti-inflammatory drugs, and orthotic control of the hypermobile calcaneus are used. If the subcutaneous bursa is involved, heel counter collar modification should also be employed (Fig. 9–55). Shoe selection should place a high priority on a stable heel counter. Structural predisposition may be alleviated by a heel lift; surgical excision of bony spurs in chronic conditions that do not respond to conservative management may be necessary.

PLANTAR FASCIITIS

The plantar fascia is a dense band of fibrous connective tissue that originates from the calcaneal tuberosity and runs forward to insert on the metatarsal heads. As a tension band, it supports the medial longitudinal arch and assists in the push-off power of running and jumping.[44] Biomechanical abuse of this tissue results in microtrauma and inflammation. Chronic overuse and irritation can

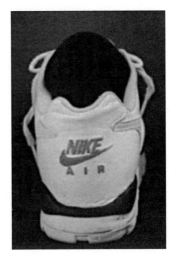

Figure 9–55. Notched heel collar on athletic shoe.

lead to bone formation in response to the traction forces of the plantar fascia and the muscles attaching to the calcaneal tuberosity.

This condition is most often seen in the running athlete who hyperpronates or has a rigid cavus foot and tight Achilles tendon. In both instances, excessive traction is placed on the fascia, which can be magnified with uphill or hard-surface training terrain. Creighton and Olson[12] have noted that decreased active and passive ranges of motion at the first MTP joint correlates with the onset of plantar fasciitis. Inadequate or inappropriate MTP motion can alter the windlass effect of the plantar fascia and decrease the inherent stability of the foot as the heel comes off the ground.

There is a gradual, insidious onset of pain, which can radiate along the path of the fascia, along the plantar aspect of the foot. Tenderness to palpation can be found at the medial aspect of the calcaneal tuberosity, in the medial arch, and occasionally at the distal insertion of the fascia on the metatarsal heads. The most consistent finding is that of exquisite pain with weight-bearing forces of the first few steps in the morning. The phenomenon of "physiologic creep," in which the tissues contract during the non–weight-bearing period at night and then are forcefully stretched with initial morning weight bearing, may explain this common complaint. Because the great toe is a noncontractile structure, its active or passive dorsiflexion usually elicits the symptoms. These signs and symptoms can mimic those of other pathologies but should be differentiated from medial plantar nerve irritation, tarsal tunnel syndrome, and infracalcaneal bursitis.

Treatment should initially be directed at controlling the inflammatory response and then at alleviating or reducing the excessive tension being placed on the plantar fascia and its associated structures, which have their origin at the calcaneal tuberosity. During the acute state, ice massage, anti-inflammatory medications, and rest from aggravating activities are prescribed. A cold soda bottle with ridges can be used like a rolling pin under the arch of the foot to provide gentle stretch and cryomassage to the plantar fascia. Sponge-rubber heel lifts with a doughnut-shaped cutout may provide weight-bearing relief on the injured structures. In the subacute stage, pulsed phonophoresis, cross-fiber friction massage, and heel cord stretching are used to manage symptoms. A night splint will hold the ankle joint in dorsiflexion and the subtalar joint in the neutral position to reduce plantar fascia contracture. Correction of abnormal stresses can be provided through Low-Dye taping for the hyperpronator (Fig. 9–56), shock-absorbing inserts for the rigid cavus foot, and joint mobilization for the hypomobile first MTP joint (Fig. 9–57).

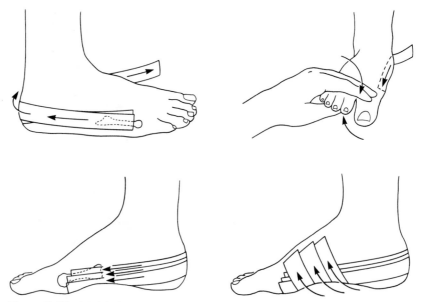

Figure 9–56. Modified Low-Dye taping technique to decrease traction stress on plantar fascia. (Steven Roy/Richard Irvin, Sports Medicine: Prevention, Evaluation, Management, and Rehabilitation, 1983, p. 58. Reprinted by permission of Prentice-Hall, Inc., Englewood Cliffs, New Jersey.)

Foot Injuries

TARSOMETATARSAL INJURIES

The tarsometatarsal joint is an articulation (Lisfranc's joint) that consists of the three cuneiforms and the cuboid as they articulate with the five metatarsals. Transverse ligamentous supports span the base of the metatarsals with the exception of the first and second metatarsals. Midfoot sprains, dislocations, and fracture-dislocations, although not common, can occur in athletic competition. The joint can be injured through direct and indirect mechanisms. The direct crushing type of injury is less common and predictable in its pathology. Indirect injuries usually occur with an axial load to the heel with the foot in plantar flexion causing a hyperextension stress on the joint (Fig. 9–58).

Midfoot sprains have subtle examination findings that make diagnosis difficult. Swelling is usually mild. Pain with passive pronation-supination and tenderness on palpation are reliable indicators of this injury. The athlete will have

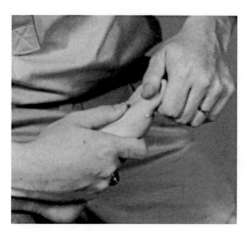

Figure 9–57. Traction-translation mobilization of first metatarsophalangeal joint to increase mobility.

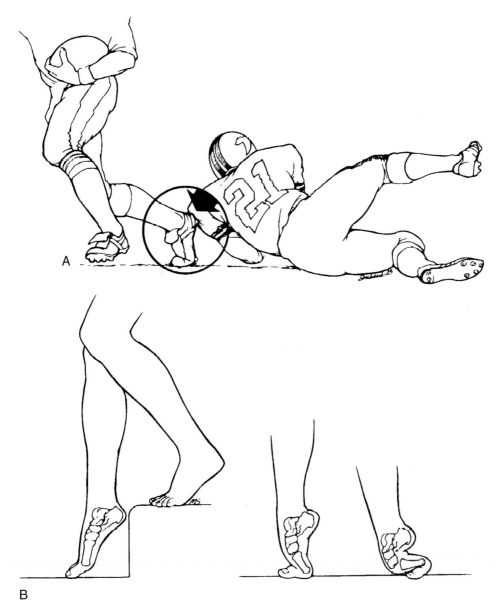

Figure 9–58. Mechanism of Lisfranc's fracture-dislocation. *A*, Axial load applied to heel with foot fixed in equinus. *B*, Axial load applied by body weight with ankle in extreme equinus. (From Heckman, J.D. [1991]: Fractures and dislocations of the foot. *In:* Rockwood, C.A. Jr., Green, D.P., and Bucholz, R.W. [eds.]: Rockwood and Green's Fractures in Adults, 3rd ed. Philadelphia, J.B. Lippincott, p. 2143.)

pain or inability to perform unilateral heel raises, jumps, or cutting maneuvers. After the acute injury, initial evaluation should also include a circulatory assessment of the dorsalis pedis pulse and a neurologic screen for abnormal toe sensation.

Following open or closed reduction, the foot is immobilized for a period of time depending on the severity of the injury. Rehabilitation and weight-bearing progression can commence after immobilizaton with a gradual progression of functional activities on the toes. Medial midfoot sprains tend to progress at a slower rate and take longer to return to full activity.[32]

TARSAL TUNNEL SYNDROME

Tarsal tunnel syndrome is an entrapment neuropathy of the posterior tibial nerve as it passes through the osseofibrous tunnel between the flexor retinaculum and medial malleolus (Fig. 9–59). The typical mechanism of injury in athletes is excessive pronation, which causes a tightening of the flexor retinaculum. Hyperpronation of the forefoot can also cause the calcaneonavicular ligament to compress the medial plantar branch of the posterior tibial nerve. Direct trauma or chronic inflammation in this area produces a space-occupying lesion that can alter neurologic function.

The athlete reports intermittent burning, pain, tingling, and numbness in the medial foot, which are aggravated by weight bearing. A positive Tinel's sign may be elicited with tapping or compression over the affected nerves to reproduce the symptoms. In advanced stages, weakness in toe flexion and atrophy of the abductor hallucis may be evident.

The athlete should be placed in a neutral-position orthosis to control pronation and should be instructed in activity modifications. Therapeutic modalities such as ultrasound phonophoresis and ice massage may be tried to reduce edema and fibrosis in the area of entrapment. Resistant cases may require surgical release of the tissue that is causing compression.

CUBOID SYNDROME

Cuboid syndrome describes a partial displacement of the cuboid bone by the pull of the peroneus longus. The onset can be gradual or traumatic. Acute pain and hypomobility can be induced with trauma or with a powerful contraction, with the foot in a plantar-flexed and inverted position. Gradual onset is more typical in the hyperpronated foot. Under these circumstances the peroneus longus is at a mechanical disadvantage, and it pulls the lateral portion of the cuboid dorsally and the medial portion in a plantar direction.[51]

The signs and symptoms of this injury include decreased or abnormal accessory motion of the calcaneocuboid joint and tenderness along the cuboid, peroneus longus, and lateral metatarsal heads. Treatment is directed at restoring normal osteokinematics and protecting against further trauma or aggravation. Following ice massage or a cold whirlpool bath, the athlete is prepared for bony manipulation. With the athlete prone, with the knee mildly flexed to protect against excessive traction of the superficial peroneal nerve, a downward thrust of the thumbs is used to relocate the cuboid into its appropriate position (Fig. 9–60). Following restoration of bony anatomy, a segmental balance pad may be used to unload stress on the fourth metatarsal and its cuboid articulation.[51] In

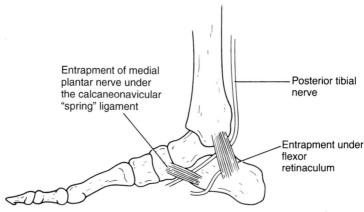

Entrapment of medial plantar nerve under the calcaneonavicular "spring" ligament

Posterior tibial nerve

Entrapment under flexor retinaculum

Figure 9–59. Tarsal tunnel syndrome (medial view).

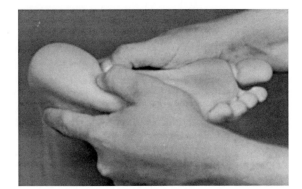

Figure 9–60. Cuboid mobilization.

athletes with chronic hyperpronation, Low-Dye taping or medial heel wedges can be used to counteract the damaging pull of the peroneus longus.

METATARSAL STRESS FRACTURES

Metatarsal stress fractures occur when osteoclastic activity is greater than osteoblastic activity. Stress overload caused by prolonged pronation and excessive hypermobility of the first ray can begin a cycle of injury (Fig. 9–61). Hughes[23] has noted that predisposition to stress fractures is greatest in the presence of forefoot varus and decreased ankle dorsiflexion range of motion. Both these conditions result in pronation during the propulsive phase of gait, placing considerable stress on the central three metatarsals, especially the second. Metatarsal stress fractures are most likely to occur at the beginning of the season

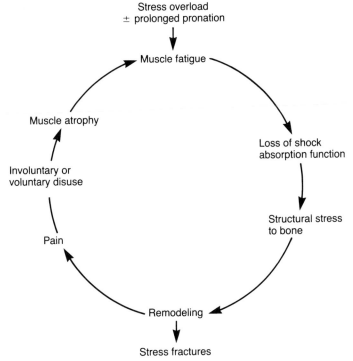

Figure 9–61. Stress fracture injury cycle. (From Taunton, J.E., Clement, D.B., and Webber, D. [1981]: Lower extremity stress fractures in athletes. Physician Sportsmed., 9:85.)

in the deconditioned athlete or with sudden changes in training surfaces or athletic footwear.

There is localized pain and swelling over the metatarsal, which increase with activity and decrease with rest. Percussion and active flexion-extension of the toes also exacerbate the complaint.

Treatment is straightforward. The athlete must rest from weight-bearing or aggravating activities and find alternative methods of conditioning. In those in whom pain is present with ambulation or in whom there is suspicion of noncompliance with reducing activity levels, a short-leg walking cast may be appropriate. On return to activity, orthoses, tape, or a felt cutout to float the affected metatarsal should be used to relieve osteoclastic stresses.

During the subacute phase it is important for the athlete to correct the muscular, flexibility, and conditioning deficits that may have led to the initial injury.

PROXIMAL DIAPHYSIS FRACTURE OF THE FIFTH METATARSAL

Weight-bearing forces are great on the fifth metatarsal because of its many soft-tissue attachments. Tension on the bone from the peroneus brevis, cubometatarsal ligament, lateral band of the plantar fascia, and peroneus tertius can lead to stress reactions, which can become a complete fracture with inversion trauma or a nonunion stress fracture with repetitive forces.[14] These lesions normally occur just distal to the base of the fifth metatarsal and are notoriously unpredictable in healing (Fig. 9–62). Nonunion and reinjury are frequent. Management is therefore controversial and must be customized to the athlete. Some clinicians recommend early, aggressive surgical intervention with the use of percutaneous intermedullary screw fixation across the fracture site, whereas others simply use non–weight-bearing immobilization. The screw-fixation method has shown predictable healing and return to full athletic competition in an average of 8 weeks.[34] Conservative management allows 4 to 6 weeks of healing; the cast is

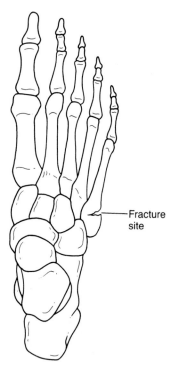

Fracture site

Figure 9–62. Proximal diaphysis fracture of fifth metatarsal (dorsal view).

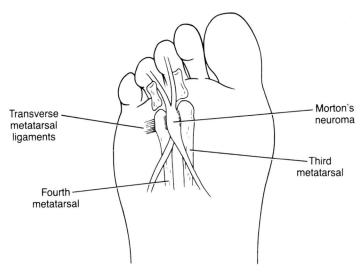

Figure 9–63. Plantar view of interdigital neuroma.

then removed to determine whether the athlete can function with a nonfibrous union. Full athletic participation is contraindicated until there is full consolidation of the fracture site. When healing is complete, orthotic therapy should be considered to redistribute injurious forces.

INTERDIGITAL NEUROMA

Compression and shearing forces at the bifurcation of the neurovascular bundle between the metatarsal heads can result in the formation of a benign tumor of fibrous tissue, called Morton's neuroma (Fig. 9–63). Pinching and squeezing of the neurovascular bundle between the metatarsal heads and transverse metatarsal ligament occur in the hypermobile foot during midstance and propulsion.

The chief complaint is that of a burning or electric-shock sensation in the forefoot that radiates into the toes. The lesion is usually located between the third and fourth metatarsals and is often mistaken for a stone in the shoe by the athlete. Pain can be relieved by removal of shoes and is aggravated by manual metatarsal head compression. A clicking or reproduction of symptoms can be elicited with simultaneous compression of the metatarsal heads in the transverse plane and plantar flexion of the affected MTP joints (Fig. 9–64).

Some success has been achieved with a metatarsal pad placed just proximal to the metatarsal heads, which increases their spatial spread and increases toe

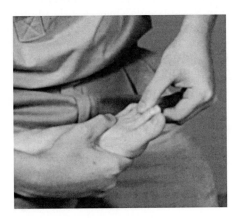

Figure 9–64. Metatarsal head compression in combination with plantar-dorsal glide to elicit pain from an interdigital neuroma.

flexion. Shoe selection should ensure a wide toe box, and orthotic inserts may be used to control hypermobility. Corticosteroid and anesthetic injections or oral anti-inflammatory medications can also be tried. Surgical excision of the neuroma is indicated when conservative measures fail.

STAIRCLIMBER'S TRANSIENT PARESTHESIA

With the increase in popularity of stationary stair-climbing devices, a relatively new injury has become more common. In a study by Vereschagin and colleagues,[46] 39% of the individuals using these exercise machines experienced mild to moderate numbness or paresthesia in their feet during stair-climbing exercise. The symptoms are a result of persistent and prolonged weight-bearing compression of the interdigital nerve. It has been postulated that these transient paresthesia symptoms are magnified because there is no swing phase during the exercise movement to unload compressive forces under the foot. The following suggestions are offered to minimize neurologic irritation: (1) avoid repetitive MTP dorsiflexion by reducing step height and maintaining a flat-foot position on the pedals; (2) ensure proper footwear with ample toe-box depth, looser shoe lacing, and shock-absorbing insoles; and (3) limit the duration of the stair-climbing exercise according to the severity of the symptoms.

TURF TOE

Acute hyperdorsiflexion injuries to the first MTP joint occur as the toes are pressed down into an unyielding surface just prior to toe-off. This force causes hyperextension of the MTP joint as the phalanx is jammed into the metatarsal.[47] Repetitive trauma of this nature results in plantar capsule tears, articular cartilage damage, and possible fracture of the medial sesamoid bone. Chronic trauma can lead to metatarsalgia, with ligamentous calcification and hallux rigidus.[38]

Sudden acceleration under high loads against unyielding AstroTurf is the usual mechanism of injury. Athletes who wear shoes that are extremely flexible and offer minimal support are especially prone to this injury. Also, athletes who wear a longer shoe to achieve greater width effectively lengthen the lever arm forces acting on the joint and subject the feet to repetitive trauma.

The athlete presents with a tender, red, and swollen first MTP joint that has increased pain with passive toe extension. Initial management calls for rest, ice, compression, elevation, and support to the injured joint. Tape immobilization can be used to limit excessive extension and valgus stresses that irritate the joint (Fig. 9–65). Rehabilitation procedures may include whirlpool range-of-motion exercises, ultrasound to mobilize scar tissue, and active range-of-motion exercises with the first ray stabilized. Figure 9–66 demonstrates exercise to increase active range of motion for the hypomobile first MTP joint.

In the subacute stage, gentle plantar-dorsal glides of the first phalanx may be indicated to improve arthrokinematic mobility. On return to activity, the athlete should possess at least 90° of painless passive toe extension and have been screened for appropriate shoe selection.[38] A steel spring plate in the toe box or rigid taping into plantar flexion should be used initially when resuming full participation.

SESAMOIDITIS

The two small sesamoid bones of the foot are present on the plantar surface of the first metatarsal head, embedded within the tendon of the flexor hallucis brevis. The sesamoid bones enhance the windlass mechanism and help distribute and disperse weight-bearing forces during propulsion. The medial or tibial sesamoid is often bipartite, and its appearance can be confused with a fracture.[48]

Step 1:   Prepare the plantar surface of the foot and toe with tape adherent. Encircle the first phalanx and midfoot with anchor strips. Do not extend the anchor strip to the IP joint as this will cause the MTP joint to extend during the taping technique.

Step 2:   Using precut moleskin or 1″ white tape, run a checkrein on the plantar-medial surface of the foot to limit dorsiflexion and adduction of the first MTP joint. Enclose the checkrein with elastic tape.

Step 3:   Modify the athletic shoe. Ensure proper length to decrease the lever arm effect on the joint. Place a spring steel, polyethylene, or orthoplast insert in the shoe to increase the rigidity of the distal forefoot.

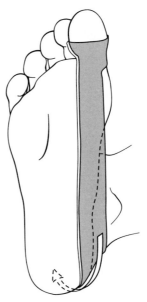

Figure 9–65. Turf toe taping technique to prevent excessive hyperextension of the first metatarsophalangeal (MTP) joint. IP, interphalangeal.

Sesamoiditis describes an inflammatory condition of the tissues surrounding the sesamoids.

The athlete most prone to medial sesamoid pathology is the one with a rigid cavus foot, tight Achilles tendon, and plantar-flexed first ray.[2] Sesamoid pain also occurs in athletes with normal foot structure but whose activities require maximal dorsiflexion of the first MTP joint, which allows excessive impact loading stresses on the sesamoids.

The athlete usually presents with tenderness and swelling of the first metatarsal head and pain with passive dorsiflexion. Pressure from improperly placed cleats on the athletic shoe may be a source of further aggravation.

Initial treatment in the acute stage involves ice massage, anti-inflammatory medications or cortisone injections, and rest. Pulsed phonophoresis and iontophoresis are alternative methods of combating the inflammatory response, which may be of value in reducing symptoms. Definitive treatment must include relief of weight-bearing stresses on the affected area. A semirigid orthosis with the first ray cut out or a Morton's extension can provide this relief.

ORTHOTIC THERAPY

The intent of orthotic therapy is to allow the subtalar joint to function near and around its neutral position. This is accomplished by balancing the forefoot

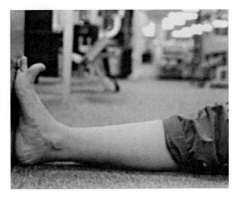

Figure 9–66. Active range of motion of first metatarsophalangeal joint, with first metatarsal head stabilized.

to the rearfoot and by balancing the rearfoot with its supporting surface. There are a number of indications for the use of biomechanical orthoses:

1. Support and correction of intrinsic rearfoot and forefoot deformities
2. Support or restriction of range of motion
3. Treatment of postural problems
4. Dissipation of excessive ground reaction forces
5. Decrease of shear forces or tender spots on the plantar surface of the foot by redistributing weight bearing to more tolerant areas
6. Control of abnormal transverse rotation of the lower extremity

Contraindications to the use of orthotic therapy in the management of lower extremity injuries include the following:

1. Lack of intrinsic structural foot abnormality
2. Correction of soft-tissue–induced equinus
3. Incomplete lower quarter biomechanical examination

The orthosis consists of the module (shell) and the post (Fig. 9–67). The module is the body of the orthosis, which conforms to the foot's plantar contours. The post is the "shim"; this is placed on the front or rear of the module, which brings the ground up to the foot and places the subtalar joint in its neutral position.

Two main types of orthoses are used. The biomechanical orthosis is constructed of rigid materials such as high-density plastic or of semirigid materials called thermoplastics (Fig. 9–68). Biomechanical orthoses control and resist abnormal foot forces. Accommodative orthoses are constructed of soft materials, such as Plastazote.* These orthoses allow the foot to compensate, and the materials used in construction yield to abnormal foot forces. Posting on accom-

*Available from Alimed, Dedham, Massachusetts

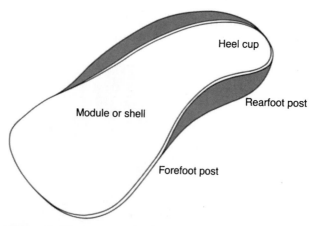

Figure 9–67. Anatomy of orthosis.

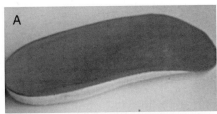

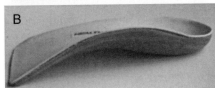

Figure 9–68. Orthoses. *A,* Semirigid. *B,* Rigid.

modative orthoses is referred to as bias. Table 9–15 offers the rationale and considerations for selecting the specific type of orthotic device that would be most appropriate for any particular athlete.

The post is the corrective portion of the orthosis and is analogous to the corrective lens of an eyeglass. Posts can be located in the rearfoot or forefoot and can be constructed intrinsically or extrinsically to provide a varus (medial) or valgus (lateral) angulation. For the biomechanical orthosis to be effective and for the athlete to comply in its use, it must meet the following requirements:

1. It must conform precisely to all contours of the foot, especially the heel seat and calcaneal and forefoot inclinations
2. It must be rigid enough to maintain the shape, contour, and imposed angular relationships of the foot
3. It must control abnormal motion, allow normal motion, and provide proper sequencing and timing of motion
4. It must be able to withstand stress and wear
5. It must be comfortable and ensure wearer compliance
6. It must be adjustable
7. It must end proximal to the weight-bearing surfaces of the metatarsal heads
8. It must be narrow enough to fit on the shoe last and allow the first and fifth rays to function independently

Table 9–15. Primary Considerations for Selecting an Orthosis

Physiologic age	Not chronologic age; the older the foot, the softer the orthosis
Foot type	The more mobile the foot, the more rigid the orthosis
Primary activity	Straight-ahead movements vs pivoting or cutting
Chief complaint/diagnosis	Dictates need for specific accommodations (clips, extensions, metatarsal pads, etc.)
Subtalar motion	Control with more rigid device vs. bias with softer orthotic device
Shock absorbancy	Softer orthosis to protect against proximal injuries up the chain or to improve dissipation of ground reaction forces
Weight of patient	Lower durometer for rigidity and firmness or for larger athlete

If an athlete is using orthoses, shoe selection should be appropriate. Criteria for shoe selection include a straight-last shoe with a snug, deep, and stable heel counter. The shoe should have minimal heel height and adequate shoe depth. For the narrow-shank shoe, the insoles and arch cookies may have to be removed and replaced with a "cobra pad" orthosis,[31] in which the entire insert consists of posting (Fig. 9–69). Feet that are high-arched or have an equinus attitude are difficult to fit with orthotic inserts.

Once the orthosis has been fabricated, it should be placed in the athlete's shoe for a 5- to 10-minute running trial. Areas of irritation may have to be ground down, and correction of gait deviations will have to be assessed. The athlete should be instructed about gradually breaking in the orthosis, with the wear time not to exceed one additional hour of wear for each day the orthosis has been worn.

RETURN TO COMPETITION

The final component of lower leg rehabilitation is the functional progression and testing program, which must precede return to athletic competition. The concept of functional progression mandates a logical and ordered sequence of rehabilitative activities leading back to previous performance. Athletes must be educated to appreciate that they cannot simply resume the activities that led to the initial injury when pain and swelling have subsided. Even the return of normal strength, flexibility, and endurance does not automatically ensure safe resumption of activity. Exercise programs cannot duplicate the speeds, forces, and stresses that normal high-speed athletic activities demand.

For these reasons, the athlete must be guided gradually back to activity by breaking down the component movements of the sport and addressing them in inverse order of difficulty. An example of this progression for an athlete with a lower extremity injury might be the following:

Non–weight-bearing exercise
Partial weight-bearing exercise
Full weight-bearing exercise
Stable surface balance training
Walking
BAPS or balance board activities
Rebounder running
Jogging
Running
Jumping and hopping
Backpedaling
Figure-eight running
Cutting and twisting
Zigzag running
Plyometrics

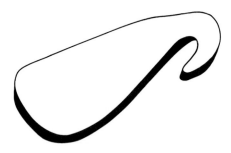

Figure 9–69. "Cobra pad" orthosis.

FOOT AND ANKLE FUNCTIONAL TESTING

Name _____ Involved Extremity _____ Date _____

HOP TESTS

TEST	PARAMETER	UNINVOLVED	INVOLVED	% DEFICIT
Unilateral standing long jump Unilateral standing triple jump	Distance in inches	Trial 1 _____ Trial 2 _____ Trial 3 _____ Mean = _____	Trial 1 _____ Trial 2 _____ Trial 3 _____ Mean = _____	
Single-leg 20-foot hop Single-leg 20-foot crossover hop	Time in seconds	Trial 1 _____ Trial 2 _____ Trial 3 _____ Mean = _____	Trial 1 _____ Trial 2 _____ Trial 3 _____ Mean = _____	
4-square hop	# of hops in ___ seconds	Trial 1 _____	Trial 1 _____	
Single-leg vertical jump	Distance in inches	Trial 1 _____ Trial 2 _____ Trial 3 _____ Mean = _____	Trial 1 _____ Trial 2 _____ Trial 3 _____ Mean = _____	

STRENGTH TESTS

TEST	PARAMETER	UNINVOLVED	INVOLVED	% DEFICIT
Single-leg squats @75% BW	# of repetitions Level __	_____ reps	_____ reps	
Unilateral heel raises	# of repetitions Level __	_____ reps	_____ reps	
Unilateral toe raises	# of repetitions Level __	_____ reps	_____ reps	

FUNCTIONAL TESTS

TEST	PARAMETER	RESULTS	EXPECTATIONS/SYMMETRY
T run			
Box run: (R) (L)			
Carioca test			
Landing			
Shuttle run			
___ -yard dash			

BALANCE TESTS

Stork stand:_____ Surface _____
BAPS board: _____ Surface _____ Level _____ Overload _____
Functional tasks : Deep knee bending _____ Squats _____ Stair descent _____

AEROBIC TESTING: Harvard step test: _____ Submaximal bicycle ergometry evaluation: _____

VIDEO GAIT ANALYSIS:

SUMMARY:

RECOMMENDATIONS:

FUNCTIONAL SCORE= ___% ___Full participation ___Participation with restrictions ___ No restrictions

Therapist _____

Figure 9–70. Sample form for functional evaluation of lower leg injuries.

The program is structured according to the specific demands of the athlete's sport. Modifications are appropriate, depending on the goals and aspirations of the athlete. Specific criteria that dictate graduation from one functional level to the next must be defined precisely. It is the responsibility of the rehabilitation professional to provide the framework and specifics by which the athlete will function and progress.

Once the athlete has completed the functional progression program and is psychologically prepared to return to competition, an objective evaluation of physical readiness should be performed. Criteria for return to activity should include absence or control of pain, swelling, and spasm; isokinetic symmetry in peak torque, total work, and average power; and functional normality with appropriate control, carriage, and confidence. Figure 9–70 is a sample functional evaluation form for lower leg injuries. It contains testing maneuvers and activities that can be used to judge an athlete's readiness to perform with symmetric functional normality.

References

1. American Academy of Orthopaedic Surgeons (1965): Joint Motion: Methods of Measuring and Recording. Chicago, American Academy of Orthopaedic Surgeons.
2. Axe, M., and Ray, R. (1988): Orthotic treatment of sesamoid pain. Am. J. Sports Med., 16:411–416.
3. Brandel, B.K., and Williams, K. (1974): An analysis of cinematographic and electromyographic recordings of human gait. In: Nelson, R., and Morehouse, C. (eds.): Biomechanics, Vol. IV. Baltimore, University Park Press.
4. Bouche, R.T., and Kuwanda, K.T. (1984): Equinus deformity in the athlete. Physician Sportsmed., 12:81–91.
5. Bosien, W.R. (1955): Residual disability following acute ankle sprains. J. Bone Joint Surg. [Am.], 37:1237–1243.
6. Bullock-Saxton, J.E. (1994): Local sensation and altered hip muscle function following severe ankle sprain. Phys Ther., 74:17–31.
7. Boytin, M.J., Fischer, D.A., and Neuman, L. (1991): Syndesmotic ankle sprains. Am. J. Sports Med., 19:294–298.
8. Carter, T.R., Fowler, P.J., and Blokker, C. (1992): Functional postoperative treatment of Achilles tendon repair. Am. J. Sports Med., 20:459–462.
9. Cetti, R., Christensen, S., Ejsted, R., et al. (1993): Operative versus nonoperative treatment of Achilles tendon rupture. Am. J. Sports Med., 21:791–799.
10. Clancy, W.G., Neidhart, D., and Brand, D.L. (1976): Achilles tendinitis in runners. A report of five cases. Am. J. Sports Med., 4:46–57.
11. Clement, D.B., Taunton, J.E., and Smart, G.E. (1984): Achilles tendinitis and peritendinitis: Etiology and treatment. Am. J. Sports Med., 12:179–184.
12. Creighton, D., and Olson, V. (1987): Evaluation of range of motion of first metatarsophalangeal joint in runners with plantar fasciitis. J. Orthop. Sports Phys. Ther., 8:357–361.
13. Cyriax, J. (1978): Textbook of Orthopedic Medicine, 7th ed. London, Bailliere Tindall.
14. Dameron, T.B. (1975): Fractures and anatomical variations of the proximal portion of the fifth metatarsal. J. Bone Joint Surg. [Am.], 57:788–792.
15. Donatelli, R. (1985): Normal biomechanics of the foot and ankle. J. Orthop. Sports Phys. Ther., 7:91–95.
16. Davies, G. (1984): A Compendium of Isokinetics in Clinical Usage. La Crosse, WI, S & S.
17. Eiff, M.P., Smith, A.T., and Smith, G.E. (1994): Early mobilization versus immobilization in the treatment of lateral ankle sprains. Am. J. Sports Med., 22:83–87.
18. Elveru, R.A., Rothstein, J.M., and Lamb, R.L. (1988): Goniometric reliability in a clinical setting: subtalar and ankle joint measurements. Phys. Ther., 68:672–677.
19. Freeman, M.A.R., Dean, M.R.E., and Hanham, I.W.F. (1965): The etiology and prevention of functional instability of the foot. J. Bone Joint Surg. [Br.], 47:678–685.
20. Friedman, M. (1986): Injuries to the leg in athletes. In: Nicholas, J., and Hershman, E. (eds.): The Lower Extremity and Spine in Sports Medicine. St. Louis, C.V. Mosby.
21. Garth, W., and Miller, S. (1989): Evaluation of toe claw deformity, weakness of foot intrinsics, and posteromedial shin pain. Am. J. Sports Med., 17:821–827.
22. Gray, G. (1984): When the Foot Hits the Ground Everything Changes. Toledo, OH, American Physical Rehabilitation Network.
23. Hughes, L.Y. (1985): Biomechanical analysis of the foot and ankle to developing stress fractures. J. Orthop. Sports Phys. Ther., 7:96–101.
24. James, S.L., and Brubaker, C.E. (1973): Biomechanics of running. Orthop. Clin. North Am., 4:605–615.

25. Kapandji, I.A. (1970): The Physiology of Joints, Vol. II. Edinburgh, Churchill Livingstone.
26. Keene, S. (1985): Ligament and muscle-tendon unit injuries. *In:* Gould, J., and Davies, G. (eds.): Orthopedic and Sports Physical Therapy. St. Louis, C.V. Mosby, pp. 135–165.
27. Kisner, C., and Colby, L.A. (1985): Ankle and foot. *In:* Therapeutic Exercise: Foundation and Techniques. Philadelphia, F.A. Davis.
28. Klein, K. (1990): Biomechanics of running. Presented at Metroplex Trainer's Meeting, Fort Worth, TX, January 1990.
29. Lattanza, L., Gray, G., and Katner, R. (1988): Closed vs. open kinematic chain measurements of subtalar joint eversion: Implications for clinical practice. J. Orthop. Sports Phys. Ther., 9:310–314.
30. Magee, D.J. (1987): Orthopedic Physical Assessment. Philadelphia, W.B. Saunders.
31. McPoil, T., and Brocato, R. (1985): The foot and ankle: Biomechanical evaluation and treatment. *In:* Gould, J., and Davis, G. (eds.): Orthopedic and Sports Physical Therapy. St. Louis, C.V. Mosby, pp. 313–341.
32. Meyer, E.A., Callaghan, J.J., Albright, J.P., et al. (1994): Midfoot sprains in collegiate football players. Am. J. Sports Med., 22:392–400.
33. Miller, W.A. (1977): Rupture of musculotendinous junction of medial head of gastrocnemius. Am. J. Sports Med., 5:191–193.
34. Mindrebo, N., Shelbourne, K.D., Van Meter, C.D., and Rettig, A.C. (1993): Outpatient percutaneous screw fixation of the acute Jones fracture. Am. J. Sports Med., 21:720–723.
35. Picciano, A.M., Rowlands, M.S., and Worrell, T. (1993): Reliability of open and closed kinetic chain subtalar joint neutral positions and navicular drop test. J. Orthop. Sports Phys. Ther., 18:553–558.
36. Rebman, L. (1986): Suggestions from the clinic: Ankle injuries: Clinical observations. J. Orthop. Sports Phys. Ther., 8:153–156.
37. Root, W.L., Orient, W.P., and Weed, J.N. (1977): Clinical Biomechanics, Vol. II: Normal and Abnormal Function of the Foot. Los Angeles, Clinical Biomechanics.
38. Sammarco, G.J. (1988): How I manage turf toe. Physician Sportsmed., 16:113–199.
39. Seibel, M.O. (1988): Foot Function. Baltimore, Williams & Wilkins.
40. Sell, K.E., Verity, T.M., Worrell, T.W., et al. (1994): Two measurement techniques for assessing subtalar joint position: A reliability study. J. Orthop. Sports Phys. Ther., 19:162–167.
41. Smart, G.W., Tauton, J.E., and Clement, D.B. (1980): Achilles tendinitis and peritendinitis. Med. Sci. Sports Exerc., 17:731–743.
42. Smith-Oricchio, K., and Harris, B.A. (1990): Intertester reliability of subtalar neutral, calcaneal inversion, and eversion. J. Orthop. Sports Phys. Ther., 12:10–16.
43. Subotnick, S. (1989): Sports Medicine of the Lower Extremity. New York, Churchill-Livingstone.
44. Tanner, S., and Harvey, J. (1988): How we manage plantar fasciitis. Physician Sportsmed., 16:39–48.
45. Tatro-Adams, D., McGann, S.F., and Carbone, W. (1995): Reliability of the figure-of-eight method of ankle measurement. J. Orthop. Sports Phys., 22:161–163.
46. Vereschagin, K.S., Firtch, W.L., Caputo, L.J., and Hoffman, M.A. (1993): Stairclimber's transient paraesthesia. Physician Sportsmed., 21:63–69
47. Visnick, A. (1987): A playing orthosis for turf toe. Athl. Train., 22:215.
48. Vogelbach, D. (1989): The foot and ankle. Presented at HEALTHSOUTH Continuing Education Program. Birmingham, AL.
49. Wallace, L. (1986): Lower quarter pain: Mechanical evaluation and treatment. Presented at Seventh Annual Conference of the Sports Physical Therapy Section, Williamsburg, VA.
50. Whittle, H.P. (1994): Fractures of the foot in athletes. Op. Tech. Sports Med., 2:43–57.
51. Woods, A., and Smith, W. (1983): Case report: Cuboid syndrome and the techniques for treatment. Athl. Train., 18:64–65.

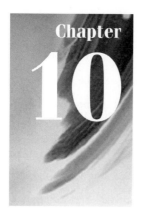

Knee Rehabilitation

Mark D. Weber, M.S., A.T.,C., P.T., S.C.S., and
A. Nelson Ware, A.T.,C., P.T.

The knee joint is one of the most frequently injured joints in the body, especially in those engaging in athletic activity. The incidence of permanent and progressively residual instability is higher from knee injury than from any other traumatic joint injury sustained in sports.[196] Even though the knee appears to be a relatively simple joint, the biomechanics of the knee and treatment of the injured knee have long been subjects of discussion in the literature and professional circles. The advent of arthroscopy has led to a greater understanding of these topics. Concurrently, the field of rehabilitation has also grown, and many traditional ideas and methods have been abandoned. Indications and contraindications for specific exercises are now research based. Rehabilitation programs are goal oriented, modified by time instead of being driven by it. This chapter emphasizes knee rehabilitation of the entire kinetic chain, early controlled motion, return to participation along a functional progression, and restoration of lower extremity muscular strength, power, endurance, and neuromuscular control.

FUNCTIONAL ANATOMY AND ARTHROKINEMATICS

To understand the arthrokinematics of the knee joint one must understand the functional anatomy of the joint (Fig. 10–1). The following sections will address the more important anatomic aspects of the knee as they relate to the function of the knee.

Bony Anatomy

The knee is a synovial joint and is typically classified as a hinge joint.[159] The joint consists of three articulations,[159, 207] the two tibiofemoral articulations and the patellofemoral articulation. All three articulations are contained within a single synovial joint capsule.[166] Although classically considered a hinge joint, the tibiofemoral joint actually has 6° of freedom in a three-axis system (Table 10–1).[84]

Internal and external rotation of the leg at the knee does not normally occur once the knee is in complete extension because of the screw-home locking mechanism of the knee.[166] The patellofemoral joint, while appearing to act simply as a plane joint, is actually a sellar joint[207] and undergoes an intricate combination of flexion, slide, tilt, and rotation during motion of the knee.[78] For the sake of

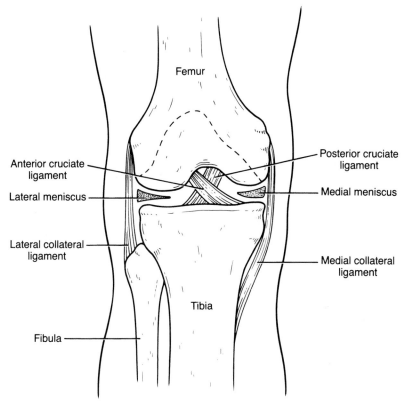

Figure 10–1. Static knee restraints.

clarity, throughout the biomechanics section, the tibiofemoral and patellofemoral components of the knee will be described separately. However, any rehabilitation program for the knee must consider the impact of the exercise on both articulations.

TIBIOFEMORAL ARTICULATION

The femoral condyles are convex in their articulation with the tibia and have a decreasing radius of curvature from anterior to posterior. This change in curvature is suggested to cause the axis of motion for flexion and extension to shift in a posterior and superior direction during flexion. During extension, the axis follows the same path in reverse.[165] The normal shift in the axis position is often disrupted when the constraints to the joint are injured.[165] This can lead to the abnormal wear of the articular cartilage.

The articular surface of the medial femoral condyle is longer than the lateral articular surface.[166] Corresponding to this, the medial tibial articular surface is larger than the lateral tibial articular surface.[166] This asymmetry between the medial and lateral compartments of the tibiofemoral joint is a minor factor

Table 10–1. Three-Axis System

AXIS	ROTATION	TRANSLATIONS
Transverse	Flexion/extension	Medial/lateral
Anteroposterior	Abduction/adduction	Anterior/posterior
Longitudinal	Internal/external rotation	Compression/distraction

involved in the screw-home or locking mechanism of the knee.[77] The screw-home mechanism is the automatic rotation that occurs in the knee during the final 30° of knee extension. The major bony influence to the screw-home mechanism is the curvature of the semilunar area on the medial side of the femoral intercondylar notch.[77] In an open kinetic chain (OKC) activity, the tibia will laterally rotate on the relatively fixed femur, whereas in a closed kinetic chain (CKC) activity, the femur will medially rotate on the relatively fixed tibia.[165, 166] This involuntary mechanism "locks" the knee into its close-packed position.[207]

PATELLOFEMORAL ARTICULATION

The patellofemoral joint is a major source of pain and dysfunction at the knee joint. The primary functions of the patella are to increase the efficiency of the quadriceps muscles and to provide anterior bony protection to the femur. The posterior surface of the patella articulates with the femoral sulcus.[207] The patellar articular surface has a vertical ridge that splits the articular surface into medial and lateral facets. Each facet can be further subdivided into three facets on the lateral side and four (including the odd facet) on the medial side.[223] The vertical ridge of the patella fits in the groove of the femoral sulcus. Normally, the femoral sulcus angle should be between 130° and 145°, with the lateral ridge being higher.[1, 157] Varying shapes of the patella and the femoral sulcus predispose individuals to patellofemoral dysfunctions.[228] The higher lateral ridge of the sulcus is one of the important restraining mechanisms against lateral subluxation or dislocation of the patella.[223]

The contact points between the patella and the femur change during flexion and extension of the tibiofemoral joint (Fig. 10–2).[76, 81, 99, 102, 214] From a starting position of full extension, as flexion is initiated, the inferior portion of the patellar articular surface engages the femoral sulcus first. This occurs at approximately 10° of knee flexion. By 45° of knee flexion the midportion of the patellar

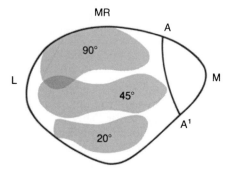

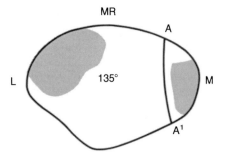

Figure 10–2. Patellofemoral contact pattern during knee flexion. L, lateral; M, medial; MR, median ridge; A–A[1], ridge separating medial and odd facets. (From Goodfellow, J., Hungerford, D.S., and Zindel, M. [1976]: Patellofemoral joint mechanics and pathology: 1. Functional anatomy of the patello-femoral joint. J. Bone Joint Surg. [Br.], 58:287–290.)

articular surface is in contact with the femoral sulcus. At 90° of flexion only the superior portion of the patellar articular surface is in contact with the femoral sulcus, and by 120° to 135° of flexion most of the contact is between the sulcus and the odd facet and the superolateral portion of the lateral facet.[80, 99] By 120°, the quadriceps tendon is also making significant contact with the femoral sulcus.[99] The contact area between the articular surfaces of the patella and femur increases as knee flexion progresses.[99, 102, 214] The articular cartilage on the posterior surface of the patella is the thickest in the body, almost 5 mm in the central portion,[75] indicating the magnitude of the compression forces that occur in the joint.

Clinically, tibiofemoral joint motion can be limited by dysfunction of the patellofemoral joint. During knee flexion the patella must glide distally in the femoral sulcus, and during extension it must glide proximally. Therefore, when patellar glide is limited, tibiofemoral joint motion is restricted as well.

Ligaments

The knee is inherently unstable because of its location between the two longest bones in the body. Knee stability is maintained through static restraints (e.g., ligaments) and dynamic restraints (e.g., muscles). Unfortunately, the inability of dynamic restraints to maintain knee stability after loss of the anterior cruciate ligament (ACL) is evident from the small number of athletes with this deficiency who can return to full and unlimited sports participation without modifying their activity or later undergoing a surgical reconstruction of this ligament.[49] The role of the ligamentous restraints in controlling forces applied to the knee joint has been studied extensively,[77, 79, 85, 86, 119, 148, 166, 203] as has the role of secondary restraints in compensating for knee instability when a ligament is torn. In addition, the load produced by rehabilitation activities on the ligaments has been the subject of numerous recent investigations.[17, 18, 29, 46, 94, 98, 114, 178, 192, 239, 240] These studies have provided the clinician with the information needed to allow the athlete to safely progress after injury or reconstructive surgery.

ANTERIOR CRUCIATE LIGAMENT

The ACL is one of the intracapsular, extrasynovial ligaments of the knee.[207] The ACL attaches medially to the anterior intercondylar area of the tibia and to the posteromedial aspect of the lateral femoral condyle.[207] As it traverses posteriorly through the femoral intercondylar notch, it twists on itself.[207] The ligament is composed of two distinct bundles, a smaller anteromedial bundle and a larger posterolateral bundle.[207] Although there is tension in the ACL throughout tibiofemoral range of motion (ROM), the anteromedial bundle is more tense in flexion, whereas the posterolateral bundle becomes more tense in extension.[119, 166]

The ACL is the primary restraint to anterior tibial translation on the femur. Grood and colleagues[85] have reported that the ACL provides 85% of the ligamentous restraining force to anterior drawer at 30° and 90° of flexion. In addition to controlling anterior tibial translation, the ACL has several other functions that include the screw-home mechanism,[77] control of varus and valgus stresses,[216] control of hyperextension stresses,[63, 119] and a guiding function during tibiofemoral flexion-extension.[77, 137] The ACL plays a major role in causing the screw-home mechanism; in fact, if the ACL is intact one cannot manually neutralize the rotation that occurs.[77] Because of its position in the femoral intercondylar notch, if there is a valgus stress on a flexed knee, the ACL becomes a restraint to external tibial rotation.[166] In extension, the ACL also assists in the limitation of varus and valgus stresses in the knee, again by virtue of its position in the femoral intercondylar notch.[216] The posterolateral bundle of the ACL assists in the limitation of hyperextension of the knee.[119, 166]

The ACL, in combination with the posterior cruciate ligament (PCL), creates a four-bar linkage system for the tibiofemoral joint.[136] This linkage system serves to control and maintain the axis of motion for flexion-extension by controlling the roll and glide of the femoral condyles during flexion-extension. Disruption of the ACL, in particular the anteromedial bundle,[166] results in excessive femoral condyle roll during knee flexion.[136]

The stresses of rehabilitation exercises on the ACL have been studied by a number of investigators.[18, 94, 99, 239, 240] Henning and associates[94] implanted a strain gauge in two patients with grade II ACL sprains. The patients then performed various rehabilitation activities and the strain was recorded. The strain on the ACL was reported as a percentage of the strain of an 80-pound Lachman test (Table 10–2). Although conclusions should be drawn with care from a study with such a small number of subjects, it still provides some useful information with regard to the relative rank of strain on the ACL with particular rehabilitation activities.

Beynnon and colleagues[18] implanted a Hall effect transducer in the knees of 11 subjects with normal ACLs and then determined the strain on the ACLs during open-chain flexion and extension as well as during isometric contractions. They concluded that the following open-chain exercises produced either low or no strain on the ACL: isometric contractions of the hamstrings at 15°, 30°, 60°, and 90°; isometric quadriceps contractions at 60° and 90°; cocontractions of the quadriceps and hamstrings at 30°, 60°, and 90°; active knee flexion and extension between 35° and 90°; and knee flexion and extension with a 45-N (10-pound) weight between 45° and 90°. Exercises that proved to significantly increase the strain on the ACL included the following: knee extension exercise with a 45-N weight (particularly at 10° and 20° of knee flexion); isometric quadriceps contractions (at 15° and 30°); and isometric cocontractions of the quadriceps and hamstrings at 15°. During knee extension exercise the transition from the unstrained ACL to the strained ACL shifted from 35° of flexion during active unweighted knee extension to 45° under the weighted extension condition. These results were similar to those found in studies on cadavers.[46, 191]

In addition, Fleming and colleagues[65] have studied the ACL strain during the CKC squat in vivo. The investigators have noted a 1% to 2% strain from greater

Table 10–2. Strain on the Anterior Cruciate Ligament

ACTIVITY	RELATIVE ACL STRAIN*
Running downhill at 5 mph	125%
Isometric quad contraction at 22° of flexion against a 20-lb weight	62–121%
Isometric quad contraction at 0° of flexion against a 20-lb weight	87–107%
Jog on floor	89%
Leg lift with 22° of knee flexion	12–79%
Jog 5 mph on treadmill	62–64%
Isometric quad contraction at 45° of flexion against a 20-lb weight	50%
Walk without assistive device	36%
Half-squat, one leg	21%
Quad set	18%
Walk with crutches, weight bearing at 50 lb	7%
Stationary cycle	7%
Isometric hamstring contraction	−7%

Data compiled from Henning, C.E., Lynch, M.A., and Glick, K.R. (1985): An in vivo strain gauge study of elongation of the anterior cruciate ligament. Am. J. Sports Med., 13:22–26.

*Single recording indicates that the activity was reported for one subject only, while range indicates recording reported for both subjects.

than 0° to 40° of knee flexion and a 2.5% to 3.75% strain from 40° to 0° during the vertical squat. Other studies using biomechanical analysis have noted no anterior translation of the tibia on the femur during CKC squatting in the normal intact knee joint.[136, 230]

Howell[98] investigated the tibial translation that occurred during open-chain isometric knee extension exercise. Using a knee arthrometer (KT-1000), the investigators measured the tibial translation that occurred with isometric contractions of the quadriceps at 15°, 30°, 45°, 60°, and 75° of flexion. Under these conditions an anterior translation occurred at all angles tested except 75° of flexion. A posterior translation occurred at 75° of flexion. In normal knees, the anterior shear created by the quadriceps contraction was never greater than the anterior shear created by an 89-N (20-pound) pull on the arthrometer. The results of the reconstructed knee group were similar to those from the group with normal knees. The anterior translation results from the ACL-deficient knees were as great or greater than those obtained with the 89-N test. However, anterior tibial translations of the normal, ACL-deficient, and reconstructed knees were the same statistically at each angle tested. Howell concluded that because of the joint compression caused by the quadriceps contraction, the anterior shear produced is no greater than the tension produced during instrumented laxity testing. A word of caution: although open-chain isometric knee extension may indeed produce the same or less anterior shear as instrumented laxity testing, this study was not designed to determine impact of cyclic loading on the reconstructed ACL during such an exercise; therefore, one repetition may be safe but 50 may not.

Most studies investigating anterior shear during rehabilitation activities have reported the results as the strain on the ACL. A few have calculated their results relative to body weight (BW). Table 10–3 contains such data.

POSTERIOR CRUCIATE LIGAMENT

The PCL, like the ACL, is intracapsular and extrasynovial.[207] The PCL arises from the posterior intercondylar region of the tibia and attaches to the lateral aspect of the medial femoral condyle.[207] The PCL can be functionally separated into bundles. Although there does not seem to be disagreement about the separation of the ligament into bundles, there does appear to be disagreement in nomenclature for the bundles. Some sources refer to them as the anteromedial and posterolateral bundles,[166, 207] others as the anteromedial and posterior oblique bundles,[73] and still others as the anterolateral and posteriomedial bundles.[5, 103] Some authors also suggest that the meniscofemoral ligaments form a third

Table 10–3. Anterior Shear Forces Across the Tibiofemoral Joint During Various Activities

REFERENCE	ACTIVITY	KNEE POSITION AT PEAK ANTERIOR SHEAR	CALCULATED FORCE TIMES BODY WEIGHT
Ericson and Nisell[57]	Cycling, 60 RPM, 120 W workload	60–70°	0.05
Kaufman et al[114]	Isokinetic knee extension at 60°/sec	25°	0.3
	Isokinetic knee extension at 180°/sec	25°	0.2
Nisell et at[164]	Isokinetic knee extension at 30°/sec	45°	1.3
	Isokinetic knee extension at 180°/sec	40°	0.5

RPM, Rotations per minute; W, watts.

bundle of the PCL.[5, 69] Similarly to the ACL, the anterior bundle of the PCL becomes taut during flexion, whereas the posterior bundle becomes taut during extension.[69, 100, 166] The posterior bundle is an important restraint to knee hyperextension.[69]

The primary function of the PCL is to limit posterior translations of the tibia on the femur.[79, 86] It also assists in controlling varus and valgus stresses to the knee.[85, 109] The role of the PCL in controlling rotational forces appears to be minimal.[79, 86] The PCL also plays a role in the screw-home mechanism; however, it is not a compulsory component like the ACL.[77] The importance of the PCL in normal knee arthrokinematics is indicated by the increased compression forces that are observed in the patellofemoral joint and medial compartment in cadaveric specimens when the PCL is sectioned.[203] This correlates with the common complaints of anterior knee pain and medial compartment arthrosis in patients with a PCL-deficient knee.[5, 203, 229] Rehabilitation activities that cause large posterior shear forces include isometric hamstring contractions, jogging, ascending and descending stairs, and squats greater than 60° of knee flexion (especially as hip flexion is increased).[5, 17, 29, 178, 229] In addition, during early PCL rehabilitation, the clinician may want to avoid activities that require high forces from the gastrocnemius, because there is evidence that these activities may produce significant strain on the PCL.[46] Isokinetic testing of the hamstrings also produces significant posterior shears of the tibiofemoral joint.[114] Table 10–4 contains calculated posterior shear data for several rehabilitation exercises.

COLLATERAL LIGAMENTS

The medial collateral ligament (MCL), also commonly referred to as the tibial collateral ligament, has two portions, a superficial and a deep. The superficial portion originates from the medial femoral epicondyle, just distal to the adductor tubercle, and attaches to the medial margin of the tibia deep to the pes anserinus.[207] The anterior border of the superficial portion is distinct from the knee-joint capsule, whereas the posterior portion blends with the posterior joint capsule.[207] The superficial portion is fan shaped, with the narrow part of the fan at the tibial attachment. The deep portion of the MCL is firmly attached to the medial meniscus and blends with the knee-joint capsule.[159, 166]

The MCL provides the primary restraint against valgus stresses to the knee.[85] The MCL provides some assistance in the control of internal rotation torsional forces through the knee, but this role decreases as the knee is flexed.[148] The MCL also assists in controlling excessive external rotation.[166] The MCL is taut in extension and external rotation.[208] Because of this, as flexion is initiated, tension

Table 10–4. Posterior Shear Forces Across the Tibiofemoral Joint During Various Activities

REFERENCE	ACTIVITY	KNEE POSITION AT PEAK POSTERIOR SHEAR	CALCULATED FORCE TIMES BODY WEIGHT
Ericson and Nisell[57]	Cycling, 60 RPM, 120 W workload	105°	0.05
Kaufman et al[114]	Isokinetic knee flexion at 60°/sec	75°	1.7
	Isokinetic knee flexion at 180°/sec	75°	1.4
Ohkoshi et al[178]	Squat	15°	<0.25
		30°	<0.3
		60°	0.25–0.5
		90°	1.0–1.25

RPM, Rotations per minute; W, watts.

within the ligament assists in reversal of the screw-home mechanism.[77] Rehabilitation activities that stress the MCL would include any adductor strengthening exercises in which the resistance is placed distal to the knee. In addition, care must be taken during CKC activities if the athlete lacks hip control, as the hip has a tendency under these conditions to adduct and internally rotate, which creates a valgus stress to the knee.

The lateral collateral ligament (LCL), or fibular collateral ligament, is a cordlike ligament that attaches to the lateral epicondyle of the femur and the head of the fibula.[207] It is fused with the joint capsule at its superior attachment but not in the middle or inferior attachment.[159] The LCL is the primary restraint to varus stresses at the knee.[85] The tendon of the biceps femoris overlaps the LCL[207] and may act as an active mechanism to bias the tension of the LCL.[85] The LCL, along with the posterolateral capsule, appears to play a large role in the control of external tibial rotation.[79, 148] Rehabilitation activities that stress the LCL would include any abductor strengthening exercises in which the resistance is placed distal to the knee.

Capsular Restraints

The posterior medial and lateral "corners" of the knee-joint capsule play an important role in the control of torsional forces through the knee. The posteromedial capsule is supported by the semimembranosus muscle and the oblique popliteal ligament, which is an expansion of the tendon of the semimembranosus.[207] The posterior medial corner provides some restraint to valgus stresses when the knee is in extension,[85] but it is primarily involved in the control of internal torsional stresses.[148]

The posterolateral capsule is reinforced by the arcuate ligament and popliteus tendon.[86] The posterior lateral corner, with the LCL, is primarily involved in the control of external rotation stresses; however, in the ACL-deficient knee it also plays a role in controlling internal rotation of the knee.[79, 86] The posterolateral corner plays a minor role in the control of varus stress to the knee when the knee is extended.[86] The posterior capsule is less prone to injury when the knee is in the flexed position because the structure is relatively slack.[85]

In vitro isolated sectioning of the ACL or PCL is generally not associated with rotational instabilities,[79, 85, 86, 127, 148] but when coupled with sectioning of either of the posterior corners, rotational instabilities become apparent. Clinically, this indicates that an athlete with an acute rotational instability probably does not have an isolated cruciate injury.[127]

THE MENISCI

Interposed between the tibia and the femur are the fibrocartilaginous, semilunar menisci of the knee. The superior meniscal surface in contact with the femur is relatively concave to match the convexity of the femur. The inferior meniscal surface in contact with the tibial surface is relatively planar.[207] This configuration of the meniscus improves the congruence of the tibiofemoral joint.[9] Each meniscus covers approximately two thirds of the tibial articular surface.[207] The convex peripheral portion is thick and is attached to the tibial plateau via coronary ligaments.[166] The inner portion of the meniscus tapers to a free concave border, forming a wedge-shaped structure in radial section.[207] The open ends of the menisci are referred to as the anterior and posterior horns.[166, 207] The attachments of the menisci are described in Table 10–5. The lateral meniscus is not as firmly attached as the medial meniscus, allowing it greater freedom of movement.[166]

The collagen fibers of the meniscus are arranged in three layers.[9] The superficial layer in contact with the femur has a woven appearance.[9] The collagen fibers of the middle zone are larger and primarily arranged circumferentially, running

Table 10–5. Attachments of the Meniscus

	MEDIAL MENISCUS	LATERAL MENISCUS
Anterior horn	Anterior tibial intercondylar area Anterior horn of lateral meniscus via transverse ligament	Anterior tibial intercondylar area Anterior horn of medial meniscus via transverse ligament Some fibers blend with tibial attachment of anterior cruciate ligament
Peripheral border	Tibia via coronary ligaments Patella via meniscopatellar ligaments Fibrous joint capsule Deep portion of medial cruciate ligament Semimembranosus insertion	Tibia via coronary ligaments Patella via meniscopatellar ligaments Loosely attached to fibrous joint capsule Popliteus tendon
Posterior horn	Posterior tibial intercondylar area	Posterior tibial intercondylar area Posterior cruciate ligament and medial femoral condyle via meniscofemoral ligaments

Data compiled from Arnoczky, S.P. (1994): Meniscus. *In*: Fu, F.H., Harner, C.D., and Vince, K.G. (eds.): Knee Surgery, Vol. 1. Baltimore, Williams & Wilkins, pp. 131–140; Norkin, C.C., and Levange, P.K. (1992): The knee complex. *In*: Joint Structure and Function: A Comprehensive Analysis, 2nd ed. Philadelphia, F.A. Davis, pp. 337–377; and Soames, R.W. (1995): Skeletal system. *In*: Gray's Anatomy, 38th ed. New York, Churchill Livingstone, pp. 703–704.

from anterior to posterior horns.[9, 25] This circumferential arrangement allows the meniscus to transmit the weight-bearing forces across the joint and resist tensile loads that occur during this function.[9] With weight bearing, there is a compression force between the femur and tibia. Collagen is designed to resist tensile, not compression, forces.[165] The wedge shape of the meniscus would suggest that under this compression force the meniscus would be forced toward the capsule. Because of the way the menisci are anchored, this translates into a tensile load on the circumferential fibers in the middle zone. This has been referred to as hoop stress.[154] The hoop stresses allow for early weight bearing after longitudinal meniscal repairs because the weight-bearing stress actually approximates the sutured edges.[154] In addition to the circumferential collagen fibers in the middle zone, there also some radially aligned collagen fibers that provide structural support and resist longitudinal splitting between the circumferential bundles.[9, 25] In the third layer of the meniscus (the zone next to the tibia), the collagen fibers are arranged primarily in a radial fashion[25] and probably function similarly to the radial fibers in the middle zone.

The peripheral 10% to 30% of the meniscus has a vascular supply from the perimeniscal capillary plexus.[9] The rest of the meniscus, 70% or more, receives nutrition by passive diffusion and mechanical pumping (intermittent compression during joint loading and unloading).[9] Meniscal tears in the vascular zone can be surgically repaired successfully, and this has become the norm in recent years because of the important role the meniscus plays in the health of the knee joint.[9] Extrapolating from animal studies, the tensile strength of the meniscus 12 weeks after repair is approximately 80%.[115]

The meniscus serves a number of important functions that include the following: increasing the stability and congruence of the knee joint,[9, 13, 140] load distribution and transmission,[9, 13, 74, 154] shock absorption,[9, 13] joint proprioception,[9] and aiding in joint lubrication and nutrition.[9, 13] The functions of load distribution, transmission, and shock absorption are probably the most important for joint health. The intact meniscus improves shock absorption of the knee by about 20%.[9] Removal of the meniscus reduces the contact area for the transmission of compression forces between the femur and tibia; there is subsequently a significant increase in force per unit area between the two articular surfaces.[74] This increase in force per unit area likely leads to the degenerative changes seen after removal of the meniscus. These changes include loss of joint space, flattening of femoral condyles, formation of a ridge on the lateral edge of the femoral condyle,[62] and other arthritic changes.[154]

There is some movement of the menisci during tibiofemoral motion; however, this "movement" is probably more of a distortion of the meniscus because of the fixed attachment of the horns.[166] During flexion, the menisci "move" posteriorly because of the posterior shear created by the oblique reaction force between the femur and the meniscus.[166] In addition, contraction of the semimembranosus and popliteus muscles during active knee flexion also assists in distorting the posterior portion of the meniscus posteriorly.[111, 145] During knee extension the posterior portion of the meniscus returns to the original position, whereas the anterior portion distorts anteriorly.[166] The anterior distortion occurs because the shear from the oblique reaction force between the femur and meniscus is now directed anteriorly.[166] Tension in the meniscopatellar ligaments created by contraction of the extensor mechanism also assists in this anterior distortion.[110, 111] In summary, during flexion and extension of the knee, the direction of meniscal distortion follows the direction of tibial plateau movement.

During internal and external rotation of the knee, the menisci distort in opposite directions. With internal rotation of the femur on the tibia, the medial meniscus distorts posteriorly, whereas the lateral meniscus distorts anteriorly.[110] The opposite occurs during external rotation of the femur on the tibia. The direction of meniscal distortion during rotation is determined by the direction of femoral condyle movement. This means that during combined flexion-extension and internal-external rotation movements, the distortions for the anterior and posterior portions of one meniscus are in opposite directions, whereas in the other meniscus these portions "move" primarily in the same direction. This is the reason for combined flexion and rotation being a frequent cause of injury to the meniscus.[8]

PATELLOFEMORAL BIOMECHANICS

It is important to understand patellofemoral biomechanics when prescribing knee exercises for a rehabilitation program, regardless of the diagnosis. The connection between the tibiofemoral and patellofemoral joints must not be overlooked, nor should these joints be treated independently. Ignoring important aspects of the biomechanics of the patellofemoral joint during rehabilitation of a tibiofemoral joint problem frequently creates patellofemoral joint problems and unnecessarily extends the rehabilitation process.

The function of the patellofemoral joint mechanism is strongly influenced by both the dynamic (contractile structures) and the static (noncontractile structures) stabilizers of the joint. This stability is based on the interplay among bony geometry, ligamentous-retinacular restraints, and muscles.[102] A dynamic stabilizer, the quadriceps femoris is made up of four muscles all innervated by the femoral nerve. The four muscles are the vastus lateralis (VL), vastus intermedius, rectus femoris, and vastus medialis. The vastus medialis has two heads, the more superior longus head and the more inferior obliquus head.[133] Each head of the vastus medialis has its own innervating branch from the femoral nerve.[104, 133] The vastus medialis longus (VML) is described as having fibers of a vertical orientation, deviating medially from the long axis of the femur by about 18°,[132] whereas the vastus medialis obliquus (VMO) fibers are more horizontal, with a medial deviation from the long axis of the femur of about 55°.[132] The VL fibers deviate laterally from the long axis of the femur by about 12° for the more central fibers and approximately 40° for the more lateral fibers.[104, 132] The vastus intermedius fibers lie parallel to the long axis of the femur.[104] The alignment of these muscles determines their function at the knee joint. The VL, vastus intermedius, VML, and rectus femoris all produce a knee extension torque. The VMO is incapable of producing any knee extension[132] but has an extremely important role in providing the joint with a dynamic restraint to forces that would laterally displace the patella.[68, 101, 132, 133, 183] The pes anserinus muscle group and biceps femoris also dynamically affect patellar stability, because they control tibial internal and external rotation, which can significantly influence patellar tracking.[107, 183]

The static stabilizers of the patellofemoral joint include the more anteriorly projected lateral side of the femoral sulcus, the extensor retinaculum (with the associated patellofemoral and patellotibial ligaments), iliotibial tract, quadriceps tendon, and patellar tendon (Fig. 10–3). The lateral retinaculum and iliotibial tracts provide stability against medially displacing forces, whereas the medial retinaculum and lateral side of the femoral sulcus provide stability against laterally displacing forces.[232] The passive soft-tissue structures that resist medial displacement of the patella are thicker and stronger than the passive soft-tissue structures that resist laterally displacing forces.[75] The patellar tendon controls superiorly displacing forces on the patella, whereas the quadriceps tendon resists forces causing inferior displacement of the patella.

The tracking pattern of the patella has been analyzed in cadaveric studies[78, 188, 225] as well as in in vivo studies with imaging instrumentation.[126] One in vivo investigation even used implanted intracortical pins with reflective markers that were tracked with video cameras.[121] Summarizing the above work, it appears

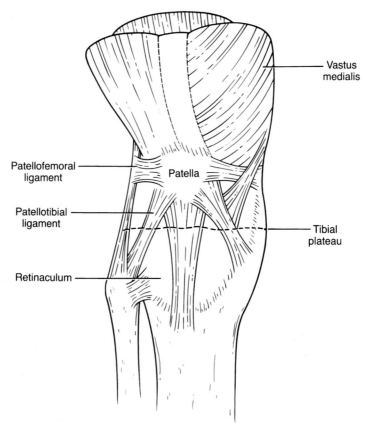

Figure 10–3. Static and dynamic supports of the patellofemoral joint. (From Woodall, W., and Welsh, J. [1990]: A biomechanical basis for rehabilitation programs involving the patellofemoral joint. J. Orthop. Sports Phys. Ther., 11:536, © by the Orthopedic and Sports Physical Therapy Section of the APTA.)

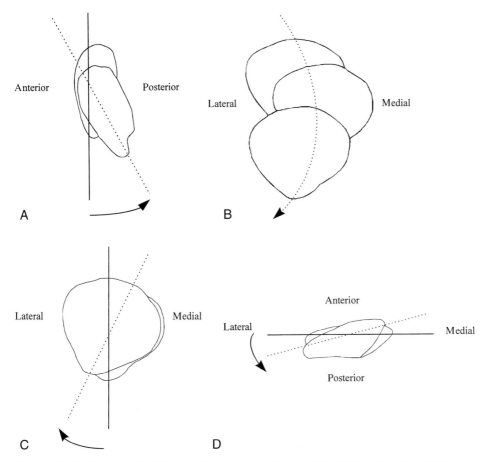

Figure 10–4. Movements of the patella during knee flexion. *A,* Sagittal section of patella demonstrating patellar flexion. *B,* Anterior view of the patella in frontal plane demonstrating patellar shift. *C,* Anterior view of the patella in frontal plane demonstrating patellar rotation. *D,* Transverse section of the patella demonstrating patellar tilt.

that in the sagittal plane the patella flexes 65° to 75° during knee flexion (Fig. 10–4*A*). This flexion lags behind the flexion of the tibia. The patella moves in a C-shaped pattern in the frontal plane, beginning in a lateral position in full knee extension, shifting medially through approximately the first 40° of knee flexion, followed by a lateral shift as flexion of the knee continues (Fig. 10–4*B*). The patella also rotates laterally in the frontal plane as flexion increases (Fig. 10–4*C*). In the transverse plane, the patella tilts laterally approximately 12° as the knee moves into flexion (Fig. 10–4*D*). Because the patella is attached to the tibial tubercle via the patellar tendon, the transverse plane position (internal-external rotation) of the tibia appears to have a strong influence on the amount of tilt, shift, and rotation of the patella.[121, 225] External tibial rotation leads to increases in lateral tilt, lateral shift, and external rotation of the patella, whereas the opposite occurs with internal tibial rotation.[225] As discussed earlier, the contact points between the patellar and femoral articular surfaces and the contact area of these points are determined by the amount of knee flexion.[99, 102, 214]

The function of the patellofemoral joint depends on the ability of the joint to control sagittal and frontal plane forces. Three factors play an important role in the sagittal plane mechanics of the patellofemoral joint: the magnitude of the posteriorly directed resultant force vector, the impact of gravity on quadriceps force, and the contact area between the patella and the femur. To fully appreciate these factors, a brief discussion of basic biomechanics is necessary. (For more comprehensive information regarding vector resolution and other subjects, see Leveau.[129a]) The contraction of the quadriceps creates a superiorly directed force that is resisted by an inferiorly directed force from the patellar tendon. Resolution of these two forces leads to a posteriorly directed resultant force vector that causes compression between the patella and femur (Fig. 10–5). The magnitude of this resultant force vector, and thus the compression force, is influenced by the angle of knee flexion and the force of the quadriceps contraction. For any constant quadriceps force, as knee flexion increases, so does the resultant force vector and, therefore, the patellofemoral compression force. At any given angle of knee flexion greater than 10°, as the quadriceps contraction force increases, so does the resultant force vector and, along with it, the patellofemoral compression force.[102, 190] The compression force is known as the patellofemoral joint reaction force (PFJR).[102, 190, 214] Therefore, the PFJR is influenced by the amount of knee flexion and the amount of force produced by the quadriceps contraction. It is important to realize that at angles less than 30° even rather large quadriceps forces do not produce tremendous compression forces because the angle between the quadriceps and the patellar tendon forces is small. This means that the posteriorly directed resultant force vector will also be small.[102, 190]

During rehabilitation activities, gravity has a profound influence on the force of the quadriceps. The force of gravity acts through the center of gravity, which, in an open-chain activity, is found on the side of the moving segment. For example, in a seated knee-extension exercise, the center of gravity will be found on the tibial side of the knee. The exact location of the center of gravity will vary with the amount of load on the leg, but for any constant load, the location of the center of gravity will remain constant for that segment. In the seated position with the knee at 90°, the center of gravity is aligned with the axis of the knee in such a way that it creates no rotation of the knee (Fig. 10–6). In other words, the quadriceps does not need to contract against the force of gravity in order to maintain the knee in this position. During knee extension, the leg moves toward a position in which it is parallel to the ground. As this occurs, the resistance by gravity will increase and reach its maximum when the leg is parallel to the ground (Fig. 10–7). Therefore, in order to extend the knee in this position, the quadriceps must produce an increasing amount of force, with the greatest force required when the resistance of gravity is greatest (knee in full extension). Experimentally, the increase in the force of the quadriceps appears

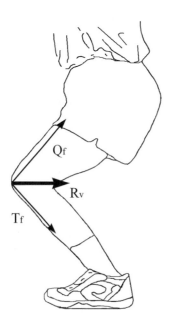

Figure 10–5. Resolution of quadriceps force (Qf) and patellar tendon force (Tf) produces a posteriorly directed resultant force (Rv).

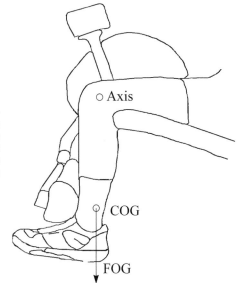

Figure 10–6. During an open-chain knee extension exercise, when the leg is perpendicular to the ground, the center of gravity (COG) is positioned such that the force of gravity (FOG) causes no rotation about the axis of the knee joint (Axis). Therefore, no quadriceps contraction is required to maintain this position.

to plateau[102] between 50° and 20° before rising to the peak force at full extension.[102, 190] During the seated knee-extension exercise, as the quadriceps force increases, so does the PFJR. While the knee is extending, the patella is moving superiorly in the femoral sulcus. Therefore, the contact area between the femur and the patella decreases as extension progresses. The combination of increasing PFJR and decreasing contact area leads to significantly higher patellofemoral joint contact stresses.[102, 190, 214] Patellofemoral joint contact stress is defined as the compression force applied per unit area of contact. The maximal contact stress peaks at approximately 35° to 40° and then declines as extension continues, because of the reduced angle of the knee.[102, 190] The contact stress is influenced by increases or decreases in the Q angle, which can produce nonuniform pressure distribution with higher peak stresses in some areas and relative unloading in others.[99] The contact stress is negligible from about 10° to full extension because of the loss of contact between the patella and the femur.[102, 214] In full extension, the patella rests on the supratrochlear fat pad.[75] Reilly and Martens[190] have calculated the compression force created by a straight leg raise to be 0.5 times

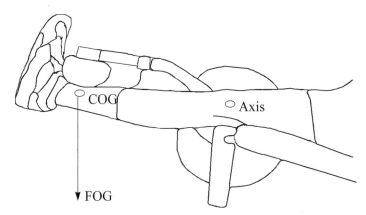

Figure 10–7. During an open-chain knee extension exercise, when the leg is parallel to the ground, the center of gravity (COG) is positioned about the knee joint axis (Axis) such that the force of gravity (FOG) creates the greatest resistance to knee extension.

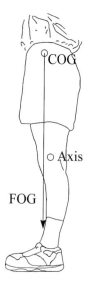

Figure 10–8. During standing, the center of gravity (COG) is normally positioned such that the force of gravity (FOG) falls just anterior to the knee joint axis (Axis). The knee can therefore be maintained in extension without contraction of the quadriceps.

BW. This compression force is absorbed between the patella, supratrochlear fat pad, and femur.

Analyzing a closed-chain activity such as a squat reveals a different result. During a squat the center of gravity is now on the femur side of the knee. The exact location of the center of gravity will vary with the load and also with the position of the body segments. For the purposes of this explanation consider the center of gravity to be just anterior to the S2 sacral body. In standing with the knee in full extension and the center of gravity positioned anterior to S2, the force line of gravity falls on or just anterior to the axis of the knee joint (Fig. 10–8).[166] This means that to maintain the knee in this position will require little or no quadriceps force. As the squat is performed, the force line of gravity will fall posterior to the axis of the knee, creating knee flexion. The greatest flexion moment created by gravity will occur when the force line of gravity is farthest from the knee-joint axis (Fig. 10–9). This typically occurs when the femur is

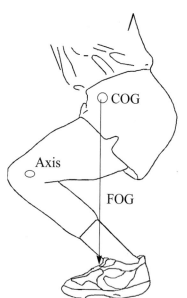

Figure 10–9. During a squat, the center of gravity (COG) and, therefore, the force of gravity (FOG) fall posterior to the knee joint axis (Axis). The farther posterior to the axis the FOG falls, the greater the resistance to knee extension.

parallel to the ground. To control knee flexion, the force of the quadriceps will have to increase as the flexion moment of gravity becomes greater. Thus during this activity, the quadriceps force increases, whereas the flexion angle increases. This causes an increase in PFJR. However, in this activity, as the PFJR is increasing, the contact area between the patella and femur is increasing. This leads to a more constant load per unit area, which the joint is better designed to tolerate.[76] The reverse occurs on return to the upright position; as the angle of knee flexion is reduced, the flexion moment of gravity decreases (force line of gravity is shifting toward the knee-joint axis) and so does the quadriceps force. This leads to a reduction in PFJR. Hungerford and Barry[102] have suggested that these relationships for closed-chain activities produce a more physiologic loading of the patellofemoral joint compared to the loading that occurs during open-chain activities.

Figure 10–10 is a graphic representation of data from several studies of the patellofemoral contact stress versus knee flexion angle for both open- and closed-chain activities.[102, 190, 214] The lines for open- and closed-chain contact stress cross at approximately 50°. These data suggest that for the athlete with an extensor mechanism problem, open-chain strengthening activities for the quadriceps are safest from 90° to 50° and 10° to 0°, whereas closed-chain activities are safest from 50° to 0°. This must be individualized for those athletes with known chondral defects of the patella or femoral sulcus. The key to choosing activities for these patients revolves around choosing activities that minimize loading in the region of the chondral defect. Mangine[141] has suggested that the rehabilitation program be oriented around the area of crepitus. Performing loaded knee extension exercises through an area of crepitus should be avoided, because frequently this is the arthrosis area, and adding weight only perpetuates the crepitus. Even use of the traditional open-chain terminal knee extension can sometimes be detrimental; it may be preferable to perform this activity in the closed-chain position (Fig. 10–11).

Table 10–6 contains the calculated PFJR data for a variety of rehabilitation

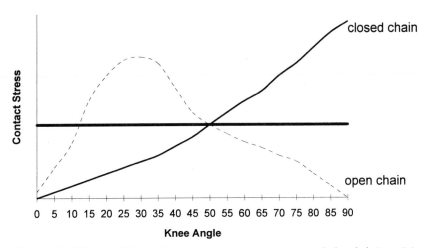

Figure 10–10. Patellofemoral contact stresses during open- and closed-chain activities. Area below horizontal line indicates relatively low contact stresses, a potentially "safe" zone. The area above the horizontal line indicates relatively high contact stresses, and therefore is potentially an "unsafe" zone. (Graph developed from data reported by Hungerford, D.S., and Barry, M. [1979]: Biomechanics of the patellofemoral joint. Clin. Orthop., 144:9–15; Reilly, D.T., and Martens, M. [1972]: Experimental analysis of the quadriceps muscle force and patellofemoral joint reaction force for various activities. Acta Orthop. Scand., 43:126–137; and Steinkamp, L.A., Dillingham, M.F., Markel, M.D., et al. [1993]: Biomechanical considerations in patellofemoral joint rehabilitation. Am. J. Sports Med., 21:438–444.)

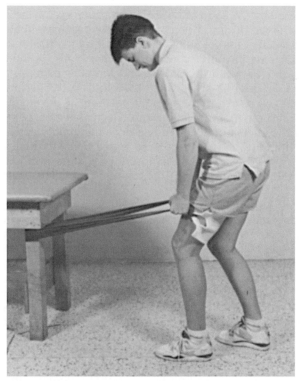

Figure 10–11. Closed-chain terminal knee extension.

Table 10–6. Patellofemoral Compressive Forces During Various Activities*

REFERENCES	ACTIVITY	KNEE POSITION AT PEAK PATELLOFEMORAL COMPRESSIVE FORCE	CALCULATED FORCE TIMES BODY WEIGHT
Dahlkvist et al[37]	Squat, slow ascent	45°	4.73
	Squat, slow descent		7.41
	Squat, fast ascent	55–60°	5.99
	Squat, fast descent	60°	7.62
Ericson and Nisell[58]	Cycling, 60 RPM, 120 W workload	83°	1.3
Flynn and Soutas-Little[67]	Forward running	35% of stance phase	5.6
	Backward running	52% of stance phase	3.0
Huberti and Hayes[99]	Squat	90°	6.5
Kaufman et al[114]	Isokinetic knee extension 60°/sec	70°	5.1
	Isokinetic knee extension 180°/sec	80°	4.9
Reilly and Martens[190]	Walking	8°	0.5
	Straight leg raise	0°	0.5
	Knee extension with 9-kg weight boot	36°	1.4
	Ascending and descending stairs	40–60°	3.3
	Deep squat	135°	7.6
Scott and Winter[199]	Running	Midstance	7.0–11.1

*Because of the change in patellofemoral contact area at different points in the range of motion, it is appropriate to compare activities that occur only in similar ranges of motion.

activities. Care must be taken in interpreting the data in this table, as these data do not account for the contact area through which the PFJR is being applied. Direct comparison of two activities should be made only between activities with peak compression forces at similar angles of knee flexion and, therefore, similar contact areas. For example, it is misleading that knee extension with a 9-kg weight boot and cycling appear to have similar PFJR values (1.4 and 1.3, respectively). Considering that the patellofemoral contact area is greater at 83° than at 36°, the patellofemoral joint contact stress will be much greater for the knee-extension exercise. In fact, the patellofemoral contact stress for knee extension with 9 kg has been calculated to be as high as eight times the contact stress during a squat at 40°.[102]

Forces between the patellar tendon and quadriceps muscle are not equal throughout the knee ROM[198]—these forces are equal only at approximately 45°.[24] During terminal extension exercises, the force developed in the patellar tendon is greater than that of the quadriceps because of the mechanical advantage of the quadriceps, so this exercise may cause local irritation of the patellar tendon. It may be necessary for the athlete to avoid exercising within this range during certain stages of patellofemoral rehabilitation.[149]

The frontal plane forces that must be balanced by the extensor mechanism also originate from forces developed by the quadriceps. As with the sagittal plane forces, the contraction of the VL, vastus intermedius, rectus femoris, and VML produces a superiorly directed force that is resisted by an inferiorly directed force from the patellar tendon. In the frontal plane these two opposing forces do not form a straight line but instead form an angle similar to the physiologic valgus angulation between the femur and the tibia (Fig. 10–12).[76] Resolving these two forces provides a resultant force that is directed laterally. This resultant force is referred to as a valgus vector.[76] Thus, when the VL, vastus intermedius, rectus femoris, and VML contract in concert, the patella has a tendency to shift laterally.[76, 78, 132] This tendency toward lateralization is dynamically balanced by the VMO[76, 78, 132] with assistance from the static restraints of the medial portion of the extensor retinaculum. Once the patella is seated in the femoral sulcus, the lateral wall of the sulcus will also assist in resisting the laterally directed resultant force vector.[76, 192]

Several factors have been suggested to influence the magnitude of this valgus

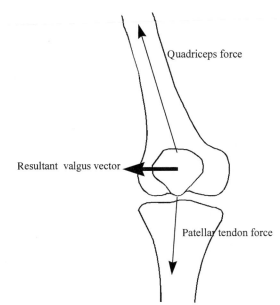

Quadriceps force

Resultant valgus vector

Patellar tendon force

Figure 10–12. Frontal plane valgus vector created by the resolution of the quadriceps and patellar tendon forces.

vector, including hip position, extensibility of lateral retinacular structures, competence of medial retinacular structures, femoral and tibial alignment, knee-joint effusion, foot position, and ineffective firing or weakness of the VMO. Excessive hip internal rotation during loading response (foot-flat) in walking or running causes a functional increase in the physiologic valgus of the femur and tibia.[16, 96] This leads to a greater valgus vector, which increases the likelihood of the patella to track laterally. Several factors can contribute to excessive hip internal rotation during gait, including weakness of the gluteus medius, tightness of the tensor fasciae latae, weakness of the hip lateral rotators, and excessive foot pronation.[16, 96] Tightness in the lateral retinaculum is associated with lateral compression syndrome of the patellofemoral joint.[16, 76] Loss of static restraint from the medial retinacular structures can also allow for an increased tendency of the patella to track laterally.[76]

Lower extremity bony malalignment can contribute to an increased valgus vector. Such malalignments would include genu valgus, anteversion of the femoral neck, and external tibial torsion.[16, 96, 104, 195] Hughston[104] referred to the combined femoral neck anteversion and external tibial torsion as the "treacherous extensor mechanism malalignment." Varus deformity of the foot that leads to excessive pronation during gait is another lower extremity alignment problem that contributes to an increased valgus vector.[16, 52] Eng and Pierrynowski[52] reported that the use of a soft foot orthosis with medial posting was effective in reducing the pain in patients with symptomatic patellofemoral pain syndrome with varus foot deformities.

Knee-joint effusion, even in absence of pain or trauma, has been documented to cause reflex inhibition of the quadriceps. The vastus medialis H-wave response is affected with as little as 20 ml of effusion, whereas the VL is not affected reflexively until there is 50 ml of effusion.[211] This would seem to suggest that the vastus medialis (Spencer et al[211] made no distinction between the VML and the VMO) is more inhibited by knee-joint effusion than is the VL. It would appear that even a relatively small amount of effusion would reduce the ability of the VMO to offset the laterally directed pull by the rest of the quadriceps, the VL in particular.

There is currently no way to test the strength of the VMO in isolation from the rest of the quadriceps, so it is impossible to directly measure isolated weakness in the VMO. Because of this, researchers have used electromyography to quantify the firing patterns and behaviors of the heads of the quadriceps. In particular, attention has centered around the firing patterns of the VMO and VL and the VMO-to-VL ratios.[30, 43, 44, 89, 92, 112, 113, 197, 226, 233] These studies have been anything but conclusive. Findings reported by Voight and Weider[226] suggested that in persons without patellofemoral pain syndrome, the VMO fires significantly faster than the VL, whereas in patients with patellofemoral pain, the VL fires first. These results were not supported in a more recent study by Karst and Willett,[113] in which no significant difference in VMO and VL firing patterns was found when symptomatic and nonsymptomatic individuals were compared. In support of their results, Karst and Willet reported a statistical power of 0.86 with an alpha level of 0.05. The VMO-to-VL ratio for both symptomatic and asymptomatic individuals engaged in a variety of open- and closed-chain activities has been reported to be approximately 1:1 in two studies[30, 197] and 2:1 in another.[233] The discrepancy between these results is due to the large individual variability in the VMO-to-VL ratio even within the normal asymptomatic population.[233] In normal individuals, Worrell and coworkers[233] reported a range of VMO-to-VL ratios from 0.35 to 17.21. In addition to the apparently wide variability within the normal population, reliability of the measurement is also problematic with reported intraclass correlation coefficients as low as 0.40.[233]

Because of the role of the VMO in balancing lateral displacement forces, the quest of patellofemoral rehabilitation has been to find activities that isolate or preferentially recruit the VMO. In this search, the results have been anything but uniform.[30, 43, 44, 89, 112, 197, 233] Reasons for this relate to differences in experimental technique, difficulty attaining reliable measures, and the apparent large variability in recruitment patterns even in normal individuals.

There is some evidence in the literature that suggests that closed-chain exercise may positively influence the tracking of the patellofemoral joint.[43, 44, 106] Ingersoll and Knight[106] compared the patellar tracking angles in a group of normal subjects trained in biofeedback and in a program using both open- and closed-chain activities with a group of normal individuals performing a program entirely of open-chain progressive-resistance exercises. The group performing the combination open- and closed-chain exercises with biofeedback had improved tracking measures, whereas the open-chain-only group actually had an increase in lateral glide. Doucette and Child[43] investigated the patellar congruency angle, using computed tomography, during an open-chain and a closed-chain activity in patients with lateral compression syndrome. In the closed-chain activity, the patellar congruence angle was improved compared to the open-chain activity at knee angles of 0°, 10°, and 20°. Their results also suggest that patellar tracking during open-chain activities improves with greater amounts of flexion. They concluded that open-chain exercise appeared to be more appropriate at angles greater than 30° of flexion, which corresponds to the "safer" ranges of patellofemoral joint contact stresses for open-chain activities.[43, 102, 214]

The preceding discussion has suggested that there are "safe" ranges to perform open- and closed-chain exercises. This would imply that there are "unsafe" ranges as well. These "safe" and "unsafe" ranges should be used only as a guide, with the truly detrimental ranges and loads being determined by the signs and symptoms of the athlete. In dealing with the extensor mechanism there are two basic caveats: the first is "if it hurts or increases effusion, don't do it" and the second is "only perform the activity in the ranges and with the loads in which the athlete has complete control." Often, the symptomatic athlete with patellofemoral problems will experience pain and an increase in symptoms if exercises are performed in the suggested "unsafe" ranges. As the athlete improves, he or she will typically tolerate loads through greater ranges without symptoms. The decision of how to progress through the exercise program should be based on what the athlete can perform without pain and symptoms and under complete control. Most athletic endeavors will require the athlete to tolerate loads through a wide ROM. Therefore, in the late stages of the rehabilitation process, it is often necessary to perform activities in the "unsafe" ranges if the athlete is to tolerate these activities upon return to competition. The use of full-arc knee extension should be used sparingly, if at all, and should be monitored closely if it is used, even in normal knees, to prevent this exercise's contributing to or perpetuating patellofemoral pathology.

MUSCLE FUNCTION

Much of the literature on muscle function has addressed the quadriceps muscles because of their importance to the function of the knee joint, but little information is available about the hamstrings because of their comparatively lesser role in knee control.[208] The hamstrings function to flex the knee and produce tibial rotation. The biceps femoris rotates the tibia externally, and the semimembranosus and semitendinosus rotate the tibia internally. Because of the insertion of the hamstrings on the tibia, they can act as dynamic restraints in ACL-deficient knees. The neuromuscular development of the hamstrings is important in helping deter tibial translation. In the presence of anterolateral rotatory instability or anteromedial rotatory instability, facilitation of enhanced neuromuscular control of the biceps femoris (anterolateral rotatory instability) and of the semimembranosus and semitendinosus (anteromedial rotatory instability), respectively, may help deter abnormal tibial excursion. Additionally, the popliteus muscle is responsible for tibial internal rotation when initial flexion occurs from knee extension, producing the unlocking of the screw-home mechanism.[139]

The quadriceps are considered the primary dynamic stabilizers of the knee and are responsible for knee extension. The isometric peak torque for the knee extensors has been recorded to be highest at 45° of flexion.[206] The influence of hip position on the rectus femoris during knee extension[32, 179] and a straight leg raise[64] has also been investigated. Electromyographic (EMG) results on the role of the rectus femoris in the sitting position conflict somewhat, but it is evident that the rectus femoris and vasti muscles act simultaneously during supine knee extension.[32, 179] It does appear from EMG studies, however, that in the sitting position the rectus femoris functions only in the terminal phase of knee extension.[32, 64] Fisk and Wells[64] have also noted high levels of EMG activity in the rectus femoris during the initial range of the straight leg raise and throughout hip flexion with the knee flexed.

The straight leg raise, isometric quadriceps contraction (quad set), and knee-extension exercise are typical therapeutic exercises prescribed after knee injury or surgery. It appears that total quadriceps activity is greatest during a quad set[82] when compared with that during the straight leg raise or unweighted knee-extension exercise.[185] Soderberg and Cook[209] have reported EMG data of the rectus femoris and vastus medialis from 40 normal subjects, in whom the straight leg raise was compared with quad sets. They noted an increase in rectus femoris activity with a straight leg raise and an increase in vastus medialis activity when a quad set was performed. Karst and Jewett[112] recorded EMG activity from the VMO, VML, vastus lateralis, and rectus femoris and noted that during the straight leg raise the activity for the rectus femoris was consistently higher than the activity of the vasti muscles. The reverse was true during the quad set. This relationship was also true for straight leg raise with the hip in external rotation or straight leg raise while resisting an abducting force, and there was no preferential recruitment of the VMO for either of these straight leg raise conditions. Their conclusion was that if the goal was to address the vasti group, the quad set was a better exercise than the straight leg raise.

Probably the most comprehensive investigation of quadriceps activity during different rehabilitation exercises was done by Cerny.[30] In this study EMG activity was measured from the VMO, VL, and adductor magnus during more than 20 exercises in both normal individuals and patients with patellofemoral pain. The exercises with the greatest quadriceps EMG activity in this study appear to be quad sets and step-downs. Cerny concluded that none of the exercises studied selectively recruited the VMO in either normal individuals or patients with patellofemoral pain syndrome.

It is extremely difficult to compare the EMG data among different studies because of differing experimental techniques. For instance, results from studies using needle EMG will probably be markedly different from results from studies using surface EMG. Another example is that for comparisons within a study, the EMG data of muscle activity during an exercise is expressed as a percentage of the EMG measurement from a maximal voluntary contraction, and unless two investigators use identical parameters to determine the maximal voluntary contraction EMG value, their data will most likely be different.

There has been much debate about the different roles of the quadriceps musculature, especially the VMO, in the various ranges of motion. Historically, it was accepted that the VMO was responsible for terminal knee extension. Some of this interpretation was based on the fact that the atrophy of the vastus medialis is more visible because of the normal prominence of the muscle and the thinness of its fascial covering compared to the fascial covering over the VL.[132] This visibility misled clinicians into believing that there was specific, rather than general, quadriceps atrophy. At the same time clinicians noted that patients had difficulty performing terminal knee extension and that an extensor lag was often present.[210] A classic study by Lieb and Perry[133] defined the role of the VMO as a dynamic stabilizer against lateral displacement of the patella. Their study determined that the VMO in isolation could not produce any extension of the knee. Each of the other parts of the quadriceps, in isolation, could produce knee extension. Interestingly, this study was performed in 1968, and confusion still lingers over the role of the VMO. Some of this confusion can be related to the subtlety of the function of the VMO in relation to the other quadriceps muscles. To place the above factors in some kind of working perspective and summarize the function of the VMO, the following section will briefly review these issues using clinically relevant questions.

Is the VMO active during terminal knee extension? Yes, but so are the other parts of the quadriceps. In fact, the VMO is active through any range of knee extension when the other parts of the quadriceps are active.

Does the VMO become more active during open-chain terminal knee extension compared to open-chain knee extension from 90° to 60°? Yes, but so do the other parts of the quadriceps. It is estimated that the terminal ranges of knee extension require twice as much quadriceps force to accomplish the last 15° of extension.[87, 212] This is because of the lessening of the quadriceps mechanical advantage and improvement in mechanical advantage of gravity.[166]

Is the VMO strengthened with terminal knee extension exercises? Yes, but so are the other parts of the quadriceps. It gets stronger through training, not because it is extending the knee, but because it is contracting against the patellar lateralizing force of the other parts of the quadriceps.

If the VMO is weak in isolation, can that weakness reduce the knee extension torque? Yes, because without the VMO functioning to stabilize the patella, the extension torque created by the other parts of the quadriceps is not being applied through an efficient patellofemoral mechanism.

BIOMECHANICS OF STATIONARY CYCLING

The stationary bicycle has long been advocated for use in knee rehabilitation. It has proven effective in restoring ROM and muscle strength, particularly after knee injury or surgery, and is helpful for cardiovascular conditioning. The bike is generally used long before running can begin, because it subjects the knee to lower tibiofemoral forces than does running. The athlete can strengthen the quadriceps and gastrocnemius using the bicycle.[155] With proper instruction, athletes can be taught to bring into action the hamstrings, hip flexors, and anterior tibialis muscles.

Investigators have examined the compression and shear forces around the tibiofemoral joint during cycling,[57] muscular function during cycling,[56] and the effects of varying seat height and pedal position on muscular forces around the knee.[155] The effect of different exercises on compression and shear forces across the tibiofemoral joint has long been a concern, particularly after ACL reconstruction. Many surgeons fear potential graft failures if these forces are too large and do not recommended early therapeutic exercise. Shear forces acting on the ACL have been studied, however. Henning and Lynch[94] reported that ACL elongation is approximately five times greater during walking on a normal floor than during stationary cycling, and they proposed that rehabilitation progress accordingly in the following sequence: crutch walking, cycling, normal walking, slow running, and fast running. Ericson and colleagues[61] have concluded that the load on the MCL of the knee is also very low during exercise on a bicycle ergometer.

Many investigators have studied compression forces during various types of activity and have estimated tibiofemoral joint compression forces to be two to four times BW during normal walking,[160] four times BW during stair climbing,[7] three to seven times BW when rising from a normal chair,[49, 50] and 2.3 times BW when lifting a 12-kg burden.[48] A maximum tibiofemoral compression force of almost nine times BW was reported during isokinetic knee extension.[163, 164] Ericson and Nisell[57] investigated tibiofemoral shear and compression forces during cycling and reached a number of conclusions:

1. Tibiofemoral joint forces induced during standardized ergometer cycling are low compared with those induced during other daily activities, such as level walking, stair climbing, rising from a chair, and lifting.
2. Compression force is reduced by a decrease in workload or an increase of seat height.
3. Stress on the ACL during cycling is low, and therefore, cycling should be a beneficial exercise in early rehabilitation after ACL repair or reconstruction.
4. The ACL load is decreased by a reduction in workload or by using an anterior rather than a posterior foot position.[57]

Others have examined the effects of muscle force during cycle ergometry. Houtz and Fischer[97] reported that the tensor fasciae latae, sartorius, quadriceps femoris, and tibialis anterior muscles are considered the most important for the cycling motion. More recently, Ericson and associates[60] have quantified quadriceps activity during ergometer cycling and found that the vastus medialis and VL peak activities are 54% and 50% of their respective maximum isometric EMG activity. Rectus femoris muscle activity determined in this study was lower (12% maximum EMG activity) than that of the vastus medialis and VL, probably because of its two-joint function. Ericson and associates[59] also analyzed the net mechanical muscular power output from stationary cycling (Table 10–7). It can be seen that the vasti muscles of the quadriceps benefit the most from stationary cycling, but other muscle groups also benefit.

Table 10–7. Mean Peak Concentric Muscle Power Output During Cycling

MUSCLES	POWER (W)	PERCENTAGE OF TOTAL WORK
Knee extension	110.1	39
Hip extension	74.4	27
Ankle plantar flexors	59.4	20
Knee flexors	30.0	10
Hip flexion	18.0	4

Compiled from data in Ericson, M.O., Bratt, P., Nisell, R., et al. (1986): Power output and work in different muscle groups during ergometer cycling. Eur. J. Appl. Physiol., 55:229.

Table 10–8. Effect of Bicycle Seat Height and Pedal Position on Knee Structures

SEAT HEIGHT AND PEDAL POSITION	EFFECTS OF POSITION ON KNEE STRUCTURES
Normal (high seat and no instruction in pedaling)	Increased gastrocnemius activity; no hamstring activity
Seat low, pedaling with ball of foot	Relies on patellofemoral force to stabilize the femoral tibial position
Low seat, pedaling with heel	Load transmitted to femur posteriorly, through anterior cruciate ligament and meniscotibial ligament to tibia; the greater the posterior angle of the tibia, the greater the load applied to the ligaments
Normal seat height, pedaling with ball of foot	Increased knee extension; ball of foot increases gastrocnemius activity, which enhances the load applied to the anterior cruciate ligament and meniscotibial ligaments; no hamstring activity
Normal seat height, pedaling with heel	No hamstring activity; no increased gastrocnemius activity; increased stress on ligaments
Low seat, pedaling with ball of foot using toe clips	Athlete instructed to pedal by pulling the pedal through at the bottom of the stroke, resulting in increased hamstring activity; this could provide some protection from stress applied to anterior cruciate ligament and meniscotibial ligament

*Compiled from McLeod, W.D., and Blackburn, T.A. (1980): Biomechanics of knee rehabilitation with cycling. Am. J. Sports Med., 8:175–180.

McLeod and Blackburn[155] have studied variations of the inclination of the tibial plateau during cycling and its possible consequences on knee load (Table 10–8). They demonstrated that changing seat height and pedal positions can alter the forces placed on ligaments and other static restraints. They also noted that an insignificant load is transmitted throughout most of the crank angle by the quadriceps. It was concluded that ligaments can be protected from stress if the athlete is taught to pedal so that hamstring activity is enhanced, whereas gastrocnemius activity is reduced. As ligament healing progresses, this situation can be reversed, so that gastrocnemius activity is enhanced and hamstring activity reduced. This allows for controlled stresses to be applied to the ligaments and other connective tissues so that these structures can be strengthened gradually over the rehabilitation period.

The forces transmitted through the tibiofemoral joint are low, but what about the forces transmitted through the patellofemoral joint during ergometric cycling? Ericson and Nisell[58] have calculated forces on the patellofemoral joint and found that patellofemoral joint forces increase with increased workload or decreased seat height. Different pedaling rates or foot positions do not significantly change these forces.

There is a comparatively low compressive load acting about the knee joint during cycling, as long as the following guidelines are observed (Fig. 10–13):

1. The seat is high and the knee is flexed 15° to 30°.
2. The workload is low to moderate.
3. Pedaling is with ball of the foot using toe clips and a pull-through motion is used at the bottom of the stroke.

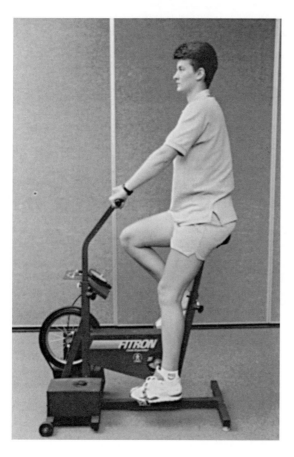

Figure 10–13. Stationary bicycle. This should be adjusted so that the knee is flexed 15° to 30°, and the resistance is low to moderate.

A number of conclusions have been drawn from the results of bicycle ergometer studies in regard to tibiofemoral compression and shear forces and muscular activity:

1. An increased ergometer workload significantly increases compression and shear forces across the patellofemoral joint.
2. Stress on the ACL and other knee ligaments is low but can be further decreased in an anterior foot position.
3. Seat height should be high so that the knee lacks 15° to 30° of extension to decrease patellofemoral compression forces.
4. Controlled stress can be applied to healing ligament restraints to promote collagen strengthening.
5. Seat height and pedal position affect tibiofemoral compression and shear forces.

A high seat height and a low to moderate workload are recommended to decrease patellofemoral compression forces, particularly when the stationary bike is used for conditioning or for athletes with patellofemoral pain. A seat that is too high, however, results in rocking of the pelvis during pedaling.[155] Additionally, when implemented to restore knee ROM, plantar flexing the ankle is a common response to help facilitate a revolution on the cycle and should be considered "cheating." Although this ankle substitution may be used in early stages of restoring motion, it is not recommended in the later stages.

Studies tend to support the efficacy of implementing stationary cycling in early stages of rehabilitation after knee surgery or injury. This excellent therapeutic rehabilitation modality can be used to control tibiofemoral forces, promote strengthening of collagen fibers, restore knee and ankle ROM, enhance muscle strengthening and endurance, and improve cardiovascular conditioning.

AN OVERVIEW OF KNEE REHABILITATION PRINCIPLES

Rehabilitation of the knee has changed drastically over the last 10 years. The greatest change has been to allow for controlled motion and selective strengthening earlier in the rehabilitation process, which ultimately leads to a faster return to athletics. Although this process has been speeded up in most instances, there are certain basic rehabilitation principles that must be followed to ensure optimum results.

Time frames are important in any rehabilitation program to allow for proper healing, but certain goals must be reached within each time frame before the athlete can progress. Throughout this overview, an attempt will be made to address goals that will help determine progression of the athlete during the rehabilitation process instead of relying on specific time frames.

After trauma to the knee, whether from surgery or injury, the initial inflammation process must be addressed, followed by muscle re-education, patella mobility and protection, ROM, strengthening, proprioception, and eventual return to function. Although certain areas can be addressed at the same time, it is critical not to advance the athlete too fast, which would lead to development of additional pain and inflammation as seen with patellofemoral dysfunction. The initial inflammation process can be treated with ice, compression, and elevation. Ice will help in reducing the inflammatory process as well as the pain. A transcutaneous electrical nerve stimulator (TENS) may also be helpful in controlling the pain, especially postsurgically.[109] Anti-inflammatory medications such as nonsteroidal anti-inflammatory drugs may be beneficial in reducing effusion and general synovial inflammation. If the athlete is unable to walk without a limp, he or she should be placed on crutches. If full weight bearing is allowed too soon, an increase in effusion could result, which could delay progression in ROM and quadriceps recruitment.

Early quadriceps recruitment is extremely important and can be initiated as one of the first exercises in a knee rehabilitation program. It has been shown that quadriceps recruitment is severely inhibited after surgery or injury to the knee. Kennedy and colleagues[117] determined that 60 ml of normal saline in the joint will diminish quadriceps recruitment by 30% to 50%. If quadriceps contraction is difficult, electrical stimulation can be used to assist in producing a maximum contraction. Quadriceps recruitment can be monitored by the use of a biofeedback device once recruitment has been established with electrical stimulation. The Myotrac* is an example of a portable biofeedback device that uses surface electrodes to monitor electrical activity in a particular muscle.

Spencer and coworkers[211] suggest that as little as 20 ml of effusion may selectively shut down the vastus medialis, and therefore, the medialis should be the muscle that is targeted when utilizing a biofeedback device. Because of this extreme sensitivity to trauma, contraction of the vastus medialis will ensure contraction of the entire quadriceps group.

Early knee motion after surgery or injury is critical to help prevent joint fibrosis, provide nutrition to the articular cartilage,[137] and initiate controlled

---

*Available from Thought Technology Ltd., Montreal, Quebec, Canada

stress. This stress will help align collagen fibers, providing for a flexible, strong scar promoting the return of normal joint mechanics.[93, 221] Following surgery, continuous passive motion (CPM) devices have been used to assist in the return of motion. It has been reported that CPM devices help increase motion initially, but by the 14th day, knees that did not receive CPM had the same outcome.[175] It is suggested that for a CPM device to be effective, it must be used 8 hours a day.[181] Active ROM can be started as soon as pain allows. Supine heel slides can be performed, but these are sometimes painful because of the contraction of the rectus femoris to assist in flexion of the hip. Seated knee flexion can be performed as well as side-lying flexion. Active-assisted exercise can be very effective because it allows for continued active involvement by the athlete, but he or she can be assisted by an outside force such as a rope and pulley, a towel with supine heel slides, or the clinician. A bike can also be used to assist with ROM, but caution should be used to avoid irritating the patellofemoral joint because of the overall decrease in patellar mobility after trauma. The knee requires approximately 105° to 110° of flexion to complete a revolution on the bike when substitution is not allowed.

Joint mobilization should be initiated at the patellofemoral joint during the early motion phase to help restore normal arthrokinematics.[187] The patella should be mobilized superiorly, inferiorly, medially, and laterally. A decrease in superior and inferior glide will decrease active extension and flexion, respectively. Stretching of the lateral patella retinaculum as described by McConnell[151] will help to decrease the incidence of patellofemoral pain by restoring the normal tilt of the patella. The athlete can be taught these mobilization techniques, and this is sometimes more successful than mobilization by the clinician because the athlete is more relaxed when performing independently.

As the athlete's active ROM is maximized and soft-tissue resistance is felt by the clinician before the athlete feels pain, aggressive passive ROM exercises can be performed (Table 10–9). Extension is usually the most difficult motion to restore, and it is critical in achieving a normal gait. Assistance in gaining extension can be obtained by placing the athlete prone with the thigh resting on the table, just proximal to the patella. A weight can be added to the lower leg so that a gradual stretch is achieved (Fig. 10–14). Following each therapy session, the knee can be placed on ice while the athlete is in the supine position with the heel elevated to assist with extension (Fig. 10–15). These two methods provide a slow, gradual stretch that will assist in plastic deformation of the tissues that is required to restore motion.[93] Dynamic splinting may be useful in achieving and maintaining motion. There are numerous spring-loaded splints on the market such as Dynasplint* and Ultraflex† (see Chap. 6) that are commonly used to assist with extension but that may also help with regaining flexion. Flexion may

---

*Available from Dynasplint Systems, Inc., Baltimore, Maryland
†Available from Empi, Inc., Clear Lake, South Dakota

Table 10–9. Pain Resistance Sequence

REACTION TO MOVEMENT*	JOINT STATUS	TREATMENT ACTION
Pain before resistance	Acute	Red light—No attempt should be made to gain ROM.
Pain with resistance	Subacute	Yellow light—Gentle attempt can be made to regain ROM, but should be done cautiously. (Vigorous attempts may revert to acute state.)
Resistance before pain	Chronic	Green light—Vigorous intervention may be necessary to restore ROM.

From Wallace, L.A., Mangine, R.E., and Malone, T. (1985): The knee. *In:* Gould, J.A. III, and Davies, G.J. (eds): Orthopaedic and Sports Physical Therapy. St. Louis, C.V. Mosby.
*Refers to passive movement through physiologic range.

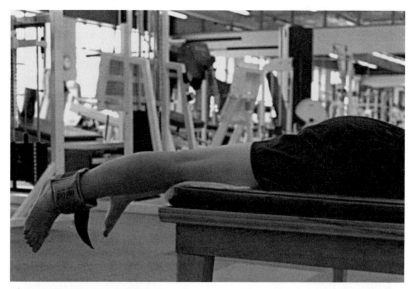

Figure 10–14. Prone passive knee extension with weight.

be increased with the use of supine wall slides (Fig. 10–16). Once the athlete achieves approximately 110° of flexion, supine wall slides are not effective because of the position of the knee and the loss of the effect of gravity. Passive flexion can also be performed by the athlete using his or her BW while sliding forward from a seated position (Fig. 10–17). Isokinetic machines can be used by manually pushing the athlete's leg back as far as pain will allow and then locking the machine in an isometric mode. This will allow for a prolonged sustained stretch. The authors believe the Total Gym* is an excellent way to assist with flexion limitations (Fig. 10–18). The amount of stress that is applied to the knee can be controlled by the athlete's hands, the position of the slide of the board, or the range-limiting protection strap. Joint mobilization by the use of inferior glides of the patella, as previously mentioned, and posterior glides of the tibiofemoral joint may assist in decreasing pain as well as increasing ROM.

Once ROM and recruitment of the vastus medialis are sufficient, strengthening can be initiated. Strengthening should be progressed in a manner that provides

*Available from Engineering Fitness International, San Diego, California

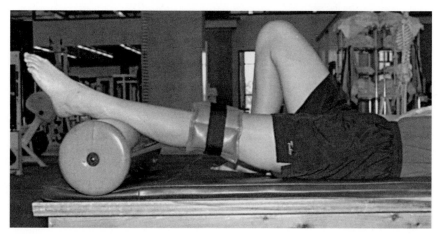

Figure 10–15. Supine passive knee extension with weight.

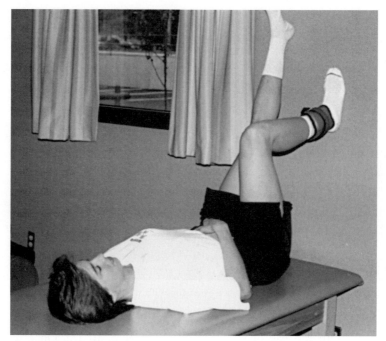

Figure 10–16. Supine wall slides.

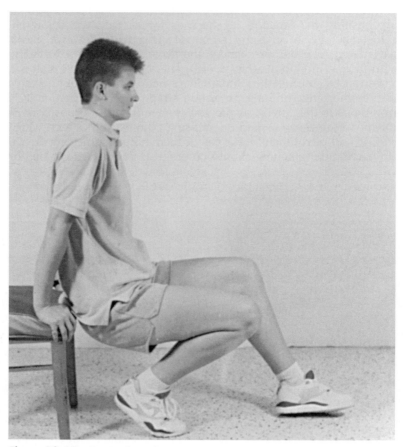

Figure 10–17. Passive knee flexion using body weight.

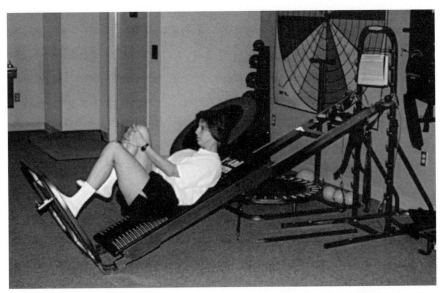

Figure 10–18. Total gym. Passive flexion is controlled by the angle of the slide board or by the range-limiting protection strap.

protection to the healing structures. Initial exercises may consist of four-quadrant leg lifts, multiple-angle isometrics,[218] and supine, as well as prone, terminal knee-extension exercises (Fig. 10–19). Close attention must be paid to the amount of active extension achieved with straight leg raises and supine terminal knee extension. If the athlete is unable to achieve full extension with these exercises, weight should not be added in the open-chain position. Open-chain exercises allow for muscle isolation. This is seen with active leg-extension exercises in which the quadriceps group is primarily responsible for performing the task. As the leg begins to straighten, the mechanical advantage of the patella is lost, and maximum contraction is required to gain full extension. If weight is added too early, strengthening will not occur through the full ROM, and proper quadriceps strengthening will not occur.

When weight bearing is allowed, the athlete can begin performing closed-chain exercises. This type of exercise uses muscles that cross joints both proximally and distally to assist with motion at the desired joint. During a minisquat, the quadriceps as well as the gluteals and soleus assist in extension of the knee, and therefore, less strength is required by the quadriceps to gain full extension.

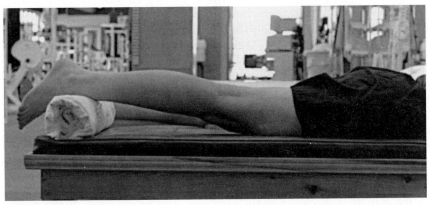

Figure 10–19. Prone terminal knee extension. The quadriceps are assisted in performing knee extension by the hip extensors.

Table 10–10. Example of Closed-Chain Progression of the Minisquat

Weight shifts with support
↓
Weight shifts without support
↓
Bilateral minisquats with support
↓
Bilateral minisquats without support
↓
Bilateral minisquats against wall
↓
Bilateral minisquats against wall with weights in hands
↓
One-legged minisquats with support
↓
One-legged minisquats without support
↓
One-legged minisquats against wall
↓
One-legged minisquats against wall with weight in hands
↓
Bilateral minisquats with tubing
↓
One-legged minisquats with tubing
↓
Gradually increase tubing strength and speed of movement

This allows the athlete to strengthen throughout the full ROM but does not provide for isolated strengthening of a particular muscle. Owing to this lack of isolation, both closed- and open-chain exercises should be used in a manner that provides optimum strengthening of the desired muscle while protecting the healing structures.

The Total Gym, weighted leg press type of machine, and swimming pool all allow the athlete to begin closed-chain exercises when full weight bearing is not permitted. When weight bearing is allowed, a closed-chain progression of the minisquat can be used (Table 10–10). When the athlete begins full weight bearing and there is adequate strength of the quadriceps to achieve full knee extension in the open-chain position, weight can be added with both closed- and open-chain exercises. The daily adjustable progressive-resistance exercise programs as proposed by Knight[120] can be applied if high repetition and low weight are not required to protect the joint and healing structures after surgery (see Chap. 7).

As weight increases with closed-chain exercises, close attention must be paid to the proper performance of the exercises. During closed-chain exercises, each joint is dependent on other joints both proximally and distally to assist in proper body alignment. Examples of this can be seen when an athlete performs a lateral step-up (Fig. 10–20), minisquat, or leg press type of exercise (Fig. 10–21). If the hip is not strong enough to control adduction and internal rotation, the knee will assume a valgus alignment, and the foot will be pronated. This alignment increases the Q angle and predisposes the athlete to patellofemoral pain.

With increased strength of the lower extremity, proprioception exercises can be started. Proprioception, as defined by Sherrington, refers to all neural input from joints, muscles, tendons, and associated deep tissues.[194] Proprioception, also referred to as joint position sense, seems to be primarily determined by muscle spindle receptors. These muscle receptors are assisted in a lesser degree by the cutaneous and joint receptors, thereby providing the neuromuscular control required for a joint to perform efficiently.[194] Proprioception was addressed with the initiation of closed-chain exercises. The progression of the minisquat (see Table 10–10) is an excellent way to introduce the athlete to proprioception

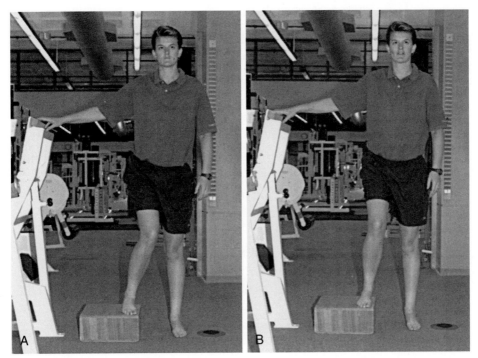

Figure 10–20. Lateral step-up. *A,* Performed incorrectly, allowing the hip to adduct and rotate internally. *B,* Performed correctly.

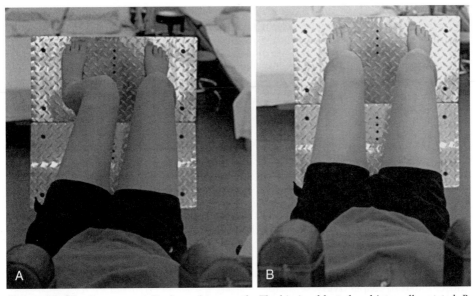

Figure 10–21. Leg press. *A,* Performed incorrectly. The hip is adducted and internally rotated. *B,* Performed correctly.

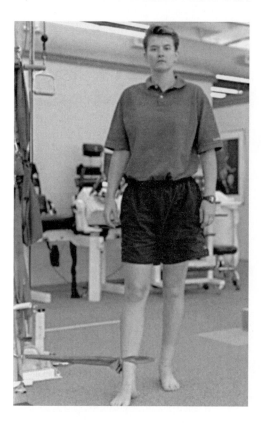

Figure 10–22. Proprioceptive exercise with use of a Thera-Band. The athlete stands on the involved leg and attaches the Thera-Band to the uninvolved ankle. The Thera-Band is pulled in each direction with the uninvolved leg while the involved leg attempts to maintain balance.

exercises. A Thera-Band* attached to the opposite extremity can add an outside force, making the balancing more difficult (Fig. 10–22).

Devices such as the Biomechanical Ankle Platform System (BAPS)† (Figs. 10–23 to 10–25), Slide Board‡ (Fig. 10–26), and Medi-Ball Rebounder,§ can be helpful in assisting the development of proprioception. The Medi-Ball Rebounder can be used by having the athlete stand on the injured leg (stork stand) and bounce the ball off the rebounder. Exercises can become more sport specific as the athlete progresses and comes closer to returning to athletics.

As ROM, strength, and proprioception continue to advance, cardiovascular and muscular endurance must be addressed. The bike can be used to help increase endurance once ROM at the knee is sufficient. Swimming with the use of kickboards, flippers, and resistive paddles can also be helpful in promoting cardiovascular and muscular endurance. Threlkeld and colleagues[218] determined that backward running avoids the rapid initial loading of the knee that occurs with forward running because of the absence of heel strike. This may benefit an athlete who has pain with forward running because of lack of lower extremity control.

Isokinetic equipment may be useful in the development of muscular power and endurance near the end of the rehabilitation process. Caution must be used because of the increase in patellofemoral compression forces as well as the tibial translatory effects seen in open-chain exercises. It is suggested that the last 5° at the end of both flexion and extension be blocked to help prevent hyperflexion and extension, respectively.[221]

Rehabilitation of the knee should offer every possible option to help the

---

*Available from Smith-Nephew, Roylan Inc., Menomonee Falls, Wisconsin
†Available from Camp International, Jackson, Michigan
‡Available from Don Courson Enterprises, Birmingham, Alabama
§Available from Engineering Fitness International, San Diego, California

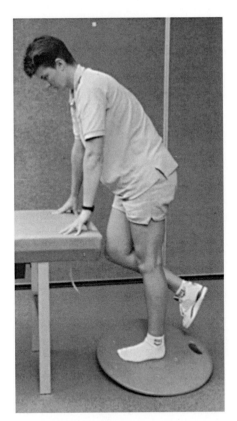

Figure 10–23. Biomechanical ankle platform system. One leg with support.

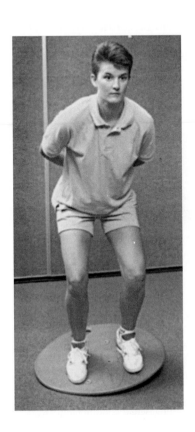

Figure 10–24. Biomechanical ankle platform system. Bilateral balancing.

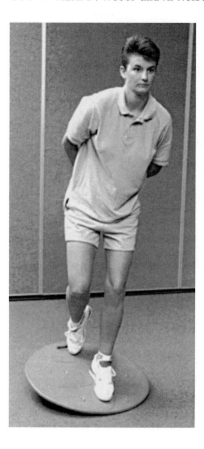

Figure 10–25. Biomechanical ankle platform system. One leg without support.

athlete return to the preinjury level. Each athlete should be constantly evaluated throughout the rehabilitation process so that he or she can progress accordingly. No injuries are identical because every athlete's physical, mental, and healing capabilities are different. Therefore, there are no specific "cookbook" approaches, and each rehabilitation program should be designed to maximize the athlete's potential as quickly and as safely as possible.

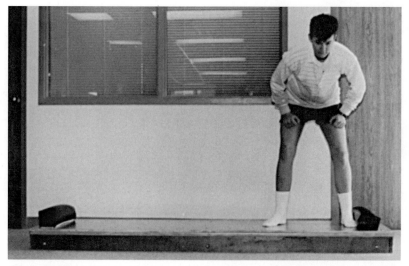

Figure 10–26. Slide board. This can be used to develop muscular strength, proprioception, eccentric firing of the hamstring muscles, and cardiovascular conditioning.

REHABILITATION FOR SPECIFIC KNEE INJURIES

Anterior Cruciate Ligament Injuries

Treatment after ACL injury continues to be one of the most controversial issues in sports medicine. Because of the variability in rehabilitation reported in the literature, we will present an overview using the most accepted guidelines.

Following an injury to the ACL, immediate attention must be given to the hemarthrosis and general inflammatory process. The athlete should be placed on crutches and instructed in partial weight bearing. A brace is not required unless there are other associated injuries such as an MCL sprain. Motion exercises should be started immediately, concentrating on passive extension to help prevent rapid scarring in the intercondylar notch. Full extension also allows for greater ease in quadriceps recruitment, which is extremely important after ACL injury. Friden stated that there is a decrease in quadriceps strength after injury because of defects in afferent inflow from the ACL-deficient knee.[72] It is also thought that the lack of voluntary contraction after ACL injury may be due to reflex inhibition or arthrogenous muscle inhibition.[205] Weight bearing should be increased as pain, effusion, and quadriceps control allow. The athlete can progress to full weight bearing once these goals have been accomplished.

Rehabilitation should progress, with concentration on quadriceps strengthening as well as on neuromuscular control of the hamstrings. Emphasis has previously been placed on strengthening the hamstrings because of their role as the primary dynamic restraint in controlling anterior tibial translation.[88] Recently, however, emphasis has been placed instead on increasing general muscular control. A study by Friden,[72] in which 26 patients with ACL-deficient knees were tested before and after rehabilitation, suggests that there is minimum loss of strength of the hamstrings, and the greatest gains are obtained when both general muscular strength and coordination are addressed. Studies indicate that athletes with complete tears of the ACL experience a decrease in proprioception at the knee.[137] The loss in proprioception may be due to the "ACL-mechanoreceptor reflex arc" to the hamstrings.[137] Beard and colleagues found that the latency of reflex hamstring contraction was twice that of the contralateral limb.[70] Improving recruitment time of the hamstrings may place less stress on the ACL during functional activities.[137] It has been reported that active hamstring control, reducing the pivot shift with an ACL injury, may be the key to successfully avoiding surgery. Therefore, rehabilitation should concentrate on facilitating control of the hamstrings, as opposed to just strengthening in the sagittal plane. Engle and Canner[53–55] have reported success in treating ACL-deficient knees with a program that employs proprioceptive neuromuscular facilitation (PNF) for the hamstrings. PNF and seated Thera-Band exercises (Fig. 10–27) help to incorporate the tibial rotation component of hamstring function. Also, the use of the Slide Board, BAPS, and Medi-Ball Rebounder helps to facilitate hamstring control and knee proprioception, thereby limiting anterior tibial translation during functional activities.

Following an ACL injury, the athlete must decide whether a reconstructive procedure is the treatment of choice. Whether to reconstruct the ACL or treat conservatively continues to be a subject of debate. Noyes and colleagues[177] have used subjective and objective measurements to clinically evaluate 84 individuals with documented ACL lesions. Their conclusion was that an ACL tear leads to functional disability for the majority of patients. They found that one third of the population compensated, knew their limits, and did well; one third compensated (although they could tolerate the condition, they found it aggravating); and one third became worse and needed surgery to correct their instability. Within 12

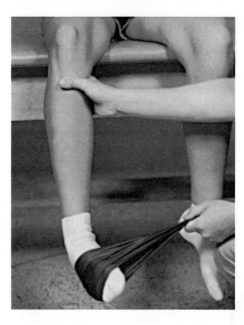

Figure 10–27. External rotation of tibia with tubing to isolate the biceps femoris muscle.

months, 51% of the 84 subjects had a significant "giving-way" episode, 64% had an episode within 24 months, and 44% had multiple reinjuries.[176] With each giving-way episode, the possibility of a meniscal tear or chondral degeneration wear exists.

In a study on the prognosis of partial ACL tears, it was determined that tears of 25% or less, 50%, or 75% of the ligament have a chance of 12%, 50%, or 86%, respectively, of progressing to complete tears. A lack of full active extension may indicate a partial ACL tear.[169]

It is recommended that to have the best knee possible, competitive or recreational athletes need surgical intervention, whereas light recreational athletes who are willing to limit sports may avoid surgery.[167] The nonathlete, who can easily limit activities, may also choose not to have surgery. Clinically, it appears that the competitive athlete does not perform well with an ACL-deficient knee. There are no specific identifying factors that indicate which athletes will function well without surgery.[220, 227] ACL-deficient knees demonstrate abnormal joint kinematics during gait[134] and functional activities,[171] leading to early degenerative changes.[167]

When surgery is the treatment of choice after injury, the ACL must be reconstructed because of the lack of success with a direct repair. Initial concerns include the timing of surgery, graft selection, and surgical technique. Fowler has suggested that surgery should not be performed until knee inflammation has diminished and a full ROM is present.[70]

The ACL can be reconstructed by an extra-articular, an intra-articular, or a combined surgical technique. Extra-articular procedures, which are rarely used, are designed to eliminate the pivot shift but cannot restore normal arthrokinematics through the axis of the normal ACL. These procedures are becoming obsolete as a result of the low success rate in regard to retaining knee stability over time. These poor results are due to a gradual stretching of the tissue. Extra-articular procedures are now mostly used in adolescents with open physis, in whom bone tunnels cannot be drilled through the epiphysis for intra-articular graft placement or for augmenting an intra-articular procedure.

Initial rehabilitation after an extra-articular procedure involves slow restoration of extension. Aggressive extension may cause elongation of the tissues around the repair, resulting in early failure. Most adolescents who underwent an extra-articular repair return for an intra-articular surgical procedure after their physis close. Some surgeons use an intra-articular procedure when the epiphysis is open, drilling smaller holes through the tibia and routing the graft over the top of the femur.

Many types of tissues have been used for intra-articular repairs of the ACL, including autografts (tissue transferred from one part of a person's body to another), allografts (human donor tissue), and prosthetic (synthetic) ligaments. The various types of autografts have different strength characteristics (Table 10–11). Currently, reconstructing the ACL is most commonly performed under arthroscopic guidance using the middle third of the patellar tendon with bone plugs as a free graft. This tissue provides a graft of high tensile strength to compensate for the ACL. Amiel and colleagues,[3] using a rabbit model, showed that after being placed in this ACL environment, the patellar tendon undergoes a "ligamentization" process. By 4 weeks the bone plugs have healed sufficiently for rehabilitation to progress, but 8 weeks may be required if fixation was not adequate.[28] Animal studies on autograft strength over time indicate that most failures occur at the bone attachment site in the first 2 months after surgery. This failure may be at the soft tissue–bone interface or at the bone-to-bone fixation site. After 2 months, failures begin to be predominately in the midsubstance of the tissue.[28]

There has been much debate about the times and percentages of graft strength and revascularization. Initial measurements by Noyes et al,[172] who used on average a 14-mm-wide central-third patellar tendon graft, showed that the grafts averaged 168% of the strength of the ACL at graft harvest. More recently, Cooper et al,[35] who tested 10-mm-wide central-third patellar tendon grafts, reported this graft to be 174% of the strength of the ACL at harvest. A 10-mm-wide graft was used because most surgeons prefer to use this graft width to avoid the problem of graft impingement in the intercondylar notch. Additionally, if the graft is twisted 90°, the ultimate tensile strength in the Cooper model could be increased.[35] On the basis of data from animal models it is generally accepted that the bone–patellar tendon–bone autografts undergo a "ligamentization" process that results in a graft whose vascular and histologic appearance resembles that of a normal ACL at 1 year. [3, 10, 31, 45, 152] The patellar tendon autograft is stronger at implantation than at 4 to 8 weeks after surgery because of avascular necrosis. As revascularization and ligamentization occur, the graft regains strength but does not approach the initial strength advantage over an ACL it had at harvest. Using the medial one third of the patellar tendon in rhesus monkeys, Clancy et al [31] reported transplanted patellar tendon graft strength to be 53% at 3 months, 52% at 6 months, 81% at 9 months, and 81% at 12 months, as compared to an ACL. Noyes[172] suggests that in most strenuous activities, the ACL is seldom exposed to more than 50% of its maximum load.

Patellar tendon allografts appear to undergo the same avascular necrosis

Table 10–11. Strength of Anterior Cruciate Ligament (ACL) Substitutes

GRAFT	PERCENTAGE OF ACL STRENGTH
Patellar tendon	168
ACL	100
Semitendinosus	70
Gracilis	49
Iliotibial band	44
Fascia lata	36
Retinaculum	21

*Compiled from data in Noyes, F.R., Butler, D.L., and Grood, E.S., et al. (1984): Biomechanical analysis of human ligament repairs and reconstruction. J. Bone Joint Surg. [Am.], 66:344.

followed by revascularization and cellular proliferation.[11] Grood[83] believes that the patellar tendon autograft is 35% as strong as the original ACL at 1 year. Patellar tendon allografts are weaker throughout the rehabilitation process, thereby accounting for the differences in the rehabilitation protocols.

Rehabilitation after ACL reconstruction with bone–patellar tendon–bone autograft varies tremendously from surgeon to surgeon. Numerous protocols have been developed, concentrating on early motion, the initiation of closed-chain exercises, full passive extension, and controlled weight bearing. Table 10–12 and Table 10–13 represent protocols for ACL reconstruction using a bone–patellar tendon–bone autograft. Previously, extension exercises were avoided in the terminal ranges of extension in an open-chain position because of the possible stresses that were placed on the graft. The terminal ranges that were avoided varied from 0° to 30°,[47] 0° to 45°,[48] and 0° to 60°.[26]

Accelerated rehabilitation protocols, concentrating on closed-chain exercises as suggested by Shelborne and Nitz, have significantly speeded up the rehabilitation process (Table 10–14).[200] The selection of exercises that produce decreased stress on the ACL is crucial. Henning and colleagues[94] and Beynnon and colleagues[18] have documented exercises that cause different amounts of stress on the ACL, as seen in Tables 10–2 and 10–3. This information is useful in developing exercises at different time frames in the rehabilitation program.

Howell has suggested that active isometric contractions at 15°, 30°, 45°, and 60° produce no more stress on the ACL than does instrumented laxity testing using the KT-1000 (see section on arthrometers later in this chapter) with an 89-N force.[26] Mangine and colleagues have used the KT-1000 7 days postoperatively and throughout the rehabilitation process to document changes in anterior translation as a means of progressing through a rehabilitation program.[144] Although the forces produced by the KT-1000 and by isometric contractions were similar, it is not known what repetitive stress created by exercising at these angles will do over time.

The time frame for progression in rehabilitation of the ACL is quite variable; however, there are areas that must be addressed before the athlete can be allowed to progress, regardless of time. Immediately after surgery, emphasis should be placed on controlling inflammation, maintaining full passive extension, promoting patellar mobility, and increasing quadriceps recruitment. Facilitation of quadriceps recruitment early will help promote increased patellar mobility and prevent patella infra syndrome.[144] Early in the rehabilitation process, the patellar area may be too tender, because of the incision from the graft harvest site, to allow for productive mobilization. Electrical stimulation can be extremely valuable in facilitating a quadriceps contraction great enough to allow for superior mobilization of the patella. During electrical stimulation to assist with patella mobility, the knee should be placed in maximum comfortable extension. Electrical stimulation of minimal to moderate intensity for the purpose of patellar mobility should not be used until the athlete achieves close to full passive extension, because with the knee in flexion and with ROM limitations, a cocontraction of the thigh musculature, rather than quadriceps isolation, may be facilitated. Isolated quadriceps recruitment with the knee in full extension (quad sets) has been established only when there is no active involvement of the hamstrings or gluteals when a quadriceps-setting exercise is performed. If electrical stimulation is being used for quadriceps strengthening, instead of quadriceps re-education and recruitment, flexing of the knee to approximately 65° has been advocated.[204] Active involvement of the vastus medialis and inactivity of the gluteals and hamstrings during a quad set can be confirmed by palpation or with biofeedback devices. If a commercially produced biofeedback device is not available, an ordinary blood pressure cuff can be used. A minimally inflated cuff should be placed under the athlete's heel when quad sets are attempted (Fig. 10–28). When a quad set is performed incorrectly, the pressure reading on the sphygmomanometer will increase because of the activity of the

Text continued on page 374

Table 10–12. Rehabilitation Protocol After Anterior Cruciate Ligament Reconstruction Using Bone–Patellar Tendon–Bone Autograft

	WEEK 1	WEEKS 2–4	WEEKS 5–8	3 MONTHS	4–6 MONTHS	6–12 MONTHS
Functional progression Criteria	Begin PWB with two crutches As postoperative pain allows	Begin WB with one crutch or FWB Full extension during gait Good quadriceps control No increased effusion/edema	Advance strengthening exercises No increased effusion AROM 0–125° Patellar mobility normal	Begin full ROM open-chain quadriceps strengthening Full AROM Normal patellar mobility No increased effusion No patellofemoral pain	Begin jogging No effusion with aerobic exercise Absence of pain	Return to athletics Athlete feels comfortable 85% test results
Evaluation	Pain Effusion Patellar mobility AROM Passive extension Quadriceps recruitment	Pain Gait AROM/PROM Effusion/edema Patellar mobility Quadriceps recruitment Incision/portals	Effusion Patellar mobility AROM/PROM Gait Flexibility Standing balance	AROM Patellar mobility Effusion	Functional testing Isokinetic testing Leg press strength test (1 and 10 RM)	Functional testing Isokinetic testing Leg press strength test (1 and 10 RM)
Treatment	Pain management Control of effusion/edema Mobilization of patella Passive extension Quadriceps electrical stimulation/biofeedback AROM exercises	Pain management Control of effusion/edema Mobilization of patella AROM/PROM Quadriceps electrical stimulation/biofeedback Closed-chain exercise General strengthening exercises (hamstrings, hip, etc.) Scar massage	Flexibility exercises Mobilization of patella AROM/PROM exercise Proprioceptive exercises Endurance exercises Increase resistance with closed-chain exercises	Increase isotonic exercise Aerobic conditioning Isokinetic exercise	Isotonic exercise Aerobic conditioning Sport-specific proprioceptive exercises Isokinetic exercise	Isotonic exercise Aerobic conditioning Sport-specific proprioceptive exercises Isokinetic exercise
Goals	AROM 20–80° Passive extension, 10° 50% WB	AROM 0–110° 75–100% WB Full passive extension	Full AROM No gait deviations Increase strength and endurance	Absence of pain with increased resistance through full ROM 20–30 min biking or ambulation without increased effusion	85% with functional, isokinetic, and isotonic testing	Return to athletics

Adapted from Mangine, R.E., Noyes, F.R., and DeMaio, M. (1992): Minimal protection program: Advanced weight bearing and range of motion after ACL reconstruction: Weeks 1 to 5. Orthopedics, 15:504–515, and DeMaio, M., Mangine, R.E., and Noyes, F.R. (1992): Advanced muscle training after ACL reconstruction: Weeks 6 to 52. Orthopedics, 15:757–767.
AROM, Active range of motion; FWB, full weight bearing; PROM, passive range of motion; PWB, partial weight bearing; RM, repetition maximum; ROM, range of motion; WB, weight bearing.

Table 10–13. Rehabilitation Protocol After Anterior Cruciate Ligament–Patellar Tendon Graft

I. **Phase I: Immediate Postoperative Phase**
  A. Postoperative Day 1
    1. Brace at 0° extension immediately postoperatively
    2. Weight bearing: Two crutches as tolerated (less 50%)
    3. Exercises
      • Ankle pumps
      • Passive knee extension to 0°
      • Straight leg raises
      • Quad sets, gluteal sets
      • Hamstring stretch
    4. Muscle stimulation: Muscle stimulation to quadriceps (4 hours/day) during quad sets
    5. Continuous passive motion (CPM): 0 to 90° as tolerated
    6. Ice and elevation: Ice 20 minutes out of every hour and elevate with knee in extension
  B. Postoperative Days 2–4
    1. Brace locked at 0° extension
    2. Weight bearing: Two crutches as tolerated
    3. Range of motion: Athlete out of brace four to five times daily to perform self ROM
    4. Exercises
      • Multiangle isometrics at 90, 60, and 30°
      • Intermittent ROM exercises continued
      • Patellar mobilization
      • Ankle pumps
      • Straight leg raises (all four directions)
      • Standing weight shifts and minisquats (0–30° ROM)
      • Hamstring curls
      • Continue quad sets/gluteal sets
    5. Muscle stimulation: Electrical muscle stimulation to quadriceps (6 hours per day) during quad sets, multiangle isometrics, and straight leg raises
    6. CPM: 0–90°
    7. Ice and elevation: Ice 20 minutes out of every hour and elevate with knee in extension
  C. Postoperative Days 5–7
    1. Brace locked at 0° extension
    2. Weight bearing: Two crutches as tolerated
    3. Range of motion: Remove brace to perform ROM four to five times daily
    4. Exercises
      • Multiangle isometrics at 90, 60, and 30°
      • Intermittent passive ROM (PROM) exercises
      • Patellar mobilization
      • Ankle pumps
      • Straight leg raises (all four directions)
      • Standing weight shifts and minisquats (0 to 30°)
      • Passive knee extension to 0°
      • Hamstring curls
      • Active knee extension 90–40°
    5. Muscle stimulation: Electrical muscle stimulation (continue 6 hours daily)
    6. CPM: 0–90°
  Criteria for discharge from hospital
      • Quadriceps control (ability to perform good quad set and single leg raise)
      • Full passive knee extension
      • PROM 0–90°
      • Good patellar mobility
      • Minimal effusion
      • Ambulation with crutches
II. **Phase II: Maximum Protection Phase (Weeks 2 to 3)**
  Goals
      • Obtain absolute control of external forces and protect graft
      • Nourish articular cartilage
      • Decrease fibrosis
      • Stimulate collage healing
      • Decrease swelling
      • Prevent quadriceps atrophy
  A. Week 2
    1. Goals: Prepare athlete for ambulation without crutches
    2. Brace: Locked at 0° for ambulation only, unlocked for self ROM (four to five times daily)

Table 10–13. Rehabilitation Protocol After Anterior Cruciate Ligament–Patellar Tendon Graft *Continued*

    3. Weight bearing: As tolerated (goal is to discontinue crutches 7 to 10 days postoperatively)

    4. Range of motion: Self ROM (four to five times daily), emphasis on maintaining 0° passive extension

    5. KT-2000 test: 15-lb anterior test only

    6. Exercises
- Multiangle isometrics at 90, 60, and 30°
- Straight leg raises (all four directions)
- Hamstring curls
- Knee extension 90–40°
- Minisquats (0–40°) and weight shifts
- PROM 0–105°
- Patellar mobilization
- Hamstring and calf stretching
- Proprioception training
- Well-leg exercises
- Passive resistance exercise program: Start with 1-lb weight, progress by 1 lb per week

    7. Swelling control: Ice, compression, elevation

  B. Week 3

    1. Brace: Locked at 0° for ambulation only, unlocked for self ROM (four to five times daily)

    2. Range of motion: Self ROM (four to five times daily), emphasis on maintaining 0° of passive extension

    3. Weight bearing: Full weight bearing, no crutches

    4. Exercises
- Same as week 2
- PROM, 0–115°
- Bicycle for ROM stimulus and endurance
- Pool walking
- Initiate eccentric quads, 40 to 100° (isotonic only)
- Leg press (0 to 60°)
- StairMaster
- Nordic Track

III. Phase III: Controlled Ambulation Phase (Weeks 4–7)

Criteria to enter phase III
- Active ROM (AROM) 10–115°
- Quadriceps strength 60% or more of the contralateral side (isometric test at 60° knee flexion angle)
- Unchanged KT test (1 or less)
- Minimal effusion

    1. Goal: Control forces during walking

    2. Brace: Discontinued

    3. Range of motion: Self ROM (405 times daily), emphasis on maintaining 0° of passive extension

    4. KT-2000 test: Week 4, 20-lb anterior, 15-lb posterior test only
                     Week 6, 20- and 30-lb anterior and posterior test

    5. Exercises:
- Same as week 3
- PROM 0–130°
- Initiate swimming program
- Initiate step-ups (start with 2 in. and gradually increase)
- Increase closed kinetic chain rehabilitation
- Increase proprioception training

IV. Phase IV: Moderate Protection Phase (Weeks 7 to 12)

Criteria to enter phase IV
- AROM 0–125°
- Quadriceps strength, 60% of contralateral leg (isokinetic test)
- No change in KT scores ($+2$ or less)
- Minimal effusion
- No patellofemoral complaints
- Satisfactory clinical examination

    1. Goals: Protect articular cartilage of patellofemoral joint quadriceps Maximallly strengthen, lower extremity

    2. KT-2000 test: Week 10, total displacement at 20 lb and 30 lb, manual maximal test

    3. Isokinetic test: Week 10

Table continued on following page

Table 10–13. Rehabilitation Protocol After Anterior Cruciate Ligament–Patellar Tendon Graft *Continued*

    4. Exercises
- Emphasize eccentric quadriceps work
- Continue closed-chain exercises, step-ups, minisquats, leg press
- Continue knee extension 90–40°
- Hip abduction and adduction
- Hamstring curls and stretches
- Calf raises
- Bicycle for endurance
- Pool running (forward and backward)
- Walking program
- StairMaster
- Initiate isokinetic work 100–40°

V. **Phase V: Light Activity Phase (Months 2.5–3.5)**
Criteria to enter phase V
- AROM 0° to more than 125°
- Quadriceps strength, 70% of contralateral side, knee flexor/extensor rated 70% to 79% of contralateral side
- No change in KT scores (+2 or less)
- Minimal or no effusion
- Satisfactory clinical examination

    1. Goals: Develop strength, power, and endurance
            Begin preparation or return to functional activities
    2. Tests: Isokinetic test (weeks 10–12 and 16–18)
    3. Exercises
- Continue strengthening exercises
- Initiate plyometric program
- Initiate running program
- Initiate agility drills
- Sport-specific training and drills

Criteria to initiate running program
- Satisfactory isokinetic test
- Unchanged KT resuts
- Functional test, 70% or more of contralateral leg
- Satisfactory clinical examination

VI. **Phase VI: Return-to-Activity Phase (Months 3.5–4.5)**
Criteria for return to activities
- Isokinetic test that fulfills criteria
- KT-2000 test unchanged
- Functional test, 80% or more of contralateral leg
- Proprioceptive test, 100% of contralateral leg
- Satisfactory clinical examination

    1. Goals: Achieve maximal strength and further enhance neuromuscular coordination and endurance
    2. Tests: Isokinetic test prior to return, KT-2000 test, functional test
    3. Exercises
- Continue strengthening program
- Continue closed-chain strengthening program
- Continue plyometric program
- Continue running and agility program
- Accelerate sport-specific training and drills

VII. **Phase VII: 6-Month Follow-up**
- Isokinetic test
- KT-2000 test
- Functional test

VIII. **Phase VIII: 12-Month Follow-up**
- Isokinetic test
- KT-2000 test
- Functional test

Note: The protocol may be accelerated by discontinuing the brace at 2 weeks postoperatively rather than at weeks 4 to 7 postoperatively.

From HealthSouth Sports Medicine and Rehabilitation Center, Birmingham, Alabama.

Table 10–14. Accelerated Rehabilitation Protocol After Anterior Cruciate Ligament–Patellar Tendon Graft Reconstruction

I. 1 Day
   A. Continuous passive motion (CPM)
   B. Rigid knee immobilizer in full extension for walking
   C. Weight bearing: As tolerated without crutches
II. 2 to 3 Days
   A. CPM: Continue
   B. Passive ROM: 0–90° (emphasis on full extension)
   C. Weight bearing: As tolerated without crutches
III. 2 to 4 Days
   A. Discharge from hospital
   B. CPM at home
   Prerequisites to discharge
   • Satisfactory pain management
   • Full extension symmetric to nonoperated knee
   • Able to do single leg raise for leg control
   • Full weight bearing with or without crutches
IV. 7 to 10 Days
   A. Exercises
   • ROM terminal extension
   • Prone hangs (2 lb) if athlete has not achieved full extension
   • Towel extension
   • Wall slides
   • Heel slides
   • Active-assisted flexion
   • Knee bends
   • Step-ups
   • Calf raises
   B. Weight bearing: Gradual elimination of required use of knee immobilizer
V. 2 to 3 Weeks
   A. ROM: 0–110°
   B. Exercises
   • Unilateral knee bends
   • Step-ups
   • Calf raises
   • StairMaster 4000
   • Leg press
   • Quarter-squats
   • Calf raises in the squat rack
   • Stationary bicycling
   • Swimming
   C. Brace: Custom-made functional knee brace with no preset limits (to be used at all times out of the home for the next 4 weeks)
VI. 5 to 6 Weeks
   A. ROM: 0–130°
   B. Isokinetic evaluations with 20° block at 180 and 240°/sec
   C. When strength is 70% or greater than the opposite unoperated knee, begin lateral shuffles, cariocas, light jogging, jumping rope, agility drills, weight-room activities, stationary bicycling, and swimming
   D. Brace: Discontinue functional brace (except for sports activities) when muscle tone and strength are sufficient
VII. 10 Weeks
   A. Full ROM
   B. Isokinetic evaluation at 60, 180, and 240°/sec
   C. KT-1000 test
   D. Increased agility workouts and sport-specific activities
VIII. 16 Weeks
   A. Isokinetic evaluation
   B. KT-1000 test
   C. Increased agility workouts
IX. 4–6 Months
   A. Return to full sports participation if patient has met criteria of full ROM, no effusion, and good knee stability and has completed the running program

From Shelbourne, K.D., and Nitz, P. (1990): Accelerated rehabilitation after anterior cruciate ligament reconstruction. Am. J. Sports Med., 18:292–299.

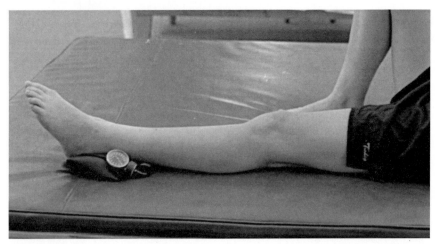

Figure 10–28. Use of a blood pressure cuff for biofeedback during performance of quad sets.

hamstrings and gluteals during hip extension. When a quad set is performed correctly, the pressure reading will stay the same or will decrease slightly. Once an isolated quadriceps contraction is present, table exercises such as straight leg raises can be progressed as pain and muscle control allow.

Maintaining full passive extension usually becomes increasingly difficult during the first 2 weeks after surgery. Emphasis should be placed on gaining and maintaining extension, because flexion will increase as pain and effusion decrease. While maintaining extension, quadriceps recruitment should be closely monitored and the table exercises advanced for motion and general strengthening. Active terminal knee-extension exercises can be started as soon as incisional pain allows. Terminal active ROM exercises historically have been limited early because of the stress placed on the graft but have been allowed 4 to 6 weeks postoperatively. The graft loses strength over the first few weeks, and therefore, performing active extensions early may not be as harmful as initiating them later in the program. These active terminal extension ROM exercises help facilitate quadriceps recruitment and patellar mobility. If the athlete has difficulty performing supine terminal active ROM exercises, they can be performed in the prone position with the assistance of hip extensors.

Once the incision is adequately healed, mobilization and desensitization of the scar can be performed. The use of gentle transverse friction massage will help mobilize the scar and prevent adhesions that may be painful during progressive ROM. The scar may remain sensitive if it continues to be protected and massage is not initiated.

The athlete can discontinue the use of crutches when full active extension is achieved during gait and good quadriceps control is present. Commonly, the athlete will hold the knee in slight flexion at heel strike and will lack full active extension in the stance phase of gait.[204] This lack of extension in gait may be due to a lack of strength or may simply be an adaptation that was learned before surgery when the knee was unstable.[204] When this gait abnormality is due to lack of strength, electrical stimulation will help in the return of a normal gait. A study by Snyder-Mackler and colleagues[204] involving 110 patients found that high-intensity electrical stimulation (performed at 65° of knee flexion) combined with closed-chain exercises resulted in a 70% recovery of quadriceps strength 6 weeks postreconstruction, whereas the group performing closed-chain exercises alone showed only a 57% recovery. The high-intensity electrical stimulation group also had superior knee control during midstance 6 weeks after surgery when compared to the closed-chain exercise–only group.[204]

Once gait has normalized, crutches can be discontinued and strengthening should be progressed in a closed-chain fashion. Closed-chain exercises allow for strengthening of the lower extremity without creating stresses that are harmful to the graft. The decreased stress that is afforded by the use of closed-chain exercises is due to the compression forces at the tibiofemoral joint and the cocontraction of other muscles to help control motion at the hip, knee, and ankle. An excellent initial closed-chain exercise is terminal knee extensions in the standing position using a Thera-Band (see Fig. 10–11). The athlete must concentrate on performing a quadriceps contraction instead of simply extending the hip while performing this exercise. If the athlete continues to use the hip to gain knee extension, the athlete should be positioned with the back and heel against a wall with the knee slightly flexed. A blood pressure cuff can be placed behind the knee, and the athlete is asked to straighten the knee, putting pressure on the cuff (Fig. 10–29). This exercise will introduce the athlete to closed-chain exercises, making sure that the quadriceps is being used. It will also help the athlete gain active extension because of the feedback provided by the blood pressure cuff.

Hip strength should be addressed in order to decrease excessive frontal plane motion as weight is increased with closed-chain exercises (see Fig. 10–20A). Lack of control at the hip can contribute to patellofemoral pain. The initiation of weighted leg extension and isokinetics in the terminal range of extension varies greatly with each protocol but is usually allowed at 3 to 6 months.

The athlete can be advanced through a functional progression program as seen in Table 10–15. Running is most often allowed at 4 to 6 months, with a return to athletics at 6 to 12 months.

Several types of allografts that are commonly used in reconstructive procedures are the fascia lata, Achilles tendon, and bone–patellar tendon–bone. Noyes

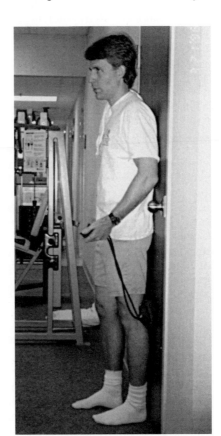

Figure 10–29. Use of a blood pressure cuff for biofeedback during terminal knee extension exercise in standing position.

Table 10–15. Functional Progression Program

Jogging in place	Jogging figure eights (large to small)
Jumping rope	Jogging to sprinting
Jogging	Sprinting/reversing/cutting on command
Jogging forward/reversing on command	Sport-specific drills
Side-to-side sliding	

reported on 66 knees receiving allografts after a failed previous reconstruction. The results determined that bone–patellar tendon–bone allografts helped to decrease symptoms and abnormal displacement in the majority of patients.[171]

Rehabilitation after an allograft will be dictated by the type of graft that is used. Generally, rehabilitation progression after reconstruction with an allograft is slower than with an autograft. Usually, weight bearing is not allowed for 4 to 6 weeks. When weight bearing is allowed, the order of progression for the athlete is similar to that for an athlete with an autograft. The goals that were stressed in the overview of this chapter must be achieved, regardless of the graft used.

Posterior Cruciate Ligament Injuries

Injury to the PCL remains relatively uncommon in the athletic population. Studies suggest that 2% to 20% of all knee injuries involve the PCL; the literature on rehabilitation after injury is, therefore, limited.[5]

A PCL-deficient knee can lead to tibiofemoral and patellofemoral articular cartilage damage.[5] Retropatellar pain may be the most disabling symptom after injury. This increase in patellofemoral pain may be due to the posterior tibial sag, resulting in increased pressure through the quadriceps mechanism.[5]

Noyes has stated that there are incomplete data to date demonstrating the ability of any operative procedure to restore posterior stability at all angles of knee flexion.[5] Presently, the most common technique for PCL reconstruction is the bone–patellar tendon–bone autograft, although semitendinosus, medial head of the gastrocnemius, and PCL allografts have been used.[5, 66] As with the ACL, primary repair is not possible, and optimum placement and fixation of the graft is crucial to allow for early motion and a successful outcome.

After surgery, the greatest concern is the posterior shear forces that are created beyond 60° of flexion. Motion is limited from 0° to 60° for 4 weeks, and hamstring strengthening is also prohibited for a minimum of 8 weeks after surgery to prevent any posterior translation that may jeopardize the graft.[229] Partial weight bearing is allowed for the first 6 to 8 weeks, and full weight bearing may not be allowed for 10 weeks. Because of the lack of success after reconstructive procedures for isolated PCL injures, most injuries continue to be treated conservatively until lack of function dictates operative management. Tables 10–16 and 10–17 represent examples of PCL rehabilitation protocols. If other structures are involved, leading to rotational instability, surgery may be indicated initially.

Medial Collateral Ligament Injuries

The attention received by MCL injuries in the early days of sports medicine is similar to that received by ACL injuries today. MCL injuries receive less attention today because of their nonoperative management and because of their frequent involvement with ACL injuries, which receive more attention.

Table 10–16. Rehabilitation Protocol for Posterior Cruciate Ligament Reconstruction

	WEEKS 1–3	WEEKS 4–6	WEEKS 7–20
Functional progression	WB with two crutches	WB with one crutch	Independent ambulation
Criteria	Postoperative pain and hemarthrosis are controlled ROM 0–70° Patellar mobility is normal Voluntary quadriceps contraction/straight leg raise	Pain is controlled without narcotics Effusion is controlled ROM 0–90° Muscle control throughout ROM	Pain is controlled Effusion is controlled ROM 0–135° by week 16 Muscle control throughout ROM
Evaluation	Pain Effusion/edema Muscle strength/control/ spasm ROM Patellar mobility	Pain Effusion/edema Muscle strength/control spasm ROM Patellar mobility	Pain Effusion/edema Muscle strength/control/ spasm ROM Patellar mobility
Treatment	Pain management Control of effusion/edema Mobilization of patella Quadriceps recruitment/ biofeedback ROM exercises No hamstring exercises No stairs during ambulation Rehabilitation brace	Pain management Control of effusion/ edema Mobilization of patella Quadriceps strengthening Minisquats ROM activities No hamstring exercises No stairs during ambulation	Pain management Control of effusion/ edema Mobilization of patella Quadriceps strengthening Begin hamstring exercise 12 weeks postoperatively No deep squats past 60° Endurance exercises ROM activities
Goals	ROM 0–90° Adequate quadriceps recruitment Control of inflammation and effusion 25–50% WB Early recognition of complications	ROM 0–100° Muscle control Control of inflammation and effusion 50–75% WB Early recognition of complications	Muscle endurance 100% WB with normal gait pattern 7–10 weeks postoperatively ROM: Weeks 7–8: 0–110° Weeks 9–12: 0–120° Weeks 12–16: 0–135° Return to sports at 9–12 months

Adapted from Anderson, J.K., and Noyes, F.R. (1995): Principles of posterior cruciate ligament rehabilitation. Orthopedics 18:493–500.
ROM, Range of motion; WB, weight bearing.

Several studies report excellent results with emphasizing early motion after nonsurgical management of grade III MCL injuries.[105, 189] When ACL disruption is present with a grade III MCL tear, the ACL is reconstructed, and the MCL is left to heal on its own. The only exception is if the posterior oblique ligament is also ruptured, in which case some physicians may opt to reconstruct or repair the MCL. When injuries to both structures have occurred, rehabilitation follows the ACL protocol.

Rehabilitation after isolated injuries to the MCL varies greatly, as do protocols with any ligamentous injury to the knee, but with all protocols early motion and protection from valgus stress are emphasized. Full ROM and vigorous quadriceps recruitment exercises should be employed with each MCL injury. Most of the differences in treatment arise from the use of rehabilitation braces to protect against valgus stress and in initiation of weight bearing. Tables 10–18 and 10–19 represent examples of rehabilitation protocols for MCL sprains. With grade III MCL sprains, some residual valgus laxity may be present, but it should not cause any functional limitations.

Table 10–17. Rehabilitation Protocol After Posterior Cruciate Ligament–Patellar Tendon Graft

---

I. **Phase I: Immediate Postoperative Phase**
    A. Postoperative Day 1
        1. Brace: Locked at 0° of extension
        2. Weight bearing: Two crutches as tolerated (less than 50%)
        3. Exercises
            • Ankle pumps
            • Quad sets
            • Straight leg raises (three-way) hip flexion, abduction, adduction
            • Knee extension 60–0°
        4. Muscle stimulation: Muscle stimulation to quadriceps
           (4 hours/day) during quad sets
        5. Continuous passive motion 0–60° as tolerated
        6. Ice and elevation: Ice 20 minutes out of every hour and elevate with knee in extension
II. **Phase II: Maximum Protection Phase (Weeks 2–6)**
    Goals
        • Gain absolute control of external forces to protect graft
        • Nourish articular cartilage
        • Decrease swelling
        • Decrease fibrosis
        • Prevent quadriceps atrophy
    A. Week 2
        1. Brace: Locked at 0° continue to perform intermittent ROM exercises
        2. Weight bearing: As tolerated (50% or greater)
        3. KT test: Performed with 15-lb maximum force at 70° of flexion
        4. Exercises
            • Multiangle isometrics 60, 40, and 20°
            • Quad sets
            • Knee extension 60–0°
            • Intermittent ROM 0–60° (405 times daily)
            • Patellar mobilization
            • Well-leg bicycle
            • Proprioception training squats (0–45°)
            • Continue electrical stimulation to quadriceps
            • Leg press (0–60°)
            • Continue ice and elevation
    B. Week 4
        1. Brace: Locked at 0°
        2. Full weight bearing, no crutches (one crutch if necessary)
        3. KT-2000 test performed
        4. Exercises
            • Weight shifts
            • Minisquats 0–45°
            • Intermittent ROM 0–90°
            • Knee extension 60–0°
            • Pool walking
            • Initiate biking for ROM and endurance
    C. Week 5
        1. Initiate pool exercises
        2. Fit for functional posterior cruciate ligament brace
III. **Phase III: Controlled Ambulation Phase (Weeks 7–12)**
    Goals
        • Control forces during ambulation
        • Increase quadriceps strength
    A. Week 7
        1. Brace: Opened 0–125°; discontinue locked brace
        2. Criteria for full weight bearing with knee motion
            • Active-assisted range of motion, 0–115°
            • Quadriceps strength, 70% of contralateral side (isometric test)
            • No change in KT-2000 test
            • Decrease joint effusion
        3. Ambulation: With functional brace

Table 10–17. Rehabilitation Protocol After Posterior Cruciate Ligament–Patellar Tendon Graft *Continued*

    4. Exercises
- Continue all exercises stated above
- Initiate swimming
- Initiate vigorous stretching program
- Increase closed kinetic chain rehabilitation

  B. Week 8
    1. Perform KT-2000 test
    2. Exercises
- Continue all exercises stated above

  C. Week 12
    1. Ambulation: Discontinue brace
    2. Brace: Use for strenuous activities
    3. KT-2000 test performed
    4. Exercises
- Begin isokinetic 60–0° ROM
- Continue minisquats
- Initiate lateral step-ups
- Initiate pool running (forward only)
- Initiate hamstring curls (0–60°, low weight)
- Bicycle for endurance (30 min)
- Begin walking program

IV. Phase IV: Light Activity Phase (3–4 Months)
  Goals
- Develop strength, power, and endurance
- Begin to prepare for return to functional activities

    1. Exercises
- Begin light running program
- Continue isokinetic tests (light speed, full ROM)
- Continue minisquats/lateral step-ups
- Initiate hamstring curls (0–60°, low weight)
- Bicycle for endurance (30 min)
- Begin walking program

    2. Tests
- Isokinetic test (week 15)
- KT-2000 test (prior to running program)
- Functional test (prior to running program)

    3. Criteria for running
- Isokinetic test interpretation satisfactory
- KT-2000 test unchanged
- Functional test 70% of contralateral leg

V. Phase V: Return to Activity (5–6 Months)
  Advance rehabilitation to competitive sports
  Goal
- Achieve maximal strength and further enhance neuromuscular coordination and endurance

    1. Exercises
- Closed-chain rehabilitation
- High-speed isokinetics
- Running program
- Agility drills
- Balance drills
- Plyometrics initiated

VI. 6-Month Follow-up
- KT-2000 test
- Isokinetic test
- Functional test

VII. 12-Month Follow-up
- KT-2000 test
- Isokinetic test
- Functional test

From HealthSouth Sports Medicine and Rehabilitation Center, Birmingham, Alabama.

Table 10–18. Rehabilitation Protocol for Isolated Medial Collateral Ligament Sprains Grades I, II, and III

	WEEK 1	WEEKS 2–3	WEEKS 4–8
Functional progression	Begin WB without crutches, grades I and II	Progress strengthening exercises	Return to athletics, grades I and II
Criteria	Full knee extension present during gait No limp No pain at MCL No increased effusion Quadriceps control	VMO recruitment present Full active extension ROM No pain with exercises No increased effusion/edema Patellar mobility normal	Full AROM No tenderness Functional testing 85% Quadriceps strength 85%
Evaluation	Pain Effusion/edema Quadriceps recruitment ROM Patellar mobility	Effusion/edema Patellar mobility Quadriceps recruitment Active ROM Standing balance, grades I and II	Functional testing Isokinetic testing
Treatment	Pain management Control of effusion/edema Quadriceps recruitment/biofeedback ROM exercises Flexibility exercises NWB, grade III only Rehabilitation brace, grades II and III	Pain management Control of effusion/edema Mobilization of patella Quadriceps strengthening AROM exercises Proprioception exercises Endurance exercises	Strengthening exercises Endurance exercises Sport-specific drills
Goals	Maximize ROM Good quadriceps recruitment Control valgus stress 75–100% WB, grades I and II	Full ROM Absence of pain FWB, grades I and II Normal patellar mobility	Discontinue brace, grade II Begin WB, grade III and progress through criteria beginning week 1 Discontinue brace, week 6, grade III Return to sports, grades I and II

AROM, Active range of motion; FWB, full weight bearing; MCL, medial collateral ligament; NWB, non–weight bearing; ROM, range of motion; VMO, vastus medialis obliquus; WB, weight bearing.

Meniscal and Articular Cartilage Injuries

Meniscal lesions have been treated by total meniscectomy, partial meniscectomy, and most recently, meniscal repair. Total meniscectomy by arthrotomy quickly alleviates the mechanical symptoms, and short-term results have usually been good.[41] Long-term outcomes have been disappointing because of the degenerative articular changes that occur in knees after a total meniscectomy.[108, 125, 153] Currently, total meniscectomy is rarely indicated.

Meniscal lesions are now repaired, or a partial meniscectomy is performed. The rationale behind partial meniscectomy is the removal of the torn portion of the meniscus. As much meniscus tissue as possible is retained in the hope that it will continue to perform, to some extent, the essential function of the meniscus.[41] Meniscal lesions are often associated with other intra-articular pathology, usually an ACL disruption. Some studies[108, 138] have reported poor results in those patients after meniscectomy in whom the ACL was not reconstructed. Patients complained of increased knee symptoms and developed progressive degenerative changes. The extent of the degenerative changes was directly proportional to the amount of meniscus removed. A rehabilitation protocol for a partial meniscectomy is given in Table 10–20.

Table 10–19. Rehabilitation Protocol for Isolated MCL Sprains

This program may be accelerated for grade I MCL sprains or may be extended depending on the severity of the injury. The following schedule serves as a guideline to help in the expediency of returning an athlete to the preinjury state.

Any increase in pain, swelling, or loss of ROM is a sign that the progression of the athlete may be too rapid.

I. **Phase I: Maximal Protection Phase**

Goals
- Begin early protected ROM
- Prevent quadriceps atrophy
- Decrease effusion/pain

A. Day 1
1. Ice, compression, elevation
2. Hinged-knee brace, nonpainful ROM, if needed
3. Crutches: Weight bearing as tolerated
4. Passive ROM/active-assisted ROM (AAROM) to maintain ROM
5. Electrical muscle stimulation to quadriceps (8 hours/day)
6. Isometrics quads: quad sets, straight leg raises (flex)
7. Emphasize hamstring stretches and AAROM of knee flexion, stretching to tolerance

B. Day 2
1. Continue above exercises and add
   - Quad sets
   - Straight leg raises (flexion and abduction)
   - Hamstring isometric sets
   - Well-leg exercises
2. Use whirlpool for ROM (cold for first 3–4 days, then warm)
3. Apply high-voltage galvanic stimulation to control swelling

C. Days 3–7
1. Continue above exercises and begin
   - Eccentric quad work
   - Bicycling for ROM stimulus
   - Resisted knee extension with electrical muscle stimulation
   - Hip adduction and extension
   - Minisquats
   - Leg press isotonics
2. Use weight-bearing crutches as tolerated
3. Wear brace at night; brace during day as needed
4. Continue ROM and stretching exercises; progress ROM as tolerated

II. **Phase II: Moderate Protection Phase**

Criteria for progression
- No increase in instability
- No increase in swelling
- Minimal tenderness
- PROM 10–100°

Goals
- Perform full painless ROM
- Restore strength
- Ambulate without crutches

A. Week 2
1. Continue strengthening program with passive resistance exercises
2. Continue electrical muscle stimulation to quadriceps during isotonic strengthening
3. Continue ROM exercises and stretching
4. Emphasize closed kinetic chain exercises: lunges, squats, lateral lunges, wall squats, lateral step-ups
5. Bicycle for endurance and ROM stimulus
6. Perform full ROM exercises
7. Perform flexibility exercises, hamstrings, quadriceps, iliotibial band, etc.
8. Perform water exercises, running in water forward and backward
9. Do proprioception training (balance drills)
10. Use StairMaster for endurance work

B. Days 11–14
1. Continue all exercises in week
2. Passive resistance exercises with emphasis on quadriceps, medial hamstrings, and hip abduction
3. Initiate isokinetics, submaxial to maximal, fast contractile velocities
4. Begin running program if full, painless extension and flexion are present

Table continued on following page

Table 10–19. Rehabilitation Protocol for Isolated MCL Sprains
Continued

III. **Phase III: Minimal Protection Phase**
  Criteria for progression
  • No instability
  • No swelling/tenderness
  • Full painless ROM
  Goal
  • Increase strength and power
  A. Week 3
    1. Continue strengthening program
      • Wall squats
      • Vertical squats
      • Lunges
      • Lateral lunges
      • Step-ups
      • Leg presses
      • Knee extensions
      • Hip abduction/adduction
      • Hamstring curls
      • Emphasis:
          Functional exercise drills
          Fast-speed isokinetics
          Eccentric quads
          Isotonic hip adduction, medial
            hamstring
      • Isokinetic test
      • Proprioception training
      • Endurance exercises
      • Stationary bike 30–40 min
      • Nordic Track, swimming, etc.
      • Initiate agility program, sport-specific activities
IV. **Phase IV: Maintenance Program**
  Criteria for return to competition
  • Full ROM
  • No instability
  • Muscle strength, 85% of contralateral side
  • Proprioception ability satisfactory
  • No tenderness of MCL
  • No effusion
  • Quadriceps strength; torque/body weight ratio that fulfills criteria
  • Lateral knee brace (if necessary)
  Maintenance program
  • Continue isotonic strengthening exercises
  • Continue flexibility exercises
  • Continue proprioceptive activities

From HealthSouth Sports Medicine and Rehabilitation Center, Birmingham, Alabama.

Meniscal repairs have increased over the past several years because of a greater understanding of the overall function of the meniscus. Repairs can be performed through a small incision or with an arthroscope and usually involve only the peripheral third of the meniscus because of its vascularity. No clear difference in the healing rates supports one type of repair over the other.[13]

Rehabilitation after meniscal repair is of longer duration, with return to participation 4 to 6 months after surgery. Tables 10–21 and 10–22 represent examples of rehabilitation protocols after meniscal repair. Although rehabilitation takes longer with a meniscal repair, many surgeons feel it is a worthwhile procedure because of the protection the meniscus lends to the articular cartilage. In cases of ACL reconstruction and associated meniscus repairs, the ACL protocol is followed to help prevent overall morbidity, although caution must be used when performing closed-chain exercises. After a meniscal repair, the athlete is allowed to gradually increase weight bearing over a 4-week period. Axial load-

Table 10–20. Rehabilitation Protocol for Partial Meniscectomy

	WEEK 1	WEEKS 2–3	WEEKS 4–8
Functional progression	Begin FWB without crutches	Progress strengthening exercises	Return to athletics
Criteria	Full extension present during gait No limp No increased effusion/edema No increased pain Quadriceps control	VMO recruitment present Full active extension ROM Absence of pain No increased effusion/edema	Full AROM No effusion Functional testing, 85% Quadriceps strength, 85%
Evaluation	Pain Gait Quadriceps recruitment Active ROM Patellar mobility Surgical incisions/portals	Surgical incisions/portals Gait Effusion/edema Quadriceps recruitment AROM Patellar mobility Standing balance	Functional testing Isokinetic testing
Treatment	Pain management Control of effusion/edema Quadriceps recruitment ROM exercises Flexibility exercises	Effusion/edema reduction Strengthening exercises Endurance exercises Proprioception exercises Flexibility exercises	Strengthening exercises Endurance exercises Sport-specific drills
Goals	Maximum ROM Good quadriceps recruitment Normal patellar mobility Full passive extension FWB	Full ROM No pain with strengthening exercises	Return to athletics

AROM, Active range of motion; FWB, full weight bearing; ROM, range of motion; VMO, vastus medialis obliquus.

ing compresses the meniscus, approximating the margins of the repair. The athlete may be placed in a brace, keeping the knee locked in full extension during gait, for 4 weeks to help prevent flexion of the knee under a load that could damage the repair. Full ROM is usually allowed in a non–weight-bearing position, although flexion is not aggressively addressed to allow for continued protection of the meniscus. As effusion decreases, active flexion will continue to progress, but if it plateaus, aggressive passive flexion can be initiated at 4 weeks. Closed-chain exercises can be started as soon as knee flexion is allowed during gait. Stair-climbing machines may be used after 3 months.[154] Running may be allowed at 3 months, with cutting and jumping activities at 6 months.

Rehabilitation after damage to the articular cartilage is similar to that after meniscus repair, except that the athlete is kept non–weight-bearing for 6 weeks. At present, surgery for osteochondritis, abrasion chondroplasty, involves drilling of the defect to promote bleeding and chondrosis in the involved area. Keeping the athlete non–weight-bearing allows the normal healing process to occur without disruption.

Autologous chondrocyte transplantation for the treatment of osteochondritis is being investigated. A biopsy specimen from healthy cartilage is cultured and injected into the defect.[22] Brittberg and associates suggest that treatment of chondromalacia patellae with the use of chondrocyte transplantation is less successful than is treatment of femoral condylar defects.[22] Rehabilitation after this type of procedure, although not documented, should concentrate on protecting the transplanted defect by keeping the athlete non–weight-bearing and preventing ROM across the defect.

Table 10–21. Rehabilitation Protocol for Meniscus Repair

	WEEKS 0–3	WEEKS 4–11	WEEKS 12–15	WEEKS 16–24
Functional progression	Begin partial to full WB with brace locked in full extension	Begin full WB without brace	Begin jogging	Begin cutting and jumping activities
Criteria	As postoperative pain allows No increased effusion	Good quadriceps contrtol present Effusion continues to decrease Full extension during gait	Absence of effusion Absence of patellofemoral pain No gait deviations	No increased effusion with running No pain
Evaluation	Pain Effusion Patellar mobility Quadriceps recruitment AROM Passive extension Incision/portals	Pain AROM/PROM Quadriceps recruitment Patellar mobility Effusion Standing balance	Gait Patellar mobility Isokinetic testing Functional testing	Effusion
Treatment	Pain control Control of effusion/edema Patellar mobility AROM Quadriceps recruitment with biofeedback/electrical stimulation Passive extension FWB in brace locked at 0°	AROM/PROM Quadriceps recruitment/strengthening General strengthening Progress closed-chain exercises (no flexion greater than 60°) Endurance exercise Proprioception exercises	Strengthening exercises Endurance exercises Proprioception exercises	Strengthening exercises Endurance exercises Sport-specific drills
Goals	AROM 10–90° Full passive extension FWB in brace Good quadriceps recruitment	Full AROM No gait deviations	Absence of effusion No pain	Return to athletics

Adapted from McLaughlin, J., DeMaio, M., Noyes, F.R., et al. (1994): Rehabilitation after meniscus repair. Orthopedics, 17:463–471.
AROM, Active range of motion; FWB, full weight bearing; PROM, passive range of motion; WB, weight bearing.

Patellofemoral Dysfunction

Anterior knee pain, or more commonly patellofemoral pain that is related to dysfunction of the patellofemoral joint, is one of the most prevalent knee pathologies seen in athletes.[113] Patellofemoral pain is used to describe many conditions associated with patellofemoral dysfunction, including patella malalignment syndrome, chondromalacia patellae, and subluxating or dislocating patella; often, even patellar tendinitis falls under this broad diagnosis.

Pain in the patellofemoral region can be due to trauma or may be of insidious onset, as seen in overuse injuries. After surgery or injury to the hip, knee, or ankle, patellofemoral pain can be present because of changes in the mechanics of the lower extremity; it is one of the most prevalent complications after knee surgery. The need for a comprehensive lower extremity evaluation is paramount in athletes complaining of patellofemoral pain. The functioning of the patella depends on a fine balance between ligaments and muscles because of its lack of inherent bony stability. When this balance is disrupted, improper tracking, or more commonly lateral tracking, of the patella occurs.[30] Complications from lateral tracking occur more often in women and may be due to the slight increase

Table 10–22. Rehabilitation Protocol After Meniscus Repair

Key factors in meniscal repair
- Anatomic site of tear
- Suture fixation: can lead to failure if too vigorous
- Location of tear: anterior or posterior
- Other pathology: PCL, MCL, ACL

I. **Phase I: Maximum Protection (Weeks 1–6)**
  A. Stage I: Immediate postsurgery day 1 through week 3
    1. Ice, compression, elevation
    2. Electrical muscle stimulation
    3. Brace locked at 0°
    4. Range of motion (ROM), 0–90°; motion is limited for the first 7 to 21 days, depending on the development of scar tissue around repair site; gradual increase in flexion ROM based on assessment of pain (0–30° to 0–50° to 0–70° and to 0–90°)
    5. Patellar scar tissue mobilization
    6. Passive ROM
    7. Exercises
      - Quadriceps isometrics
      - Hamstring isometrics (if posterior horn repair, no hamstring exercises for 6 weeks)
      - Hip abduction/adduction
    8. Weight bearing: As tolerated with crutches with brace locked at 0°
    9. Proprioceptive training
  B. Stage II: Weeks 4–6
    1. Weight bearing: Full, without assistive device, with brace locked at 0°
    2. Exercises
      - Passive resistance exercise program initiated
      - Limited-range knee extension (end-ROM less likely to impinge or pull on repair)
      - Toe raises
      - Minisquats
      - Cycling
      - Surgical tubing exercises—diagonal patterns
      - Flexibility exercises

II. **Phase II: Moderate Protection Phases (Weeks 6–10)**
  Goals
    - Increase strength, power, endurance
    - Normalize knee ROM
    - Prepare athlete for advanced exercises
  Criteria to progress to phase II
    - ROM 0–90°
    - No change in pain or effusion
    - Good quadriceps control
    1. Exercises
      - Strength: Passive resistance exercise program continues
      - Flexibility exercises emphasized
      - Lateral step-ups: 30 sec × 5 sets progressing to >60 sec × 5 sets
      - Minisquats
      - Isokinetic exercises
    2. Endurance program
      - Swimming
      - Cycling
      - Nordic Track
      - StairMaster
      - Pool running
    3. Coordination program
      - Balance board
      - High-speed bands
      - Pool sprinting
      - Backward walking
    4. Plyometric program

Table continued on following page

in lateral pull from the quadriceps mechanism. VMO dysfunction, tight lateral structures, including iliotibial band and patella retinaculum, and increased subtalar pronation leading to an increased Q angle all are possible causes for lateral tracking of the patella.

Chondromalacia patellae is described as a softening of the articular cartilage.

Table 10–22. Rehabilitation Protocol After Meniscus Repair *Continued*

III. **Phase III: Advanced Phase (Weeks 11–15)**
  Goals
  • Increase power and endurance
  • Emphasize return to skill activities
  • Prepare to return to full unrestricted activities
  Criteria to progress to phase III
  • Full nonpainful ROM
  • No pain or tenderness
  • Satisfactory isokinetic test
  • Satisfactory clinical examination
  Exercises
  • Continue all exercises in phase II
  • Increase tubing program, plyometrics, pool program
  • Initiate running program
  Criteria for return program
  • Full nonpainful ROM
  • Satisfactory clinical examination
  • Satisfactory isokinetic test

From HealthSouth Sports Medicine and Rehabilitation Center, Birmingham, Alabama.

This diagnosis can be made only with surgical procedures in which the articular cartilage is observed. Crepitus of the patellofemoral joint does not necessarily indicate chondromalacia, but every effort should be made to not exercise the athlete in a way that increases the crepitation of the joint.

Rehabilitation of patellofemoral dysfunction, after a comprehensive evaluation, should concentrate on recruiting the VMO, normalizing patellar mobility, and increasing general flexibility and muscular control of the entire lower extremity. There are no specific exercises that have been proven to isolate the VMO. Knee extension with internal tibial rotation, hip adduction with quadriceps contraction, and hip external rotation with quadriceps contraction have all been proposed for isolating the VMO, but no proof exists of their efficacy.[30] Ensuring that the exercises are pain free should be the biggest concern in choosing exercises for the athlete with patellofemoral dysfunction. This should be continually emphasized to the athlete to prevent the "no pain, no gain" attitude.

Multiple-angle isometrics and straight leg raises are often initially recommended to restore muscle function, but if the VMO is not monitored through the use of biofeedback devices, proper recruitment is difficult to determine. Closed-chain exercises are often the treatment of choice because of the decrease in patellofemoral compression forces, but the entire lower extremity must be closely observed to ensure proper performance. Strengthening of the hip musculature to help prevent hip adduction and internal rotation may be crucial in allowing the progression of closed-chain exercises. Restoration of proprioception is extremely important in re-establishing neuromuscular control.

Several authors have reported other techniques that may be beneficial in the treatment of lateral compression syndrome and subluxating patella. Kramer[124] has reported success with manual lateral retinaculum stretching in conjunction with a traditional patellofemoral program. It was noted that in the patellar malalignment syndrome there is excessive pressure on the lateral aspect of the patellofemoral joint, with resultant damage to the articular cartilage. Kramer has proposed two types of manual maneuvers: (1) medial patellar glide with the knee extended, held for 1 minute to stretch the lateral retinaculum; and (2) patellar compression with tracking.[124] With the athlete sitting and the knee flexed to 90°, the patella is compressed against the patellofemoral articular surface and tracked medially by the clinician as the athlete extends the knee.

McConnell[150] has reported a 96% success rate with a patellofemoral treatment regimen. This not only emphasizes closed-chain exercises but attempts to correct the glide, tilt, and rotation components of the patella with tape. Initially, quadriceps isometrics or functional exercises such as lateral step-ups are performed. If pain can be alleviated by manually gliding the patella medially while performing the same exercise that elicited the pain, the individual will probably respond well to the treatment regimen. After the evaluation, tape is used to correct patellar orientation. The lateral tilt component is corrected by pulling the tape from the midline of the patella medially (Fig. 10–30A). This lifts the lateral border and provides a passive stretch to the lateral retinacular structures. Excessive lateral tracking is corrected by pulling the patella medially (Fig. 10–30B). Excessive lateral tracking is the most frequent dysfunction seen clinically. The external rotation component is corrected by taping from the middle inferior patellar pole upward and medially (Fig. 10–30C). The superior and inferior poles of the patella should be in line with the longitudinal axis of the femur. The rotational component must be corrected before any of the other components are corrected. Finally, anteroposterior tilt is corrected by attempting to tilt the inferior pole of the patella anteriorly by placing a strip of tape at the superior pole of the patella and pulling the tape medially (Fig. 10–30D). Pain at the inferior pole of the patella in athletes performing quadriceps contractions with the knee extended may be due to a posterior tilt of the inferior pole of the patella. McConnell has suggested that taping the patella or tensor fasciae latae medially

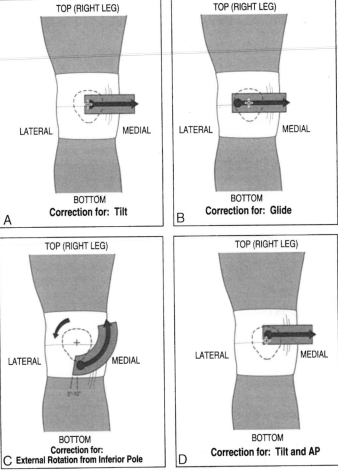

Figure 10–30. Tape correction. *A,* For lateral patellar tilt. *B,* For lateral patellar shift. *C,* For external rotation of the patella. *D,* For anteroposterior (AP) tilt of the patella. (Illustration courtesy of Smith & Nephew DonJoy Inc., Carlsbad, California.)

improves patellar tracking, decreases pain, and increases the VMO-to-VL muscle activity ratio.[30]

Recently, several studies have examined the effectiveness of taping to reposition the patella. Larsen and colleagues[128] noted that patellar taping was ineffective in maintaining the repositioned patella after an exercise program. Brockrath and colleagues [23] noted no significant change in patellar position after taping of the patella. Kowall and colleagues[123] compared two treatment programs in which one group underwent a conventional patellofemoral rehabilitation program and the other group was taped and performed the same rehabilitation program. The investigators found no significant differences between the two groups in their rate of improvement. Therefore, we are unsure regarding the effect of patellar taping and its long-term efficacy.

Patellofemoral braces are commonly used in treating patellofemoral dysfunction, but clinically they offer only minimum support and pain relief when compared to taping techniques. If malalignment of the feet is noted, orthoses may be beneficial. Patellofemoral pain that is often seen in runners may be due to increased pronation from a compensated forefoot varus condition. Before expensive orthoses are fabricated, Low-Dye arch taping may be beneficial in reducing the pain and confirming the cause. If taping consistently helps, some orthosis is usually beneficial.

If conservative treatment fails, surgery may be indicated. One of the most common procedures is a lateral retinaculum release in which the lateral retinaculum is cut, thus freeing the patella medially. Table 10–23 shows a lateral release rehabilitation protocol. If the line of pull of the VMO is vertical, the VMO may be advanced in conjunction with the lateral release. Although this surgical technique was popular in the past, the procedure is presently performed after greater scrutiny.

Sometimes a distal realignment is performed, which involves transferring the patellar tendon and tibial tubercle to decrease the Q angle. The main concern with this procedure is progression of knee motion and weight bearing. A progressive running program can begin at 16 to 20 weeks, with a progression to full activity by 6 months after surgery. Rehabilitation of the knee should emphasize all forms of exercises that allow for a safe progression of the athlete. Early controlled motion, muscle recruitment, and a restoration of joint arthrokinematics should be the focus of any program regardless of injury. These goals must be accomplished independently of time frames that are established with each rehabilitation protocol. Once these goals are accomplished, strength, proprioception, power, and endurance can be developed so that the athlete can return to competition. Objective measurements should be taken after rehabilitation with all means available to ensure that the athlete returns to competition safely.

FUNCTIONAL KNEE BRACES

Many authors[15, 21, 33, 34, 158] have investigated the effect of functional knee braces for controlling instability in individuals with ACL-deficient knees. In vivo measurements have generally shown that braces reduce anterior tibial displacement at low loads, but the low forces used in laxity testing probably do not reveal the absolute excursions that result from higher physiologic loads.[33, 173] Markolf and colleagues[147] have stated that forces in excess of 200 N are required to produce an accurate measurement of absolute laxity. Other experts have stated that to function at physiologic levels, braces must control stresses of at least 400 N.[224] In a study of 10 different braces on surrogate knees, none of the braces were able to control anterior translation at forces greater than 300 N (67 pounds).[224] Seven braces (three custom and four off-the-shelf) have been tested in vivo with a Hall effect transducer implanted on the ACL.[19] Only two of the braces, an off-the-shelf DonJoy four-point ACL sport brace and a custom Townsend brace,

Table 10–23. Rehabilitation Protocol for Lateral Release

	WEEK 1	WEEKS 2–4	WEEKS 4–6	WEEKS 6
Functional progression	Begin WB and four-quadrant lifts	Begin WB without crutches	Begin strengthening	Return to athletics
Criteria	As pain allows Quadriceps recruitment sufficient to maintain extension with SLR	Full extension in gait No limp No increase in pain No increase in edema/effusion Good quadriceps control	VMO recruitment is present Full active extension ROM Absence of pain No increase in edema/effusion	Full ROM No effusion Functional testing, 85% Quadriceps strength, 85%
Evaluation	Pain Incision Effusion/edema Active flexion Quadriceps recruitment Passive extension Patellar mobility Hamstring flexibility Iliotibial band flexibility	Pain Gait Incision/scar Effusion/edema ROM/patellar mobility Quadriceps recruitment	ROM Quadriceps recruitment Patellar mobility Standing balance	Functional testing Strength testing
Treatment	Pain management Effusion/edema control Active flexion exercise Quadriceps recruitment exercise Passive extension Patellar mobilization Hamstring stretching IT band stretching	Pain management Effusion/edema control Scar massage Active ROM exercise Patellar mobilization Quadriceps recruitment General strengthening Flexibility exercise	Strengthening Endurance exercise Proprioception exercise	Strengthening Endurance exercise Sport-specific drills
Goals	75% weight bearing Increase patellar mobility Full passive extension Good quadriceps recruitment	WB without crutches AROM 10–110° Normal patellar mobility	Full AROM Strengthening without pain	Return to athletics

AROM, Active range of motion; IT, iliotibial; ROM, range of motion; VMO, vastus medialis obliquus; WB, weight bearing.

provided any strain shielding of the ACL with an anterior shear load of 100 N.[19] Four braces, the DonJoy, the Lennox-Hill, the Townsend, and the CTi, provided strain shielding of the ACL under conditions of a 5-Nm internal rotation torque applied to the leg.[19]

It is clinically evident, however, that some patients with a functional brace perform well, whereas others do not. The major subjective determinant in the success of a brace is a reduction in the number of giving-way episodes reported. Subjective improvements while wearing a brace have been hypothesized to be a result of heightened proprioception.[21, 34, 158] Tibone and associates[220] have found EMG evidence of a longer duration of medial hamstring muscle activity in the unbraced, ACL-deficient knees of subjects engaged in running. The vastus medialis showed an earlier onset of activity during swing phase in the involved limb.

This evidence of "out-of-phase" muscle activity, coupled with the observation of Cook and coworkers[34] that weaker patients perform much better in their braces, supports the increased proprioception theory, especially because braces do not prevent abnormal tibial displacement at physiologic force levels.

Bracing after ACL injury or reconstruction is an acceptable practice. Although bracing probably does not prevent tibial displacement at physiologic loads, there is some evidence that it leads to improved proprioception function for some athletes. However, research in this area has to overcome two major hurdles. The first is the lack of a standard definition for proprioception.[135] The second is the current inability to directly measure proprioception during a physiologic activity and correlate that measure to improved performance.[135, 224] Keeping this in mind, and being aware of the growing number of off-the-shelf functional braces on the market, physicians and clinicians must decide whether the custom-made brace is worth the extra cost to the athlete if the protection offered is only proprioceptive. Another decision the clinician and the athlete must make relates to the effect of the brace on other parameters of athletic performance. There is evidence that bracing increases energy expenditure and decreases maximal torque output from the quadriceps.[182]

INSTRUMENTED AND FUNCTIONAL TESTING

Arthrometer Tests

Clinical tests for ligament instability are hard to quantify and difficult to reproduce. The physical examination allows for only a rough estimation of translation and rotation. Wroble and associates[237] evaluated 11 expert examiners with regard to grading anterior-posterior and internal-external rotation and varus-valgus displacement. Only 4 of 11 examiners (36%) estimated the induced displacements in all 3° of freedom within an acceptable range. There were large differences between starting flexion angles and the amount of displacement induced.

An objective method of testing provides quantitative and reproducible data. The first objective attempt to determine knee ligament laxity was made by Kennedy and Fowler,[116] who in 1971 used a clinic stress machine for in vivo measurements of anterior-posterior laxity using serial radiography after external forces had been applied to the tibia. Torzilli and colleagues[222] further refined this technique in 1978. Markolf and associates,[146] in 1978, presented a knee-testing device that measured anterior-posterior forces versus displacement-response curves; this was referred to as the UCLA instrumented clinical knee testing apparatus. In 1983, Daniel and coworkers[39] introduced the KT-1000,* which measures anterior-posterior laxity (Fig. 10–31). Since then other devices have been introduced to measure knee laxity in various planes, including the Genucom† (Fig. 10–32), the Knee Signature System (KSS),‡ and the Stryker knee laxity tester.§

Many investigations have been undertaken since these arthrometers have become available to evaluate their validity and inter- and intraexaminer reliability and to make comparisons among devices.[4, 38, 40, 51, 91, 118, 156, 162, 180, 201, 237] It appears that knee ligament arthrometers can detect ACL disruption with a high degree of reliability.[4, 38, 180] Detection of PCL deficiency varies a little more, with the KT-1000 and Genucom appearing to perform best in this respect.[4] Varus-valgus laxity can be tested only by the Genucom, which appears to do so reliably.[51]

---

*Available from Medmetric, San Diego, California
†Available from Faro Medical Technologies, Inc., Montreal, Quebec, Canada
‡Available from Orthopaedic Systems, Hayward, California
§Available from Stryker, Kalamazoo, Michigan

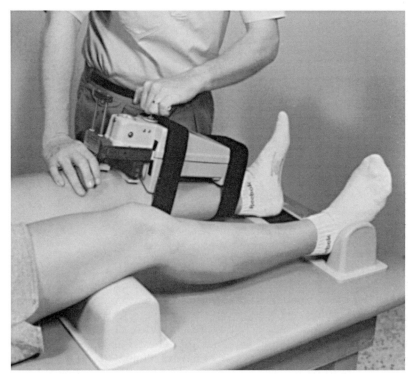

Figure 10–31. KT-1000 arthrometer.

However, the ability of these arthrometers to reproduce reliable displacement readings within and among testers on the same and different days varies widely, and displacement forces as measured by different arthrometers is highly variable. Several investigators have calculated 90% confidence intervals.[4, 162, 235] The

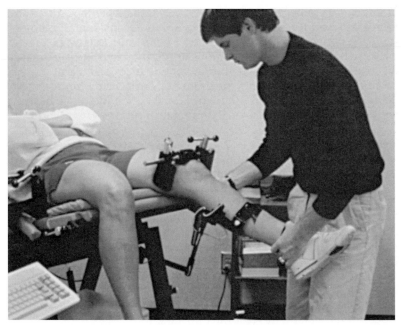

Figure 10–32. Genucom arthrometer.

Table 10–24. Comparison of Three Types of Arthrometers

	REPRODUCI- BILITY	COST	EASE OF OPERA- TION	SPEED	PORTA- BILITY	EASE OF MAINTE- NANCE	DEGREE OF FREEDOM
KT-1000	+ + +	+	+ + +	+ + +	+ + +	+ +	1
KSS	+ +	+ +	+ +	+ +	+ +	+	4
Genucom	+	+ + +	+	+	−	+	6

*From Wroble, R.R. (1990): Practical rules for objective ligament assessment: KT-1000 and other devices. *In:* 1990 Advances on the Knee and Shoulder. Cincinnati, Cincinnati Sports Medicine and Deaconess Hospital.

following confidence intervals (90%) have been reported for normal knees in total anterior-posterior translations:

KT-1000: ± 1.6 mm[238]
KSS: ± 2.7 mm[193]
Genucom: ± 3.4 mm[236]

These results suggest that the KT-1000 has the lowest error in measurement. It is also better than or equal to other arthrometers when considering interexaminer and intraexaminer reliability on the same and different days.[91, 235, 237] Hanten and Pace[91] have reported relatively high reliability coefficients of 0.85 for interexaminer and 0.83 for intraexaminer reliability. The KT-1000 is also the easiest to operate, is portable, and is the least expensive (Table 10–24).[237] Therefore, the KT-1000 appears to be the arthrometer used most often for clinical testing and research.[2, 26, 27, 71, 90, 140, 174, 202, 215, 219] The KT-2000 has also been shown to be more reliable for both between-day measures (intraclass correlation coefficient [ICC] = 0.94) and intertester ratings (ICC = 0.92) than the KSS or the Genucom machine.[186] For the KT-2000, 95% confidence intervals for side-to-side differences in normal individuals have been reported. The intervals range from ± 1.11 mm to ± 1.68 mm, depending on the applied testing force for different-day intratester measures.[161]

The KT-1000, Stryker, and KSS systems seem to be somewhat similar in displacement readings,[4, 168] whereas the Genucom system produces higher absolute values than the other three devices.[156, 180, 236] Usually, with most arthrometers, a difference between the two knees of 2 to 3 mm is considered pathologic.

Examiner experience is a large source of error and decreases the reliability among and within examiners. Meticulous application and measuring techniques must be used to determine whether potential increased tibial translation is induced from ligament deficiency or examiner error. Error can also result from the patient or instrument itself. Guidelines for the examiner have been compiled from various studies to enhance an arthrometer's accuracy:

1. Use total anteroposterior translations. This eliminates the need to identify the neutral position of the knee, thereby eliminating this as a source of error.[235]
2. Report right-left differences with each test, rather then individual knee measurements. This helps account for day-to-day changes, such as anxiety and patient relaxation. Also, single-knee measurements ignore simultaneously occurring changes in the contralateral knee that may appear during training, disuse, or rehabilitation.[237] All these are potential sources of error.
3. Repeat initial testing at least once to take into account the "learning effect."

4. A 30-pound force has been found to provide more discrimination between the ACL-deficient and the normal knee[95] and has been adopted as the standard force by the International Knee Documentation Committee.[42] For testing during the first 8 weeks after reconstructive surgery, the 20-pound force is still being recommended.[42] In addition, the manual maximum is a popular force level for KT testing, especially in the long-term follow-up of ACL reconstructions.
5. Carry out multiple examinations on different days.
6. Use meticulous examination technique. The KT-1000 must be placed accurately over the joint line, and the anterior pull must be in line with the vertical bar of the arthrometer handle.[122]
7. Carefully assess patient relaxation.

If these guidelines are followed, the ability to reproduce tibial displacements with an arthrometer is greatly enhanced and the potential for the results' being caused by chance is diminished. The arthrometer can be used as a diagnostic instrument but may be more valuable as a rehabilitation tool. Some investigators use the arthrometer to determine advancement through an ACL rehabilitation program.[42, 142] For instance, increased tibial translation early in rehabilitation results in a decrease in exercise intensity, modification of the rehabilitation program, or possible continuance of or regression back to crutch ambulation. If used wisely, the arthrometer can provide quantitative information about the surgical and rehabilitation techniques being employed. Also, by detecting increased tibial translation early, the arthrometer may help head off early graft and knee problems that may not be detected by physical examination. Arthrometry also provides important prognostic information. KT-1000 mean maximal differences of greater than 3 mm are significantly correlated with positive pivot shifts, lower scores using the Hospital for Special Surgery knee scoring system, and greater patient dissatisfaction with the reconstructive surgery.[12]

Isokinetic Tests

The knee has been studied isokinetically more than has any other joint.[47] Isokinetic testing can provide the clinician with valuable information regarding the isolated strength of muscles groups, either those damaged by injury or those that provide support to injured joints. Isokinetic testing of the knee has been shown to be extremely reliable, with ICCs as high as 0.99[130] for concentric contraction in asymptomatic subjects. Most of the studies reviewed by Perrin[184] had ICCs between 0.80 and 0.99. For eccentric contraction measures, isokinetic testing is still reliable but not to the same degree that concentric testing is, especially in subjects with knee injuries.[213] With eccentric testing, Steiner and colleagues[213] reported ICCs ranging from 0.58 to 0.96 for average peak torque, with the symptomatic subjects scoring lower. Joint angle at peak torque eccentric testing has not been found to be a reliable measure. At test speeds of 180° per second, ICCs have been reported to be as low as 0.01 for subjects with knee injuries.[213] To ensure high retest reliability the clinician should make sure that the dynamometer axis is closely matched to the knee joint axis and that the athlete is positioned identically each time the test is performed.[184] This includes the accurate replacement of the resistance pad of the dynamometer on the leg. The joint should be tested only through pain-free motion. Allowing the athlete to warm up and perform practice repetitions at the testing speed also improves the reliability of the test.[184]

Isokinetic testing generally provides information on torque (peak or average), total work, and power. When comparing test results of the quadriceps to the hamstrings (agonist-to-antagonist comparisons), it is important to apply a gravity correction factor.[184] The often-quoted concentric normal peak torque hamstring-to-quadriceps ratio is 60%. This ratio for gravity-corrected measures is fairly accurate for slower testing velocities (60° per second), but as testing velocities increase, the ratio is usually greater than 60%. This occurs because the decrease in hamstring torque with increasing velocities is usually less than that of the quadriceps.[47, 184] Dvir[47] has suggested that the hamstring-to-quadriceps ratio is generally not as important as the ratio developed by dividing the involved side measure by the uninvolved side measure. To illustrate this point, if an athlete produces 100 Nm of torque with the right quadriceps and 60 Nm of torque with the right hamstrings, the hamstring-to-quadriceps ratio is 60%. If an athlete produces a left quadriceps torque of 200 Nm and left hamstring torque of 120 Nm, then the left side hamstring-to-quadriceps ratio is also 60%. A side-to-side comparison between the hamstring-to-quadriceps ratios would suggest that the legs were equal, but there is certainly a large deficit with regard to the right thigh musculature torque production. Therefore, in most instances, the injured-side test results should be compared to the uninjured-side test results.

In making side-to-side comparisons it is important to consider the following testing principles. The placement of the dynamometer resistance pad must be the same on both legs, and both knees should be tested through the same ROM. If an antishear device (Fig. 10–33) is used to protect the injured knee, it must be used when testing the uninjured side for a valid comparison to be made. A study on normal subjects revealed a statistically and clinically significant decrease in quadriceps measures when using an antishear device compared to using the normal resistance pad.[131] The hamstring measures were not affected by the antishear attachment.[131] It is also important to test the injured and noninjured sides through the same ROM. For instance, the isokinetic total work measure is determined by the area under the torque curve. The y-axis for this measure is torque and the x-axis is ROM. Thus, if the noninjured side is tested through a greater ROM, the total work for that side could be higher merely because it was performed through a greater ROM and not because it produced a higher torque curve.[184]

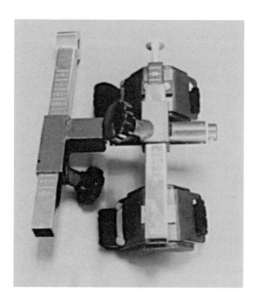

Figure 10–33. Johnson antishear device. This provides a dual-pad placement to reduce tibiofemoral shear.

Using isokinetic testing with injured athletes does have to be done with caution and with an understanding of the joint forces produced during testing. Kaufman and associates[114] studied the joint forces during dynamic isokinetic testing and found significant compression forces for both the patellofemoral and the tibiofemoral joint. Patellofemoral joint compression forces were calculated to reach approximately 5.1 times BW at a knee angle of 70° to 75° during concentric testing at 60° per second. During concentric testing at 180° per second, the compression force was almost as high at 4.9 times BW. This suggests that the common premise that tests at higher speeds produce less joint compression is false. Fortunately at angles less than 20°, the patellofemoral compression forces dropped to less than BW. In this study tibiofemoral compression forces during knee extension peaked at approximately 55° of knee flexion during the 60° per second test and produced a force four times BW. The 180° per second test produced a force of 3.8 times BW. During knee extension, anterior shear of the tibiofemoral joint was greatest at about 25° of flexion and was calculated to be 0.3 times BW for testing at 60° per second and 0.2 times BW for the 180° per second test. Posterior shear force of the tibiofemoral joint during knee flexion peaked at approximately 75° of flexion measured 1.7 times BW for the 60° per second test and 1.4 times BW for the 180° per second test. Again, it is important to note that testing at 180° per second did very little to reduce the anterior and posterior shear forces compared to those that occurred at 60° per second.

It must be stressed that while isokinetic testing provides accurate measures of muscle torque, work, and power, this is not the only information that should be used to determine the readiness of an athlete to return to play. Results are mixed in studies examining the relationship between function and isokinetic tests.[6, 36, 129, 231, 234] For example, Lephart and coworkers[129] reported very low, nonsignificant correlations between isokinetic tests and functional tests in ACL-deficient athletes. This study was designed to explore the differences between athletes who were able to return to sports with an ACL-deficient knee and those who were not. The scores on the functional tests in this study were significantly higher for those who returned versus those unable to return.[129] On the other hand, Wilk and colleagues[231] have reported correlation coefficients of 0.71 and 0.67 for the relationship between subjective knee scores and isokinetic scores in 50 patients with ACL reconstruction. They also reported significant correlations as high as 0.69 for the relationship between isokinetic performance and functional tests.

Functional Tests

Objective test data that can be used in making rehabilitation progression and return-to-play decisions after knee injury or surgery include arthrometry and isokinetic, proprioception, and functional testing. Objective functional testing of the lower extremity aids in determining the functional capabilities of the knee joint during sports activities.[168] Functional tests can be used to determine functional limitations, which cannot be determined through muscle testing alone. This is evidenced by a report from Tibone and colleagues,[220] who examined functional abilities in ACL-deficient individuals. They reported isokinetic peak torque data for quadriceps and hamstrings of 86% and 96%, respectively, but this was not sufficient to eliminate the subjective need for ACL reconstruction.

Several functional tests have been used to assess functional performance objectively after ACL injury. Tegner and associates[217] have used one-legged hopping, figure-eight running, running up and down a spiral staircase, and running up and down a slope to evaluate functional knee integrity. They found that athletes with ACL injuries perform significantly worse than do uninjured players.

Barber and coworkers[14] have evaluated the effectiveness of five-hopping, jumping, and cutting-type tests (shuttle runs) in determining lower extremity functional limitations in athletes with ACL-deficient knees, including the one-legged hop for distance, the one-legged vertical jump, the one-legged timed hop test, and two types of shuttle runs. The shuttle runs and vertical jump test did not consistently detect functional limitations. In the one-legged hop tests, 50% of patients performed normally, but all reported giving-way episodes, indicating a lack of sensitivity of these tests in defining functional limitations. Also, their data showed that 60% of the athletes with ACL-deficient knees performed abnormally (could not jump and land on the involved limb without significant difficulty) on at least one out of two tests in the combined test analysis. Therefore, the authors[14] recommended that clinicians use two one-legged hop tests as a screening procedure to determine lower limb function, in addition to subjective complaints of giving-way. Individuals who score abnormally on the two functional tests have a significant functional limitation for sports activities. Those who score normally may still have giving-way episodes under uncontrolled sports situations.

Noyes and Mangine[143, 168, 170] have reported four tests for appraising functional stability (Fig. 10–34): (1) one-legged hop for distance; (2) one-legged hop for time; (3) one-legged triple hop for distance; and (4) one-legged crossover hop for distance. From their results, the one-legged hop for distance and the one-legged crossover hop for distance appear to be the most consistent in determining functional stability.[143] Mangine[143] has noted that the one-legged hop for distance may be normal, but the one-legged crossover hop for distance may be abnormal if the posterolateral knee complex is involved.

Although it is apparent that functional testing is an important part of the information needed to determine an athlete's status, the reliability of only a few of these tests has been established. The one-legged hop for distance appears to be the most reliable, with ICC reported as high as 0.99.[20] The single-legged 6-m hop for time has a reported ICC of 0.77.[20] The ICC for a 30-m single-legged agility hop has been reported to be 0.09.[20] However, Booher and associates[20] still contend that the agility hop is a stable measure for clinical use because in their study there was a mean difference between trials of less than 0.5 second. Based on their 95% confidence intervals for the agility hop, a clinical difference of greater than ± 2 seconds is probably significant. When using any of the functional tests for clinical assessment, it is suggested that the measure be repeated at least once and the average score of the repeated tests be used as the measure-

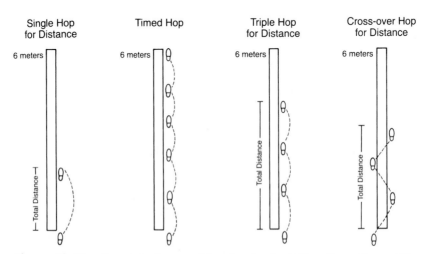

Figure 10–34. Four tests for appraising functional stability. (From Noyes, F.R., Barber, S.D., and Mangine, R.E. [1991]: Abnormal lower limb symmetry determined by function hop tests after anterior cruciate ligament rupture. Am. J. Sports Med., 19:513–518.)

ment.[20] The reliability of functional tests must be established so clinicians can use the tests to serially evaluate the athlete with the confidence that the change in test result is a true change and does not arise from random error in measurement.

Functional testing allows the athlete to be tested in a CKC, rather than in the traditional OKC isokinetic testing environment. It is hoped that the combined data from arthrometer, isokinetic, and functional testing can be used to extrapolate how an individual will perform on the field and thus reduce the risk of reinjury.

SUMMARY

Rehabilitation of the lower extremity should incorporate the appropriate balance of closed- and open-chain exercises along an increasing continuum of difficulty. The determination of the appropriate balance requires a thorough understanding of the biomechanical behavior of the knee and lower extremity during both of these types of activities. Early controlled motion, muscle recruitment, restoration of joint arthrokinematics, and understanding of the relationship of the tibiofemoral to the patellofemoral joint help deter arthrofibrosis after knee injury or surgery. Normal knee-joint kinematics must be understood so that a safe rehabilitation program that emphasizes restoration of joint motion, muscle strength, power, endurance, and proprioception can be developed. Progression should be guided by the athlete's ability to meet specific criteria and not simply by time alone. Functional testing and other objective measurements, such as arthrometry and isokinetic testing, should be used to assist in the determination of when an athlete can return to competition.

References

1. Aglietti, P., and Ceralli, G. (1979): Chondromalacia and recurrent subluxation of the patella: A study of malalignment with some indications for radiography. Ital. J. Orthop. Traumatol., 5:187–190.
2. Aglietti, P., Buzzi, R., and Bassi, P.O. (1988): Arthroscopic partial meniscectomy in the anterior cruciate-deficient knee. Am. J. Sports Med., 16:597–602.
3. Amiel, D., Kleiner, J.B., and Akeson, W.H. (1986): The natural history of the anterior cruciate ligament autograft of patellar tendon origin. Am. J. Sports Med., 14:449–462.
4. Anderson, A.F., and Lipscomb, A.B. (1989): Preoperative instrumented testing of anterior and posterior knee laxity. Am. J. Sports Med., 17:387–392.
5. Anderson, J.K., and Noyes, F.R. (1995): Principles of posterior cruciate ligament rehabilitation. Orthopedics, 18:493-500.
6. Anderson, M.A., Gieck, J.H., Perrin, D., et al. (1991): The relationship among isometric, isotonic, and isokinetic concentric and eccentric quadriceps and hamstring force and three components of athletic performance. J. Orthop. Sports Phys. Ther., 14:114-120.
7. Andriacchi, T.P., Anderson, G.B.J., Ferlier, R.W., et al. (1980): A study of lower-limb mechanics during stair-climbing. J. Bone Joint Surg. [Am.], 62:749–757.
8. Arnheim, D.D. (1989): The knee and related structures. In: Modern Principles of Athletic Training, 7th ed. St. Louis, Times Mirror/Mosby College Publishing.
9. Arnoczky, S.P. (1994): Meniscus. In: Fu, F.H., Harner, C.D., and Vince, K.G. (eds.): Knee Surgery, Vol 1. Baltimore, Williams & Wilkins, pp. 131–140.
10. Arnoczky, S.P., Tarvin, G.B., and Marshall, J.L. (1982): Anterior cruciate ligament replacement using patellar tendon. J. Bone Joint Surg. [Am.], 64:217–224.
11. Arnoczky S.P., Warren R.F., and Ashlock MA. (1986): Replacement of the anterior cruciate ligament using a patellar tendon allograft. J. Bone Joint Surg. [Am.], 68: 376–385.
12. Bach, B.R., Jones, G.T., Hager, C.A., et al. (1995): Arthrometric results of arthroscopically assisted anterior cruciate ligament reconstruction using autograft patellar tendon substitution. Am. J. Sports Med., 23:179–185.
13. Barber, F.A. (1994): Accelerated rehabilitation for meniscus repairs. Arthroscopy, 10:206–210.
14. Barber, S.D., Noyes, F.R., Mangine, R.B., et al. (1990): Quantitative assessment of functional limitations in normal and anterior cruciate ligament-deficient knee. Clin. Orthop., 255:204–214.
15. Beck, C., Drez, D., and Young, J., et al. (1986): Instrumented testing of functional knee braces. Am. J. Sports Med., 14:253–256.

16. Beckman, M., Craig, R., and Lehman, R.C. (1989): Rehabilitation of patellofemoral dysfunction in the athlete. Clin. Sports Med., 8:841–861.
17. Berchuck, M., Andriacchi, T.P., Bach, B.R., et al. (1990): Gait adaptations by patients who have a deficient anterior cruciate ligament. J. Bone Joint Surg. [Am.], 72:871–877.
18. Beynnon, B.D., Fleming, B.C., Johnson, R.J., et al. (1995): Anterior cruciate ligament strain behavior during rehabilitation exercises in vivo. Am. J. Sports Med., 23:24–34.
19. Beynnon, B.D., Pope, M.H., Wertheimer, C.M., et al. (1992): The effect of functional knee-braces on strain on anterior cruciate ligament in vivo. J. Bone Joint Surg. [Am.], 74:1298–1312.
20. Booher, L.D., Hench, K.M., and Worrell, T.W. (1993): Reliability of three single-leg hop tests. J. Sports Rehabil., 2:165–170.
21. Branch, T., Hunter, R., and Reynolds, P. (1988): Controlling anterior tibial displacement under static load: A comparison of two braces. Orthopedics, 11:1249–1252.
22. Brittberg, M., Lindahl, A., and Nilsson, A. (1994): Treatment of deep cartilage defects in the knee with autologous chondrocyte transplantation. New Engl. J. Med., 11:889–895.
23. Brockroth, K., Wooden, C., Worrell, T., et al. (1993): The effects of patellar taping on patellar position and perceived pain. Med. Sci. Sports Exerc. 25:989–992.
24. Brownstein, B., Mangine, R.E., Noyes, F.R., and Kryger, S. (1988): Anatomy and biomechanics. In: Mangine, R.E. (ed.): Physical Therapy of the Knee. New York, Churchill Livingstone.
25. Bullough, P.G., Munuera, L., Murphy, J., et al. (1970): The strength of the menisci of the knee as it relates to their fine structure. J. Bone Joint Surg. [Br.], 52:564–570.
26. Burks, R.T., and Leland, R. (1988): Determination of graft tension before fixation in anterior cruciate ligament reconstruction. J. Arthrosc. Rel. Surg., 4:260–266.
27. Burks, R., Daniel, D., and Losse, G. (1984): The effect of continuous passive motion on anterior cruciate ligament reconstruction stability. Am. J. Sports Med., 12:323–327.
28. Butler, D.L. (1994): Biomechanics of graft fixation, changes in tension over time. In: Advances on the Knee and Shoulder. Cincinnati, Cincinnati Sports Medicine and Deaconess Hospital.
29. Castle, T.H., Noyes, F.R., and Grood, E.S. (1992): Posterior tibial subluxation of the posterior cruciate-deficient knee. Clin. Orthop., 284:193–202.
30. Cerny, K. (1995): Vastus medialis oblique/vastus lateralis muscle activity ratios for selected exercises in person with and without patellofemoral pain syndrome. Phys. Ther., 75:672–683.
31. Clancy, W.G., Narechania, R.G., Rosenberg, T.D., et al. (1981): Anterior and posterior cruciate ligament reconstruction in rhesus monkeys. J. Bone Joint Surg. [Am.], 63:1270–1284.
32. Close, J.R. (1964): Motor Function in the Lower Extremity: Analyses by Electronic Instrumentation. Springfield, IL, Charles C Thomas.
33. Colville, M.R., Lee, C.L., and Ciullo, J.V. (1986): The Lenox Hill brace: An evaluation of effectiveness in treating knee instability. Am. J. Sports Med., 14:257–261.
34. Cook, F.F., Tibone, J.E., and Redfern, F.C. (1989): A dynamic analysis of a functional brace for anterior cruciate ligament insufficiency. Am. J. Sports Med., 17:519–524.
35. Cooper, D.E., Deng, X.H., Burstein, A.L., and Warren, R.F. (1993): The strength of the central third patellar tendon graft: A biomechanical study. Am. J. Sports Med., 21: 818–824.
36. Cordova, M.L., Ingersoll, C.D., Kovaleski, J.E., et al. (1995): A comparison of isokinetic and isotonic predictions of a functional task. J. Athl. Train., 30:319–322.
37. Dahlkvist, N.J., Mayo, P., and Seedhom, B.B. (1982): Forces during squatting and rising from a deep squat. Engineering Med., 11:69–76.
38. Daniel, D.M., Malcom, L.L., and Losse, G., et al. (1985): Instrumented measurement of anterior laxity of the knee. J. Bone Joint Surg. [Am.], 67:720–726.
39. Daniel, D.M., Stone, M.L., and Malcom, L., et al. (1983): Instrumented measurement of ACL disruption. Orthop. Res. Soc., 8:12–17.
40. Daniel, D.M., Stone, M.L., Sachs, R., and Malcom, L. (1985): Instrumented measurement of anterior knee laxity in patients with acute anterior cruciate ligament disruption. Am. J. Sports Med., 13:401–407.
41. DeHaven, K.E. (1985): Rationale for meniscus repair or excision. Clin. Sports Med., 4:267–273.
42. DeMaio, M., Mangine, R.E., and Noyes, F.R. (1992): Advanced muscle training after ACL reconstruction: Weeks 6 to 52. Orthopedics, 15:757–767.
43. Doucette, S.A., and Child, D.D. (1996): The effect of open and closed chain exercise and knee joint position on patellar tracking in lateral patellar compression syndrome. J. Orthop. Sports Phys. Ther., 23:104–110.
44. Doucette, S.A., and Goble, E.M. (1992): The effect of exercise on patellar tracking in lateral patellar compression syndrome. Am. J. Sports Med., 20:434–440.
45. Drez, D.J., DeLee, J., Holden, J.P., et al. (1991): Anterior cruciate ligament reconstruction using bone-patellar tendon-bone allografts. Am. J. Sports Med., 19:256–263.
46. Dürselen, L., Claes, L., and Kiefer, H. (1995): The influence of muscle forces and external loads on cruciate ligament strain. Am. J. Sports Med., 23:129–136.
47. Dvir, Z. (1995): Isokinetics: Muscle Testing Interpretation and Clinical Applications. Edinburgh, Churchill Livingstone.
48. Ekholm, J., Nisell, R., and Arborelius, U.P., et al. (1984): Load on knee joint structures and muscular activity during living. Scand. J. Rehabil. Med., 16:1–9.
49. Ellis, M.I., Seedhom, B.B., Amis, A.A., et al. (1979): Forces in the knee joint whilst rising from normal and motorized chairs. N. Engl. J. Med., 8:33–40.

50. Ellis, M.I., Seedhom, B.B., and Wright, V. (1984): Forces in the knee joint whilst rising from seated positions. J. Biomed. Eng., 6:113–120.
51. Emery, M., Moffroid, M., and Boerman, J., et al. (1989): Reliability of force/displacement measures in a clinical device designed to measure ligamentous laxity at the knee. J. Orthop. Sports Phys. Ther., 10:441–447.
52. Eng, J.J., and Pierrynowski, M.R. (1993): Evaluation of soft foot orthotics in the treatment of patellofemoral pain syndrome. Phys. Ther., 73:62–68.
53. Engle, R.P. (1988): Hamstring facilitation in anterior instability of the knee. Athl. Train., 23:226–228, 285.
54. Engle, R.P., and Canner, G.G. (1989): Proprioceptive neuromuscular facilitation (PNF) and modified procedures for anterior cruciate ligament (ACL) instability. J. Orthop. Sports Phys. Ther., 11:230–236.
55. Engle, R.P., and Canner, G.C. (1989): Rehabilitation of symptomatic anterolateral knee instability. J. Orthop. Sports Phys. Ther., 11:237–244.
56. Ericson, M.O. (1988): Muscular function during ergometer cycling. Scand. J. Rehabil. Med., 20:35–41.
57. Ericson, M.O., and Nisell, R. (1986): Tibiofemoral joint forces during ergometer cycling. Am. J. Sports Med., 14:285–290.
58. Ericson, M.O., and Nisell, R. (1987): Patellofemoral joint forces during ergometer cycling. Phys. Ther., 67:1365–1369.
59. Ericson, M.O., Bratt, P., and Nisell, R., et al. (1986): Power output and work in different muscle groups during ergometer cycling. Eur. J. Appl. Physiol., 55:229.
60. Ericson, M.O., Nisell, R., Arborelius, U.P., and Ekholm, J. (1985): Muscular activity during ergometer cycling. Scand. J. Rehabil. Med., 17:53.
61. Ericson, M.O., Nisell, R., and Ekholm, J. (1984): Varus and valgus loads on the knee joint during ergometer cycling. Scand. J. Sports Sci., 6:39–45.
62. Fairbank, T.J. (1948): Knee joint changes after meniscectomy. J. Bone Joint Surg. [Br.], 30:664–670.
63. Fiebert, I., Gresly, J. Hoffman, S., et al. (1994). Comparative measurements of anterior tibial translation using a KT-1000 knee arthrometer with the leg in neutral, internal rotation, and external rotation. J. Orthop. Sports Phys. Ther. 19:331–334.
64. Fisk, R., and Wells, J. (1980): The quadriceps complex in bipedal man. J. Am. Osteopath. Assoc., 80:291–294.
65. Fleming, B.C., Beynnon, B.D., Pevia, G.D., et al. (1995). Anterior cruciate ligament strain during open and closed kinetic chain exercise: an in vivo study. Trans. Orthop. Res. Soc. 20:631–636.
66. Fleming, R.E., Blatz, D.J., and McCorroll, J.R. (1981): Posterior problems in the knee. Am. J. Sports Med., 9:107–113.
67. Flynn, T.W., and Soutas-Little, R.W. (1995): Patellofemoral joint compressive forces in forward and backward running. J. Orthop. Sports Phys. Ther., 21:277–282.
68. Fowler, P.J. (1984): Functional anatomy of the knee. In: Hunter, L.Y., and Funk, F.J. (eds.): Rehabilitation of the Injured Knee. St. Louis, C.V. Mosby.
69. Fowler, P.J., and Lubliner, J. (1995): Functional anatomy and biomechanics of the knee joint. In: Griffin, L.Y. (ed.): Rehabilitation of the Injured Knee. St. Louis, C.V. Mosby.
70. Fowler, P.S. (1994): The ACL injury. In: 1994 Advances on the Knee and Shoulder. Cincinnati, Cincinnati Sports Medicine and Deaconess Hospital.
71. Fox, J.M., Sherman, O.H., and Markolf, K. (1985): Arthroscopic anterior cruciate ligament repair: Preliminary results in instrumented testing for anterior stability. J. Arthrosc. Rel. Surg., 1:175–181.
72. Friden, T., Zatterstrom, R., Anders, L., et al. (1991): Anterior cruciate-insufficient knees treated with physiotherapy. Clin. Orthop., 263:190–199.
73. Friederich, N.E., and O'Brien, W.R. (1992): Functional anatomy of the cruciate ligaments. In: Jakob, R.P., and Staubli, H.U. (eds.): The Knee and the Cruciate Ligaments. Berlin, Springer-Verlag, pp. 80–81.
74. Fukubayashi, T., and Kurosawa, H. (1980): The contact area and pressure distribution pattern of the knee. Acta Orthop. Scand., 51:871–879.
75. Fulkerson, J.P., and Hungerford, D.S. (1990). Normal anatomy. In: Disorders of the Patellofemoral Joint, 2nd ed. Baltimore, Williams & Wilkins, pp.1–22.
76. Fulkerson, J.P., and Hungerford, D.S. (1990). Biomechanics of the patellofemoral joint. Disorders of the Patellofemoral Joint, 2nd ed. Baltimore, Williams & Wilkins, pp. 25–39.
77. Fuss, F.K. (1992): Principles and mechanisms of automatic rotation during terminal extension in the human knee joint. J. Anat., 180: 297–304.
78. Goh J.C., Lee P.Y.C., and Bose K. (1995): A cadaver study of the function of the oblique part of vastus medialis. J. Bone Joint Surg. [Br.], 77: 225–231.
79. Gollehon, D.L., Torzilli, P.A., and Warren, R.F. (1987): The role of the posterolateral and cruciate ligaments in the stability of the human knee. J. Bone Joint Surg. [Am.], 69:233–242.
80. Goodfellow, J., Hungerford, D.S., and Woods, C. (1976): Patello-femoral joint mechanics and pathology. J. Bone Joint Surg. [Br.], 58:291–299.
81. Goodfellow, J., Hungerford, D.S., and Zindel, M. (1976): Patellofemoral joint mechanics and pathology: 1. Functional anatomy of the patello-femoral joint. J. Bone Joint Surg. [Br.], 58:287–290.

82. Gough, J.V., and Ladley, G. (1971): An investigation into the effectiveness of various forms of quadriceps exercises. Physiotherapy, 57:356–361.
83. Grood, E.S. (1994): Patellar tendon autograft and allograft healing. *In:* Advances on the Knee and Shoulder. Cincinnati, Cincinnati Sports Medicine and Deaconess Hospital.
84. Grood, E.S., and Suntay, W.J. (1983). A joint coordinate system for the clinical description of three-dimensional motions: application to the knee. J. Biomech. Eng., 105: 101–107, 1983.
85. Grood, E.S., Noyes, F.R., Butler, D.L., and Suntay, W.J. (1981): Ligamentous and capsular restraints preventing straight medial and lateral laxity in intact human cadaver knees. J. Bone Joint Surg. [Am.], 63:1257–1269.
86. Grood, E.S., Stowers, S.F., and Noyes, F.R. (1988): Limits of movement in the human knee. J. Bone Joint Surg. [Am.], 70:88–97.
87. Grood, E.S., Suntay, W.J., Noyes, F.R., and Butler, D. (1984): Biomechanics of the knee-extension exercise. J. Bone Joint Surg. [Am.], 66:725–733.
88. Gross, M.T., Tyson, A.D., and Burns, C.B.B. (1993): Effect of knee angle and ligament insufficiency on anterior tibial translation during quadriceps muscle contraction: A preliminary report. J. Orthop. Sports Phys. Ther., 17:133–143.
89. Gryzlo, S.M., Patek, R.M., Pink, M., et al.(1994): Electromyographic analysis of knee rehabilitation exercises. J. Orthop. Sports Phys. Ther., 20:36–43.
90. Hanley, S.T., and Warren, R.F. (1987): Arthroscopic meniscectomy in the anterior cruciate ligament-deficient knee. J. Arthrosc. Rel. Res., 3:159–165.
91. Hanten, W.P., and Pace, M.B. (1987): Reliability of measuring anterior laxity of the knee joint using a knee ligament arthrometer. Phys. Ther., 67:357–359.
92. Hanten, W.P., and Schulthies, S.S. (1990): Exercise effect on electromyographic activity of the vastus medialis oblique and vastus lateralis muscles. Phys. Ther., 70:561–565.
93. Hardy, M.A. (1989): The biology of scar formation. Phys. Ther., 69:1014–1024.
94. Henning, C.E., Lynch, M.A., and Glick, K.R. (1985): An in vivo strain gauge study of elongation of the anterior cruciate ligament. Am. J. Sports Med., 13:22–26.
95. Highgenboten, C.L., Jackson, A.W., Jansson, K.A., et al. (1992): KT-1000 arthrometer: Conscious and unconscious test results using 15, 20, and 30 pounds of force. Am. J. Sports Med., 20:450–454.
96. Host, J.V., Craig, R., and Lehman, R.C. (1995): Patellofemoral dysfunction in tennis players. Clin. Sports Med., 14:177–203.
97. Houtz, S.J., and Fischer, F.J. (1959): An analysis of muscle action and joint excursion during exercise on a stationary bicycle. J. Bone Joint Surg. [Am.], 41:123.
98. Howell, S.M. (1990): Anterior tibial translation during a maximum quadriceps contraction: Is it clinically significant? Am. J. Sports Med., 18:573–578.
99. Huberti, H.H., and Hayes, W.C. (1984): Patellofemoral contact pressure. J. Bone Joint Surg. [Am.], 55:715–724.
100. Huiskes, R., and Blankevoort, L. (1992): Anatomy and biomechanics of the anterior cruciate ligament: A three-dimensional problem. *In:* Jakob, R.P., and Staubli, H.U. (eds.): The Knee and the Cruciate Ligaments. Berlin, Springer-Verlag, pp. 80–81.
101. Hungerford, D.S. (1983): Patellar subluxation and excessive lateral pressure as a cause of fibrillation. *In:* Pickett, J.C., and Radin, E.L. (eds.): Chondromalacia of the Patella. Baltimore, Williams & Wilkins, pp. 24–42.
102. Hungerford, D.S., and Barry, M. (1979): Biomechanics of the patellofemoral joint. Clin. Orthop., 144:9–15.
103. Hughston, J.C. (1993): Knee Ligaments: Injury and Repair. St. Louis, C.V. Mosby, p. 16.
104. Hughston, J.C., Walsh, W.M., and Puddu G. (1984). Patellar Subluxation and Dislocation. Philadelphia, W.B. Saunders, pp. 1–20.
105. Indelicato, P.A., Hermansdorfer, J., and Huegel M. (1990): Nonoperative management of complete tears of the medial collateral ligament of the knee in intercollegiate football players. Clin. Orthop., 256:174–177.
106. Ingersoll, C.D., and Knight, K.L. (1991): Patellar location changes following EMG biofeedback or progressive resistive exercises. Med. Sci. Sports Exerc., 23:1122–1127.
107. James, S.L. (1979): Chondromalacia of the patella in the adolescent. *In:* Kennedy, J.C. (ed.): The Injured Adolescent Knee. Baltimore, Williams & Wilkins, pp. 205–251.
108. Johnson, R.J., Kettelkamp, D.B., and Clack, W., et al. (1974): Factors affecting late results after meniscectomy. J. Bone Joint Surg. [Am.], 56:719–729.
109. Kahn, J. (1987): Transcutaneous electrical nerve stimulation. *In:* Principles and Practice of Electrotherapy. New York, Churchill Livingstone.
110. Kannus, P., and Jarvinen, M. (1987): Conservatively treated tears of the anterior cruciate ligament. J. Bone Joint Surg. [Am.], 69:1007–1012.
111. Kapandji, I.A. (1987): The Physiology of the Joints, Vol 2, 5th ed. New York, Churchill Livingstone.
112. Karst, G.M., and Jewett, P.D. (1993): Electromyographic analysis of exercises proposed for differential activation of medial and lateral quadriceps femoris muscle components. Phys. Ther., 73:286–295.
113. Karst, G.M, and Willett, G.M. (1995): Onset timing of electromyographic activity in the vastus medialis oblique and vastus lateralis muscle in subjects with and without patellofemoral pain syndrome. Phys. Ther., 75:813–823.

114. Kaufman, K.R., An, K., Litchy, W.J., et al. (1991): Dynamic joint forces during knee isokinetic exercise. Am. J. Sports Med., 19:305–316.

115. Kawai, Y., Fukubayashi, T., and Nishino, J. (1989): Meniscal suture: An experimental study in the dog. Clin. Orthop., 243:286–293.

116. Kennedy, J.C., and Fowler, P.M. (1971): Medial and anterior instability of the knee. An anatomical and clinical study using stress machines. J. Bone Joint Surg. [Am.], 53:1257.

117. Kennedy, J.C., Alexander, I.J., and Hayes, K.C. (1982): Nerve supply of the human knee and its functional importance. Am. J. Sports Med., 10:329–335.

118. King, J.B., and Kumar, S.J. (1989): The Stryker knee arthrometer in clinical practice. Am. J. Sports Med., 17:649–650.

119. King, S., Butterwick, D.J., and Cuerrier, J.P. (1986): The anterior cruciate ligament: A review of recent concepts. J. Orthop. Sports Phys. Ther., 8:110-122.

120. Knight, K.L. (1985): Guidelines for rehabilitation of sports injuries. Clin. Sports Med., 4:405-416.

121. Koh, T.J., Grabiner, M.D., and De Swart, R.J. (1992): In vivo tracking of the human patella. J. Biomech., 25:637-643.

122. Kowalk, D.L., Wojtys, E.M., Disher, J., et al. (1993): Quantitative analysis of the measuring capabilities of the KT-1000 knee ligament arthrometer. Am. J. Sports Med., 21:744-747.

123. Kowall, M.G., Kolk, G., Nuber, G.W., et al. (1996). Patellar taping in the treatment of patellofemoral pain. A prospective radiographic study. Am. J. Sports Med., 24: 61-66.

124. Kramer, P.G. (1986): Patella malalignment syndrome: Rationale to reduce excessive lateral pressure. J. Orthop. Sports Phys. Ther., 8:301–309.

125. Krause, W.R., Pope, M.H., Johnson, R.J., et al. (1976): Mechanical changes in the knee after meniscectomy. J. Bone Joint Surg. [Am.], 58:599–604.

126. Kujala, U.M., Osterman, K., Kormano, M., et al.(1989): Patellar motion analyzed by magnetic resonance imaging. Orthop. Scand., 60:13–16.

127. Lane, J.G., Irby, S.E., Kaufman, K., et al. (1994): The anterior cruciate ligament in controlling axial rotation. Am. J. Sports Med., 22:289–293.

128. Larsen B.J., Anderson, E., Unfer, A., et al. (1995). Patellar taping: A radiographic examination of the medial glide technique. Am. J. Sports Med., 23:465–471.

129. Lephart, S.M., Perrin, D.H., Fu, F.H., et al. (1992): Relationship between selected physical characteristics and functional capacity in the anterior cruciate ligament-insufficient athlete. J. Orthop. Sports Phys. Ther., 16:174–181.

129a. Leveau, R.F. (1992): Williams and Lissner's Biomechanics of Human Motion, 3rd ed. Philadelphia, W.B. Saunders.

130. Levene, J.A., Hart, B.A., Seeds, R.H., et al. (1991): Reliability of reciprocal isokinetic testing of the knee extensors and flexors. J. Orthop. Sports Phys. Ther., 14:1221–1227.

131. Li, C.K., Chan, K.M., Hsu, S.Y., et al. (1993): The Johnson anti-shear device and standard shin pad in the isokinetic assessment of the knee. Br. J. Sports Med., 27:49–52.

132. Lieb, F.J., and Perry, J. (1968): Quadriceps function: An anatomical and mechanical study using amputated limbs. J. Bone Joint Surg. [Am.], 50:1535–1548.

133. Lieb, F.J., and Perry, J. (1971): Quadriceps function: An electromyographic study under isometric conditions. J. Bone Joint Surg. [Am.], 53:749–758.

134. Limbird, T.J., Shiavi, R., Frazer, M., and Borra, H. (1988): EMG profiles of knee joint musculature during walking: Changes induced by anterior cruciate ligament deficiency. J. Orthop. Res., 6:630–638.

135. Liu, S.H., and Mirzayan, R. (1995): Current review: Functional knee bracing. Clin. Orthop., 317:273–281.

136. Lutz, G.A., Palmitier, R.A., and An, K.N. (1993): Comparison of tibiofemoral joint forces during open and closed kinetic chain exercises. J. Bone Joint Surg. [Am.], 75:732–739.

137. Lutz, G.E., Stuart, M.J., and Sim, F.H. (1990): Rehabilitative techniques for athletes after reconstruction of the anterior cruciate ligament. Mayo Clin. Proc., 65:1322–1329.

138. Lynch, M.A., Henning, C.E., and Glick, K.R. (1983): Knee joint surface changes. Long-term follow-up meniscus tear treatment in stable anterior cruciate ligament reconstructions. Clin. Orthop., 172:148–153.

139. MacConnail, M.A. (1953): The movement of bone and joints. 5. The significance of shape. J. Bone Joint Surg. [Br.], 35:290–297.

140. Malcom, L.L., Daniel, D.M., Stone, M.L., and Sachs, R. (1985): The measurement of anterior knee laxity after ACL reconstructive surgery. Clin. Orthop., 196:35–41.

141. Mangine, R. (1989): Knee flexion-extension exercise. In: 1989 Advances on the Knee and Shoulder. Cincinnati, Cincinnati Sports Medicine and Deaconess Hospital.

142. Mangine, R. (1990): Post-surgical management following PCL surgery. In: 1990 Advances on the Knee and Shoulder. Cincinnati, Cincinnati Sports Medicine and Deaconess Hospital.

143. Mangine, R. (1990): Rules for management, functional testing, braces. In: 1990 Advances on the Knee and Shoulder. Cincinnati, Cincinnati Sports Medicine and Deaconess Hospital.

144. Mangine, R.E., Noyes, F.R., DeMaio, M. (1992): Minimal protection program: Advanced weight bearing and range of motion after ACL reconstruction—Weeks 1 to 5. Orthopedics, 15:504–515.

145. Markolf, K.L., Bargar, W.L., Shoemaker, S.C., and Amstutz, H.C. (1981): The role of joint load in knee stability. J. Bone Joint Surg. [Am.], 63:570–585.

146. Markolf, K.L., Graff-Radford, A., and Amstutz, H.C. (1978): In vivo knee stability: A quantitative assessment using instrumented clinical testing apparatus. J. Bone Joint Surg. [Am.], 60:664.

147. Markolf, K.L., Kochan, A., and Amstutz, H. (1984): Measurement of knee stiffness and laxity in patients with documented absence of the anterior cruciate ligament. J. Bone Joint Surg. [Am.], 66:242.

148. Markolf, K.L., Mensch, J.S., and Amstutz, H.C. (1976): Stiffness and laxity of the knee—the contributions of the supporting structures. J. Bone Joint Surg. [Am.], 58, 583.

149. Marshall, J., Girgis, F.G., and Zelko, R.R. (1972): The biceps femoris tendon and its functional significance. J. Bone Joint Surg. [Am.], 54:1444.

150. McConnell, J. (1986): The management of chondromalacia patellae: A long-term solution. Aust. J. Physiother., 32:215–223.

151. McConnell J. (1991): McConnell Patellofemoral Treatment Plan. Santa Ana, CA, McConnell Seminars.

152. McFarland, E.G., Morrey, B.F., An, K.N., and Wood, W.B. (1986): The relationship of vascularity and water content to tensile strength in a patellar tendon replacement of the anterior cruciate in dogs. Am. J. Sports Med., 14:436–448.

153. McGinty, J.B., Guess, L.F., and Marvin, R.A. (1977): Partial or total meniscectomy: A comparative analysis. J. Bone Joint Surg. [Am.], 59:763–766.

154. McLaughlin, J., DeMaio, M., Noyes, F.R., et al. (1994). Rehabilitation after meniscus repair. Orthopedics 17:463–471.

155. McLeod, W.D., and Blackburn, T.A. (1980): Biomechanics of knee rehabilitation with cycling. Am. J. Sports Med., 8:175–180.

156. McQuade, K.J., Sidles, J.A., and Larson, R.V. (1989): Reliability of the Genucom knee laxity system. Clin. Orthop., 245:216–219.

157. Merchant, A.C., Mercer, R.L. Jacobsen, R.H.J., and Cool, C.R. (1974): Roentgenographic analysis of patellofemoral congruence. J. Bone Joint Surg. [Am.], 56:1391–1398.

158. Mishra, D.V., Daniel, D.M., and Stone, M.L. (1989): The use of functional knee braces in the control of pathologic anterior knee laxity. Clin. Orthop., 241:213–220.

159. Moore, K.L. (1992): Clinically Oriented Anatomy, 3rd ed. Baltimore, Williams & Wilkins.

160. Morrison, J.B. (1968): Bioengineering analysis of force actions transmitted by the knee joint. Biomed. Eng., 3:164–170.

161. Myer, J.W., Schulthies, S.S., Fellingham, G.W. (1996): Relative and absolute reliability of the KT-2000 arthrometer for uninjured knees. Am. J. Sports Med., 24:104–108.

162. Neuschwander, D.C., Drez, D., Paine, R.M., and Young, J.C. (1990): Comparison of anterior laxity measurements in anterior cruciate-deficient knees with two instrumented testing devices. Orthopedics, 13:299–302.

163. Nisell, R., and Ekholm, J. (1985): Patellar forces during knee extension. Scand. J. Rehabil. Med., 17:63–74.

164. Nisell, R., Ericson, M.O., Nemeth, G., and Ekholm, J. (1989): Tibiofemoral joint forces during isokinetic knee extension. Am. J. Sports Med., 17:49–54.

165. Nordin, M., and Frankel, V.H. (1989): Basic Biomechanics of the Musculoskeletal System. Philadelphia, Lea & Febiger.

166. Norkin, C.C. and Levange, P.K. (1992): The knee complex. In: Joint Structure and Function: A Comprehensive Analysis, 2nd ed. Philadelphia, F.A. Davis, pp. 337–377.

167. Noyes, F.R. (1989): Rules for surgical indications in ACL surgery. In: 1989 Advances on the Knee and Shoulder. Cincinnati, Cincinnati Sports Medicine and Deaconess Hospital.

168. Noyes, F.R. (1990): Objective functional testing. In: Noyes, F.R. (ed.): The Noyes Knee Rating System. Cincinnati, Cincinnati Sports Medicine Research and Education Foundation.

169. Noyes, F.R. (1994): ACL deficient knee: Natural history, indications, surgery, risk analysis. In: 1994 Advances on the Knee and Shoulder. Cincinnati, Cincinnati Sports Medicine and Deaconess Hospital.

170. Noyes, F.R., Barber, S.D., and Mangine, R.E. (1991): Abnormal lower limb symmetry determined by function hop test after anterior cruciate ligament rupture. Am. J. Sports Med., 19:513–518.

171. Noyes, F.R., Barber-Westin, S., and Roberts, C. (1994): Use of allografts after failed treatment of rupture of the anterior cruciate ligament. J. Bone Joint Surg. [Am.], 76:1019–1031.

172. Noyes, F.R., Butler, D.L., Grood, E.S., et al. (1984): Biomechanical analysis of human ligament frafts used in knee-ligament repairs and reconstructions. J. Bone Joint Surg. [Am.], 66:344–352.

173. Noyes, F.R., Grood, E.S., Butler, D.L., and Malek, M. (1980): Clinical laxity tests and functional stability of the knee: Biomechanical concepts. Clin. Orthop., 146:84–89.

174. Noyes, F.R., Mangine, R.E., and Barber, S. (1987): Early knee motion after open and arthroscopic anterior cruciate ligament reconstruction. Am. J. Sports Med., 15:149–160.

175. Noyes, F.R., Mangine, R.E., and Barber, S.D. (1992): The early treatment of motion complications after reconstruction of the anterior cruciate ligament. Clin. Orthop., 277:217–228.

176. Noyes, F.R., Matthews, D.S., Mooar, P.A., and Butler, D.L., (1983): The symptomatic anterior cruciate-deficient knee. Part I: The long term functional disability in athletically active individuals. J. Bone Joint Surg. [Am.], 65:163–174.

177. Noyes, F.R., Matthews, D.S., Mooar, P.A., and Grood, E.S. (1983): The symptomatic anterior cruciate-deficient knee. Part II: The results of rehabilitation, activity modification, and counseling on functional disability. J. Bone Joint Surg. [Am.], 65:154–162.

178. Ohkoshi, Y., Yasuda, K., Kaneda, K., et al. (1991): Biomechanical analysis of rehabilitation in the standing position. Am. J. Sports Med., 19:605–611.

179. Okamoto, T. (1969): Electromyographic study of the function of muscle rectus femoris. Res. J. Phys. Educ., 12:175–182.
180. Oliver, J.H., and Coughlin, L.P. (1987): Objective knee evaluation using the Genucom Knee Analysis System. Am. J. Sports Med., 15:571–578.
181. O'Meara, P.M. (1993): Rehabilitation following reconstruction of the anterior cruciate ligament. Orthopedics, 16:301–306.
182. Ott, J.W., and Clancy, W.G. (1993): Functional knee braces. Orthopedics, 16:171–175.
183. Paulos, L., Rusche, K., Johnson, C., and Noyes, F. (1980): Patellar malalignment: A treatment rationale. Phys. Ther., 60:1624–1632.
184. Perrin, D.H. (1993): Isokinetic Exercise and Assessment. Champaign, IL, Human Kinetics Publishers.
185. Pocock, G.S. (1963): Electromyographic study of the quadriceps during resistive exercise. J. Am. Phys. Ther. Assoc., 43:427–434.
186. Queale, W.S., Snyder-Mackler, L., Handling, K.A., et al. (1994): Instrumented examination of knee laxity in patients with anterior cruciate deficiency: A comparison of the KT-2000, Knee Signature System, and Genucom. J. Orthop. Sports Phys. Ther., 19:345–351.
187. Quillen, W.S., and Gieck, J.H. (1988): Manual therapy: Mobilization of the motion restricted knee. Athl. Train., 23:123–130.
188. Reider, B., Marshall, J.L., and Ring, B. (1981): Patellar tracking. Clin. Orthop., 157:143.
189. Reider, B., Sathy, M.R., Talkington, J., et al. (1993): Treatment of isolated medial collateral ligament injuries in athletes with early functional rehabilitation. Am. J. Sports Med., 22:470–477.
190. Reilly, D.T., and Martens, M. (1972): Experimental analysis of the quadriceps muscle force and patellofemoral joint reaction force for various activities. Acta Orthop. Scand., 43:126–137.
191. Renström, P., Arms, S.W., Stanwyck, T.S., et al. (1986): Strain within the anterior cruciate ligament during hamstring and quadriceps activity. Am. J. Sports Med., 14:83–87.
192. Reynolds, L., Levin, T.A., Medeiros, J.M., et al. (1983): EMG activity of the vastus medialis oblique and the vastus lateralis in their role in patellar alignment. Am. J. Phys. Med., 62:61–70.
193. Riederman, R., Wroble, R.R., Grood, E.S., et al. (1991): Reproducibility of the Knee Signature System. Am. J. Sports Med., 19:660–664.
194. Rowinski, M.J. (1985): Afferent neurobiology of the joint. In: Gould, J.A., and Davies, G.J. (eds.): Orthopedic and Sports Physical Therapy. St. Louis, C.V. Mosby.
195. Ruffin, M.T., and Kiningham, R.B. (1993):Anterior knee pain: The challenge of patellofemoral syndrome. Am. Fam. Phys., 47:185–194.
196. Rusche, K., and Mangine, R. (1988): Pathomechanics of injury to the patellofemoral and tibiofemoral joint. In: Mangine, R. (ed.): Physical Therapy of the Knee. New York, Churchill Livingstone.
197. Schaub, P.A., and Worrell, T.W. (1995): EMG activity of six muscles and VMO:VL ratio determination during a maximal squat exercise. J. Sports Rehabil., 4:195–202.
198. Schultz, R.A., Miller, D.C., Kerr, C.S., and Micheli, L. (1984): Mechanoreceptors in human cruciate ligaments. J. Bone Joint Surg. [Am.], 66:1072–1076.
199. Scott, S.H, and Winter, D.A. (1990): Internal forces at chronic running injury sites. Med. Sci. Sports Exerc., 22:357–369.
200. Shelbourne, D.K., and Nitz, P. (1990): Accelerated rehabilitation after anterior cruciate reconstruction. Am. J. Sports Med., 18:292–299.
201. Sherman, O.H., Markolf, K.L., and Ferkel, R.D. (1987): Measurement of anterior laxity in normal and anterior cruciate-absent knees with two instrumented test devices. Clin. Orthop., 215:156–161.
202. Shields, C.L., Silva, I., Yee, L., and Brewster, C. (1987): Evaluation of residual instability after arthroscopic meniscectomy in anterior cruciate-deficient knees. Am. J. Sports Med., 15:129–131.
203. Skyhar, M.J., Warren, R.F., Ortiz, G.J., et al. (1993): The effects of sectioning the posterior cruciate ligament and posterolateral complex on the articular pressures within the knee. J. Bone Joint Surg. [Am.], 75:694–699.
204. Snyder-Mackler, L., DeLitto, A., Bailey, S.I., et al. (1995): Strength of the quadriceps femoris muscle and functional recovery after reconstruction of the anterior cruciate ligament. J. Bone Joint Surg. [Am.], 77:1166–1173.
205. Snyder-Mackler, L., DeLuca, P.F., Williams, P.R., et al. (1994): Reflex inhibition of the quadriceps femoris muscle after injury or reconstruction of the anterior cruciate ligament. J. Bone Joint Surg. [Am.], 76:555–560.
206. Smidt, G.L. (1973): Biomechanical analysis of knee flexion and extension. J. Biomech., 6:79–92.
207. Soames, R.W. (1995): Skeletal system. In: Gray's Anatomy, 38th ed. New York, Churchill Livingstone.
208. Soderberg, G.L. (1986): Kinesiology: Application to Pathological Motion. Baltimore, Williams & Wilkins.
209. Soderberg, G.L., and Cook, T.M. (1983): An electromyographic analysis of quadriceps femoris muscle setting and straight leg raising. Phys. Ther., 63:1434–1438.
210. Speakman, H.G.B., and Weisberg, J. (1977): The vastus medialis controversy. Physiotherapy, 63:249–254.
211. Spencer, J.D., Hayes, K.C., and Alexander, I.J. (1984): Knee joint effusion and quadriceps reflex inhibition in man. Arch. Phys. Med. Rehabil., 65:171–177.

212. Sprague, R.B. (1982): Factors related to extension lag at the knee joint. J. Orthop. Sports Phys. Ther., 3:178–181.

213. Steiner, L.A., Harris, B.A., and Krebs, D.E. (1993): Reliability of eccentric isokinetic knee flexion and extension measurements. Arch. Phys. Med. Rehabil., 74:1327–1335.

214. Steinkamp, L.A., Dillingham, M.F., Markel, M.D., et al. (1993): Biomechanical considerations in patellofemoral joint rehabilitation. Am. J. Sports Med., 21:438–444.

215. Straub, T., and Hunter, R.E. (1988): Acute anterior cruciate ligament repair. Clin. Orthop., 227:238–250.

216. Takeda, Y., Xerogeanes, J.W., Livesay, G.A., et al. (1994): Biomechanical function of the human anterior cruciate ligament. Arthroscopy, 10:140–147.

217. Tegner, Y., Lysholm, J., Lysholm, M., and Gillquist, J. (1986): A performance test to monitor rehabilitation and evaluate anterior cruciate ligament injuries. Am. J. Sports Med., 14:156–159.

218. Timm, K. (1994): Knee. In: Richardson, J.K., and Iglarsh, A.Z. (eds.): Clinical Orthopedic Physical Therapy. Philadelphia, W.B. Saunders.

219. Threlkeld, A.J., Horn, T.S., Wojtowicz, G.M., et al. (1989): Kinematics, ground reaction force, and muscle balance produced by backward running. Orthop. Sports Phys. Ther., 11:56–63.

220. Tibone, J.E., and Antich, T.J. (1988): A biomechanical analysis of anterior cruciate ligament reconstruction with the patellar tendon. Am. J. Sports Med., 16:332–333.

221. Tibone, J.E., Antich, T.J., and Fanton, G.S., et al. (1986): Functional analysis of anterior cruciate ligament instability. Am. J. Sports Med., 14:276–284.

222. Torzilli, P.A., Greenberg, R.L., and Install, J. (1981): An in vivo biomechanical evaluation of anterior-posterior motion of the knee. Roentgenographic measurement technique, stress machine, and stable population. J. Bone Joint Surg. [Am.], 63:960.

223. Tria, A.J., Palumbo, R.C., and Alicea, J.A. (1992): Conservative care for patellofemoral pain. Orthop. Clin. North Am., 23:545–554.

224. Vailas, J.C., and Pink, M. (1993): Biomechanical effects of functional knee bracing. Sports Med., 15:210–218.

225. van Kampen, A., and Huiskes. R. (1990). The three-dimensional tracking pattern of the human patella. J. Orthop. Res., 8:372–382.

226. Voight, M.L., and Wieder, D.L. (1991): Comparative reflex response times of vastus medialis obliquus and vastus lateralis in normal subjects and subjects with extensor mechanism dysfunction. Am. J. Sports Med., 19:131–137.

227. Walla, D.J., Albright, J.P., and McAuley, E., et al. (1985): Hamstring control and the unstable ligament-deficient knee. Am. J. Sports Med., 13:34–39.

228. Wiberg, G. (1941): Roentgenographic and anatomic studies on the femoropatellar joint. With special reference to chondromalacia patella. Acta Orthop. Scand., 12:319–410.

229. Wilk, K.E. (1994): Rehabilitation of isolated and combined posterior cruciate ligament injuries. Clin. Sports Med., 13:649–677.

230. Wilk, K.E., Escamilla, R.F., Flesig, G.S, et al. (1996). A comparison of the joint forces and EMG activity during open and closed kinetic chain exercises. Am. J. Sports Med., 24:518–527.

231. Wilk, K.E., Romaniello, W.T., Soscia, S.M., et al. (1994): The relationship between subjective knee scores, isokinetic testing, and functional testing in the ACL-reconstructed knee. J. Orthop. Sports Med., 20:60–73.

232. Woodall, W.R., and Welsh, J. (1990): A biomechanical basis for rehabilitation programs involving the patellofemoral joint. J. Orthop. Sports Phys. Ther., 11:535–542.

233. Worrell, T.W., Connelly, S., and Hilvert, J. (1995): VMO:VL ratios and torque comparisons at four angles of knee flexion. J. Sports Rehabil., 4:264–272.

234. Worrell, T.W., Perrin, D.H., Gansnelder, B.M., et al. (1991): Comparison of isokinetic strength and flexibility measures between hamstring injured and noninjured athletes. J. Orthop. Sports Med., 13:118–125.

235. Wroble, R.R. (1990): Practical rules for objective ligament assessment: KT-1000 and other devices. In: 1990 Advances on the Knee and Shoulder. Cincinnati, Cincinnati Sports Medicine and Deaconess Hospital.

236. Wroble, R.R., Grood, E.S., Noyes, F.R., et al. (1990): Reproducibility of Genucom knee analysis system testing. Am. J. Sports Med., 18:387–395.

237. Wroble, R.R., Van Ginkel, L.A., Grood, E.S., et al. (1990): In: Noyes, F.R. (ed.): The Noyes Knee Rating System. Cincinnati, Cincinnati Sports Medicine Research and Education Foundation.

238. Wroble, R.R., VanGinkel, L.A., and Grood, E.S. (1990): Repeatability of the KT-1000 arthrometer in a normal population. Am. J. Sports Med., 18:396–399.

239. Yack, H.J., Collins, C.E., and Whieldon, T.J. (1993): Comparison of closed and open kinetic chain exercise in the anterior cruciate ligament-deficient knee. Am. J. Sports Med., 21:49–54.

240. Yack, H.J., Riley, L.M., and Whieldon, T.R. (1994): Anterior tibial translation during progressive loading of the ACL-deficient knee during weight-bearing and nonweight-bearing isometric exercise. J. Orthop. Sports Phys. Ther., 20:247–253.

Chapter 11

Hamstring, Quadriceps, and Groin Rehabilitation

James B. Gallaspy, M.Ed., A.T.,C.

The quadriceps, hamstrings, adductor group, sartorius, and tensor fasciae latae constitute the thigh muscles and are subject to extreme forces as they propel the body under various degrees of resistance.[16] Muscle strains are the most common injury to the hamstrings and adductors, whereas contusions rank as the primary injury to the quadriceps.[3] Strains involving the quadriceps occur less frequently than do hamstring strains because of the great strength and size of the quadriceps muscle.[8] Strains involve injury to the muscle, tendon, musculotendinous junction, or tendon-bone attachment. They can result from muscle imbalance, poor flexibility, overstretching, violent muscle contraction against heavy resistance, idiosyncrasy of nerve innervation, or leg length discrepancy.[2–4, 8, 11, 14]

Strains are graded by their degree of severity. Each is determined by the amount of muscle or tendon damage and is labeled as mild, moderate, or severe (or first, second, or third degree). Athletes suffering a muscle strain present with the signs and symptoms shown in Table 11–1.

The goals in treating muscle strains are to reduce pain, restore muscle function, and reduce the likelihood of reinjury. Restoration of muscle length is important in reinjury prevention, because a shortened muscle is more susceptible to strains.[1, 4, 15]

Initial treatment of strains and contusions consists of ice, compression, elevation, and rest, along with the use of nonsteroidal anti-inflammatory drugs (NSAIDs) to decrease inflammation.[3, 7, 8] Additional modalities such as pulsed ultrasound to decrease hematoma formation, without the adverse effects of increasing tissue temperature (as with continuous ultrasound in the early stages of healing), and electrical stimulation to decrease pain and inflammation can be beneficial.[18] The use of deep-water pool exercises is excellent during the early phases of the rehabilitation program (see Chap. 16). An elastic wrap (e.g., Tubi-Grip*) or other supporting orthosis should be used in the early stages of treatment to provide compression and should be continued throughout the rehabilitation program to support the thigh.

The restoration of muscle length precedes muscle strengthening unless the length of the injured muscle is equal to or greater than that of the uninjured muscle.[5] The decision to begin restoring muscle length depends on the athlete's response to stretching. If intense or moderate pain develops in the injured muscle before the athlete perceives a stretch, the injured muscle is not ready for stretching.[5] Once the athlete can feel the muscle stretch before or with pain, stretching may begin. In mild to moderate strains, stretching can begin within 2

*Available from SePro, Montgomeryville, Pennsylvania

Table 11–1. Signs and Symptoms of Muscle Strains

SEVERITY	SYMPTOMS	SIGNS
Mild (first degree)	Local pain, mild pain on passive stretch and active contraction of the involved muscle; minor disability	Mild spasm, swelling, ecchymosis; local tenderness; minor loss of function and strength
Moderate (second degree)	Local pain; moderate pain on passive stretch and active contraction of the involved muscle; moderate disability	Moderate spasm, swelling, ecchymosis; local tenderness; impaired muscle function and strength
Severe (third degree)	Severe pain; disability	Severe spasm; swelling, ecchymosis; hematoma; tenderness, loss of muscle function; palpable defect may be present

to 7 days of injury. Muscle strengthening can begin when the muscle can tolerate strengthening with light resistance that is pain free. The rehabilitation program should include active and passive stretching, proprioceptive neuromuscular facilitation (PNF) stretching and strengthening techniques, and isometric, isotonic, and isokinetic strengthening exercises.

If low-grade muscle spasm is present, the use of cryostretching, as described by Knight,[12] may be beneficial. This technique consists of cold applications and the PNF technique of hold-relax and can be summarized as follows[12]:

I. Numb with ice (20 minutes maximum)
II. Exercise
    A. First exercise bout (65 seconds total)
        1. Static stretch (20 seconds)
        2. Isometric contraction (5 seconds)
        3. Static stretch (10 seconds)
        4. Isometric contraction (5 seconds)
        5. Static stretch (10 seconds)
        6. Isometric contraction (5 seconds)
        7. Static stretch (10 seconds)
    B. Rest (20 seconds)
    C. Second exercise bout (65 seconds total; same as first exercise bout)
III. Renumb with ice (3 to 5 minutes)
IV. Exercise—two bouts and rest as in step II
V. Renumb with ice (3 to 5 minutes)
VI. Exercise—two bouts and rest as in step II

Although it is similar to cryokinetics in that exercise is performed while the body part is numbed, cryostretching differs with regard to the number of exercise sets and the exercise itself.[12] During cryostretch the affected muscle is alternately stretched statically and contracted isometrically.[12]

Knight[12] has also proposed a neuromuscular training session before the first initial exercise session; this may be done prior to or immediately after ice application but before the first exercise bout. The purpose of this session is to help the athlete "get the feel" of contracting the proper muscle group. Sometimes, without this session, the athlete contracts both the agonist and the antagonist muscle group when asked to contract the muscle with the spasm. During the neuromuscular training session the clinician moves the appropriate body part in a direction that elongates the muscle in spasm. The athlete is then asked to return the body part to the anatomic position, which requires contracting the affected muscle. This is repeated three to four times, always within a comfortable range of motion.

The stretchings consist of 65-second exercise bouts, with a static stretch interspersed with three isometric contractions of about 5 seconds each, as outlined above. The exercise is begun by stretching the affected muscle until pain or tightness is incurred; the athlete backs off just a little until the pain disappears and holds the limb in that position for 20 seconds. The athlete then begins a slow contraction of the muscle with the spasm, building up to a maximal muscle contraction. A second stretch is held for 10 seconds, followed by a second isometric contraction of about 5 seconds. The athlete moves forward again so that tightness or slight pain is felt in the traumatized area, and a 10-second stretch is repeated. Finally, the body part is rested in the anatomic position for 20 seconds, and the 65-second exercise bout is repeated as outlined above. Second and third renumbing sequences are also carried out.

Once muscle spasm begins to abate (often within 2 or 3 days) a combination of cryostretching and cryokinetics can be implemented, as follows[12]:

I. Numb with ice for 15 to 20 minutes
II. Perform cryostretch exercise
III. Renumb
IV. Perform cryokinetic exercise
V. Renumb
VI. Perform cryokinetic exercise
VII. Renumb
VIII. Perform cryokinetic exercise
IX. Renumb
X. Perform cryostretch exercise

Cryokinetic exercise should begin with manual, resisted muscle contractions through a full range of motion and progress to isotonic, isokinetic, and functional drills. The use of cryostretch and cryokinetic techniques should not be overlooked in the early phases of rehabilitation as methods to return muscular strength and endurance to their preinjury level sooner. Progressive-resistance exercise (PRE) can begin when tolerated, with an emphasis on eccentric exercises.[3, 7, 8]

HAMSTRING REHABILITATION

Hamstring strain is one of the most common and frustrating injuries that an athlete can incur; it can also recur frequently.[8, 10, 11, 16, 19] The biceps femoris, laterally, and the semitendinosus and semimembranosus, medially, compose the hamstring muscle group. These muscles function in knee flexion, hip extension, and internal and external rotation of the tibia and antagonistically resist knee extension.[1, 2, 6] The semimembranosus also dynamically reinforces the posterior and medial knee capsular structures, retracts the medial meniscus posteriorly, and supports the anterior cruciate ligament to prevent anterior tibial translation.[21] The tendons of insertion of the semitendinosus, sartorius, and gracilis form the pes anserinus, which inserts on the proximomedial aspect of the tibia.[21] Cumulatively, the hamstrings support the anterior cruciate ligament to help prevent anterior excursion of the tibia on the femur and to assist the medial capsule and medial collateral ligament.[6] The hamstrings perform an important role in walking and assume an extensor action with heel strike.[10, 21] During running, the hamstrings are active longer during the swing and early stance phases of gait.[10]

Hamstring injuries usually occur during sprinting or high-speed exercises (e.g., in a sprinter leaving the block, in the lead leg of a hurdler, in a jumper's takeoff leg).[10, 14] Hamstring strains can have various causes: (1) a sudden change from a stabilizing flexor to an active extensor, combined with muscle imbalance between the quadriceps and hamstrings; (2) poor flexibility; (3) faulty posture; and (4) leg length discrepancy. All are potential mechanisms for hamstring injuries.[2, 3, 8, 11, 14] The short head of the biceps femoris is most often injured; it is believed to contract simultaneously with the quadriceps muscle as a result of an idiosyncrasy in nerve innervation, thus contributing to the high injury rate of this hamstring muscle.[3, 6, 11, 15] It has been suggested that hamstring strength should be 60% to 70% that of the antagonist quadriceps to help prevent hamstring injuries.[1, 3, 14]

The clinician should perform active, passive, and resisted knee flexion and hip extension tests to determine injury severity. Usually, the amount of knee extension the athlete can achieve while prone indicates injury severity. Once severity has been ascertained, treatment can proceed as follows:

I. Initial phase
  A. RICE (rest, ice, compression, elevation)
  B. Tubi-Grip for effusion
  C. Modalities
    1. Pulsed ultrasound
    2. Electrical stimulation
    3. Ice postexercise
  D. Cryostretching and cryokinetics with the following exercises:
    1. Hamstring setting
    2. Cocontractions
    3. Heel slides (seated and supine)
    4. Active hamstring curls
    5. Active hip extensions
    6. Single-leg hamstring stretches to tolerance
  E. Aquatic therapy
  F. Active range of motion, as tolerated
II. Intermediate phase
  A. Stationary bike, StairMaster
  B. Modalities
    1. Continuous ultrasound
    2. Moist heat
  C. Hamstring stretching
    1. Single-leg hamstring stretches
    2. Straddle groin and hamstring stretches
    3. Side straddle and hamstring stretches
    4. Supine assisted hamstring stretches
  D. PRE
    1. Hamstring curl
    2. Hip extensions
    3. Hip adduction and abduction
    4. Straight leg raises
  E. Proprioceptive exercise
  F. Prophylactic cryotherapy
  G. Increased pool program
  H. PNF patterns
  I. Beginning of functional activity progression
    1. Forward and backward walking or jogging (use neoprene sleeve for support)
III. Advanced phase
  A. High-speed isokinetic exercise (seated and prone)
  B. Eccentric hamstring curls
  C. Functional drills
    1. Jogging or running (forward and backward)
    2. Jogging or running (uphill, backward)
    3. Slide Board, if available
    4. Lateral drills

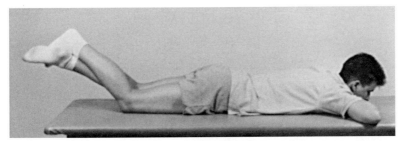

Figure 11–1. Use of the prone position and the uninvolved leg to promote hamstring elasticity. This can be used in conjunction with cryotherapy techniques.

    D. High-speed surgical tubing exercises in hip flexion, extension, abduction, and adduction and in knee flexion and minisquats

    E. Protective wrapping

In the acute stage emphasis is on reducing inflammation, pain, and spasm through the use of appropriate modalities. Depending on injury severity, at about day 2 to 4 postinjury, athletes can begin a stretching program within their pain-free range. Initially, the injured extremity can be stretched in the prone position using the uninvolved extremity to control the amount of hamstring stretch achieved (Fig. 11–1). As pain decreases and elasticity increases, a more aggressive stretching program can be implemented (Figs. 11–2 and 11–3). The exercise session should be terminated with cryotherapy, and a traction weight should be used above the knee to facilitate lengthening of the hamstring muscle with the spasm (Fig. 11–4).

Later in the rehabilitation process, isokinetic equipment can be used at higher speeds because of the high percentage of type II or fast-twitch muscle fibers located in the hamstrings.[10, 21] The hamstrings can be isolated isokinetically to a greater degree by having the athlete lie prone (Fig. 11–5A) or by having the athlete lean forward while in the traditional seated position (Fig. 11–5B). Isokinetic equipment can also be used to obtain data that can aid in determining

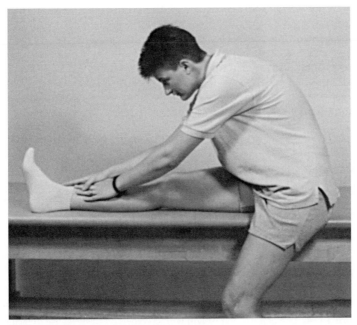

Figure 11–2. Single-leg hamstring stretch.

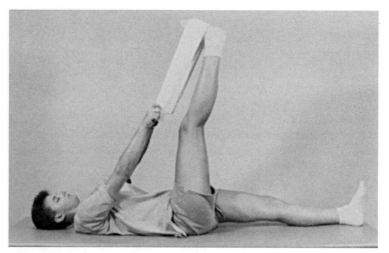

Figure 11-3. Single-leg hamstring stretch with towel. The uninvolved leg is kept flat on the table.

when the athlete has reached the optimal hamstring-to-quadriceps ratio for deterring injury.

The athlete can also use surgical tubing (Fig. 11–6) for high-speed resistance exercise to fatigue in hip flexion, extension, abduction, and adduction and in knee flexion (hamstring curls) or can use the Inertia machine,* if available, in the above planes.

The athlete may return to unlimited participation, wearing a neoprene sleeve for support and proprioception, when the following criteria are met:

1. Hamstring flexibility is equal bilaterally.
2. Muscular strength, power, endurance, and time to peak torque, as measured by an isokinetic dynamometer, are 85% to 90% of those of the contralateral limb.
3. Hamstring strength is 60% to 70% that of the quadriceps.
4. No symptoms are noted with functional activities.

*Available from E.M.A., Newnan, Georgia

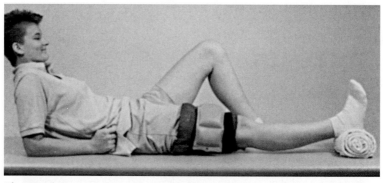

Figure 11-4. Use of a traction weight with cryotherapy postexercise to facilitate the return of hamstring length.

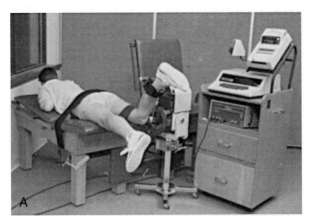

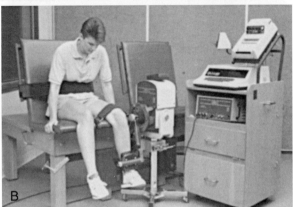

Figure 11–5. The athlete can accentuate hamstring muscle activity by lying prone *(A)* or by leaning forward while in the traditional seated position *(B)*.

QUADRICEPS REHABILITATION

Quadriceps injuries are a common occurrence in sports. The quadriceps muscle is subject to both strains and contusions, with the latter having a higher incidence.[2, 3] The quadriceps is composed of the rectus femoris, vastus medialis, vastus lateralis, and vastus intermedius muscles. Its static role is to prevent knee buckling while standing, and its dynamic function is to extend the knee forcefully, as in running or jumping exercises. The rectus femoris is a biarticular muscle, functioning in knee extension and hip flexion. The tensor fasciae latae and the sartorius are also considered part of the anterior thigh.

Contusions

The quadriceps is constantly exposed to direct contact in various vigorous sports such as football, soccer, and basketball.[2, 3] A quadriceps contusion can vary from a mild bruise to a large, deep hematoma that may take months to heal.[2] The mechanism of injury is usually a direct blow to the relaxed thigh, compressing the muscle against the femur. The anterior or anterolateral aspect of the quadriceps is most often involved, because the medial aspect is protected by the athlete's contralateral leg.[14, 16, 19] A quadriceps contusion displays standard signs and symptoms of other muscle injuries, but the symptoms are less localized than those in a more subcutaneous area.[16] The athlete may exhibit local pain, stiffness, pain on passive stretching, disability that varies with the site and extent of injury, tenderness, ecchymosis, hematoma formation, and loss of active

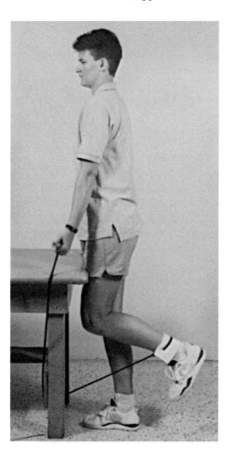

Figure 11–6. Hamstring curls with surgical tubing can be performed at varying rates to fatigue to help increase muscle endurance.

extension.[2–4, 14, 16, 19] Injury severity can usually be determined by the degree of limitation of active knee flexion.

Moderate to severe quadriceps contusions should be treated nonaggressively to prevent the development of myositis ossificans, and exercise is progressed according to the athlete's tolerance. Some authors[3, 8] have advocated the use of cryotherapy with simultaneous prolonged knee flexion at 20-minute intervals to help prevent the transitory loss of knee flexion that usually accompanies a quadriceps contusion. The degree of active knee flexion is determined by the athlete's pain tolerance. Modalities such as massage, heat, and forced stretching of the muscle during the acute phase are contraindicated.[2, 16, 19, 20] Quadriceps setting can be performed and electrical muscle stimulation can be used to help deter muscle atrophy and to increase quadriceps re-education if these treatments cause no pain.[1, 3, 9] Also, passive range-of-motion devices can be useful in the early stages of injury. Figures 11–7 to 11–14 depict stretching exercises that can be used at various stages of the healing process to increase the elasticity of the quadriceps muscle. The following protocol outlines the progression of rehabilitation after quadriceps injury:

I. Initial phase
   A. RICE
   B. Modalities
      1. Pulsed ultrasound
      2. Electrical muscle stimulation
      3. Ice postexercise
   C. Tubi-Grip for effusion
   D. Active range of motion, as tolerated

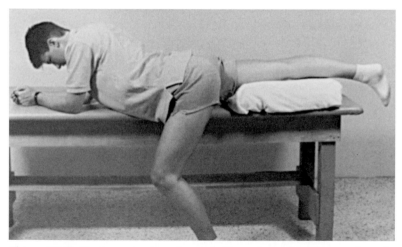

Figure 11-7. Passive rectus femoris stretch. The amount of passive stretch can be modified by the amount of hip extension, which is based on the athlete's tolerance to stretch. It can be used in conjunction with cryotherapy techniques.

    E. Cryostretch and cryokinetics with the following exercises:
       1. Active straight leg raises
       2. Active terminal knee extensions
       3. Active hip flexion
       4. Heel slides (seated and supine)
       5. Quadriceps sets
       6. Cocontractions
    F. Aquatic therapy
II. Intermediate phase
    A. Stationary cycling

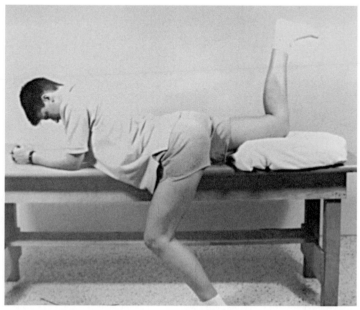

Figure 11-8. Passive hip flexor stretch. The amount of passive stretch can be modified by the amount of hip extension, which is based on the athlete's tolerance to stretch. It can be used in conjunction with cryotherapy techniques.

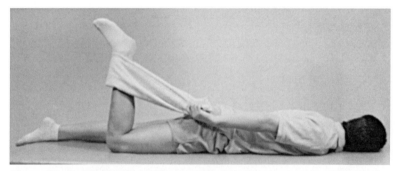

Figure 11-9. Single-leg quadriceps stretch. A towel is used to stretch the quadriceps muscle gradually. In the later stages of rehabilitation the proprioceptive neuromuscular facilitation contract–relax technique can be used to facilitate the range of motion.

 B. Modalities
  1. Continuous ultrasound
  2. Moist heat
 C. Increase in aquatic program
 D. Quadriceps stretching
 E. Concentric 90° to 45° knee extensions
 F. PNF patterns
 G. Proprioception exercises
 H. PRE with exercises initiated in initial phase
 I. Active-assisted flexion
 J. Closed-chain exercises
  1. Terminal knee extensions with Thera-Band
  2. Lateral step-ups
III. Advanced phase
 A. High-speed isokinetic exercises (seated and supine)

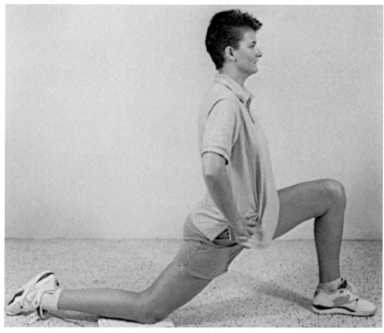

Figure 11-10. Iliopsoas stretch.

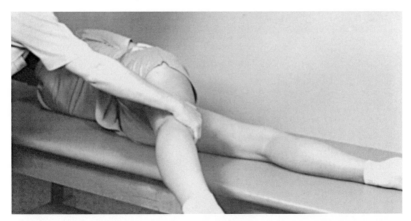

Figure 11–11. Manual iliopsoas stretch. This can later be adapted into the proprioceptive neuromuscular facilitation contract–relax technique or into other proprioceptive neuromuscular facilitation patterns.

B. Functional drills
C. Eccentric 90° to 0° knee extensions
D. High-speed surgical tubing exercises in hip flexion, extension, abduction, and adduction and in minisquats
E. Protective wrapping

In contusions, if the hematoma is not readily resolved, the clinician should suspect the development of myositis ossificans. Third-degree injuries need protective rest—cryotherapy, isometric exercise, and gentle active range of motion, as tolerated, before aggressive rehabilitation can begin. With severe thigh contusions, the use of massage, heat, and forced stretching or running is contraindicated in the early phases of healing.

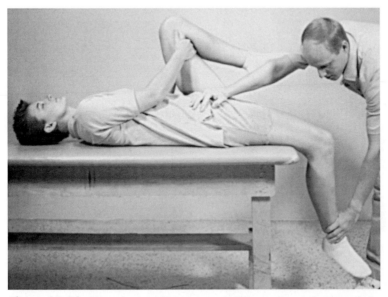

Figure 11–12. Manual rectus femoris stretch. This can be used to stretch the rectus femoris muscle and can also be used as a test to determine its length.

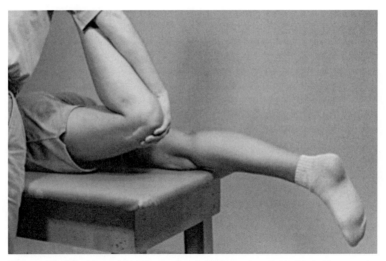

Figure 11-13. Manual hip flexor stretch. This can be adapted into the proprioceptive neuromuscular facilitation contract–relax technique to increase the range of motion.

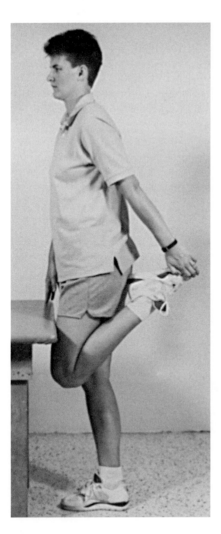

Figure 11-14. Single-leg standing quadriceps stretch. The athlete can also pull the hip into extension to accentuate the stretch.

The athlete may return to unlimited participation when the following criteria are met:

1. Quadriceps flexibility is equal bilaterally.
2. Muscular strength, power, endurance, and time to peak torque, as measured by an isokinetic dynamometer, are 85% to 90% of those of the contralateral limb.
3. Minimal or no tenderness is present in the quadriceps.
4. No symptoms are noted with functional activities at full speed.
5. The traumatized area is protected. Use of a pad made of Orthoplast*, with a raised section over the injured area, is recommended.

Strains

Quadriceps strains usually involve the rectus femoris muscle.[8, 19] Strains to this area occur less frequently than do hamstring strains because of the great strength, size, and flexibility of the quadriceps muscle group.[8] The injury is usually a result of insufficient warm-up, poor stretching, tight quadriceps, bilateral quadriceps imbalance, or a short leg.[19] Signs and symptoms vary with injury severity but are characterized by pain down the entire length of the rectus femoris and tenderness in the area of the strain. The athlete exhibits pain on active quadriceps contraction and passive stretching. If the muscle is ruptured, swelling may initially mask a muscle defect, but a permanent bulge in the thigh is present as the swelling subsides.[1, 8, 9]

Rehabilitation for a quadriceps strain is similar to that for strains of other muscles. The severity of injury determines when active rehabilitation may begin, and all exercises should be performed within a pain-free range of motion. Static stretching is begun as tolerated (see Figs. 11–7 to 11–9) along with passive range-of-motion exercises. Progression should be made to active range-of-motion and resistive exercises with emphasis on knee extension and hip flexion.

In the late phases of rehabilitation, isokinetic equipment can be used, at higher speeds, with the athlete in the supine position to accentuate the quadriceps muscle (Fig. 11–15A) or in the traditional seated position (Fig. 11–15B).

Additionally, surgical tubing can be used for exercising in the planes of hip flexion, extension, adduction, abduction, and knee extension at high contractile speeds to fatigue for endurance (Fig. 11–16). The quadriceps rehabilitation protocol outlined above can be used as a guideline for quadriceps strains. Although designed for quadriceps contusions, the program can be accelerated to accommodate quadriceps strains, because this injury can usually be rehabilitated more quickly than a quadriceps contusion.

The athlete may return to unlimited participation, wearing a neoprene sleeve for support and proprioception, when the following criteria are met:

1. Muscular strength, power, endurance, and time to peak torque, as measured by an isokinetic dynamometer, are 85% to 90% of those of the contralateral limb.
2. Quadriceps flexibility is equal bilaterally.
3. No symptoms are noted with functional activities at full speed.

---

*Available from Johnson & Johnson, New Brunswick, New Jersey

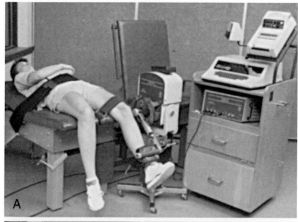

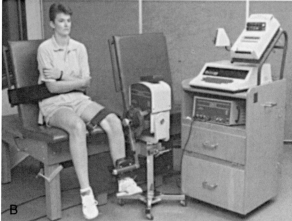

Figure 11-15. The athlete can accentuate quadriceps activity by lying supine *(A)* or by exercising in the traditional seated position *(B)*.

GROIN REHABILITATION

The groin is the depressed region that lies between the thigh and abdominal area. The muscles of this region include the adductor group, rectus femoris, and iliopsoas. The adductor group is composed of the adductor longus, adductor brevis, adductor magnus, pectineus, and gracilis. These muscles adduct the thigh and flex and externally and internally rotate the hip.[21] The adductors function dynamically to adduct the thigh and serve as hip flexors and extensors, depending on their anterior or posterior relationship to the flexion-extension axis of the hips. During walking and running, contraction of the adductors contributes to the forward and backward swing motion of the leg. The static effect of these muscles is to stabilize the trunk by constantly adjusting the position of the pelvis. Twisting of the pelvis is prevented by the adducting and the internal-external rotating components of the adductor group.[21]

Groin strains can result from any forced adduction, overextension, twisting, running, or jumping with external rotation.[2, 3, 8, 16, 17] This stretching usually occurs when the muscular unit is overloaded during the eccentric phase of muscular contraction.[9, 13, 22] The athlete complains of a sudden, sharp pain located along the ischiopubic ramus, the lesser trochanter, or the adductor's musculotendinous junction.[1, 6, 7] The athlete complains of pain on passive abduction and resisted adduction. The pain may begin at the origin of the traumatized muscle and radiate along the medial aspect of the thigh into the rectus abdominis area.[20]

The injury should be assessed by administering active, passive, and resisted tests in hip flexion, extension, adduction, abduction, and internal and external

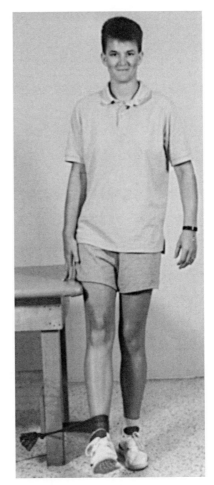

Figure 11-16. Hip flexion and extension using a Thera-Band at varying speeds. The knee is straight, and the athlete flexes and extends the hip at varying speeds. In the final stages of rehabilitation, the athlete performs this exercise as fast as possible to fatigue, but not at the expense of good mechanics.

rotation and in knee extension.[3] The use of a hip spica with the hip internally rotated may help to alleviate some of the pain and discomfort experienced with activities of daily living and during the rehabilitation program (Fig. 11–17). Lateral movements and abduction with external rotation should be avoided until symptoms subside. The following protocol outlines a rehabilitation program for groin strains:

I. Initial phase
   A. RICE
   B. Modalities
      1. Pulsed ultrasound
      2. Electrical stimulation
      3. Ice postexercise
   C. Cryostretch and cryokinetics with the following exercises:
      1. Active hip abduction
      2. Active straight leg raises
      3. Active hip flexion
      4. Isometric hip adduction
   D. Hip active range of motion
   E. Aquatic therapy
   F. Stationary cycling
II. Intermediate phase
   A. Modalities

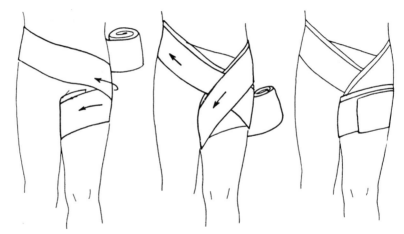

Figure 11-17. Hip spica. With the leg internally rotated to relax the adductor muscles, a 6-inch extra-long elastic bandage is used to help support the groin area. (From Arnheim, D. [1989]: Modern Principles of Athletic Training, 7th ed. St. Louis, C.V. Mosby, p. 341.)

      1. Continuous ultrasound
      2. Moist heat
  B. Proprioceptive exercises
  C. PRE with active exercises initiated in initial phase
  D. Active adduction
  E. Groin stretching
      1. Straddle groin and hamstring stretches
      2. Side straddle groin and hamstring stretches
      3. Groin stretches
      4. Wall groin stretches
  F. Increase of aquatic program
  G. Prophylactic cryotherapy
  H. PNF patterns
  I. Stationary cycling
III. Advanced phase
  A. Concentric and eccentric hip abduction and adduction
  B. High-speed surgical tubing exercises in hip abduction, adduction, flexion, and extension
  C. Functional drills
      1. Running
      2. Cariocas
      3. Cutting
      4. Lateral movements
      5. Slide Board, if available
  D. Protective wrapping—hip spica

The athlete may return to unlimited participation when the following criteria are met:

    1. Muscular strength is equal bilaterally, as determined by manual muscle testing.
    2. Full, pain-free hip range of motion is present.
    3. The athlete can perform the sport-specific functional activities required, asymptomatically, at full speed.

Most injuries to the thigh region usually result in trauma to the soft tissue, particularly muscle. Although fractures can occur to this area, they are not as prevalent as muscle strains and contusions. Strains are most often produced indirectly though poor muscle flexibility, abnormal agonist-to-strength or antagonist-to-strength ratios, or eccentric muscle contraction. Contusions are generally incurred more in contact sports and result from a direct blow to the soft tissue.

Soft-tissue injuries of the thigh are treated initially with emphasis on decreasing pain, spasm, and inflammation of the traumatized region. Early range-of-motion and stretching exercises can be instituted as tolerated, except for quadriceps contusions, in which the potential for myositis ossificans exists. Early aggressive motion, stretching, heat, and massage to quadriceps contusions are contraindicated.

As muscle elasticity is restored and inflammation subsides, the athlete can begin active PRE, as tolerated. Later stages of rehabilitation should concentrate on high functional speed and eccentric exercise. Isokinetic machines can be used at higher speeds, and surgical tubing can be used for exercises at varying speeds to aid in reconditioning the type II muscle fibers. The athlete should also perform sport-specific functional activities at 50%, 75%, and then full speed. This allows the clinician to judge how the athlete performs in the sport. The athlete should be able to perform these functional activities asymptomatically before returning to participation. Once the athlete returns to competition, the area should be supported or protected with an appropriate orthosis. Most muscular strains to this region can be prevented through an adequate stretching and warm-up program before participation.

APPLICATION

Hamstring and Groin Exercises

Hamstring Stretch. The athlete lies on a table, and an object is placed under the foot to apply a gentle stretch of the hamstring. The quadriceps should be relaxed.

Straddle Groin and Hamstring Stretch. The athlete sits on the floor with the legs spread and the back straight (Fig. 11–18). The athlete then leans forward until a stretch is felt, holds for 10 seconds, relaxes, and repeats the exercise.

Side Straddle Groin and Hamstring Stretch. The athlete sits on the floor with the legs spread and the back straight (Fig. 11–19). The athlete leans to the left and tries to grasp as far down the leg as possible, holds 10 seconds, relaxes, and repeats on the opposite side.

Supine Assisted Hamstring Stretch. With the help of a partner or towel, the athlete raises the leg until a stretch is felt in the hamstring, holds for 10 seconds, relaxes, and then repeats the exercise (see Fig. 11–3). PNF contract-relax can also be performed easily in this position.

Single Hamstring Stretch. The athlete straightens the supported leg with the other leg off to the side (Fig. 11–20) and slowly leans forward until a stretch is felt in the back of the hamstring. This is held for 10 seconds, and then the athlete relaxes and repeats the exercise. The stretch is performed with the chin up and the back straight and without bouncing.

Groin Stretch. In the sitting position, with the back straight, the athlete bends the knees, places the feet together, and pulls the feet toward the groin (Fig. 11–21). The elbows are placed on the knees and pressed down. This position is held for 10 seconds, followed by the athlete's relaxing and repeating the exercise.

Wall Groin Stretch. The athlete lies on the back with the buttocks and legs against the wall. The legs are spread enough so that a stretch is felt in the groin region (Fig. 11–22). A small amount of weight can be used around the ankles to

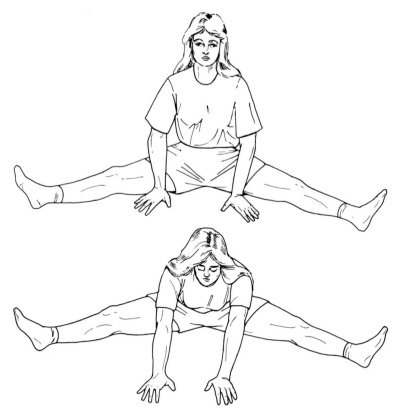

Figure 11–18. Straddle groin and hamstring stretch.

increase the stretch and allow it to be more passive. This is held for 10 seconds. The athlete then relaxes and repeats the exercise.

Quadriceps Exercise

Standing Quadriceps Stretch. The athlete holds on with one arm for balance, grasps the foot of the injured extremity with the hand, and brings the heel to the buttocks (Fig. 11–23). While standing up straight, the athlete slowly extends the leg, maintaining the hold on the foot, and holds for 10 seconds. A stretch should be felt in the quadriceps. The athlete then relaxes and repeats the exercise.

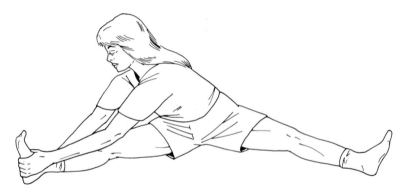

Figure 11–19. Side straddle groin and hamstring stretch.

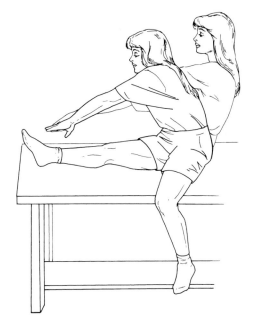

Figure 11–20. Single hamstring stretch.

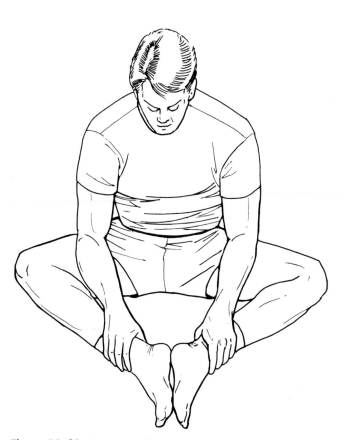

Figure 11–21. Groin stretch.

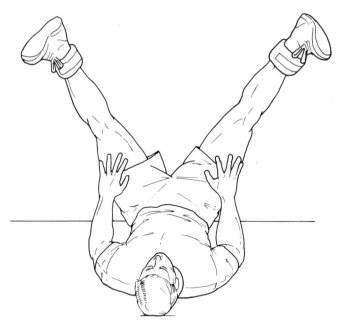

Figure 11–22. Wall groin stretch.

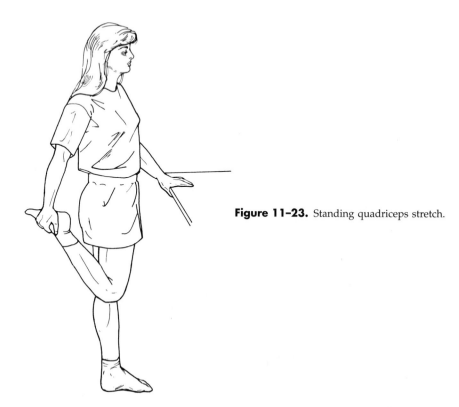

Figure 11–23. Standing quadriceps stretch.

References

1. Agre, J.C. (1985): Hamstring injuries: Proposed etiological factors, prevention, and treatment. Sports Med., 2:21–33.
2. American Academy of Orthopaedic Surgeons (1984): Athletic Training and Sports Medicine. Chicago, American Academy of Orthopaedic Surgeons.
3. Arnheim, D.H., and Prentice, W.E. (1993): Modern Principles of Athletic Training, 8th ed. St. Louis, C.V. Mosby, pp. 586–617.
4. Booher, J.M., and Thibodeau, G.A. (1989): Athletic Injury Assessment, 2nd ed. St. Louis, C.V. Mosby, pp. 171–172.
5. Cibulka, M.T. (1989): Rehabilitation of the pelvis, hip, and thigh. Clin. Sports Med., 8:777–803.
6. Distefano, V. (1978): Functional anatomy and biomechanics of the knee. Athl. Train., 13:113–118.
7. Estwanik, J.J., Sloane, B., and Rosenberg, M.A. (1990): Groin strain and other possible causes of groin pain. Physician Sportsmed., 18:54–65.
8. Fahey, T.D. (1986): Athletic Training: Principles and Practice. Palo Alto, CA, Mayfield, pp. 77, 340–343.
9. Gardner, L. (1977): Hip abductors and adductors in rehabilitation. Physician Sportsmed., 5:103–104.
10. Garrett, W.E., Califf, J.C., and Gassett, F.H. (1984): Histochemical correlates of hamstring injuries. Am. J. Sports Med., 12:98–103.
11. Heiser, T.M., Weber, J., Sullivan, G., et al. (1984): Prophylaxis and management of hamstring muscle injuries in intercollegiate football. Am. J. Sports Med., 12:368–370.
12. Knight, K.L. (1995): Cryotherapy in Sports Injury Management. Champaign, Human Kinetics Publishers, pp. 233–239.
13. Knight, K.L. (1985): Strengthening hip abductors and adductors. Physician Sportsmed., 13:161–163.
14. Kulund, D.N. (1982): The Injured Athlete. Philadelphia, J.B. Lippincott, pp. 356–358.
15. Liemohn, W. (1978): Factors related to hamstring strains. J. Sports Med. Phys. Fitness, 18:71–75.
16. O'Donoghue, D.H. (1984): Treatment of Injuries to Athletes, 4th ed. Philadelphia, W.B. Saunders, pp. 433–442.
17. Peterson, L., and Renstrom, P. (1986): Sports Injuries. Chicago, Year Book Medical Publishers, pp. 440–443.
18. Prentice, W.E. (1994): Therapeutic Modalities in Sports Medicine. St. Louis, C.V. Mosby, pp. 7, 268–269.
19. Roy, S., and Irvin, R. (1983): Sports Medicine: Prevention, Evaluation, Management, and Rehabilitation. Englewood Cliffs, NJ, Prentice-Hall, pp. 299–305.
20. Torg, J.S., Vegso, J.J., and Torg, E. (1987): Rehabilitation of Athletic Injuries. Chicago, Year Book Medical Publishers, pp. 97–101, 110–115.
21. Weineck, J. (1986): Functional Anatomy in Sports. Chicago, Year Book Medical Publishers, pp. 102–115.
22. Zarins, B., and Ciullo, J.V. (1983): Acute muscle and tendon injuries in athletes. Clin. Sports Med., 2:167–182.

Chapter 12

Low Back Rehabilitation

Tim Holbrook, P.T., Cert. MDT

Low back pain (LBP) affects 70% to 80% of the population at some point in life and is the most common cause of limited activity in persons 45 years of age and younger. The anatomic location of LBP in the general population is as follows: cervical pain, 36%; thoracic pain, 2%; and lumbar pain, 62%, with the L4-L5 and L5-S1 vertebral levels being the most frequently involved in the lumbar area. LBP is self-limiting, with 44% of people with LBP improving in 1 week, 86% in 1 month, and 92% in 2 months.[4, 47, 57] In 90% of the population LBP is recurrent, and 35% of individuals with recurrent LBP develop sciatica.[77]

Incidence of back pain in athletes has been reported to be between 10% and 85%,[22, 32, 67, 73] depending on the athlete's age and sport. Episodes of LBP are usually related to an acute traumatic event or to overuse and ordinarily resolve within a few weeks, with or without treatment. Athletes with persistent LBP, however, will often be found to have acquired or predisposing conditions that account for their pain.[34] Most conditions causing LBP in athletes can be treated nonsurgically.

The incidence of LBP for specific sports has been reported. For instance, 29% of professional golfers have reported a history of LBP.[76] In a retrospective study of LBP in racquet sports, 10% of badminton players, 15% of squash players, and 15% of tennis players reported low back injuries.[9] Ferguson and colleagues[22] reported that 12 out of 25 (48%) football lineman sought medical help for LBP during a 1-year period. Of 506 football players' records reviewed during an 8-year period, Semon and Spengler[67] reported that 135 (27%) had complained of LBP. Back pain associated with gymnastics has been the most investigated. Spinal injuries account for 12.2% of all injuries incurred by female gymnasts.[24] Of 100 gymnasts, with a mean age of 14, 25% reported LBP of significant enough magnitude to interfere with training.[32] Similarly, Szot and colleagues[75] reported that of 41 male gymnasts (ages 15 to 31) sampled, 49% reported back pain. Sward and associates[73, 74] also noted that male gymnasts had a significantly increased incidence (85%) and severity of back pain compared with female gymnasts, wrestlers, soccer players, tennis players, and nonathletes. Also, the incidence of lumbar spondylolysis has been reported to be much higher in gymnasts than in the general population.[32, 33, 40]

Radiographic investigations have shown an increased frequency of spinal abnormalities in wrestlers (55%), gymnasts (42%),[25, 73, 74] and swimmers (15.8%).[25] Radiographic changes in the lumbar spine in 11% of athletes with back pain were reported by Cannon and James.[8] Jackson also found degenerative changes in almost all athletes with back pain that persisted for more than 3 months.[31] Sward and colleagues[73] reported that 36% to 55% of subjects in their study of 142 top Swedish wrestlers, gymnasts, soccer, and tennis players had radiographic abnormalities that included reduced disc height, Schmorl's nodes, and configuration changes of the vertebral body. Additionally, Sward and colleagues[74] found a greater prevalence of disc degeneration in 75% of elite male gymnasts compared with a prevalence of 31% in nonathletes, as determined by magnetic resonance imaging. Athletes who engage in sports that place a great demand on the back have more radiographic abnormalities[29] in the thoracolumbar spine then do nonathletes and more back pain than do other athletes.[73]

Factors that predispose an individual to LBP include a poor sitting posture, which duplicates the fully flexed standing posture; frequent flexion; and loss of extension range of motion. Movement and activity can precipitate LBP and therefore contribute to its incidence and recurrence. It is often the unexpected or unguarded movement that causes a sudden episode of LBP. Whenever predisposing factors are present, very little provocation can precipitate a sudden onset of LBP. Finally, poor lifting position and fatigue can precipitate LBP. Athletic endeavors that place a great demand on the spine subject the athlete to an increased risk of symptomatic spinal damage.[73] This chapter will address the biomechanics of the spine, the importance of the evaluation process in determining the treatment of LBP, various treatment interventions, and rehabilitation for specific low back pathologies.

BIOMECHANICS

The spine consists of five regions: cervical (7 vertebrae), thoracic (12 vertebrae), lumbar (5 vertebrae), sacral (5 fused vertebrae), and coccygeal (4 vertebrae). This gives a total of 33 vertebrae, with 24 of these forming distinct regions: the cervical, thoracic, and lumbar regions. The vertebrae increase in size from the cervical to the lumbar region and decrease in size from the sacral to the coccygeal region. The spine consists of four curves. The two curves that have a posterior convexity (anterior concavity) are referred to as kyphotic curves (thoracic and sacral regions). The cervical and lumbar regions have posterior concavities (anterior convexity) that are referred to as lordotic curves. It is believed that the lordotic curves develop as a result of the accommodation of the skeleton in the upright posture.[56] It has also been reported that the cervical, thoracic, and lumbar curves function to increase the ability of the spine to withstand axial compression.[21, 35] Additionally, calculations have determined that a three-curve spine can withstand more compressive forces than a straight spine can.[35, 66] Dynamic stabilization of the spine depends on muscular, capsular, and ligamentous systems and their interplay with the facets to allow movement yet to remain stable during weight bearing.[26]

Motion between any two vertebrae is extremely limited and consists of a small amount of gliding. The motions available to the spine may be likened to that of a joint with three degrees of freedom, permitting flexion and extension, lateral flexion, and rotation.[56] The type and the amount of motion that is available differ from region to region and depend on the orientation of the articulating facets and the fluidity, elasticity, and thickness of the intervertebral disc (IVD).[56]

Facet or zygapophyseal joints guide and limit spinal motions of flexion, extension, lateral flexion, and rotation. These joints are diarthrodial joints, complete with synovial membrane and joint capsule, and are highly innervated. The plane of the facet joints determines the direction and amount of movement possible between spinal segments.[56]

Specifically, the lumbar spine provides support for the weight of the upper part of the body.[56] The lumbar vertebrae are the largest, which helps in supporting this additional weight. A change in the lumbar curve or in the vertebrae themselves will result in a redistribution of the normal compressive and shear stresses across the lumbar region. For example, an increase in lordosis of the lumbar curve will increase the shearing forces acting on the lumbar vertebrae and will increase the likelihood of anterior displacement of the fifth lumbar vertebra. Also, an increased lumbar curvature will increase the compressive forces on the posterior aspect of the vertebral structures, which can lead to injury as a result of excessive stress.[56]

Because the lumbar facets lie in a sagittal plane, the lumbar spine from L1 to L4 favors flexion and extension and limits lateral flexion and rotation.[15] At the L5-S1 junction the facets change their orientation from a sagittal plane to being oriented somewhat obliquely in the frontal plane.[64] This results in a closer approximation of the facet joints at the lumbosacral junction, resulting in further restriction of lateral flexion and rotation, with no additional restriction of flexion and extension.[15] It has been reported that as much as 75% of the total amount of lumbar flexion-extension takes place at the lumbosacral joint, with 20% at the L4-L5 level and the remaining 5% of motion at the other segments, namely, L1 to L3.[7]

Major ligamentous support is provided to the spine by the anterior longitudinal ligament and the posterior longitudinal ligament. The anterior longitudinal ligament is a very broad and strong ligament that extends the full length of the spine. It is attached to the vertebral bodies and IVD anteriorly, thus providing support to both of these structures. The anterior longitudinal ligament's main function is to provide support and reinforcement to the anterior aspect of the intervertebral disc during the lifting of heavy loads. The posterior longitudinal ligament is also very strong and runs the full length of the spine but becomes very narrow as it descends. In the lower lumbar region it is so narrow that it is of little protective value for the lumbar discs.[26] It is also highly innervated and is on constant stretch in the flexed position.

The IVD has been the focus of many investigations because of its perceived significance in LBP. The IVD absorbs and helps distribute forces that are applied to the spine. Although the IVD is considered avascular, it receives nutrients from diffusion as well as from its contact with the cartilaginous end-plate, at which blood vessels ramify close to the nucleus and annulus.[12, 59] The inner two thirds of the annulus fibrosus is denervated; however, the point at which the annulus fibrosus inserts on the vertebral periosteum is innervated, and therefore any strain of the outer annulus fibers will be registered as painful.[26]

The IVD has two distinct components: a tough outer fibrocartilaginous covering called the annulus fibrosus serves as a retaining wall for the second component, the nucleus pulposus. The annulus fibrosus consists of concentric rings of cartilaginous fibers that run obliquely to each other at an angle of about 30° to the plane of the disc.[80] The annulus fibers are attached to the cartilaginous end-plates above and below, except posteriorly, where the peripheral attachment of the annulus is not so firm.[47] Additionally, the annulus fibrosus fibers are thicker and more numerous anteriorly than posteriorly. The lack of ligament support and reduced annulus fibrosus thickness combine to make the posterior part of the annulus the weakest, particularly posterolaterally.[68]

The nucleus pulposus is a mucopolysaccharide gel that is centrally located within the annulus fibrosus. It is hydrophilic and behaves like a highly viscous fluid. It has been reported that in young adults, as much as 80% of the nucleus pulposus is water,[2, 6, 27, 37] with a gradual reduction in the water content to about 70% as a result of degeneration[74] and aging.[2, 6] Because of the high water content of the nucleus pulposus, it is nearly incompressible and therefore acts in force distribution.[26] The pressure within the disc is equally distributed in all directions of the intervertebral compartment.[47] When the IVD is compressed, the pressure within the disc increases, with a resultant loss of water from the nucleus pulposus.[42] This loss of water from the disc causes a decrease in disc height of about 1 cm over the course of a day.[20] When compressive forces are reduced or absent, the nucleus absorbs water from the vertebral body, restoring the height of the IVD.[39] This water-absorbing capacity is lost with age.

The position of the nucleus pulposus within the annulus fibrosus during sustained or dynamic flexion and extension of the lumbar spine has been documented.[13, 42, 47, 56] Static or repeated flexion will result in gradual movement of the nucleus pulposus in a posterior direction, resulting in tension forces posteriorly (at the least protected and weakest aspect of the IVD) and compressive forces anteriorly on the IVD. Because individuals are in the flexed position most of the time, the nucleus pulposus is not given the opportunity to migrate anteriorly. Instead, greater stresses are placed on the IVD posteriorly, resulting in microtrauma to the annular fibers, with eventual fiber tearing and disc bulging or herniation, which can impinge on nerve roots or other innervated structures, causing pain. The opposite has been shown to be true with static or repeated extension: there is gradual movement of the nucleus pulposus anteriorly, where the IVD is stronger, causing anterior tension forces and posterior compressive forces on the IVD. It is this concept of nucleus pulposus movement during flexion and extension that is the basis for extension exercises. However, once the annular wall has been compromised and nuclear material has escaped, the hydrostatic mechanism is no longer intact.

The effect of body position and activities on intradiscal pressures has been investigated extensively by Nachemson and colleagues.[49-55] Of note here is that the intradiscal pressure is greatest in the sitting and forward flexed positions. This is true with activities of daily living (Fig. 12–1) or with therapeutic exercises (Fig. 12–2). The nucleus pulposus distributes pressure in all directions of the annulus fibrosus, which can exceed the applied load.[52] Axial compression is the most common form of spine loading, which forces water out of the disc, but compression in itself is not a significant factor in damage of a healthy disc.[30, 42] Compression forces do increase the pressure in the nucleus pulposus, and over time, the collagen fibers of the inner annulus wall can stretch, resulting in fissuring.[5] Virgin[78] demonstrated in vitro that discs subjected to very high compressive loads showed permanent strain (deformation) after removal of the load but no herniation of the nucleus pulposus. A more common sequel of compressive forces is that the pressure is transmitted to the cartilaginous end-plates and subsequently to the vertebral bodies. When vertical compression is applied, the discs and spongy bone are able to undergo a greater amount of deformation without failure than the cartilaginous end-plate or cortical bone can. The cartilaginous end-plates are able to undergo the least deformation and will be the first to fail under high compressive loading.[42, 52, 59, 78] The discs will be the last structure to fail. The anterior longitudinal ligament and posterior longitudinal ligament

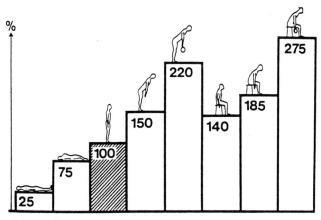

Figure 12–1. Relative change in pressure (or load) in the third lumbar disc in various positions in living subjects. (From Nachemson, A.L. [1976]: The lumbar spine: an orthopaedic challenge. Spine, 1:59–71.)

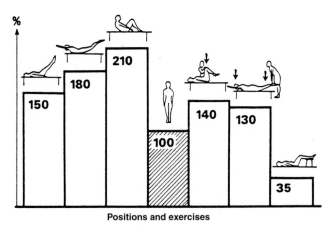

Figure 12–2. Relative change in pressure (or load) in the third lumbar disc in various muscle-strengthening exercises in living subjects. (From Nachemson, A.L. [1976]: The lumbar spine an orthopaedic challenge. Spine, 1:59–71.)

reinforce the anterior and posterior aspects of the discs and intervertebral joints, thereby assisting in maintaining stability in static and dynamic situations.

Lu and associates[42] describe two types of IVD prolapse: a nuclear extrusion, in which nuclear material escapes from the disc, and an annulus protrusion, in which displaced nuclear material causes the outer annulus to bulge. Generally, a single-axis force, such as pure compression, does not cause a disc prolapse.[42] The IVD disc is most prone to injury during the transition stage from one direction of rotation to the other. This occurs in the lumbar spine when the individual flexes and sidebends, picks up a load, or tries to come to the upright position while maintaining a sidebent position.[28, 42, 48] This particular movement places the lumbar disc in a precarious situation. Because of facet and ligamentous restraints during sidebending, the vertebra will rotate to the same side as the sidebend. As a result of this rotatory movement, the annular fibers oriented in the direction of the movement become taut, whereas the fibers oriented in the opposite direction tend to slacken. Then, as the upright position is assumed, there is a point between the flexed and upright positions at which the annular fibers are at their weakest. At the midpoint of movement, should there be a weakness in the annulus fibrosus, the contents of the nucleus pulposus may protrude, causing herniation or extrusion of the nuclear contents.[26, 64] Although this component of rotation with sidebending occurs in all regions of the spine, the shift in the direction of rotation in flexion and in the upright position is unique to the lumbar area.[26] Table 12–1 describes the injury mechanism for sudden and gradual disc prolapse.

Disc saturation has also been reported to have a role in disc prolapse. During sleep, the spine is unloaded and will absorb water. At waking, the disc is saturated with fluid and is at its maximum volume and height. As the day progresses, the disc proceeds to lose height and volume because of fluid loss

Table 12–1. Mechanisms of Injury for Disc Prolapse

Sudden disc prolapse	High compressive forces applied suddenly to a spine in an unfavorable postural position (i.e., forward bending combined with twisting)
Gradual disc prolapse	Prolapse is a slow progressive injury resulting from compressive force of lesser magnitude applied repetitiously to a spine in flexion (i.e., frequent bending and lifting)

Description from Lu, Y.M., Hutton, W.C., and Gharpuray, V.M. (1996): Do bending, twisting, and diurnal fluid changes in the disc affect the propensity of prolapse? A viscoelastic finite element model. Spine, 21:2570–2579.

from compression.[42] Therefore, because the disc is at its maximum saturation in the morning, the disc may be more prone to prolapse, if subjected to high enough compression forces with flexion and twisting, earlier in the morning compared with later in the day when the disc has lost water.[1, 42] Several factors are involved in the initiation and propagation of annulus failure: axial compressive load, bending and twisting, and disc saturation. Absence of even one of these factors makes it less easy for the annulus to fail.[28, 42, 48]

EVALUATION AND TREATMENT PHILOSOPHIES

Several approaches to LBP and its treatment, encompassing innumerable evaluation and treatment techniques, have been recommended. These include conservative measures of therapeutic exercise, modalities, massage, mobilization, manipulation, back education, training in body mechanics, and the most nonconservative approach to LBP, surgical intervention. The two most common methods of treating LBP are those proposed by Williams[81, 82] and McKenzie.[47] These two philosophies toward LBP are in direct contradiction to each other. Williams recommends performance of exercises and adherence to postural principles that serve to decrease the lumbar lordosis to a minimum, and he has introduced a set of exercises called William's Flexion Exercises.[81, 82] McKenzie's concept of treatment is based on the migrating movement of the nucleus pulposus as a result of spinal flexion and extension, as described in the previous section. McKenzie recommends exercises and postural instructions that restore or maintain the lumbar lordosis.[47] Exercises involving lumbar spine extension, particularly in the early stages of treatment, are the cornerstone of this treatment philosophy. However, lumbar flexion exercises are usually added at a later time so that the athlete has full range of spinal flexion and extension. McKenzie's treatment is also based on an extensive mechanical evaluation, in which the clinician determines which movements centralize or abolish the athlete's pain and which exercises should, therefore, be part of the treatment plan. Movements that increase or peripheralize the pain or symptoms are avoided. There are several studies that have addressed the effectiveness of the McKenzie treatment approach in patients with acute[3, 13, 14, 16, 18, 36, 44, 58, 60, 70–72] or chronic[63] LBP. It has been my experience that LBP resulting from mechanical stresses responds well to the McKenzie approach, and this approach therefore serves as an outline for the rest of this chapter.

EVALUATION

The evaluation includes necessary observations that will provide the clinician with a "mechanical picture" of the lumbar spine and a path of treatment. Many opinions and approaches for evaluation of LBP exist. Often clinicians become frustrated in assessing the athlete with low back complaints. Unlike with a knee assessment, efforts to diagnose the specific causes of pain or the decrease in function in the low back are often futile. In fact, the precise diagnosis is unknown in 80% to 90% of cases of LBP.[52] A more effective approach is to consider in the evaluation the athlete's current symptoms, the response of those symptoms with activities of daily living, and the response of symptoms after stressing the lumbar spine in weight-bearing and non–weight-bearing positions. It is assumed that the athlete's LBP is suspected to be of mechanical origin and that all other serious pathologies have been excluded by a physician.

History

The history is that part of the evaluation in which the clinician should become informed about the current condition of the athlete, the behavior of the injury, and any past treatments the athlete has received for LBP. Each question asked should have a purpose and should help the clinician discern mechanical from nonmechanical sources of pain when the information is combined with the information gained in the objective part of the evaluation. The clinician should keep the athlete "on track" in discussing the current low back condition and should discourage conversation about "old injuries" that are not pertinent to the current complaints. Both the clinician and the athlete should be seated during the interview, and the following questions should be asked:

1. *What are the current symptoms or complaints?* The clinician should develop a good understanding of the current symptoms, which can be marked on a body diagram that shows both anterior and posterior views (Fig. 12–3). The clinician should note whether the athlete's symptoms are symmetric, asymmetric, unilateral, or bilateral and whether any numbness, tingling, or sensory changes are present in the spine, buttocks, or extremities. Centralization is an excellent indicator that the current position or exercise is the correct direction of movement.[19, 47] Distal symptoms should move

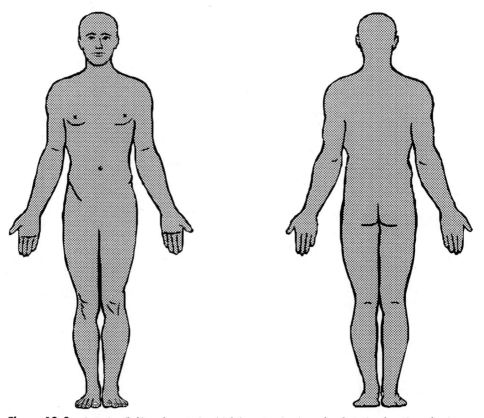

Figure 12–3. Anterior (left) and posterior (right) anatomic views for denoting location of pain.

proximally. Centralization is discussed in more detail in the treatment part of this chapter. The most distal symptoms should be noted, as these are the indicators of improvement. There are many adjectives to describe LBP and any referred symptoms that may exist. The Oswestry Low Back Pain Questionnaire includes over 60.[11] LBP symptoms often change rapidly.

2. *When did the current onset begin? Are the symptoms improving, remaining unchanged, or worsening?* Athletes will often answer these questions with the response, "I've had LBP for months or even years." The clinician should note this in the "previous episodes" section of the history. The clinician should question the athlete about when the most recent exacerbation of symptoms occurred, and the athlete should be as specific as possible. The answer will assist the clinician in classifying the current condition as acute (of 0 to 14 days' duration), subacute (of 2 to 8 weeks' duration), or chronic (of more than 8 weeks' duration) in onset. Because of soft-tissue healing time and inflammatory processes, individuals with acute low back injuries should be assessed with much greater care.

3. *How did this most recent onset of LBP commence?* Identifying the mechanism of injury is important in the individual with acute, subacute, and even chronic LBP. The clinician should direct the athlete to describe the reason for the most recent exacerbation or episode of LBP. Present complaints may not always be due to "old injuries." Often, athletes will not be able to pinpoint a specific episode of trauma. The athlete may report that the LBP appeared for no apparent reason.

4. *What were the symptoms at onset? Did the athlete experience only LBP initially? How much time elapsed before referred symptoms began?* Comparing onset of symptoms to current symptoms should assist the clinician in determining if indeed the athlete's condition is improving, remaining unchanged, or worsening since onset.

5. *Is the pain constant or intermittent?* Constant pain can be of mechanical or chemical origin. The differentiation between mechanical and chemical pain will be discovered in the repeated movements portion of the evaluation. McKenzie[47] states that "movements may superimpose mechanical forces on an existing chemical pain and enhance it, but they will never reduce or abolish chemical pain." The nociceptive system responsible for chemical pain does not turn off and on like a switch. Thus, intermittent pain must be the result of mechanical deformation.

6. *Do the symptoms get better, get worse, or remain the same with activities such as sitting, bending, walking, standing, or lying? Are they less severe in the morning*

or as the day progresses? Sitting is a sustained flexion activity, whereas walking is an extension activity. Difficulty standing upright from a seated position indicates a curve reversal block from flexion to extension. Curve reversal block is the inability of the athlete to move immediately from a kyphotic lumbar spine position (sitting) to a more lordotic position (standing). Often individuals will attest to having to take 2 or 3 steps walking before they were able to stand upright from a seated position. The answer to these important questions should hint at a possible treatment plan for the athlete because of the very different stresses placed on the lumbar spine with these activities.

7. *Does the LBP disturb sleep? What sleeping position is comfortable for the athlete?* Often individuals with asymmetric or unilateral signs and symptoms are unable to sleep on the affected side. Pain that is worse upon awakening may indicate a faulty sleeping position or a mattress that is too soft or too firm.

8. *Are there any bowel or bladder problems?* These are indicative of cauda equina injury or other ominous pathology that necessitates further referral.

9. *What is the athlete's current sport or activity level?* Basketball players transmit large forces of axial loading to the spine with jumping. Gymnasts hyperextend the spine, thus greatly loading the facet joints. Golfers position the spine at extremes of unilateral side flexion and rotation in driving and repeatedly flex the lumbar spine in picking up balls. Student athletes should be questioned not only about their particular sport and its effects on their LBP but also about how the back feels while they are attending class or studying. The posture assumed after practice, rather than positions assumed in the particular sport, may be to blame for the current condition.

10. *What previous episodes of LBP has the patient suffered and what was the treatment?* An athlete's experience with treatment and relief of symptoms with previous episodes of LBP should assist the clinician in deciding the current treatment plan. The clinician's asking about previous episodes of LBP should also cue the athlete to recall previous radiographic findings and results of any special tests.

11. *What is the athlete's medical history? Have there been any recent or major surgeries?*

12. *Have radiographs or special tests been ordered?* Once a diagnosis has been made based solely on radiographic findings, the diagnosis may seem to "follow" the athlete. At least 30% of asymptomatic individuals show abnormalities in the lumbar spine as determined by myelography, computed tomography (CT), and magnetic resonance im-

aging (MRI).[13] Mechanical assessment may or may not correlate with radiographic findings.[73] Therefore, a treatment that is based solely on the radiographs of an individual is, at best, poor. Radiographs are necessary to rule out instabilities of the spine and, in some cases, encroachment of bony structures on neurologic structures. The presence of spinal instability is a contraindication for evaluation of LBP by mechanical assessment.

13. *What medications are currently being taken?* Analgesics and nonsteroidal anti-inflammatory drugs may negatively affect the mechanical assessment by masking symptoms.

Posture

Sitting. An athlete who is complaining of LBP should have the history taken while in the seated position. The clinician observes whether the athlete sits with a reduced, normal, or accentuated lumbar lordosis; whether he or she sits symmetrically or deviated to one side; and whether the athlete continually adjusts the seated position by bearing weight through the hands and arms.

Standing. Standing is observed in anterior, posterior, and side views. The clinician should note whether the athlete is standing with equal weight on the right and left lower extremities. The posterior superior iliac spines should be level, and if a lateral shift exists, it should be noted. A lateral shift is the position of the top half of the body in relation to the bottom half (Fig. 12–4). A right lateral shift indicates that the top half of the body has moved right in relation

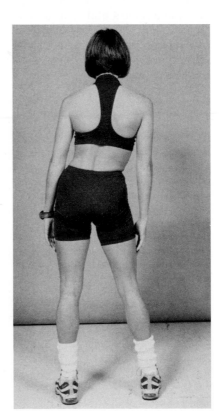

Figure 12–4. Right lateral shift.

to the bottom half. Lateral shifts are evident in about 52% of patients.[46] The standing posture should also reveal whether the lumbar lordosis is normal, reduced, or accentuated. A lateral shift may be more easily identified anteriorly by noting shoulder position. An athlete with LBP who presents with a lateral shift may have increased symptoms and may remain worse when in the flexed or extended position. Therefore, the shift should be corrected before sagittal plane exercises can be tolerated by the athlete. Correction of a lateral shift is presented later in the treatment section of this chapter.

Active Range of Motion

Flexion in Standing. With the knees straight, the athlete bends forward as far as possible, with the hands reaching toward the floor, and immediately returns to the neutral standing position (Fig. 12–5). The clinician should be positioned behind the athlete and should note range-of-motion loss, quality of lordotic curve reversal (the lordotic curve becomes kyphotic with flexion), and any deviation from the sagittal plane. Deviation during flexion may occur while the athlete is bending forward or is returning to the neutral standing position. Often individuals with suspected disc lesions will deviate away from the side of pain. Deviations toward the side of pain may occur when soft-tissue structures have adaptively shortened because of poor postural habits or previous trauma.

Extension in Standing. The athlete places both hands in the small of the back while keeping the knees straight, bends backward as far as possible, and returns immediately to the neutral standing position (Fig. 12–6). Significant deviation from the sagittal plane in extension is not very common. Anatomically, the facets in extension are in an approximated position. Therefore, any deviation from the sagittal plane in extension would be sharply opposed by the close-packed position of the facets. Again, the clinician notes any range-of-motion loss and the athlete's ability to accentuate the lumbar lordosis required with extension in standing. A loss of extension range of motion is present in 75% to 80% of people with LBP.[46] Active range-of-motion measurements of the spine can be determined specifically using a spinal inclinometer or using Schober's tech-

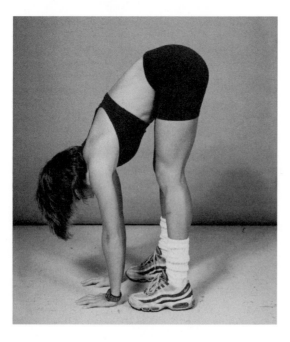

Figure 12–5. Flexion in standing.

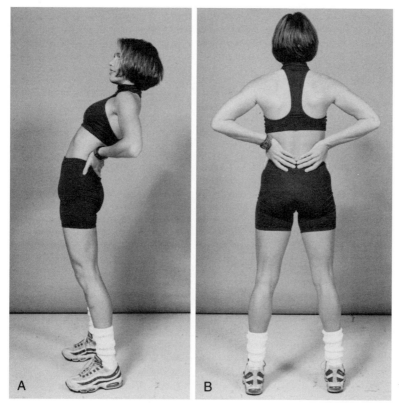

Figure 12–6. *A*, Extension in standing. *B*, Extension in standing hand placement.

nique[65] with a tape measure, or one can use a scale of range-of-motion loss such as major, moderate, minimum, or none. Regardless of the method used, the quality of curve reversal of the lumbar spine during range of motion and any deviation that occurs from the normal pathway of movement should be noted. For instance, the athlete may exhibit full flexion range of motion but uses the hands to "walk" back up the thighs to return to neutral.

Sidegliding Right and Sidegliding Left. Sidegliding combines rotation and side flexion of the lumbar spine (Fig. 12–7). It is most easily carried out by the clinician by placing one hand on the athlete's shoulder and the other hand on the opposite iliac crest. The athlete is asked to simultaneously move the shoulder and pelvis in opposite directions. The shoulders must be kept parallel to the ground. The clinician should note any range-of-motion loss to the left and then to the right and any restriction to movement. This is most easily observed if the clinician is positioned posterior to the athlete.

MEASUREMENT

Again, active range of motion of the lumbar spine can be measured in many different ways. Quantity of motion is important, just as with any joint assessment. However, the quality of motion and any difficulties of completing the motion in the lumbar spine can be more useful than quantity in bridging the information gathered during the examination to form a treatment plan. For instance, noting that an athlete's flexion is limited is important; however, of greater importance is the fact that when the athlete is allowed to deviate to the right, there is a subsequent increase in flexion range of motion.

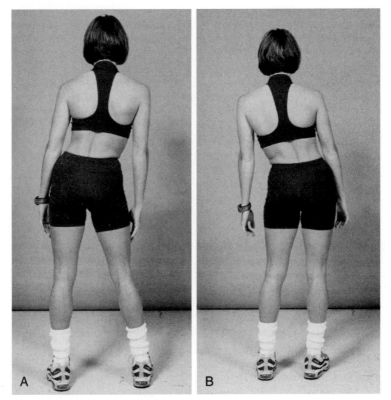

Figure 12–7. *A*, Sideglide in standing, right. *B*, Sideglide in standing, left.

The next section of the lumbar spine evaluation is vital. Often, an athlete presents with symptoms that are improving or may even be symptom free. Dixon and colleagues[7] reported that 44% of individuals with LBP were better in 1 week and 92% were better in 2 months, regardless of treatment. Other reasons an athlete may present for evaluation include spinal deformity or loss of function. The objective for the clinician is to use repeated movements or sustained positions to challenge the lumbar spine mechanically. Determining movements that reproduce symptoms has good reliability and should be considered in the assessment process.[45]

McKenzie[47] states: "If we are to relate movements to pain, the test movements must be performed in such a way that they produce a change in the patient's symptoms. If there is no change in the patient's symptoms during or immediately following the test movements, the joints have not been stressed adequately and the process should be repeated more vigorously. It may also be that the pain is not of mechanical origin, because mechanical pain must be and always is affected by movement or position."

Test Movements

The current symptoms should be noted with the athlete in the standing position, prior to beginning test movements. These symptoms may be different from symptoms recorded previously in the history, with the athlete in the sitting position. The repeated movements suggested here have been explored extensively by McKenzie[47] and others[18, 19] and are used by me daily in evaluating individuals with LBP. When performing repeated movements, the number of sets of repetitions is limited when the athlete indicates a change in signs and symptoms such as increase, decrease, or abolition of pain. The clinician may also limit sets of repetitions by noting a change in the movement pattern, such as increased difficulty in returning to the neutral position after the athlete flexes the spine.

The test movements are the following:

1. *Flexion in standing.* The clinician should note any change in signs and symptoms during and after this single movement and when the athlete is standing in the neutral position (see Fig. 12–5).
2. *Repeated flexion in standing.* If the athlete's single movement of lumbar flexion did not result in a change in baseline signs and symptoms or there was no effect, repeated flexion in standing should be performed. Flexion in standing is performed in sets of five repetitions, and symptoms are reassessed after every set. Each repetition should be performed by the athlete in a slow and controlled fashion. A progression of force may need to be incorporated by the clinician by adding overpressure at the shoulders when the athlete is at the end range of motion (Fig. 12–8).
3. *Extension in standing.* The clinician should note the quantity and quality of this single movement following flexion in standing and compare this with baseline range-of-motion data gathered in the active range-of-motion section of the evaluation (see Fig. 12–6). Often with repeated flexion of the lum-

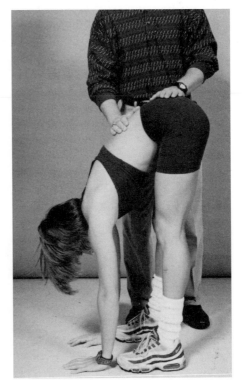

Figure 12–8. Flexion in standing with overpressure by the clinician.

bar spine, a recheck of one repetition of extension in standing will reveal blocked or decreased extension range of motion. Again, the clinician is looking for any change in symptoms during the movement and after the athlete returns to the neutral standing position.

4. *Repeated extension in standing.* If the athlete's single movement of lumbar extension did not affect the symptoms, lumbar extension should be repeated in sets of five repetitions, and the symptoms should be reassessed after every set. A progression of force with extension in standing is incorporated by the athlete's bending backward to the end range, briefly pausing while exhaling, and then immediately returning to the neutral position.

The sagittal plane must be evaluated thoroughly before the lateral or unilateral components of the spine are investigated. If there is no change, no improvement, or no worsening as a result of repeated movements of flexion and extension in standing, the clinician should investigate flexion and extension in lying before testing sidegliding in standing. The athlete is placed in a supine position, which removes the gravitational stress of a standing position. A baseline of current symptoms is once again noted.

5. *Flexion in lying.* The athlete lies supine with the hips and knees flexed so that the feet are flat on the treatment table. The athlete bends the knees onto the chest, clasping the knees with both hands, as in the double knee-to-chest position, and applies firm pressure (Fig. 12–9). The athlete then returns to the starting position. The clinician should note any change in symptoms during and after the movement.

6. *Repeated flexion in lying.* The athlete repeats the

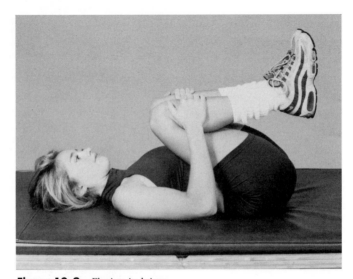

Figure 12-9. Flexion in lying.

movement as described in flexion in lying in sets of five repetitions, with the clincian reassessing signs and symptoms after every set. The clinician applies an overpressure force by adding pressure to the knees with the arms and hands.

The primary reason for testing flexion in lying rather than in standing, besides stressing of the lumbar spine in an unloaded position, involves biomechanics of the spine. Flexion in standing occurs from the upper lumbar levels initially and the lower lumbar segments last. Most mechanical problems of the lumbar spine involve the lower levels, L5-S1 and L4-L5. Therefore, flexion in lying stresses the L5-S1 segment immediately as flexion is initiated. Flexion in standing, however, will stress the L5-S1 junction only when flexion in standing is almost full.

7. *Extension in lying.* The athlete lies prone on the table with the hands placed directly under the shoulders. The clinician asks the athlete to raise the top half of the body off the table while keeping the hips, pelvis, knees, and legs on the treatment table (Fig. 12–10). This is a passive movement in the lumbar spine; therefore, the athlete must keep the paraspinals, gluteals, and hamstring muscles relaxed during the entire movement. The spine should sag at the top of the movement. The athlete then returns to the starting position. Any change in signs and symptoms during the movement and as a result of the movement should be noted.
8. *Repeated extension in lying.* The "press-up" as described in extension in lying is repeated in sets of five, and signs and symptoms are reassessed during and after each set.

Both extension in standing and extension in lying extend the lumbar spine, from upper levels (L4-L5) to lower levels (L5-S1). McKenzie[47] reports that the greatest extension stretch that a patient can apply to the back is extension in lying. The force exerted to the plane of the body with extension in lying is perpendicular and has a maximal mechanical effect.

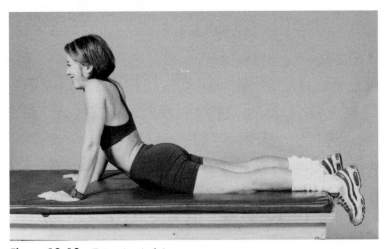

Figure 12–10. Extension in lying.

The following guidelines must be followed with repetitive movements:

1. Movements that cause the signs and symptoms to move to a proximal or to a more midline position should be part of the treatment process. This has been described as the centralization phenomenon.[47]
2. Movements that cause symptoms to peripheralize or move laterally from the midline and that remain worse as a result should be avoided.
3. Movements that create a further block in range of motion should be avoided.
4. The presence of a lateral shift should be explored if sagittal movements in both directions cause an increase and peripheralization of pain in loaded or unloaded positions or if a progression of forces, by adding overpressure with repeated movement, causes no change in initial complaints.

Reflexes and Cutaneous Distribution

The deep tendon reflexes that should be tested by the clinician with a reflex hammer are listed in Table 12–2. Any bilateral differences (asymmetry) should be recorded. The athlete's muscles or tendons must be relaxed. The quadriceps and gastrocnemius-soleus reflexes can be tested with the athlete seated. To elicit the quadriceps reflex, the athlete's knee should be flexed to a minimum of 30° and preferably 90°. The hammer should strike the tendon directly. The gastrocnemius-soleus reflex is elicited with the ankle at 90° or slightly dorsiflexed. Again, the reflex hammer should strike the tendon directly. The medial hamstring reflex is elicited by positioning the athlete prone. The clinician should flex the athlete's knee to 30° to 60°, place a thumb over the semitendinosus, and strike the thumbnail with the reflex hammer. Again, the athlete must be relaxed.

Myotomes and Dermatomes

It is important to check the dermatome patterns and cutaneous distribution of the nerve roots during the low back evaluation. The clinician should keep in mind that dermatome patterns will vary from person to person. The athlete's awareness of light touch at various points on the lower extremities should be compared bilaterally. Asymmetries that appear to be present can be further tested with a pinwheel, brush, or cotton ball to locate specific areas of sensory difference to determine the nerve root affected.

Myotomes are a group of muscles supplied by a single nerve root (Table 12–3). Each contraction should be held for a minimum of 5 seconds to determine whether weakness becomes evident. Myotomal weakness takes time to develop. Myotomes can be tested with the athlete sitting or supine. A good practice for the clinician to follow is to test, for instance, the athlete's left L2 myotome (hip flexion) and then immediately test the right L2 myotome before proceeding to

Table 12–2. Deep Tendon Reflexes

STRUCTURE	NERVE ROOT
Quadriceps	L3–L4
Gastrocnemius/soleus	S1–S2
Medial hamstrings	L5–S1

Table 12–3. Low Back Myotome Distribution

MOVEMENT/STRUCTURE	SPINAL LEVEL
Hip flexion	L2
Knee extension	L3
Ankle dorsiflexion	L4
Extensor hallucis longus	L5
Ankle eversion	S1
Knee flexion	S2

test the L3 (knee extension) myotome. Again, any differences in bilateral strength should be recorded.

Standing Neurologic Screen

At times, a bilateral strength difference may not reveal itself with the athlete in a non–weight-bearing position or in the accepted myotome testing position. Therefore, for the clinician to test the lower lumbar and upper sacral nerve roots further and in a more functional position, the athlete is asked to stand and walk first on the heels and then on the toes. Any movement control difficulty from left to right should be noted. Because myotome weakness takes time to develop and in order to test function further, the athlete is asked to repeat a unilateral calf raise 20 times without rest on first the left foot and then the right. Again, the clinician should note any movement control difficulty or complaints of fatigue on bilateral comparison. The athlete may place a hand on the wall to help with balance during the unilateral calf raise but should not use the wall to help complete the movement.

The sitting root test as described by Magee[43] is used to stretch the dura and produce symptoms of radiculopathy. The test is performed with the athlete sitting with a flexed neck. The knee is actively extended, while the hip remains flexed at 90° (Fig. 12–11). Increased pain indicates tension on the sciatic nerve. Athletes with true sciatic pain will arch backward and complain of pain into the buttock, posterior thigh, and calf when the leg is straightened, indicating a positive test.

In order to help the clinician differentiate between low back pathology and sacroiliac dysfunction, the following tests, described by Laslett and Williams[38] in their work on the reliability of provocation tests for sacroiliac joint pathology, are offered. Tests are positive when the athlete's signs and symptoms are reproduced with the forces applied.

1. *Distraction or gapping test.* This test applies pressure directed posteriorly and laterally to both anterior superior iliac spines to stretch the anterior sacroiliac ligaments (Fig. 12–12).
2. *Compression test.* This test compresses the pelvis when pressure is applied to the uppermost iliac crest, directed toward the opposite iliac crest. It stretches the posterior sacroiliac ligaments or compresses the anterior part of the sacroiliac joint (Fig. 12–13).
3. *Posterior shear or thigh thrust test.* This test applies a posterior shearing stress to the sacroiliac joint through the femur. Excessive adduction of the hip is avoided because flexion and adduction combined are normally uncomfortable or painful (Fig. 12–14).

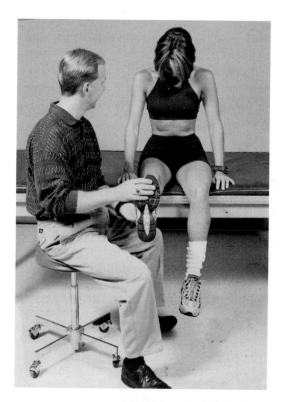

Figure 12–11. Sitting root test is used to reproduce radiculopathy symptoms.

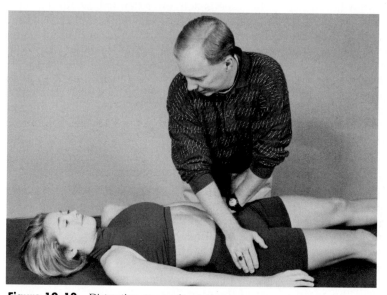

Figure 12–12. Distraction or gapping test.

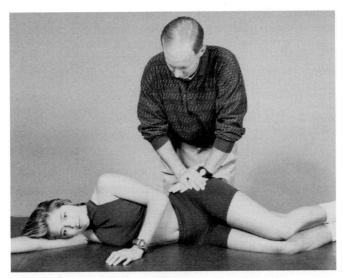

Figure 12–13. Compression test.

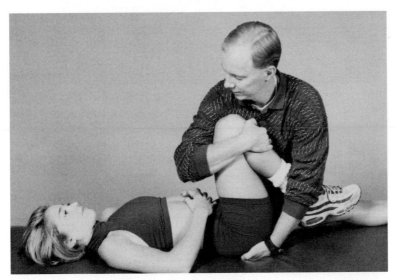

Figure 12–14. Posterior shear or thigh thrust test.

4. *Pelvic torsion–right posterior rotation.* This is some-times called Gaenslen's test. Posterior rotation of the right ilium on the sacrum is achieved by flexion of the right hip and knee and simultaneous left hip extension. Overpressure is applied to force the sacroiliac joint to its end range (Fig. 12–15A).

5. *Pelvic torsion–left posterior rotation.* This is sometimes called Gaenslen's test. Posterior rotation of the left ilium on the sacrum is achieved by flexion of the left hip and knee and simultaneous right hip extension. Overpressure is applied to force the sacroiliac joint to its end range (Fig. 12–15B).

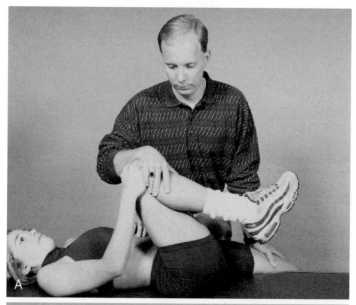

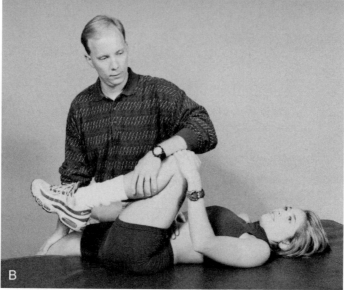

Figure 12–15. *A,* Pelvic torsion, right posterior rotation. *B,* Pelvic torsion, left posterior rotation.

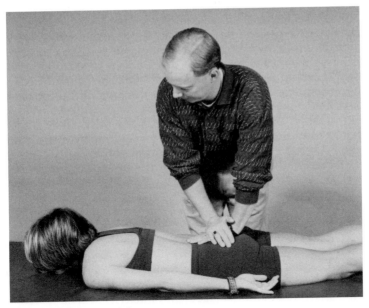

Figure 12–16. Sacral thrust test.

6. *Sacral thrust test.* Pressure is applied directly to the sacrum while the athlete lies prone. The force is directed anteriorly against the ilia, which are fixed against the table (Fig. 12–16).
7. *Cranial shear test.* Pressure is applied to the coccygeal end of the sacrum, directed cranially. The ilium is held immobile through the hip joint as the examiner holds the leg firmly with a counterpressure in the form of a traction force that is directed caudad (Fig. 12–17).

Other authors have investigated the reliability of various sacroiliac tests and have reported conflicting results.[10, 45, 61]

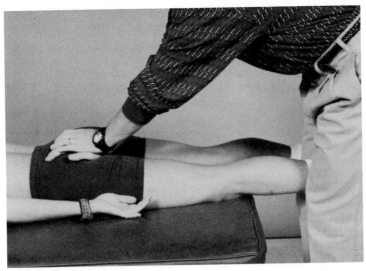

Figure 12–17. Cranial shear test.

Of the above tests, the sacral thrust and cranial shear tests were only marginally reliable, whereas the other tests showed substantial intertherapist reliability. Cibulka and colleagues,[10] who measured innominate tilt, showed that agreement was excellent if three positive tests out of four were used to indicate sacroiliac disturbances. It would seem reasonable that clinicians should not rely on any single test for sacroiliac joint problems. Only tests that have proven individual interexaminer reliability should be used for diagnostic purposes. Further studies are required to assess the sensitivity and specificity of sacroiliac tests.[61]

Once the history and repeated movements examination are complete, the clinician should be able to discern a mechanical pattern in the spine regarding the stresses that exacerbate symptoms or reduce or abolish symptoms.

TREATMENT

A method for classifying the athlete's response to repeated movements is appropriate. In 1987, at the request of the Quebec Worker's Health and Safety Commission, the Quebec Task Force on Spinal Disorders (QTFSD) published a monograph that provided a comprehensive examination of the scientific evidence for the assessment and management of activity-related spinal disorders.[69] These disorders are typically caused or exacerbated by movements or postural positions that load the spinal tissues excessively.[69] The QTFSD concluded that a specific diagnosis of low back problems is not possible in 90% of cases and recommended a classification system based on a description of pain location. The task force considered symptom duration, pain intensity, and work status as being of secondary importance.

Additionally, the QTFSD recommended that its own and any other classification system meet the following criteria[69]:

1. Biologic plausibility: the classification is compatible with current knowledge of vertebral physiopathology
2. Exhaustive classification: the classification encompasses all clinical cases seen in occupation health
3. Mutually exclusive categories: the great majority of clinical cases, at one point, fit into one and only one category; however, the patient may subsequently move into another category
4. Reliability: a given case of a vertebral disorder can be classified in the same manner by two or several clinicians
5. Clinical usefulness: the classification facilitates the making of clinical decisions as well as the evolution of care
6. Simplicity: the classification is simple and neither calls for complex paraclinical examination nor encourages superfluous investigations

The purpose of a universally accepted classification system for activity related to LBP is to allow for a better method of communication between clinicians regarding the appropriateness and efficacy of a treatment intervention and to allow scientific investigation of treatment methods.

Such a classification system, meeting all of the listed criteria of the QTFSD, was proposed by McKenzie[47] in 1972, 15 years before the publication of the QTFSD classification. The first four categories of the QTFSD classification are nearly identical to those in the McKenzie classification. The McKenzie system's basic theme of pain location and response to movement adheres to the criteria of the QTFSD. In addition, this system allows for classification of the athlete with LBP into three distinct syndromes. These are the postural, dysfunction, and derangement syndromes, each of which requires a specific treatment program developed in response to progressive repeated end-range movement testing.

Identification of the different syndromes is based on the effects that repeated movements in the evaluation and follow-up treatments have on the initiation of pain; the point in the pathway where pain is first perceived; the site of pain and subsequent change in location of pain; increasing or decreasing intensity of the pain; and finally, abolition of the pain. Treatment of the various syndromes is based on the movements and positions that decrease or abolish the LBP found in the evaluation. The classification system described in this chapter of postural, dysfunction, and derangement syndromes is the same as that described by McKenzie.[47]

The Postural Syndrome

Certain postures maintained over long periods of time will place stress on soft tissues and lead to pain. Athletes will complain of pain that develops locally, adjacent to the midline of the spinal column. Not only may prolonged end-range static loading cause LBP, but it may cause pain in the cervical and thoracic regions. Pain caused by postural syndromes is always intermittent. The evaluation of repeated movements will reveal no spinal deformity, no loss of range of motion, and no signs of pathology. The athlete's history will reveal that LBP is not present for days at a time and that no pain is present with activity or movement. The only objective finding often noted in the athlete with postural syndrome is a poor standing or sitting posture (Table 12–4).

Treatment of the athlete with postural syndrome is simply by education. The reason or cause of the discomfort is a mechanical deformation resulting from prolonged stress that eventually causes pain. For example, in the slouched seated position, the posterior soft-tissue structures of the spine are on stretch, including the ligaments, joints, capsules, muscles, and posterior annulus disc fibers. The normal resting position of the lumbar spine has an anatomic lordosis. However, a slouched or kyphotic position is often adopted, placing a stretch on the posterior structures. The clinician can use the following example to explain the reason for the athlete's LBP. After a 2- to 3-hour drive in a car, some aching is usually felt in the low back. What is the first thing people do when they get out of the car? Stretch. And which way do they stretch? Backward. This relieves posterior spinal stress and returns the lumbar spine to its more anatomic lordotic position. What happens to the back pain? It is usually abolished after bending backward only one time! Therefore, no pathology existed to cause the LBP. By relieving the stresses placed on the structures by a kyphotic sitting position, the pain is abolished.

Treatment of the postural syndrome includes correction of sitting posture, standing posture, and lying posture. A lifestyle of poor postural habits will lead to adaptive shortening of soft tissues and to eventual dysfunction or loss of

Table 12–4. Characteristics of Poor Sitting and Standing Postures

POOR SITTING POSTURE	POOR STANDING POSTURE
Head forward Shoulders rotated anteriorly Increased kyphosis of the thoracic spine Kyphosis of the lumbar spine	Flat back: decrease in lumbar lordosis; posterior tilt of the pelvis Swayback: increase in lumbar lordosis; increase in anterior tilting of the pelvis and hip flexion

movement, usually in the extension direction. Therefore, the athlete's complaints of LBP must first be reproduced by the athlete's assuming the poor postural position that was noted in the evaluation. It may take 10 to 15 minutes before the onset of pain.

The optimal position of the spine in standing, sitting, and lying includes a lordosis at the cervical and lumbar spines and a kyphosis at the thoracic spine. Swayback posture causes an approximation of the articular facets (Fig. 12–18A). The facets may become weight bearing, which may cause synovial irritation and inflammation. In this position, there is also excessive pressure on the anterior longitudinal ligament and a narrowing of the intervertebral foramen. The sway-back position will present with muscle imbalances that include tight hip flexors, back extensor muscles (erector spinae), and weak abdominal muscles. Correction of the swayback posture in standing includes cueing the athlete to lift the shoulders and rib cage, tighten the abdominals, and rotate the pelvis posteriorly. Exercises should emphasize regaining flexibility of the hip flexors and erector spinae and abdominal strengthening that includes the rectus abdominis and oblique muscles.

Flat back posture results in the spine's losing its shock-absorbing effect in the lumbar region, which can predispose the athlete to injury (Fig. 12–18B). An increase in kyphosis of the lumbar spine (flat back) will also result in a greater stretch of the posterior longitudinal ligament, which has extensive nerve innervation and can thus be a source of pain. There is also a greater stress placed on the posterior annular fibers.

Muscle imbalances noted in the flat back posture include tight trunk flexors (rectus abdominis, intercostals), hip extensor muscles, and hamstrings. Weakness may be present in the lumbar extensors and hip flexors. Correction of flat back includes lifting the shoulders and rib cage, rolling the pelvis anteriorly until a stretch is felt at about the belt line (L3-L4), and then backing off of the stretch by 10%. Exercises should emphasize restoring or increasing the normal lumbar

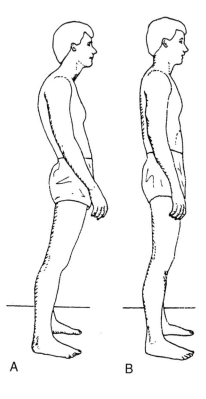

Figure 12–18. *A*, Swayback. *B*, Flat back. (From Kisner, C., and Colby, L.A. (1990): Therapeutic Exercise: Foundations and Techniques, 2nd ed. Philadelphia, F.A. Davis.)

A   B

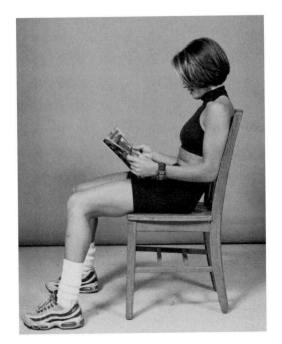

Figure 12-19. Poor sitting posture.

lordosis and decreasing the posterior stress placed on the spine that is present in the flat back position. Exercises should include stretching of the hamstrings and trunk flexors. Maintaining a small amount of lordosis in the lumbar spine while stretching the hamstrings is important in order to place a greater stretch on the hamstrings and a lesser stretch on the already flexible trunk extensors. Strengthening of the trunk extensors and press-ups in extension in lying (see Fig. 12–10) will also assist in maintaining an improved lumbar lordosis.

With athletes who complain that the LBP is worse while trying to sleep or upon awakening, an inspection of the sleeping posture and mattress quality is warranted. A firmer mattress is not necessarily better. A mattress must be flexible enough to support the curves of the spine that are naturally present but not accentuate them. The head should not be protruded in the supine position or sideflexed in side-lying but does require a pillow that supports the cervical lordosis. One pillow is usually sufficient. Suggestions for relief of acute back pain in lying include prone lying with a pillow under the abdomen, side-lying with a pillow between the knees, or supine lying with a pillow under the knees, with the knees and hips flexed.

The clinician must remember that the most frequent cause of postural pain is poor sitting posture (Fig. 12–19). Tips for correct alignment of the spine in sitting include the following:

1. The athlete should sit with the hips to the back of a chair and feet flat on the floor (Fig. 12–20*A*).
2. The athlete's knee height should be slightly lower than hip height.
3. The athlete should lean forward slightly at the hips (anterior pelvic tilt) and accentuate the lordosis at the lumbar spine (belt line) until a pinch is felt (Fig. 12–20*B*).
4. The athlete should then decrease or back off the accentuation of lordosis 10% (Fig. 12–20*C*).

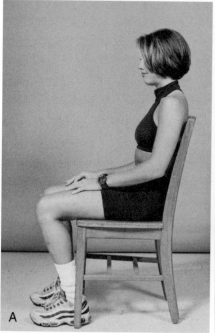
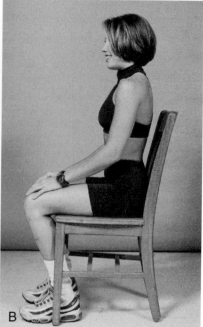
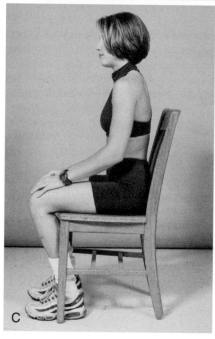

Figure 12–20. *A,* Athlete sits with hips to the back of the chair and feet flat on the floor. *B,* Athlete leans forward slightly at the hips (anterior pelvic tilt) and accentuates the lordosis at the (belt line) lumbar spine until a pinch is felt. *C,* Athlete decreases or backs off the accentuation of lordosis by 10%.

This "resting" position of the spine can be maintained actively by conscious control or passively by the addition of a lumbar roll or towel roll placed at the belt line of the athlete between the spine and the back of the chair (Fig. 12–21).

The Dysfunction Syndrome

The dysfunction syndrome is a condition in which adaptive shortening and a resultant loss of mobility cause pain prematurely, that is, before achievement of

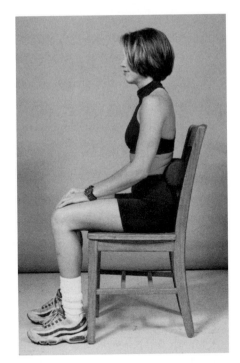

Figure 12–21. Sitting with use of lumbar roll to maintain lumbar lordosis.

full normal and end range of motion. This syndrome develops as a result of either poor postural habits or specific trauma that has involved the spine. Essentially, the condition arises because movement is performed inadequately at a time at which contraction of soft tissues is taking place. After trauma, an inextensible scar forms within or adjacent to otherwise healthy structures, and this causes reduced spinal mobility. Furthermore, the surrounding healthy structures capable of further extensibility are restricted by scar tissue. Thus, persisting pain results from the repair process itself.

From the athlete's history the clinician should be able to determine whether the LBP is intermittent. Pain will be present when positions or movements place periarticular structures on full stretch. Obviously this full stretch will occur sooner in an athlete with dysfunction than in an athlete with full spinal range of motion. The low back will feel better when the athlete is active and moving than when he or she is at rest. End range of motion is seldom required in regular activity, but during rest, end-range positions are readily assumed and may prove painful. Test movements will reveal a loss of spinal motion, which may interfere with positions that the athlete is required to assume in the sport. Test movements will reproduce pain at the end range of motion only. The LBP produced never remains once the athlete returns to the neutral standing position. For instance, when the athlete extends in standing, the presenting complaint will be reproduced at the end range of each repetition of extension but will disappear once the athlete returns to neutral. In the dysfunction syndrome, the athlete's posture will generally be poor. If there is a loss of extension, the lordosis may be reduced or the athlete may be unable to produce lordosis even if he or she strains to do so. If there is a loss of flexion, the athlete may have difficulty reaching the toes with the fingers, and during forward bending, the lumbar spine may remain in slight lordosis. Normally, the lumbar spine should become temporarily kyphotic at full flexion in standing to allow full range of motion to occur.

It is not possible to identify the specific structure causing the dysfunction pain, but any of the soft tissues adjacent to the vertebral column may adaptively shorten because of poor posture and positioning or as a result of trauma. The pain may be a result of adaptive shortening of any ligamentous structures, annular fibers of the IVD, or superficial or intrinsic muscles or attachments. Shortening of these structures would then interfere with the normal mobility or pathway of movement of facet joints during spinal movement.

The dysfunction syndrome is named according to which direction of movement is reduced. Extension dysfunction denotes a loss of extension range of motion, whereas flexion dysfunction denotes a loss of flexion range of motion. Sidegliding-right dysfunction refers to a loss of range of motion in sidegliding right or pain that is produced but not worsened when sidegliding right is completed.

Treatment of the dysfunction syndrome requires remodeling of shortened tissue structures by the regular application of stretching exercises. Rapid changes of symptoms do not occur in dysfunction. It takes weeks for soft tissues to become contracted and shortened, and likewise, it will take a long time for them to lengthen again. No benefit of stretching exercises will result unless the athlete is instructed to move to the extreme range of motion at which some, but not great, discomfort should be experienced. The "strain pain," which is mild discomfort produced by spinal movement, experienced during the recovery of lost movement is caused when contracted soft tissues are stretched enough to enhance elongation of shortened structures.

The athlete should be instructed that the "strain pain" produced with a set of exercises may worsen for up to 10 minutes after completion of the exercises. Stretching too hard or too fast will not speed the process. If pain is present 10 minutes after exercise, it is my practice to instruct the athlete to reduce the range of motion with each set to avoid further scarring. A reduction of repetitions and frequency of the exercise may even be required.

TREATMENT OF EXTENSION DYSFUNCTION

The treatment of extension dysfunction is as follows:

1. Press-ups with 10 repetitions every 2 hours (Fig. 12–22)
2. Press-ups with overpressure, either manually or with belt fixation (Fig. 12–23)
3. Postural education

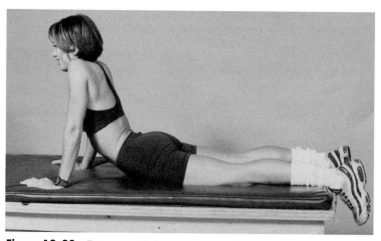

Figure 12–22. Press-up at end range of extension.

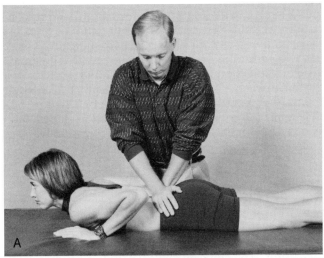

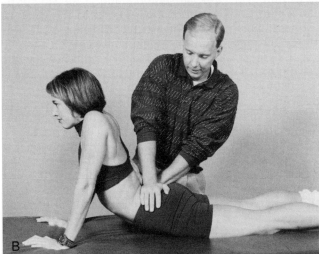

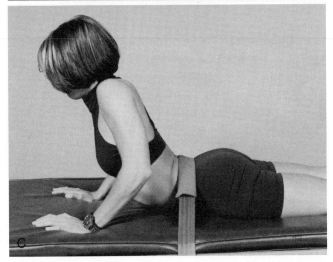

Figure 12–23. *A*, Press-up with overpressure in starting position. *B*, Press-up with overpressure in end range extension. *C*, Press-up with belt fixation.

Athletes with a loss of extension range of motion may present with a somewhat flattened lumbar spine. Therefore, a certain amount of extension range of motion will have to be gained through repeated stretching before they can be expected to sit with a lordotic curve. I have noted that treating athletes who have an extension dysfunction with the above regimen will result in 70% to 80% relief of LBP within 1 week of commencing treatment. The abolition of LBP may require continuing the press-ups (10 press-ups every 2 hours) for 4 to 6 weeks. With an athlete who plateaus with range-of-motion gains but who has not reached full end range of motion or in whom the LBP is not abolished, extension mobilization may be required.

Extension Mobilization

Athletes who cannot resolve dysfunction by self-treatment procedures may require a progression of forced extension mobilization. Extension mobilization may assist in restoring the loss of extension movement or a reduced lordosis.

Athlete's Position. The athlete should lie prone with arms by the side

Clinician's Position. The clinician should stand at the side of the athlete and place the heels of the hands (pisiform) just lateral to the spinous processes of the lumbar segment, crossing the arms. If the clinician is standing on the left side of the athlete, the right hand or fingers should be on the right side of the spine (facing cephalic), parallel to the spine. The trunk of the clinician should be aligned over the spinal column of the athlete with the elbows slightly flexed (Fig. 12–24).

Movement. Gentle pressure should be applied symmetrically, at the same spinal segment level, and should be immediately released. For example, when mobilizing L5, the clinician should make certain that the pressure of the mobilization of both hands is at L5. Each pressure is a little stronger, depending on the athlete and the pain behavior. Any peripheralization of symptoms is a warning, and the mobilization should cease immediately. Ten to 15 repetitions should be performed at each segment and at adjacent spinal segments. The clinician should never lose contact between the hands and the spine between mobilization repetitions.

TREATMENT OF FLEXION DYSFUNCTION

Treatment consists of performing flexion in lying (double knee-to-chest position), with 10 repetitions every 2 hours (see Fig. 12–9). Once full range of motion

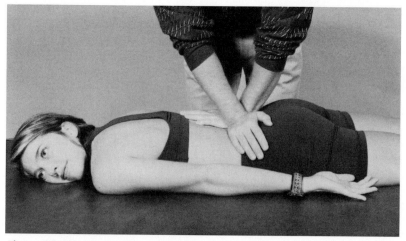

Figure 12–24. Extension mobilization.

is achieved with flexion in lying and no stretch is felt, all flexion in this position has been gained, and the athlete must now commence with flexion in standing to regain full functional range of motion. Because the force of gravity is acting during flexion in standing, this movement places the greatest stretch on the adaptively shortened structures (see Fig. 12–5).

Postural Education

Athletes with a flexion dysfunction may stand and sit with an accentuated lumbar lordosis. These athletes will reach the end range of flexion when sitting relaxed much sooner than will normal individuals.

In treating the athlete with a flexion dysfunction, the clinician must remember that flexion places tremendous stress on the posterior and posterolateral aspects of the disc. Again, anatomically, this is the weakest portion of the disc. Therefore, derangement must be suspected if flexion in standing, sitting, or lying immediately and significantly worsens symptoms. Preventing the exacerbation of a previous derangement may require the athlete to always follow flexion exercises with a set of press-ups, so that any posterior disturbance is immediately corrected.

The Derangement Syndrome

A derangement in the lumbar spine is described as an alteration of the position of the fluid nucleus within the IVD and possibly the surrounding annulus. As mentioned earlier in the biomechanics section of this chapter, the anterior annular fibers of the disc are thicker than the posterior fibers. Additionally, the thick anterior longitudinal ligament blends with the annular fibers, holding the nucleus in place. Therefore, anterior derangements account for only 10% of derangement patients. Ninety percent of low back derangements are posterior or posterolateral derangements. Once nuclear material has escaped through the annular wall, the hydrostatic mechanism is no longer intact, and internal derangement of the disc cannot be reduced significantly by movements of the spinal column. On the other hand, movements of the spinal column can be used to reverse internal derangement of the disc as long as the integrity of the disc wall is maintained.[47]

A derangement occurs when the normal resting position of the articular surfaces of the adjacent vertebrae is disturbed as a result of a change in the position of the fluid nucleus between these surfaces.[47] This change within the joint will affect the ability of the joint surfaces to move in their normal relative pathways, and departures from these pathways are frequently seen.[47] These departures from normal movement will result in losses of range of motion in flexion, extension, or slidegliding and may also result in lumbar deformities of kyphosis, lordosis, and acute scoliosis or lateral shift.

The athlete with LBP of suspected derangement origin will most likely describe the pain as constant. The pain may be symmetric, asymmetric, bilateral, or unilateral and may peripheralize into the buttock, thigh, leg, and region of the ankle and foot. During the history, the athlete will describe positions and activities that increase symptoms or peripheralize pain and positions that decrease pain and centralize peripheral signs and symptoms. Discogenic pathology should always be suspected when the athlete describes symptoms that change location after repeated movements or prolonged positioning.

Centralization as initially described by McKenzie refers to a rapid change in the perceived location of pain from a distal or peripheral location to a more proximal or central one.[19, 47] Movements that result in centralization of the pain reduce the derangement. Centralization is an excellent indicator that the correct movement or direction of mobilization has been chosen and that a positive treatment outcome can be expected.[19, 41] Conversely, nonoccurrence of centralization prognosticates poor treatment outcome and is an early predictor of the possible need for surgical intervention.[19, 41] Centralization of symptoms occurs only in the derangement syndrome.

On inspection, the athlete with derangement should always demonstrate a loss of normal range of motion in the flexion, extension, or sideglide planes of motion. Displaced tissue obstructs movements in the direction of the displacement. Further inspection may reveal an acute kyphosis of the lumbar spine (indicating a posterocentral derangement), acute scoliosis (indicating a posterolateral derangement), or acute accentuated lordosis (indicating anterior or anterolateral derangement).

The clinician is cautioned not to base treatment on the postural alignment of the spine or of the athlete. Rather, the athlete's response to the repeated movements portion of the examination is a better indicator of the correct treatment. Centralization of symptoms is the result of the correct movement reducing the derangement. Peripheralization of symptoms is contraindicated in positioning, repeated movements testing, and treatment. If test movements or positions cannot reduce or centralize symptoms, the annular wall may be breached, and spinal movements will not result in a lasting change of symptoms and will not influence the position of the nucleus.

McKenzie[47] describes seven derangements that may occur in the lumbar spine. Derangements 1 to 6 are posterocentral and posterolateral derangements, whereas derangement 7 comprises the far less common anterior and anterolateral disc disturbances.

DERANGEMENT 1

Symptoms include central or symmetric pain in the lumbar spine and rare buttock or thigh pain, with no spinal deformity. There is a minimal disturbance of disc material posteriorly, and this results in a loss of extension range of motion. Flexion movements will increase the back pain and perpetuate the loss of extension range of motion. Extension movements decrease back pain and result in a gain of extension range of motion. Treatment of derangement 1 is therefore based on the extension principle. In general, treatment of all derangements has four stages:

1. Reduction of derangement
2. Maintenance of reduction
3. Recovery of function
4. Prevention of recurrence

Derangement 1 treatment will initially begin with the athlete lying prone for 5 minutes. The athlete will then lie prone on the elbows for another 5 minutes. The athlete should then lie prone for a short while before commencing prone press-ups (extension in lying) in sets of 10 repetitions, resting approximately 2 minutes between each set. At the completion of four to five sets, the extension range of motion should be increasing and the back pain should be felt more centrally. As extension range of motion continues to increase, a reduction in LBP intensity will result. Steps should now be taken to ensure that the reduction of the derangement is maintained.

In order to maintain reduction of a posterior derangement, it is essential that lordosis be maintained at all times. Treatment will include sitting and standing with a good lordosis at all times and completing press-ups, 10 repetitions to end range, every 2 hours. Extension in standing is an acceptable replacement for extension in lying if circumstances prevent the athlete from lying prone. All athletes should be instructed that if they have severe pain that worsens or peripheralizes at the time of exercising, they should stop the exercise and seek advice from the clinician.

Reduction of the derangement can be assumed when extension is painless and full range of motion is present. If the athlete begins to plateau with range of motion gains and continues to have LBP, full end range of motion has not been achieved. To achieve full motion, the clinician may apply extension mobilization to the lumbar spine as previously described (see Fig. 12–24), 10 repetitions at each segmental level, or apply overpressure at segmental levels while the athlete is performing press-ups, either manually or with belt fixation (see Fig. 12–23)

Recovery of function with derangement 1 includes the beginning of flexion exercises. Often, because the lumbar lordosis has been maintained at all times and the principle of treatment has been extension, the athlete may have developed a flexion dysfunction or loss of range of motion in flexion. Exercise or movements to regain this flexion range of motion should begin with flexion in lying (see Fig. 12–9). If, after the athlete begins flexion, back pain returns and becomes more painful with each repetition, it is too early to begin flexion exercises, and only extension should continue. When LBP is reported, but it does not worsen or remain worse as a result of flexion, the athlete is undergoing tissue remodeling to regain flexion, and the movement may be continued. However, flexion exercises should always be followed up with extension exercises to ensure that the fluid nucleus is restored to the optimal position in the disc, thus removing the risk of recurrence of posterior derangement. When no further flexion can be gained in the lying position, the athlete should progress to flexion in standing (see Fig. 12–5). Flexion in standing should always be followed with extension in lying or extension in standing. Recovery of flexion is complete when, on performing flexion in lying and flexion in standing, full range of motion is achieved without pain.

Preventing the recurrence of derangement 1 should include continuing extension exercises twice daily to end range, for life, and flexion exercises once each day. Static or dynamic flexion positions should be interrupted frequently with extension in standing exercises. Sitting with good lumbar lordosis is encouraged, and slouched sitting should be avoided.

DERANGEMENT 2

Symptoms consist of central or symmetric pain in the lumbar spine, with or without buttock or thigh pain, with a deformity of lumbar kyphosis. There is excessive posterior accumulation of the nucleus with a major blockage of extension. Not only is extension prohibited, but the vertebrae are also forced apart, and their posterior margins cannot approximate. Any attempt to produce extension results in severe pain, and the athlete is forced to return to the flexed position, in which he or she finds some temporary relief. These athletes will present in acute distress.

Treatment of derangement 2 includes applying the extension principle. However, secondary to the kyphotic deformity, the athlete will be unable to lie prone. Therefore, prone positioning should be achieved gradually. The athlete should be placed prone, ensuring that the lumbar spine remains in flexion by placing several small pillows under the abdomen (Fig. 12–25). The pillows are then gradually withdrawn, one at a time, until the athlete reaches the prone position. It may take as long as 5 minutes before one of the pillows can be removed, and this process may take as long as 45 minutes before the athlete will be able to lie comfortably prone. Increasing extension range of motion too rapidly will cause severe pain and may provoke immediate regression. Treatment for derangement 1 can now commence. If after returning home after the initial treatment the athlete finds lying prone too painful, the athlete must be instructed to repeat the sequence of lying over pillows and then gradually lowering the body by removing the pillows until the prone position is obtained.

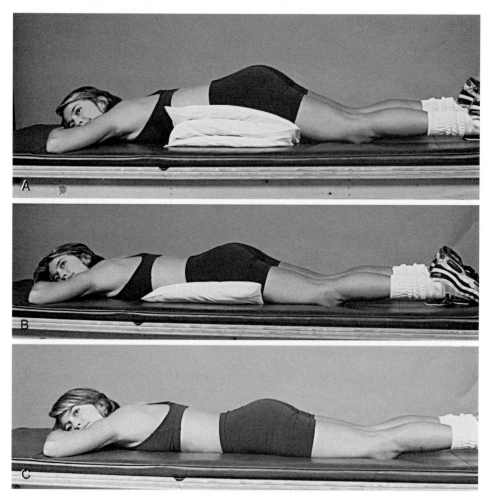

Figure 12–25. Progression of derangement 2 to end-range extension in lying. *A*, Prone trunk flexion with three pillows. *B*, Prone trunk flexion with one pillow. *C*, Prone with no pillows.

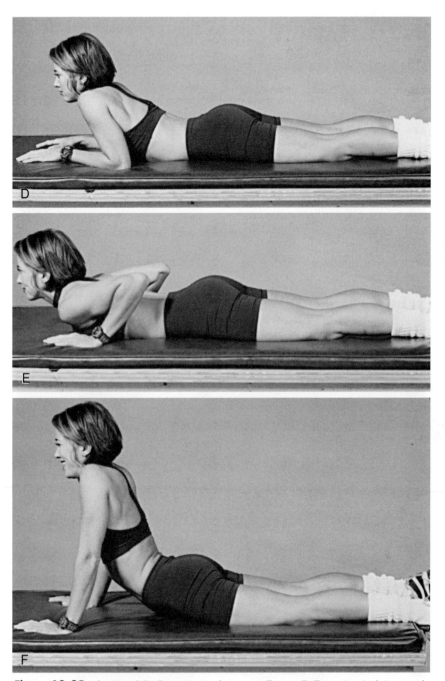

Figure 12–25 *Continued D*, Extension in lying on elbows. *E*, Extension in lying, ready to begin press-up. *F*, Full press-up to end-range extension.

DERANGEMENT 3

Symptoms consist of unilateral or asymmetric pain across the low back, with or without buttock or thigh pain (not below the knee). No spinal deformity is present. In derangement 3, the disturbance within the disc is located posterolaterally rather than posterocentrally, as in derangement 1.

Treatment for derangement 3 begins just as for the treatment for derangement 1. When an athlete's progress begins to plateau in the sagittal plane, in extension in lying, and in maintenance of the lordotic position, lateral compartment treatment may need to be incorporated. To treat the lateral compartment the athlete lies in the prone position. For right-sided LBP, the clinician will place the pelvis away from the painful side (to the left), creating a lateral shift toward the painful

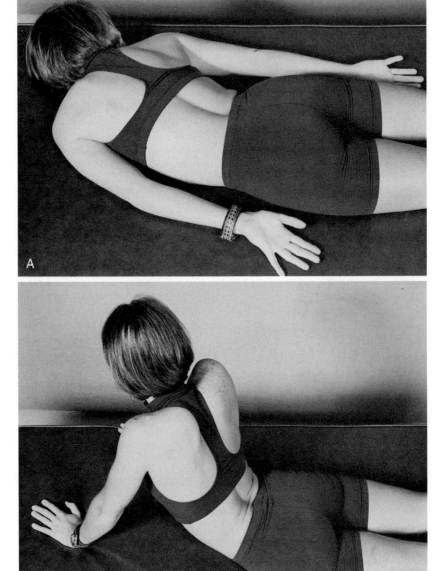

Figure 12–26. *A,* Prone lying with sideglide right. *B,* Press-up with sideglide right.

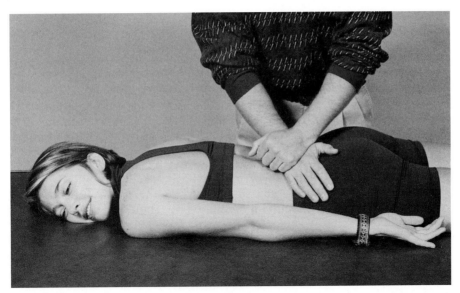

Figure 12–27. Rotation mobilization in extension.

side, which will provide a greater extension force on the right side when extension in lying is performed (Fig. 12–26A). The press-ups are completed with the hip in the off-center position (Fig. 12–26B). Ten repetitions are completed. The goal of the lateral shift press-up is centralization. Extension mobilizations (see Fig. 12–24), rotation mobilizations in extension (Fig. 12–27), or extension in lying with asymmetric overpressure by the clinician may be necessary to assist the athlete in full painless extension range of motion. Rotation mobilization in extension includes modifying the position of extension mobilization (described previously in Fig. 12–24) so that pressure is applied to one side of the transverse process and then to the other side of the appropriate segment, with a rocking effect being obtained (see Fig. 12–27).[47] The position of the clinician and athlete for the rotation mobilization in extension is the same as for extension mobilization. A more lateral component is present in a derangement 3, and therefore, centralization may be facilitated by the mobilization or pressure placed by the clinician on one side versus the other side. Repetitions should continue on the side at which a reduction in pain or centralization of pain was described by the athlete. The technique should be repeated 10 times on the involved segment. Further sets are completed as centralization progresses. Once the LBP remains centralized, treatment as for derangement 1 may commence.

DERANGEMENT 4

Symptoms consist of unilateral or asymmetric pain across the low back, with or without buttock or thigh pain (not below the knee), with a deformity of lumbar scoliosis. Lumbar scoliosis that is acute will worsen with sagittal plane movements of both flexion and extension. Ninety percent of lateral shifts are away from the painful side.[47] It is my practice not to assess the athlete's lateral shift by inspection only. Deviations of the spine are frequent and are important to the treatment of the athlete when symptoms are worsened with specific movements and when symptoms are centralized or decreased with other movements. The lateral shift becomes important to treatment when flexion or extension exercises worsen or peripheralize symptoms. Sideglide or lateral movements to one side may be full, and when assessed in the opposite direction, a marked loss of movement will be present. Correction of the lateral shift must take place before restoration of extension range of motion.

Correction of the lateral shift as described by McKenzie[47] has two parts. First, the deformity in scoliosis should be corrected, and then, the deformity in kyphosis, if present, should be reduced, and full extension restored. The athlete, standing with the feet about shoulder-width apart, should be asked to clearly define the location at which pain is currently being felt (Fig. 12–28A). The clinician should stand on the side to which the athlete is deviating and should place the athlete's near elbow at a right angle by the side. The clinician's arms should encircle the athlete's trunk, clasping the hand around the rim of the pelvis (Fig. 12–28B). The clinician should then press his or her shoulder against the athlete's elbow, pushing the athlete's rib cage and thoracic and upper lumbar spine away, while at the same time drawing the athlete's pelvis toward the clinician. In this manner, the deformity in scoliosis is reduced and, if possible, slightly overcorrected (Fig. 12–28C). As long as centralization is taking place, shift correction is safe. The first pressure in the series should be a gentle, gradual squeeze, held momentarily and then released. If well tolerated, a little more pressure is applied each time. Too much pressure, applied too fast, may result in the athlete's fainting. Restoration of the lumbar lordosis may commence once the shift has been corrected. The clinician should hold the athlete in a slightly overcorrected position while moving the athlete into the beginning of extension (Fig. 12–28D). The clinician should slowly try to reverse as much extension in standing as possible. If extension does not increase in standing, extension in lying may be commenced. I have learned that lateral shift correction is maintained much better if the athlete is corrected in standing. Shift correction in the prone position may allow restoration of lumbar lordosis and extension, but once in the standing position, the athlete often will go right back into the scoliosis or shifted position.

Self-corrections of a lateral shift can also be completed by repeated sideglides in standing, as previously described (see Fig. 12–7). When the athlete is unable to maintain reduction of derangement 4, sideglide exercises must begin during the day at regular intervals. The athlete is advised to perform a series of extension exercises after each session of self-correction (e.g., a right lateral shift equals sidegliding left, 10 repetitions every 2 hours, plus prone press-ups, 10 repetitions every 2 hours).

If full centralization is not yet achieved after a few days, the application of unilateral techniques may be indicated as outlined for derangement 3. Once the lateral shift has been corrected and full centralization has been achieved, derangement 4 can be treated according to the derangement 1 program.

DERANGEMENT 5

Symptoms consist of unilateral or asymmetric pain across the low back, with or without buttock or thigh pain, with leg pain extending below the knee, and no spinal deformity present. Derangement 5 is a progression of derangement 3 with the disc disturbance now causing impingement of the nerve root and dural sleeve. The sciatica described by the athlete will be intermittent most of the time in derangement 5.

The clinician will use the outcomes of the repeated movements examination to decide the treatment plan for derangement 5. Intermittent sciatica can be the result of current disc bulging or an athlete's recently recovering from a disc bulge whose intermittent signs and symptoms are now the result of increased nerve tension because of scarring or adherence. Flexion in standing will enhance the sciatica in both the derangement and the nerve root adherence. The revealing test movement is flexion in lying. Flexion in lying will increase and worsen pain resulting from the derangement but will not produce sciatic symptoms in the athlete with an adhered nerve root, because the nerve root is not placed on tension with flexion in lying.

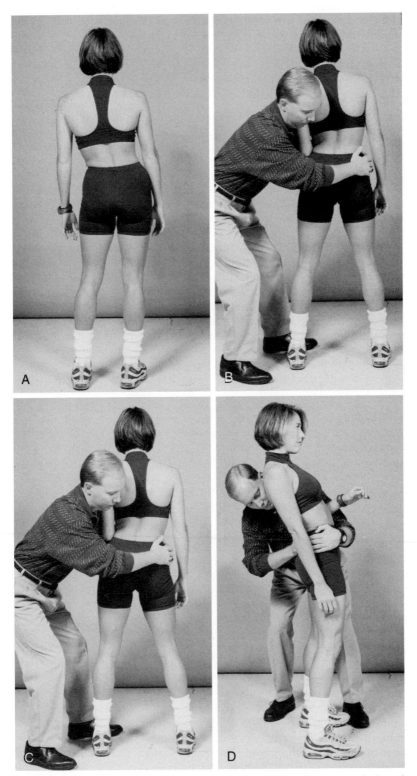

Figure 12–28. *A,* Lateral shift left. *B,* Clinician's position for correcting the lateral shift. *C,* Slight overcorrection of lateral shift, if possible. *D,* Restoration of lumbar lordosis with extension in standing.

Treatment for derangement 5 will progress as for derangement 3. Asymmetric procedures as described for derangement 3 may be necessary for the treatment of derangement 5.

DERANGEMENT 6

Symptoms consist of unilateral or asymmetric pain across the low back, with or without buttock or thigh pain, with leg pain extending below the knee and with a deformity of sciatic scoliosis or lateral shift. Sciatica is more likely to be constant in the athlete with derangement 6. Neurologic deficits such as changes in deep tendon reflexes, weakness of myotomes when compared bilaterally, and positive dural stretch signs are present. If no test movement or position is found to reduce the pain referred below the knee, there is no technique that will have a beneficial effect on the derangement. If test movements do indicate that reduction of the derangement is possible, treatment should follow the outlines for derangements 4 and 5. Any positions or movements that increase symptoms should not be a part of the treatment plan. Increased tingling or numbness in the foot must never be ignored, and if this is present, treatment should be modified immediately. The recovery of flexion in derangement 6 is a slower process than in the other derangements because of the severe sciatica. Eight to 10 weeks from the time of onset of symptoms is the recommended minimal wait before implementing flexion dysfunction procedures to maximum range of motion.[47]

DERANGEMENT 7

Symptoms consist of symmetric or asymmetric pain across the low back, with or without buttock or thigh pain, with a deformity of accentuated lumbar lordosis. In derangement 7, the disturbance within the disc appears to be located in a more anterior or anterolateral position, resulting in the increase in lumbar lordosis. The repeated movements examination will reveal a loss of flexion range of motion, with poor or no curve reversal from lordosis to kyphosis during flexion of the lumbar spine. Repeated movements in extension, both extension in lying and extension in standing, will make the condition worse.

Treatment of derangement 7 includes starting the athlete with 10 repetitions of flexion in lying every 2 hours and, after a few days, instituting flexion in standing, 10 repetitions every 2 hours, to gain full flexion and to reduce the derangement. Derangement 7 treatment rarely results in extension dysfunction, and therefore extension procedures are not indicated.

Adherent nerve root symptoms include intermittent sciatica in positions that place the nerve root on traction, such as driving or walking uphill. The history will also reveal an episode of acute LBP that has subsided and that may not have been present for years. Nerve root adherence is a result of healing and scarring from the derangement.

As described previously in derangement 6, test movements of flexion in standing will produce the athlete's familiar signs and symptoms. Flexion in lying and extension movements will have no effect.

Treatment of the adherent nerve root is done successfully by following the treatment of flexion dysfunction. Shortened structures should be stretched frequently and firmly every day until the adherence is resolved. Flexion movements should always be followed by extension in lying or extension in standing, due to the anatomic weakness of the posterior annular wall and the possibility of introducing a posterior derangement with repeated flexion movements.

Table 12–5. Absolute Contraindications for Mechanical Diagnosis and Therapy

Malignancy, primary or secondary
Infection (any type)
Active inflammatory disease
Central nervous system involvement (cord compression signs, cauda equina lesions)
Severe bone weakening disease
Fracture, dislocation, and ligament rupture
Instability
Vascular abnormality
Advanced diabetes
Increasing and peripheralizing signs or symptoms

Progression of Forces in Mechanical Diagnosis and Therapy

A progression of forces is recommended in the use of mechanical diagnosis and therapy in the treatment of LBP. In stage 1, the clinician must establish the diagnosis of derangement or dysfunction. Stage 2 includes the exploration and treatment of movements generated by the athlete. Stage 3 incorporates overpressure by the clinician in combination with movement of the athlete. Stage 4 uses mobilization and overpressure with movements to end range. This progression of forces must be strictly followed and will alert the clinician to any contraindications to movement prior to the addition of overpressure or mobilization by the clinician. Tables 12–5 and 12–6 outline the absolute and relative contraindications for mechanical diagnosis and therapy. When relative contraindications are present, these conditions may cause the clinician to delay the mechanical diagnosis process or may preclude the ability to establish a mechanical diagnosis (in which case the contraindication becomes absolute). If the mechanical diagnosis of derangement or dysfunction can be established, these conditions may cause the clinician to modify the use of clinical techniques or exclude mobilization or overpressure from the management of the athlete's problem.

Spondylolisthesis

Spondylolisthesis is a forward displacement of the fifth lumbar vertebra and spinal column upon the sacrum or, less commonly, of the fourth lumbar vertebra and spinal column upon the fifth lumbar vertebra. In approximately 85% of the cases, the fifth lumbar vertebra is displaced on the sacrum.[62] A bilateral defect in the pars interarticularis with vertebral slippage is believed in most cases to

Table 12–6. Relative Contraindications for Mechanical Diagnosis and Therapy

Mild to moderate osteoporosis (noncomplicated)
Structural or congenital anomalies
Nonactive inflammatory disease
Pregnancy (especially during the last two trimesters)
Advanced, multilevel degenerative osteoarthrosis
Psychosis, neurosis, other mental or behavioral disorder
Previous abdominal or thoracic surgery
Use of anticoagulant medication
Post-trauma status (adequate time required for healing and appropriate diagnostic work-up)
Postsurgery status (adequate time required for healing; coordinate with surgeon)
Pain medications
Severe pain, twinges, or transfixation
Spondylolisthesis

be an acquired disorder resulting from stress fractures. Although often asymptomatic, spondylolisthesis may cause LBP with or without sciatic radiation.

Inspection of the spine may reveal hyperlordosis. In more severe cases, a palpable step between the L4 and L5 spinous processes occurs when the L5 vertebra slips forward on the sacrum. Because the defect is in the pars, the posterior arch, which includes the spinous process of L5, remains in place while the anterior elements slide forward. As a result of L5's slipping forward on the sacrum, the L4 spinous process is felt to be more anterior than L5.[12] A depression above the sacrum can be seen on physical examination. Radiographs (oblique views) are necessary to confirm the diagnosis. Generally, spondylolisthesis is categorized into four grades. Grade I is characterized by 25% of the body of the lumbar vertebra slipping anteriorly, grade II by 50% of the body slipping anteriorly, grade III by 75% of the body slipping anteriorly, and grade IV by 100% of the body slipping anteriorly.[34]

A simple clinical test may determine whether the athlete's LBP is originating from the affected segment. With the athlete standing, the clinician places one hand across the sacrum and the other firmly against the abdomen.[47] Further compressing the abdomen while at the same time increasing pressure on the sacrum markedly reduces or abolishes pain in standing resulting from spondylolisthesis. On the other hand, pain resulting from derangement of any of the lumbar discs will usually be enhanced by this procedure, and postural or dysfunctional pain remains unaffected.[47]

Athletes with symptomatic spondylolisthesis will describe increased back pain with activities such as running, jumping, bending, or twisting. Other specific activities that may exacerbate symptoms of spondylolisthesis include hyperextension positions such as those required in gymnastics and contact sports or axial loading of the spine, such as squatting and the military press in weight lifting.

Rehabilitation of the athlete diagnosed with spondylolisthesis should initially include anterior lordotic abdominal strengthening exercises, pelvic stabilization or proprioception exercises, and aggressive flexibility exercises of the hip rotators, hamstrings, hip flexors and lumbosacral fascia, ligaments, and muscle-tendon units.

Contraction of the abdominal muscles acts as a "corset" for the lumbar spine, when combined with proper lumbopelvic positioning. The oblique muscles and rectus abdominis are most active during the initial head and shoulder phases of an abdominal sit-up.[79] From 45° to vertical sitting, the iliacus is the major muscle involved in the sit-up exercise (Fig. 12–29).[23] Therefore, a full sit-up is not required for optimal contraction of the rectus abdominis and internal and external obliques. Progression of the half sit-up includes half sit-ups with rotation, half sit-ups with a weight plate on the chest, and half sit-ups with various angles of incline.

Pelvic stabilization and proprioception exercises include movements that edu-

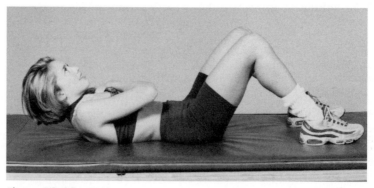

Figure 12–29. Half sit-up.

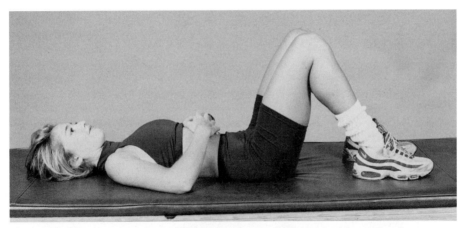

Figure 12–30. Hook lying position. Athlete is supine, with hips and knees flexed.

cate the athlete regarding the neutral spine position. This is not necessarily the spine position of 0° lordosis but is the position in which the athlete is asymptomatic and the spine most stable. The beginning position for neutral spine positioning is supine or hooklying, which is supine with the hips and knees flexed (Fig. 12–30). Suggestions for exercises in this position include pelvic tilts and "dead bug" exercises, which are performed by alternating shoulder flexion and hip flexion on opposite extremities while maintaining a neutral spine position (Fig. 12–31). The degree of difficulty for the dead bug exercise can be increased by the addition of cuff weights to the extremities. Once the athlete has mastered a neutral position in hooklying, further positions for lumbopelvic stabilization include the quadruped (Fig. 12–32), bird dog (Fig. 12–33), kneeling, half-kneeling, sitting, sitting to standing, standing, and even jumping positions. The clinician should inform the athlete that the goal of stabilization exercises is motor programming, much like various positions and postures required for an athletic skill, in which careful repetition with precise movements is required. Each exercise is designed to develop isolated and cocontraction muscle patterns that can easily be applied to the athlete's sports and training regimen.

Many young athletes develop LBP because the skeletal system is maturing and growing at a much more rapid rate than are muscles and ligaments. This imbalance predisposes athletes to a loss of flexibility in these soft-tissue structures. Therefore, a rehabilitation program must include static stretching of the muscle groups noted earlier, which includes hamstrings, hip flexors (iliopsoas and rectus femoris), hip rotators (internal and external), and lumbodorsal fascia.

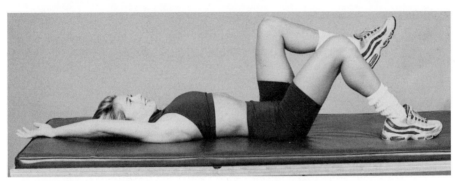

Figure 12–31. Dead bug exercise, performed by alternating shoulder flexion and hip flexion on opposite extremities while maintaining a neutral spine position.

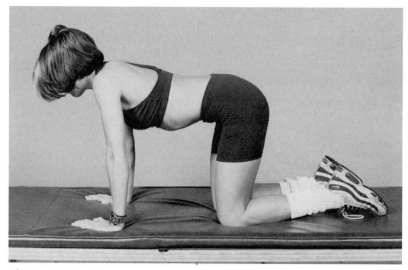

Figure 12–32. Quadruped exercise. Athlete performs a pelvic tilt in this position.

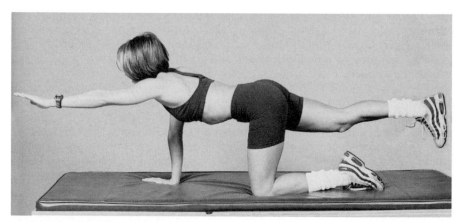

Figure 12–33. Bird dog exercise. Athlete alternates shoulder flexion and hip extension while maintaining a neutral spine position. This exercise can be progressed by adding weight to the extremities.

LOW BACK STRENGTHENING AND STABILIZATION EXERCISES

Figures 12–34 to 12–41 represent strengthening and stabilization exercises that can be added and incorporated into a rehabilitation program for the lumbar spine.

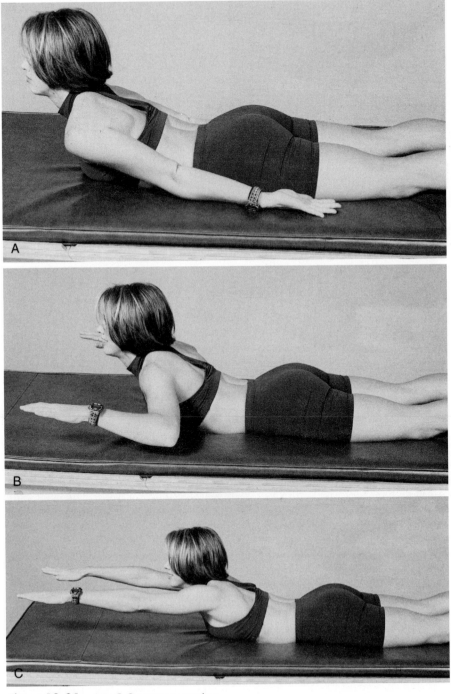

Figure 12-34. *A* to *C,* Superman exercises.

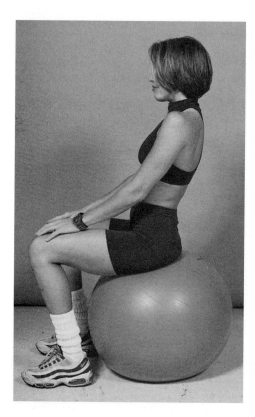

Figure 12–35. Anterior pelvic tilt on Swiss ball.

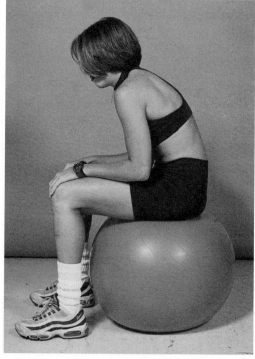

Figure 12–36. Posterior pelvic tilt on Swiss ball.

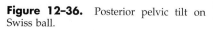

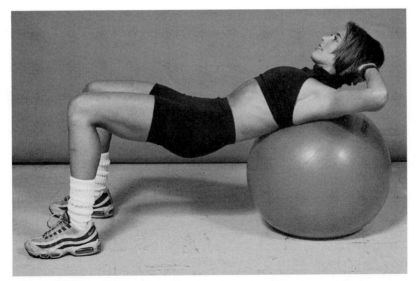

Figure 12–37. Bridging on Swiss ball.

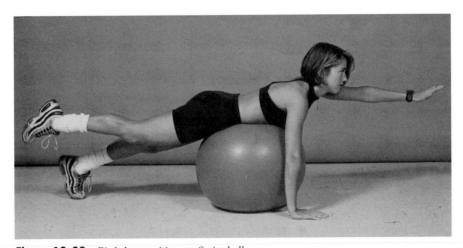

Figure 12–38. Bird dog position on Swiss ball.

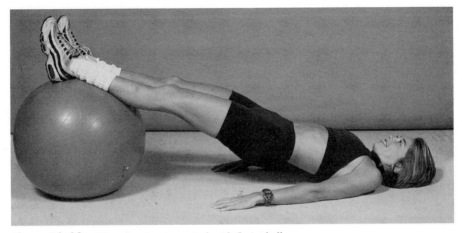

Figure 12–39. Hip extension in neutral with Swiss ball.

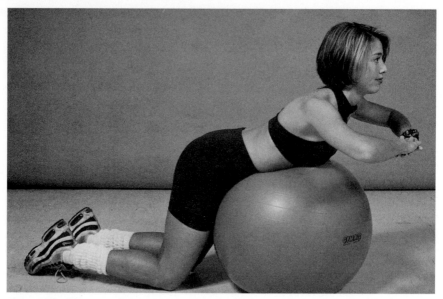

Figure 12–40. Active tall kneeling on Swiss ball.

SUMMARY

This chapter provides the clinician with an evaluation and treatment method based on a mechanical evaluation of the spine. Mechanical evaluation of the spine should be undertaken only after serious spinal pathologies have been ruled out. Mechanical evaluation is based on the centralization or peripheralization of symptoms in response to trunk movements. Those movements that peripheralize symptoms should be avoided, whereas movements that centralize the pain should be pursued and possibly incorporated into the treatment plan by the clinician. LBP can be classified into three syndromes: postural, dysfunction, and derangement. Athletes complaining of LBP can be placed into one of these syndrome categories based on the cause of their LBP. An athlete suffering from LBP as a result of poor posture would be placed in the postural syndrome category. LBP in the dysfunction syndrome category is caused by adaptive shortening of soft-tissue structures as a result of poor postural habits or trauma. Finally, those athletes with a disc prolapse, either caused by the nuclear material's escaping from the disc or caused by the nuclear material's causing

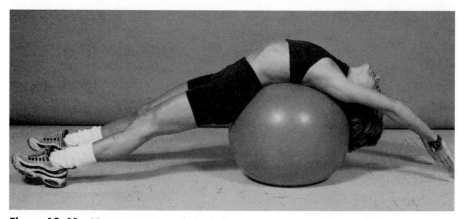

Figure 12–41. Hyperextension on Swiss ball.

the annulus wall to bulge, fall into the derangement category. Again, treatment of these three syndromes is based on what movements centralize or peripheralize the symptoms.

Movements that result in the combination of compression, flexion, and rotation should be avoided because it has been shown that these collective movements result in a greater incidence of disc prolapse. Rehabilitation of the athlete with LBP is based on the data gathered from the mechanical evaluation. Treatment interventions can consist of postural education, mobilizations, flexibility exercises, and strengthening and dynamic stabilization exercises for the trunk. Any exercise that peripheralizes the symptoms should be excluded from the rehabilitation program.

References

1. Adams, M.A., Dolan, P., and Hutton, W.C. (1987): Diurnal variations in the stresses on the lumbar spine. Spine, 12:130–137.
2. Ayad, S. and Weiss, J.B. (1987): Biochemistry of the intervertebral disc. In: Jayson, M.I.V. (ed.): The Lumbar Spine and Back Pain. New York, Churchill Livingstone, pp. 100–137.
3. Battie, M.C., Cherkin, D.C., Dunn, R., et al. (1994): Managing low back pain: Attitudes and treatment preferences of physical therapists. Phys. Ther., 74:219–226.
4. Berquist-Ullman, M., and Larsson, U. (1977): Acute low back pain in industry. Acta Orthop. Scand. Suppl., 170:105–109.
5. Brinckmann, P. (1986): Injury of the annulus fibrosus and disc protrusions: An in vitro investigation on human lumbar discs. Spine, 11:149–153.
6. Buckwalter, J.A. (1995): Aging and degeneration of the human intervertebral disc. Spine, 20:1307–1314.
7. Cailliet, R. (1982): Low Back Pain Syndrome, 2nd ed. Philadelphia, F.A. Davis.
8. Cannon, S.R., and James, S.E. (1984): Back pain in athletes. Br. J. Sports Med., 18:159–164.
9. Chard, M.D., and Lachmann, M.A. (1987): Racquet sports—patterns of injury presenting to a sports injury clinic. Br. Sports, 21:150–155.
10. Cibulka, M.T., Delitto, A., and Koldehoff, R.M. (1988): Changes in innominate tilt after manipulation of the sacro-iliac joint in patients with low back pain. Phys. Ther., 68:1359–1363.
11. Couper, J., Davies, J.B., Fairbank, J.C.T., et al. (1982): The Oswestry low back pain questionnaire. Physiotherapy, 66:220–221.
12. DeRosa, C., and Porterfield, J.A. (1994): Lumbar spine and pelvis. In: Richardson, J.K., and Iglarsh, Z.A. (eds.): Clinical Orthopaedic Physical Therapy. Philadelphia, W.B. Saunders, pp. 119–158.
13. DeRosa, C.P., and Porterfield, J.A. (1992): A physical therapy model for the treatment of low back pain. Phys. Ther., 72:261–272.
14. Dettori, J.R., Bullock, S.H., and Franklin, R.J. (1995): The effects of spinal flexion and extension exercises and their associated postures in patients with acute low back pain. Spine, 20:2303–2312.
15. Deusinger, R.H. (1989): Biomechanical considerations for clinical application in athletes with low back pain. Clin. Sports Med., 8:703–715.
16. Dimaggio, A., and Mooney, V. (1987): The McKenzie program: Exercise effective against back pain. J. Musculoskel. Med., 4:63–74.
17. Dixon, A.J. (1976): Diagnosis of low back pain. In: Jayson, M. (ed.): The Lumbar Spine and Back Pain. New York, Grune & Stratton.
18. Donelson, R., Grant, W., Camps, C., et al. (1991): Pain response to sagittal end-range spinal motion: A prospective, randomized, multicentered trial. Spine, 16:S206–S212.
19. Donelson, R., Silva, G., and Murphy, K. (1990): Centralization phenomenon: Its usefulness in evaluating and treating referred pain. Spine, 15:211–213.
20. Eckland, J.A.E., and Corlett, E.N. (1984): Shrinkage as a measure of the effect of load on the spine. Spine, 9:189–194.
21. Farfan, H.F. (1978): The biomechanical advantage of lordosis and hip extension for upright activity. Spine, 3:336–339.
22. Ferguson, R.J., McHaster, J.H., and Stanitski, C.L. (1974): Low back pain in college football lineman. J. Sports Med., 2:63–69.
23. Flint, M.M. (1965): Abdominal muscle involvement during the performance of various forms of sit-up exercise. Am. J. Phys. Med. Rehabil., 44:224–234.
24. Garrick, J.G., and Requa, R.K. (1980): Epidemiology of women's gymnastics injuries. Am. J. Sports Med., 8:261–264.
25. Goldstein, J.D., Berger, P.E., Windler, G.E., et al. (1991): Spine injuries in gymnasts and swimmers: An epidemiologic investigation. Am. J. Sports Med., 19:463–468.
26. Gould, J.A. (1990): The spine. In: Gould, J.A. (ed.): Orthopaedic and Sports Physical Therapy. St. Louis, C.V. Mosby, pp. 523–552.

27. Gower, W.E., and Pedrini, V. (1969): Age-related variations in protein-polysaccharides from human nucleus pulposus, annulus fibrosus, and costal cartilage. J. Bone Joint Surg. [Am.], 51:1154–1160.
28. Haher, T.R., O'Brien, M., Kauffman, C., et al. (1993): Biomechanics of the spine in sports. Clin. Sports Med., 12:449–464.
29. Hellstrom, M., Jaobsson, B., Sward, L., et al. (1990): Radiological abnormalities of the thoraco-lumbar spine in athletes. Acta Radiol., 31:127–132.
30. Hickey, D.S., and Hukins, D.W.L. (1990): Relation between the structure of the annulus fibrosus and the function and failure of the intervertebral disc. Spine, 5:106–112.
31. Jackson, D.W. (1979): Low back pain in young athletes: Evaluation of reaction and discogenic problems. Am. J. Sports Med., 7:364–366.
32. Jackson, D.W., Wiltse, L.L., and Cirincione, R.J. (1976): Spondylolysis in the female gymnast. Clin. Orthop., 117:68–73.
33. Jackson, D.W., Wiltse, L.L., and Dingeman, R.D. (1981): Stress reactions involving the pars interarticularis in young athletes. Am. J. Sports Med., 9:304–312.
34. Kahler, D.M. (1993): Low back pain in athletes. J. Sports Rehabil., 2:63–78.
35. Kapandji, I.A. (1974): The Physiology of the Joints, 2nd ed. Vol. III. London, Churchill Livingstone.
36. Kopp, J.R., Alexander, A.H., Turocy, R.H., et al. (1986): The use of lumbar extension in the evaluation and treatment of patients with acute herniated nucleus pulposus: A preliminary report. Clin. Orthop., 202:211–218.
37. Koreska, J., Robertson, D., Mill, R.H., et al. (1977): Biomechanics of the lumbar spine and its clinical significance. Orthop. Clin. North Am., 8:121–133.
38. Laslett, M., and Williams, M. (1994): The reliability of selected pain provocation tests for sacroiliac joint pathology. Spine, 19:1243–1249.
39. Levine, D., and Whittle, M.W. (1996): The effects of pelvic movement on lumbar lordosis in the standing position. J. Orthop. Sports Phys. Ther., 24:130–135.
40. Libson, E., Bloom, R.A., and Dinari, G. (1982): Symptomatic and asymptomatic spondylolysis and spondylolisthesis in young adults. Int. Orthop., 6:259–261.
41. Long, A.L. (1995): The centralization phenomenon: Its usefulness as a predictor of outcome in conservative treatment of chronic low back pain. Spine, 20:2513–2521.
42. Lu, Y.M., Hutton, W.C., and Gharpuray, V.M. (1996): Do bending, twisting, and diurnal fluid changes in the disc affect the propensity of prolapse? A viscoelastic finite element model. Spine, 21:2570–2579.
43. Magee, D.J. (1997): Orthopedic Physical Assessment, 3rd ed. Philadelphia, W.B. Saunders.
44. Magnusson, M.L., Spratt, K.F., and Pope, M.H. (1996): Hyperextension and spine height changes. Spine, 21:2670–2675.
45. McCombe, P.F., Fairbanks, J.C.T., and Cockersole, B.C. (1989): Reproducibility of physical signs in low back pain. Spine, 14:909–918.
46. McKenzie, R.A. (1979): Prophylaxis in recurrent low back pain. New Zealand Med. J., 89:22–23.
47. McKenzie, R.A. (1981): The Lumbar Spine: Mechanical Diagnosis and Therapy. Waikanae, New Zealand, Spinal Publications Limited.
48. McNally, D.S., Adams, M.A., and Goodship, A.E. (1993): Can intervertebral disc prolapse be predicted by disc mechanics? Spine, 18:1525–1530.
49. Nachemson, A. (1960): Lumbar intradiscal pressure. Acta Orthop. Scand. Suppl., 43:122–147.
50. Nachemson, A. (1963): The influence of spinal movements on the lumbar intradiscal pressure and on the tensile stresses in the annulus fibrosus. Acta Orthop. Scand., 33:183–207.
51. Nachemson, A. (1966): The load on lumbar disks in different positions of the body. Clin. Orthop., 45:107–122.
52. Nachemson, A. (1976): The lumbar spine, an orthopaedic challenge. Spine, 1:59–71.
53. Nachemson, A.L. (1981): Disc pressure measurements. Spine, 6:93–97.
54. Nachemson, A.L., and Elfstrom, G. (1970): Intravital dynamic pressure measurements in lumbar discs. A study of common movements, maneuvers and exercises. Scand. J. Rehabil. Med., 2(Suppl. 1):1–40.
55. Nachemson, A., and Morris, J.M. (1964): In vivo measurements of intradiscal pressure. Discometry, a method for the determination of pressure in the lower lumbar discs. J. Bone Joint Surg. [Am.], 46:1077–1092.
56. Norkin, C., and Levangie, P. (1983): Joint Structure & Functional: A Comprehensive Analysis. Philadelphia, F.A. Davis.
57. Nugent, C.C. (1996): Test development and validation of a back education posttest. J. Orthop. Sports Phys. Ther., 24:78–85.
58. Nwaga, G. and Nwage, V. (1985): Relative therapeutic efficacy of the Williams and McKenzie protocols in back pain management. Physiother. Practice, 1:99–105.
59. Oegema, T.R. (1993): Biochemistry of the intervertebral disc. Clin. Sports Med., 12:419–439.
60. Ponte, D.J., Jensen, G.J., and Kent, B.E. (1984): A preliminary report on the use of the McKenzie protocol versus Williams protocol in the treatment of low back pain. J. Orthop. Sports Phys. Ther., 6:130–139.
61. Potter, N.A., and Rothstein, J.M. (1985): Intertester reliability for selected clinical tests of the sacro-iliac joint. Phys. Ther., 65:1671–1675.

62. Raney, R.B., Brashear, H.R., and Shands, A.R. (1971): Shands' Handbook of Orthopaedic Surgery, 7th ed. St. Louis, C.V. Mosby.
63. Risch, S.V., Risch, E.D., and Graves, J.E. (1983): Lumbar strengthening in chronic low back pain patients. Spine, 18:232–238.
64. Saunders, H.D. (1985): Evaluation, Treatment and Prevention of Musculoskeletal Disorders. Eden Prairie, MN, Educational Opportunities.
65. Schober, P. (1937): Lendenwirbelsaule und Kreuzschmerzen. Munchn. Med. Wochenschr., 84:336–338.
66. Schultz, A.B., and Andersson, G.B. (1981): Analysis of loads on the lumbar spine. Spine, 6:76–80.
67. Semon, R.L., and Spengler, D. (1981): Significance of lumbar spondylolysis in college football players. Spine, 6:172–174.
68. Soderberg, G.L. (1986): Kinesiology: Application to Pathological Motion. Baltimore, MD, Williams & Wilkins.
69. Spitzer, W.O., LeBlanc, F.E., and Dupuis, M. (1987): Scientific approach to the assessment and management of activity-related spinal disorders. Spine, 12:S1–S58.
70. Stankovic, R. (1995): Conservative treatment of acute low back pain: A 5-year follow-up study of two methods of treatment. Spine, 20:469–472.
71. Stankovic, R., and Johnell, O. (1990): Conservative treatment of acute low-back pain. A prospective randomized trial: McKenzie method of treatment versus patient education in "mini back school." Spine, 15:120–123.
72. Sullivan, M.S., Kues, J.M., and Mayhew, T.P. (1996): Treatment categories for low back pain: A methodological approach. J. Orthop. Sports Phys. Ther., 24:359–364.
73. Sward, L., Hellstrom, M., Jacobsson, B., et al. (1990): Back pain and radiologic changes in the thoraco-lumbar spine in athletes. Spine, 15:124–129.
74. Sward, L., Hellstrom, M., Jacobson, B., et al. (1991): Disc degeneration and associated abnormalities of the spine in elite gymnasts: A magnetic resonance imaging study. Spine, 16:437–443.
75. Szot, Z., Boron, Z., and Galaj, Z. (1985): Overloading changes in the motor system occurring in elite gymnasts. Int. J. Sports Med., 6:36–40.
76. Tall, R.L., and DeVault, W. (1993): Spinal injury in sport: Epidemiologic considerations. Clin. Sports Med., 12:441–449.
77. Valkenburg, H.A., and Haanen, H.C.M. (1982): The epidemiology of low back pain. *In:* White, A.A., and Gordon, S.L. (eds.): American Academy of Orthopaedic Surgeons Symposium on Idiopathic Low Back Pain. St. Louis, C.V. Mosby, pp. 9–22.
78. Virgin, W.J. (1951): Experimental investigations into the physical properties of the intervertebral disk. J. Bone Joint Surg., 33B:607–611.
79. Walters, C.E., and Partridge, M.J. (1957): EMG study of the differential action of the abdominal muscles during exercise. Am. J. Phys. Med. Rehabil., 36:259–268.
80. White, A.A., and Panjabi, M.M. (1978): Clinical Biomechanics of the Spine. Philadelphia, J.B. Lippincott.
81. Williams, P. (1955): Examination and conservative treatment for disc lesions of the lower spine. Clin. Orthop., 5:28–40.
82. Williams, P. (1974): Low Back and Neck Pain: Causes and Conservative Treatment, 3rd ed. Springfield, IL, Charles C Thomas.

Shoulder Rehabilitation

Kevin E. Wilk, P.T.,
Gary L. Harrelson, Ed.D., A.T.,C.,
Christopher Arrigo, M.S., P.T., A.T.,C., and
Terri Chmielewski, M.A., P.T.

Most athletic shoulder injuries are the result of repetitive overhead activity (microtrauma) or a significant force (macrotrauma) to the shoulder region. The violent action of throwing and other overhead movements results in repeated application of high stresses to the shoulder and elbow. Most of these injuries can be classified as microtraumatic or as resulting from an overuse mechanism. Tullos and King[98] have reported that at least 50% of all baseball players experience sufficient shoulder or elbow joint symptoms to keep them from throwing for varying periods of time during their careers. The synchronous kinematics of throwing can be influenced by a number of factors including glenohumeral and scapulothoracic motions, connective tissue flexibility, osseous structure, and dynamic muscle balance and symmetry. The glenohumeral joint complex is also susceptible to traumatic injuries such as dislocations, subluxations, acromioclavicular joint sprains, soft-tissue injuries, and other types of injuries that commonly occur in contact sports. In fact, the glenohumeral joint is the joint most commonly dislocated. The shoulder region is further predisposed to athletic injury because the tremendous mobility afforded by the joint comes at the cost of inherently poor glenohumeral stability.

JOINT ARTHROLOGY

The shoulder region is composed of three synovial joints—the sternoclavicular, acromioclavicular, and glenohumeral joints—and one physiologic articulation, the scapulothoracic joint. These articulations, along with the ligaments (Fig. 13–1), musculotendinous rotator cuff, and primary mover musculature of the upper quarter, must work in unison to produce the various ranges of motion possible in the shoulder joint. Dysfunction of one of these joints or structures can result in limited function or injury to the shoulder complex.

Sternoclavicular Joint

The sternoclavicular joint is a modified saddle joint with a joint capsule, three major ligaments, and a joint disc. The joint is stabilized anteriorly and posteriorly by the sternoclavicular ligament, which serves to check anterior and posterior movements of the clavicular head. The costoclavicular ligament is the principal stabilizer of the sternoclavicular joint and serves to stabilize the clavicle against the pull of the sternocleidomastoid muscle and to check motion about the axis

478

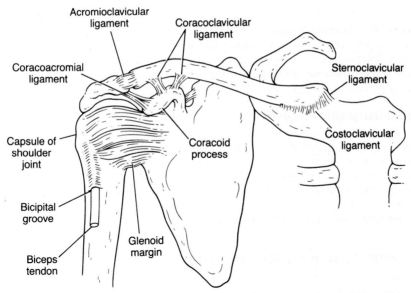

Figure 13-1. Ligamentous structures of the shoulder girdle. (From O'Donoghue, D.H. [1984]: Treatment of Injuries to Athletes, 4th ed. Philadelphia, W.B. Saunders, p. 119.)

producing elevation-depression and protraction-retraction.[77] The costoclavicular ligament also functions to check elevation of the clavicle.[21] The proximal end of the clavicle is separated from the manubrium by an intra-articular disc or meniscus, which helps absorb forces transmitted along the clavicle from its lateral end and aids in checking the tendency of the clavicle to dislocate medially on the manubrium.[69] This tendency toward dislocation is a result of the incongruence of the articular surfaces. Functionally, the sternoclavicular joint is the only bony articulation connecting the shoulder complex to the thorax.

Acromioclavicular Joint

The acromioclavicular joint is classified as a plane joint and consists of two major ligament complexes and a joint meniscus. Joint integrity is maintained by the surrounding ligaments rather than by the bony configuration of the joint. The two primary functions of the acromioclavicular joint are (1) maintaining the relationship between the clavicle and the scapula in the early stages of upper limb elevation and (2) allowing the scapula additional range of rotation on the thorax in the later stages of limb elevation.[77]

The integrity of the articulation between the acromion and the distal clavicle is maintained by the joint capsule, which is reinforced by the anterior, inferior, posterior, and superior acromioclavicular ligaments. The fibers of the deltoid and upper trapezius muscles, which attach to the superior aspect of the clavicle and acromion process, serve to strengthen the acromioclavicular ligaments and stabilize the acromioclavicular joint. However, the coracoclavicular ligaments are the primary acromioclavicular joint stabilizers. The ligaments consist of a lateral portion, the trapezoid ligament, and a medial portion, the conoid ligament. A fall onto an outstretched arm tends to translate the scapula medially, and the small acromioclavicular joint alone cannot prevent scapular motion without resulting in joint dislocation. As the scapula and its coracoid process attempt to move medially, the trapezoid ligament tightens, transferring the force of impact to the clavicle and, ultimately, to the strong sternoclavicular joint.[77] Thus, anterior-posterior stability of the acromioclavicular joint is maintained by the acromioclavicular joint capsule, and vertical stability is maintained by the coracoclavicular ligaments. The coracoclavicular ligaments are also responsible for producing the longitudinal rotation of the clavicle necessary for full unrestricted range of motion in elevation of the upper extremity.

Glenohumeral Joint

The glenohumeral joint is the most mobile and the least stable of all the joints in the human body. It is composed of the large humeral head and the shallow glenoid fossa. The glenohumeral joint capsule has a volume twice as great as that of the humeral head,[16] which allows for slightly more than 1 inch of humeral head distraction away from the glenoid fossa.[21, 31] The joint capsule is relatively thin and rather lax, contributing to the joint's mobility and lack of stability. The joint capsule is reinforced anteriorly and posteroinferiorly by distinct ligamentous structures. Because of the joint's intrinsic weakness, it is susceptible to both degenerative changes and derangement. In fact, it is the most frequently dislocated joint in the body.

Some joint stability is provided by a fibrous rim, called the glenoid labrum, which surrounds the glenoid fossa. The glenoid labrum serves several functions vital to the glenohumeral joint. First, it deepens the glenoid fossa by approximately 50%.[45] Second, the labrum serves as an attachment between the joint capsule and the glenoid rim. Third, the labrum serves as an articular surface to the humeral head during shoulder movement. The long head of the biceps brachii tendon and the superior labrum blend together at the attachment to the supraglenoid tubercle. Fourth, the inferior glenohumeral ligament blends into the inferior labrum. Cooper and colleagues recently examined the vascular supply of the labrum and noted that the superior and anterosuperior parts of the labrum were less vascular than the posterosuperior and inferior portions. The blood supply was limited to the peripheral part of the labrum, and vascularity tended to decrease with age.[82]

The anterior glenohumeral ligaments consist of three sections: superior, middle, and inferior. These ligaments form a Z on the anterior capsule. Each portion becomes taut and provides a check to certain motions of the humerus, with all portions becoming taut on external rotation.[77] The inferior glenohumeral ligament is particularly important in deterring humeral head subluxation in abduction (90°) and external rotation.[99] The anterior superior glenohumeral ligament is taut in 0° of abduction. In this position, it is the primary restraint to anterior translation of the humeral head on the glenoid. In 45° of abduction, the middle portion of the anterior glenohumeral ligament becomes taut, resisting anterior translation. O'Brien and associates[79] have demonstrated extremely wide variations in this ligamentous structure. These variations range from a robust form of the ligamentous capsule to absence of distinct ligamentous bands; therefore, the greatest variation in stability is also demonstrated at this midrange portion of arm elevation.

The inferior glenohumeral ligament complex consists of three portions: the anterior and the posterior bands, connected by the inferior pouch. This complex is primarily responsible for glenohumeral joint stability with the arm in 90° or more of shoulder abduction. Furthermore, as the arm is externally rotated in this position, the anterior band wraps around the humeral head, tightening the inferior pouch that provides resistance to anterior humeral head translation. The opposite occurs with internal rotation in 90° or more of shoulder abduction, in which the posterior band of the inferior glenohumeral ligament provides the hammock effect to posterior displacement.

The muscles surrounding the glenohumeral joint can be classified as stabilizers and prime movers. The stabilizing muscles play a significant role in dynamic glenohumeral joint stability during everyday activities, particularly during sports movements. The dynamic stabilizers of the glenohumeral joint include the supraspinatus, infraspinatus, teres minor, subscapularis, long head of the biceps brachii, and portions of the deltoid (deltoid function is dependent on arm position). Rotator cuff strength is the key to dynamic glenohumeral stability. The rotator cuff muscles are characterized by muscle fibers in proximity to the joint and tendons that blend with the joint capsule. These muscles have two functions: rotation and joint stabilization. The primary function of the stabilizing muscles is to compress the humeral head within the glenoid cavity and to counteract the significant shear forces generated by the prime movers. The muscles around the glenohumeral joint function in a force couple relationship. The primary force couple at the glenohumeral joint is between the deltoid and the rotator cuff musculature.

The glenohumeral joint is capable of four combined movements: flexion-extension, abduction-adduction, horizontal abduction-adduction, and internal-external rotation. With the arm at the side, internal and external rotation may be limited to as little as 50°. When the humerus is abducted to 90°, the arc of rotation increases to 90° to 100°.[95] Motion of the shoulder can be restricted as a result of bony restraints that are dependent on the position of the limb. For example, if the humerus is maintained in internal rotation, it cannot abduct beyond 90° because of impingement of the greater tubercle on the acromion. With the humerus in full external rotation, however, the greater tubercle passes behind the acromion process, and abduction can continue. With bony limitations eliminated by external rotation of the humerus, the capsular and muscular structures become the checkreins of motion. The extent of glenohumeral joint elevation depends primarily on the position of the humerus.

The subacromial and subdeltoid bursae are located around the glenohumeral joint. These bursae separate the supraspinatus tendon and humeral head below from the acromioclavicular joint and deltoid muscle above.[77] The bursae allow the tendons of the supraspinatus and long head of the biceps brachii to glide smoothly under the acromion process. In addition, the bursae provide nutrients to the rotator cuff muscles.

Scapulothoracic Joint

The scapulothoracic joint is not a true anatomic joint because it has none of the usual joint characteristics, such as a joint capsule. However, it is a free-floating physiologic joint without any ligamentous restraints, except where it pivots about the acromioclavicular joint.[29] According to Steindler,[95] the primary force holding the scapula to the thorax is atmospheric pressure. The ultimate function of scapular motion is to orient the glenoid fossa for optimal contact with the maneuvering arm and to provide a stable base of support for the controlled rolling and gliding of the humeral head's articular surface.[77] This relationship allows for optimal function of the upper extremity in space by continually adjusting the length-tension relationships of all vital musculature as the scapula constantly repositions itself on the thoracic wall. The muscles of the scapulothoracic joint play a significant role in maintaining optimal scapular position and posture. Five muscles directly control the scapula. These include the trapezius (upper, middle, lower), the rhomboids, the levator scapulae, the serratus anterior, and to a lesser extent, the pectoralis minor. These muscles act in a synchronous fashion, providing both mobility and stability to the scapulothoracic joint.

Coracoacromial Arch

The coracoacromial arch, or subacromial space, has also been considered a physiologic joint by some authors.[59] It provides protection against direct trauma to the subacromial structures and prevents the humeral head from dislocating superiorly. It is bordered by the acromion process and acromioclavicular joint superiorly, the coracoid process anteromedially, and the rotator cuff and greater tuberosity of the humeral head inferiorly.[29] The coracoacromial ligament, which serves as a "roof" over the greater tubercle of the humerus, rotator cuff tendons, portions of the biceps tendon, and subdeltoid bursa, further decreases the available space. The space between the humeral head on the inferior aspect of the acromion is dependent on arm position and varies from approximately 30 ± 4.9 mm (when arm is at 0° of abduction) and 6 ± 2.4 mm (when arm is at 90° of abduction).[34] Additionally, this space can be decreased in the presence of inflamed or swollen soft tissues. Soft-tissue structures, such as the supraspinatus and infraspinatus tendons, lying between the two unyielding joint borders, are at risk for impingement or compressive injuries in the presence of abnormal glenohumeral joint mechanics or trauma.

Rotator Cuff

The supraspinatus, infraspinatus, teres minor, and subscapularis muscles comprise the rotator cuff (Fig. 13–2). Collectively, each tendon blends with and reinforces the glenohumeral capsule, and all contribute significantly to the dynamic stability of the glenohumeral joint.[75] The rotator cuff muscles could be considered the fine tuners of the glenohumeral joint and shoulder girdle, whereas the latissimus dorsi, teres major, deltoid, and pectoralis muscles are the prime movers.[45] All the rotator cuff muscles contribute in some degree to

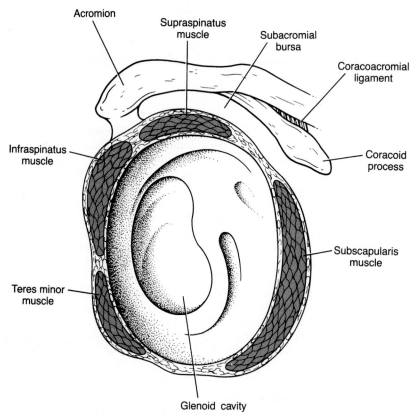

Figure 13–2. Anatomic view of the glenoid cavity with its surrounding structures. (From Hill, J.A. [1988]: Rotator cuff injuries. Sports Med. Update, 3:5.)

glenohumeral abduction, with the supraspinatus and deltoid muscles functioning as the primary abductors. The rotator cuff muscles also function to compress the glenohumeral joint and act to reduce or control vertical shear imparted onto the humeral head.[30, 88] The infraspinatus is considered the next most active rotator cuff muscle, after the supraspinatus.[47, 51, 53] Selective nerve blocks have shown that the supraspinatus and infraspinatus muscles are responsible for 90% of the shoulder's external rotation strength.[44] The teres minor also contributes to external rotation of the glenohumeral joint. The subscapularis is the primary internal rotator, with abduction activity peaking around 90°.[8]

SHOULDER ELEVATION

Most glenohumeral motion occurs around the plane of the scapula. This plane of motion is approximately 30° to 45° anterior to the frontal plane.[83] Codman[25] first reported that abduction of the humerus to 180° overhead requires that the clavicle, scapula, and humerus move through essentially their full range of motion in a specific pattern of interaction. When internally rotated, the humerus can abduct on the scapula to approximately 90° before the greater tubercle strikes up against the acromion. If the humerus is fully rotated externally, however, the greater tubercle and accompanying rotator cuff tendons clear the acromion, coracoacromial ligament, or superior edge of the glenoid fossa,[58, 63, 91] and a further 30° of abduction can be obtained (Fig. 13–3). Thus, the glenohumeral joint contributes 90° to 120° to shoulder abduction, depending on the position of humeral internal or external rotation.[21, 50, 63] The remaining 60° is supplied by scapular elevation. This combined motion between the scapula and the humerus is known as scapulohumeral rhythm. During the first 30° of glenohumeral abduction, the contribution of scapular elevation is negligible and is not coordinated with the movement of the humerus.[50, 63] This is referred to as the setting phase, during which the scapula is seeking a position of stability on the thoracic wall in relationship to the humerus.[50] The purpose of scapular rotation is two-fold[77]: (1) to achieve a ratio of motion for maintaining the glenoid fossa in an optimal position to receive the head of the humerus, thus increasing the range of motion; and (2) to ensure that the accompanying motion of the scapula permits muscles acting on the humerus to maintain a satisfactory length-tension relationship. After the initial 30° of humeral elevation, scapular motion becomes better coordinated. Toward the end range of glenohumeral elevation, however, the scapula contributes more motion and the humerus less.[49, 58] In gross terms, it is generally agreed that every 1° of scapular motion is accompanied by 2° of humeral elevation. Scapulohumeral rhythm is considered to be a ratio of 1:2.[50] If scapular movement is prevented, only 120° of passive abduction and 90° of active motion are possible.[63]

Clavicular motion at both the acromioclavicular and sternoclavicular joints is essential for full shoulder elevation. Inman and Saunders[49] have demonstrated that for full abduction of the arm to occur, the clavicle must rotate 50° posteriorly. Surgical pinning of the clavicle to the coracoid process, which has been performed in some cases in which a complete tear of the coracoclavicular ligament is present, dramatically limits shoulder abduction.

Glenohumeral elevation in abduction is the primary function of the deltoid and supraspinatus muscles. The contribution of the deltoid and supraspinatus to shoulder abduction has been extensively investigated. It was commonly assumed that abduction of the arm is initiated by the supraspinatus and is continued by the deltoid.[43] Studies in which selective nerve blocks were used to deactivate the deltoid and supraspinatus muscles have shown that complete abduction still occurs, although with a 50% loss in power, when one or the other muscle is deactivated.[26, 27] Simultaneous nerve blocks of both these muscles result in the inability to raise the arm.[26] Thus, each muscle can elevate the arm

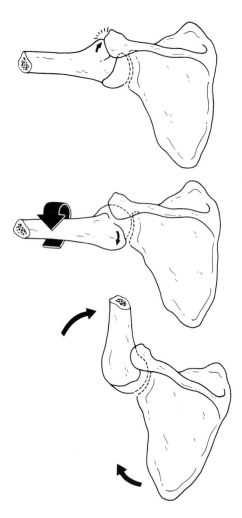

Figure 13–3. Clearing of the greater tuberosity from under the acromion to gain full abduction at the glenohumeral joint. (From Gould, J.A. [1990]: Orthopaedic and Sports Physical Therapy, 2nd ed. St. Louis, C.V. Mosby, p. 488.)

independently, but there is a resultant loss of approximately 50% of the normal power generated in abduction.[9]

Additionally, the other three rotator cuff muscles—the teres minor, the infraspinatus, and the subscapularis—are active to some degree throughout full abduction range of motion.[50] These three cuff muscles work as a functional unit to compress the humeral head to counteract the superior shear of the deltoid during arm elevation.[50, 58]

THROWING MECHANISM

Throwing is an integral part of many sports, but different techniques are required depending on the endeavor. High-speed motion analysis has allowed investigators to slow down the pitching act and examine the kinetics and kinematics involved (Fig. 13–4). The throwing act, as performed by the baseball pitcher, is a series of complex and synchronized movements involving both the upper and the lower extremities. As described by McLeod,[69] the throwing mechanism can be divided into five phases (Fig. 13–5): (1) wind-up, (2) cocking, (3) acceleration, (4) release and deceleration, and (5) follow-through. Injuries to the shoulder joint can occur during the cocking, acceleration, or deceleration phases. The overhead throw is the fastest human movement and takes approximately 0.5 second to complete (from wind-up to ball release).

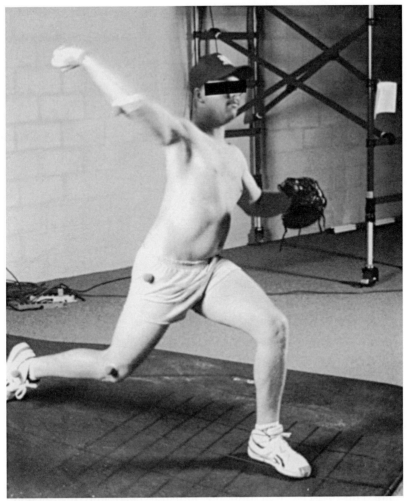

Figure 13-4. High-speed photography allows investigators to slow down the pitching act and examine the arthrokinematics involved. (Photo courtesy of Sports Medicine Update. Birmingham, Alabama. HealthSouth Rehabilitation Corporation.)

Wind-up

The purpose of the wind-up is to put the athlete in an advantageous starting position from which to throw. In addition, it can serve as a distraction to the hitter. The wind-up is a relatively slow maneuver that prepares the pitcher for correct body posture and balance while leading the body into the cocking phase (see Fig. 13–5). It can last from 0.5 to 1.0 second.[101] It is characterized by a shifting of the shoulder away from the direction of the pitch, with the opposite leg being cocked quite high and the baseball being removed from the glove.[69] It is also during this phase that the head of the humerus can wear and roughen from leverage on the posterior glenoid labrum.

Cocking

The cocking phase is most often divided into early and late cocking phases. During the cocking phase (see Fig. 13–5), the shoulder is abducted to approximately 90°, externally rotated 90° or more, and horizontally abducted to approxi-

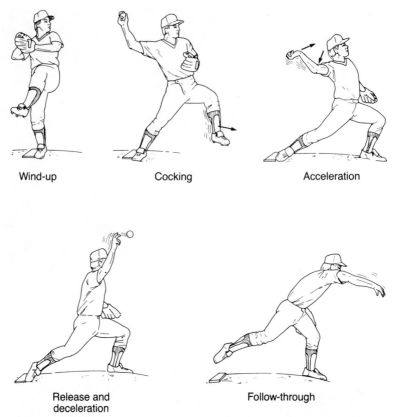

Figure 13–5. Dynamic phases of pitching. (From Walsh, D.A. [1989]: Shoulder evaluation of the throwing athlete. Sports Med. Update, 4:24.)

mately 30°.[69, 101] This is primarily accomplished by the deltoid and stabilized by the rotator cuff muscles that pull the humeral head into the glenohumeral joint.[19] The anterior, middle, and posterior deltoids reach peak electromyographic (EMG) activity in early cocking when the arm is abducted to 90°.[81] During late cocking, the activity of the deltoids decreases as the rotator cuff musculature becomes more dominant. Additionally, the pectoralis major, subscapularis, and latissimus act eccentrically to stabilize the humeral head during late cocking. This position places the anterior joint capsule and internal rotators, which are used to accelerate the ball, on maximum tension. Also, the opposite leg is kicked forward and placed directly in front of the body. Kinetic energy begins to be transferred from the lower extremities and trunk to the arm and hand in which the ball is held.[101] Because of the significant stresses placed on the anterior shoulder capsule, the capsule may "stretch out" with continuous throwing. If the anterior capsule is significantly stretched out, increased humeral head displacement during late cocking can occur, and this may clinically present as "posterior impingement," which will be discussed later.

Acceleration

The acceleration phase (see Fig. 13–5) begins at the point of maximal external rotation and ends at ball release.[70] This phase lasts an average of 50 milliseconds, approximately 2% of the duration of the pitching act.[80, 101] Muscles that once were on stretch in the cocking phase become the accelerators in a concentric muscular contraction. The body is brought forward, with the arm following behind. The energy developed by the body's moving forward is transferred to the throwing arm to accelerate the humerus.[98] This energy is enhanced via contraction of the internal rotators (primarily the subscapularis) as the humerus is rotated internally from its previously externally rotated position, and the ball is accelerated to delivery speed.[69] During this phase, the maximum internal rotation angular velocity is approximately 7365° ± 1503° per second.[35] During this phase there is also an anterior displacement force of approximately 50% of body weight. Rotatory torque at the shoulder can start at approximately 14,000 inch-pounds and builds up to approximately 27,000 inch-pounds of kinetic energy at ball release.[19]

During the acceleration phase, the pectoralis major and latissimus dorsi are the main muscles that actively generate velocity for the ball. The subscapularis muscle is active in steering the humeral head. At ball release, the throwing shoulder should be abducted about 90° or 100°, regardless of the type of pitch being thrown and the style of the thrower. The difference between the "overhead" and a "sidearm" baseball pitcher is not the degree of abduction, but rather the lateral tilt of the trunk. Because of the tremendous forces acting at the glenohumeral joint, numerous injuries can result during overhead throwing, such as instability, labral tears, overuse tendinitis, and tendon ruptures.[101]

Release and Deceleration

In the release and deceleration phases of throwing, the ball is released, and the shoulder and arm are decelerated (see Fig. 13–5). Generally, deceleration forces are approximately twice as great as acceleration forces but act for a shorter period of time (approximately 40 milliseconds).[15, 69] Initially, in the deceleration phase, the humerus has a relatively high rate of internal rotation, and the elbow rapidly extends.[69] Great forces are applied to the posterior rotator cuff muscles; these are required to slow internal rotation and horizontal adduction of the humerus and to stabilize the humeral head in the glenoid cavity. Jobe and colleagues[53, 55] analyzed the throwing mechanism using electromyography and found that the muscles of the rotator cuff are extremely active during the deceleration phase. It has been reported that the posterior rotator cuff must resist as much as 200 pounds of distraction force that is attempting to pull the arm out of the glenohumeral joint in the direction the ball has been thrown.[14] Labral tears at the attachment of the long head of the biceps, subluxation of the long head of the biceps by tearing of the transverse ligament, and various lesions of the rotator cuff, such as undersurface tearing or tensile overload, can be incurred during this phase of throwing.[101]

Follow-Through

During the follow-through phase (see Fig. 13–5) the body moves forward with the arm, effectively reducing the distraction forces applied to the shoulder.[69] This results in relief of tension on the rotator cuff muscles.

Because of the repetitive action of throwing, the baseball pitcher's shoulder undergoes adaptive changes that should be recognized and distinguished from pathologic lesions. The throwing shoulder has significantly increased external rotation and decreased internal rotation compared to that of the nonthrowing side. This is considered a functional adaptation to throwing but may lead to specific pathologies that will be discussed later.

Glousman and colleagues[40] have compared the EMG activity of the shoulder girdle muscles in pitchers with isolated anterior glenohumeral instability and in normal subjects. In pitchers, the supraspinatus and serratus anterior exhibited increased activity throughout late cocking and acceleration, the infraspinatus muscle exhibited enhanced activity during early cocking and acceleration, and the biceps brachii was noted to have an increase in activity during the acceleration phase. Additionally, the subscapularis, latissimus dorsi, and pectoralis major demonstrated less EMG activity in subjects with anterior instability during all phases.

Wick and colleagues[102] noted numerous significant differences between throwing a baseball overhead and throwing a football, the most striking differences being the following: During the acceleration phase, the angular velocity for baseball throwing was 7365° ± 1503° per second compared to 4586° ± 843° per second for throwing a football. At ball release, the shoulder was externally rotated more with the football throw—by approximately 21°. Also at ball release, shoulder abduction was calculated to be 99° during baseball throwing and 114° during football throwing. The duration of the football throw was also significantly longer (0.20 second) compared to a baseball throw (0.15 second).

OVERVIEW OF THE REHABILITATION PROGRAM

The shoulder rehabilitation program presented in this chapter is designed to restore shoulder range of motion and strength in a functional and progressive manner. The exercises may be implemented with specific limitations for certain motions, depending on the injury sustained or surgical procedure performed. Often, emphasis is placed on the rotator cuff musculature and not on the prime shoulder movers. Rehabilitation exercises that concentrate on the rotator cuff musculature are paramount after any shoulder injury but are of particular importance to throwing athletes. Shoulder rehabilitation should concentrate on increasing dynamic stability, particularly that of the rotator cuff, because of the relatively weak nature of the static restraints about the glenohumeral joint.

The entire kinematic chain should be evaluated when designing a shoulder rehabilitation program, considering the importance of proximal stability for distal mobility. The synchronous interplay among each of the joints of the shoulder complex is vital to active, balanced joint stability and normal glenohumeral function. The scapula stabilizers (e.g., latissimus dorsi, rhomboids, serratus anterior) are often overlooked when addressing shoulder injuries. The scapula stabilizers maintain the scapula–glenohumeral joint relationship, allow for normal kinematics during the pitching act, and play a large role during the deceleration phase of throwing.

Strengthening exercises for the shoulder musculature, especially the rotator cuff, have been critically analyzed by numerous investigators. Jobe and Moynes[52] first examined the effect of specific exercises on the rotator cuff musculature. They reported that the supraspinatus can best be exercised apart from the other cuff muscles with the arm abducted to 90°, horizontally adducted to 30°, and fully internally rotated—referred to as the "empty can" position (Fig. 13–6). The infraspinatus and teres minor can be exercised in the side-lying position with the arm held close to the side and the elbow flexed to 90°. The subscapularis can be strengthened with the individual in the supine position, the affected arm held close to the side, and the elbow flexed to 90°.

Since Jobe and Moynes' study,[52] Blackburn and associates[15] investigated rotator cuff activation, using intramuscular electromyography, while subjects performed specific rotator cuff exercises. Although Jobe and Moynes[52] reported that the supraspinatus is best isolated and exercised with the arm abducted to 90°, horizontally flexed 30°, and fully internally rotated (see Fig. 13–6), Blackburn and coworkers[15] noted that the supraspinatus is involved whenever the arm is elevated, whether the subject is standing or prone. Isolation of supraspinatus function appears to occur during pure abduction, with neutral rotation of the arm while standing. Also, Blackburn and coworkers[15] have noted that a signifi-

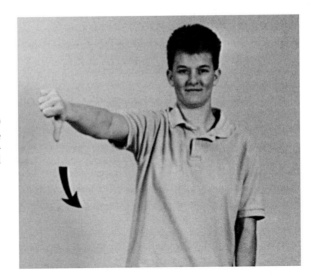

Figure 13–6. Jobe and Moynes[50] reported the supraspinatus muscle is best exercised with the arm abducted to 90°, horizontally flexed to 30°, and internally rotated.

cant increase in supraspinatus function can be achieved in the prone position, with the arm in maximal external rotation and in 100° of horizontal abduction (Fig. 13–7). Recently, Malanga and colleagues[65] analyzed the EMG activity of the rotator cuff and deltoid muscles in the empty can and the prone positions advocated by Blackburn and colleagues.[15] The empty can position produced high levels of EMG activity of the supraspinatus (107% maximum voluntary isometric contraction [MVIC]), but the middle deltoid (104%) and anterior deltoid (96%) were also extremely active. Conversely, during prone horizontal abduction (at approximately 100°) with external rotation, the most active muscles

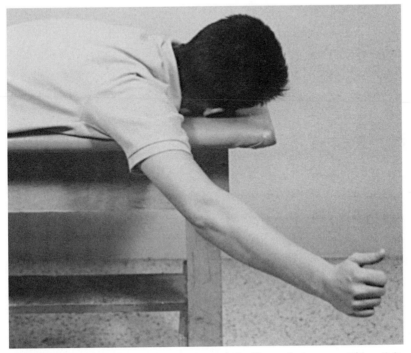

Figure 13–7. Blackburn et al.[15] have reported significant electromyographic activity of the supraspinatus in the prone position. The subject is performing horizontal abduction at 100° of abduction, with full external rotation.

were the middle deltoid (111%), the posterior deltoid (96%), and the supraspinatus (94%). The investigators concluded that neither position isolated the supraspinatus, but both positions could be used for exercising. In addition, Kelly and colleagues[56] have reported that the best test position to isolate the supraspinatus, with the least activation from the infraspinatus, is with the arm positioned at 90° of elevation in the scapular plane with 45° of humeral external rotation. This position is referred to as the "full can" position, and we recommend this position for manual muscle testing of the supraspinatus (Fig. 13–8). Townsend and associates[96] studied seven glenohumeral muscles during 17 traditional shoulder exercises and reported that certain exercises were better at recruiting selected muscles. For instance, the best exercise noted in the study to recruit the teres minor muscle was side-lying external rotation followed by prone horizontal abduction with external rotation. Table 13–1 provides detailed or specific exercises and muscle activity.

Following injury or surgery, modalities may be used as needed. Both pre-exercise and postexercise cryotherapy is recommended in the acute stages of healing to reduce the inflammatory process, and cryotherapy may be used prophylactically after the acute phase has subsided. Iontophoresis, moist heat, or ultrasound may be indicated for chronic overuse injuries of the shoulder.

Therapeutic exercises for the shoulder should address strength, endurance, and dynamic stability. A variety of machines and techniques can be used to accomplish specific goals. The upper body ergometer can be used in the early phases of rehabilitation for restoration of range of motion, and in later phases for muscular endurance (Fig. 13–9). The inertia machine (see Chap. 14) can be used for enhancing coordination and timing as well as for eccentric strengthening, particularly of the muscles involved in deceleration of the shoulder. Isokinetic equipment can be used at high speeds to help increase muscular power and endurance. Some isokinetic machines allow eccentric contraction of the

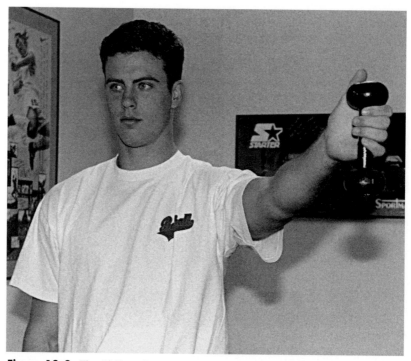

Figure 13–8. The "full can" position. This position has been suggested to be the best way to isolate the supraspinatus muscle while producing minimal activation of surrounding muscles.

Table 13–1. Electromyographic Activity of Specific Muscles During Selected Exercises

MUSCLE AND EXERCISE	ELECTROMYOGRAPHIC ACTIVITY (% MVIC ± SD)	PEAK ARC RANGE (DEGREES)
Anterior deltoid		
Scaption internal rotation	72 ± 23	90–150
Scaption external rotation	71 ± 39	90–120
Flexion	69 ± 24	90–120
Middle deltoid		
Scaption internal rotation	83 ± 13	90–120
Horizontal abduction internal rotation	80 ± 23	90–120
Horizontal abduction external rotation	79 ± 20	90–120
Posterior deltoid		
Horizontal abduction interval rotation	93 ± 45	90–120
Horizontal abduction external rotation	92 ± 49	90–120
Rowing	88 ± 40	90–120
Supraspinatus		
Military press	80 ± 48	0–30
Scaption internal rotation	74 ± 33	90–120
Flexion	67 ± 14	90–120
Subscapularis		
Scaption internal rotation	62 ± 33	90–150
Military press	56 ± 48	60–90
Flexion	52 ± 42	120–150
Infraspinatus		
Horizontal abduction external rotation	88 ± 25	90–120
External rotation	85 ± 26	60–90
Horizontal abduction internal rotation	74 ± 32	90–120
Teres minor		
External rotation	80 ± 14	60–90
Horizontal abduction external rotation	74 ± 28	60–90
Horizontal abduction internal rotation	68 ± 36	90–120

MVIC, Maximum voluntary isometric contraction

Modified from Townsend, H., Jobe, F.W., Pink, M., et al. (1992): EMG analysis of the glenohumeral muscles during a baseball rehabilitation program. Am. J. Sports Med., 19:264–269.

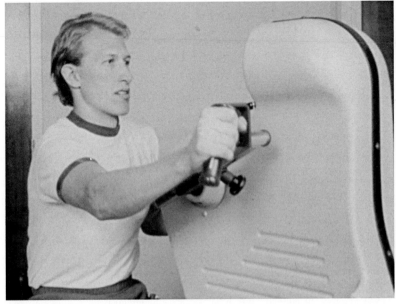

Figure 13–9. The upper body ergometer is used for range of motion and muscular endurance.

posterior cuff muscles and concentric contraction of the anterior muscles, which can be used to strengthen the muscles functionally. In addition, most isokinetic machines can be set up in functional planes, such as with proprioceptive neuromuscular facilitation (PNF) patterns (Fig. 13–10). Care must be taken when using isokinetics eccentrically at the shoulder, because the learning curve for performing this type of exercise properly is significant, and delayed-onset muscle soreness frequently results. Manual resistance exercises, such as rhythmic stabilization exercises, can be used to promote cocontractions and facilitate muscle synergies (Fig. 13–11). Finally, surgical tubing is a versatile tool that can be used to strengthen in diagonal patterns or through simulation of the throwing act (Figs. 13–12 and 13–13). The use of each of these exercises in the rehabilitation process depends on the goals of the particular phase. Specific use of each exercise will be explained in the treatment sections.

Glenohumeral mobilization techniques (see Chap. 6) are important for attaining accessory motion in the early stages of healing without subjecting the joint to the high forces of passive stretching. Grade I or II anterior-posterior, inferior-superior, and long arm distraction mobilizations can be used early in

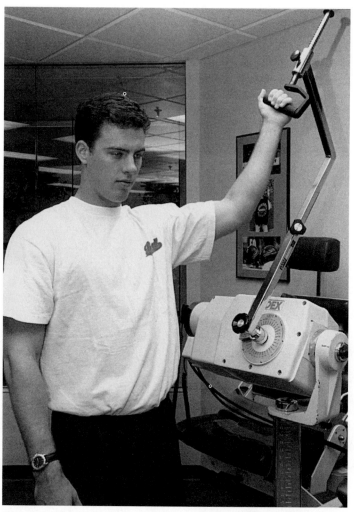

Figure 13–10. Proprioceptive neuromuscular facilitation (PNF) patterns can be used to simulate functional planes and enhance neuromuscular control of the shoulder girdle. This PNF pattern is being performed on the Biodex isokinetic device.

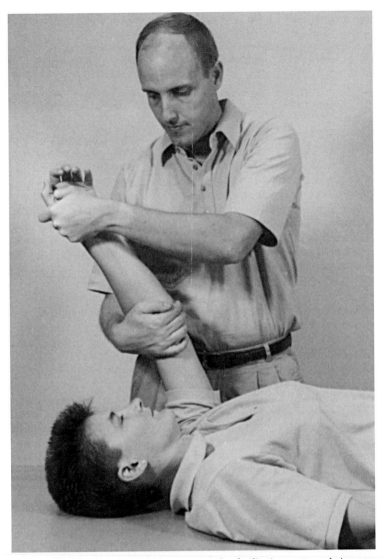

Figure 13–11. Proprioceptive neuromuscular facilitation patterns being performed against manual resistance.

the rehabilitation program to neuromodulate the patient's pain. Grade III or IV mobilizations can be added in later phases of rehabilitation to increase flexibility of the capsule.

Glenohumeral flexibility, particularly flexibility of the posterior shoulder structures, is paramount for the throwing athlete. This is particularly evident with inflexibility of the posterior capsule and musculature that presents as decreased motion in horizontal adduction and internal rotation. Tightness in the posterior shoulder leads to increased stress to the posterior shoulder structures during the follow-through phase of pitching. Tight posterior shoulder structures can also cause abnormal glenohumeral kinematics by forcing the humeral head anteriorly and superiorly into the acromial arch. The flexibility exercises illustrated at the end of this chapter (see Figs. 13–27 through 13–66) should be undertaken not only after injury or surgery but also during the off-season to help prevent posterior glenohumeral restriction and injury.

Muscular strength and endurance of the scapula stabilizer musculature are important in maintaining correct joint arthrokinematics. The role of the scapulo-

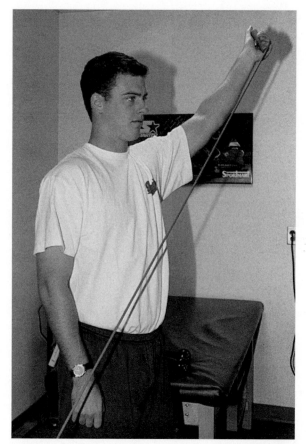

Figure 13–12. Proprioceptive neuromuscular facilitation pattern using surgical or exercise tubing.

thoracic joint and surrounding musculature in maintaining a normally functioning shoulder is critical. Muscular spasm, weakness, and poor neuromuscular coordination of these stabilizing muscles directly affect glenohumeral motion. If the scapula cannot rotate on the thoracic cage, maintain the correct length-tension muscular relationship, or properly orient the glenoid fossa with the humeral head, asynchronous motion at the shoulder complex will lead to injury. Scapula stabilizers can be strengthened by having the athlete perform push-ups, prone horizontal abduction, scapular retraction exercises, and neuromuscular control drills.

Because the rotator cuff muscles are mainly endurance-type muscles, the progressive-resistance exercise (PRE) program is based on low weight and high repetition.[10] This not only increases muscular endurance but also decreases the potential for perpetuating the inflammatory process by performing the exercises with too much weight. A common view, held by numerous clinicians, is that the PRE program should be progressed by having the athlete work from 30 to 50 total repetitions and not add weight until 50 repetitions can be performed comfortably (see Chap. 7). The PRE program is begun with a gradual progression toward more dynamic exercises as healing occurs. This decreases the chance of cuff inflammation and trauma but still produces muscle strength and endurance of the rotator cuff.

On the basis of numerous studies and their EMG results during specific movements, Wilk and Andrews[105] have developed a core exercise program for athletes who use overhead movements called the Throwers' Ten Exercise Pro-

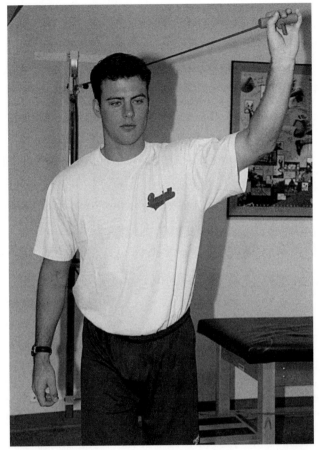

Figure 13–13. Exercise tubing being used to simulate the throwing motion.

gram (described in Appendix C). The program emphasizes the key muscles and muscle groups responsible for the throwing motion. The exercise program attempts to re-establish glenohumeral joint dynamic stability through rotator cuff musculature strength and neuromuscular control. Athletes should begin with a traditional PRE program and stretching exercises and gradually progress into eccentrics and isokinetics; this is followed by progression to a more dynamic program consisting of high-speed movements performed to muscle fatigue, proprioception exercises, use of an Inertia machine, and upper extremity plyometrics. The athlete should return to throwing gradually by progressing through the Interval Rehabilitation Programs, as outlined in Appendix D.

A plyometric exercise program can be extremely useful in the advanced phases of rehabilitation of an injured thrower. Plyometric exercise combines strength with speed of movement and has significant implications for the overhead thrower. The drills use a stretch-shortening cycle to the muscle, that is, an eccentric contraction followed by a concentric contraction. This stimulates the neurophysiologic components of the muscle to produce greater force. There are three phases to a plyometric drill: phase I is the stretch phase or the eccentric muscle loading that activates the muscle spindle; phase II is the amortization phase that represents the time between the eccentric and concentric phases; and phase III is the shortening phase or the response or concentric phase. Successful plyometric training relies heavily on the rate of stretch rather than on the length of stretch. Plyometric exercise attempts to train the neuromuscular system by using the stretch reflex, proprioceptive stimulus, and muscular activation. Plyometrics should be performed only two or three times weekly because of the microtrauma that may occur with this type of exercise. Performing plyometrics daily can result in additional trauma to a healing shoulder in some cases.

The upper extremity plyometric program is organized into four different exercise groupings: (1) warm-up drills, (2) throwing movements, (3) trunk drills, and (4) wall drills. Some of the plyometric drills are illustrated in Appendix A. For a complete description, the reader is encouraged to review several articles.[23, 38, 103, 106]

The nonoperative rehabilitation program for the overhead thrower can be divided into four distinct phases. Each phase should represent specific goals and should contain various exercises to accomplish these goals. Table 13–2 provides an overview of the program.

COMMON POSTTRAUMATIC AND POSTSURGICAL COMPLAINTS

After trauma or surgery to the shoulder joint, the athlete may report several common complaints to the clinician that may affect the rehabilitation program.

Painful Arc

A painful arc or "catching point," particularly with shoulder abduction (but also possibly present in other planes), is characterized by specific points throughout a range of motion at which pain intensifies but dissipates once past that point. There may be as many as three or four catching points through an arc of motion. The most common range of motion in which patients demonstrate a painful arc is from 70° to 120° of arm elevation. The athlete may attempt to exercise through these points of pain, which often dissipate within 5 to 7 days after initiation of treatment. Painful arcs in the young athlete can develop because of structural factors such as a hooked acromion, fracture malunion, or bursal swelling, or it may develop from a loss of dynamic humeral head stability,

---

Table 13–2. Nonoperative Rehabilitation of the Overhead Thrower

    I. Phase I: Acute Phase
      Goals
        • Diminish pain and inflammation
        • Normalize or improve motion and flexibility
        • Retard muscular atrophy
        • Enhance dynamic stabilization
    II. Phase II: Intermediate Phase
      Goals
        • Improve muscular strength and endurance
        • Maintain or improve flexibility
        • Promote concentric-eccentric muscular training
        • Maintain dynamic stabilization
    III. Phase III: Advanced Phase
      Goals
        • Initiate sport-specific training
        • Enhance power and speed (plyometrics)
        • Maintain rotator cuff strength program
        • Improve muscular endurance
    IV. Phase IV: Return to Activity
      Goals
        • Gradually return to sports activities
        • Maintain strength, power, endurance, and flexibility gains

causing the humeral head to displace superiorly during arm elevation. If the clinician determines the latter to be the cause, exercises that enhance dynamic stability should be emphasized.

Crepitus

Crepitus within the shoulder joint is a common occurrence and is usually asymptomatic. Generally, crepitus can be detected after shoulder surgery or rotator cuff tendinitis. If the crepitus remains asymptomatic, the athlete should attempt to exercise through it. Crepitus should also dissipate within 7 to 10 days after initiation of the rotator cuff exercise program.

Middle Deltoid and Elbow Pain

Middle deltoid and elbow pain can be referred from the shoulder, often from a tight shoulder capsule. It is usually exacerbated with external rotation in the supine position with 90° of abduction and 90° of elbow flexion (90/90 position). This pain is usually seen in individuals with chronic shoulder problems or in individuals who have undergone prolonged immobilization. Often, the elbow pain at the end range of shoulder external rotation may be greater than that of the actual shoulder pain. Such individuals usually respond well to moist heat and ultrasound to the shoulder capsule and to glenohumeral joint mobilization. A patient with a limitation of external rotation should not be stretched aggressively in the 90/90 position, as this will tend to exacerbate the elbow pain. Most patients can tolerate long arm distraction with imposed external rotation better than aggressive external rotation stretching in the 90/90 position. As treatment proceeds and normal synchronous glenohumeral motion is restored, the athlete should report a decrease in elbow and middle deltoid pain.

Pain Beyond 90° of Elevation

If impingement or rotator cuff tendinitis is present, pain beyond 90° of elevation is a common occurrence. Athletes with this complaint should begin active-assisted range-of-motion exercises through a full range of motion, and joint mobilization techniques should be used as indicated. The pain is often propagated by a decrease in muscular strength and usually improves with a rotator cuff therapeutic exercise program. If symptoms are severe and the athlete has radiographic changes indicative of a grade III (or hooked acromion) type of injury, the nonoperative therapeutic prognosis is poor.

SHOULDER INJURIES

Scapulothoracic Joint Lesions

The scapulothoracic joint should also be assessed after shoulder injury or surgery. Scapulothoracic pathology occurs in chronic pain conditions in which glenohumeral motion has gradually decreased or in which the glenohumeral joint has been immobilized for a long period. In most instances the scapulothoracic joint becomes involved as a secondary problem. Increased shoulder pain can result in muscle spasm in the supraspinatus, trapezius, rhomboids, latissimus dorsi, and subscapularis. As mentioned previously, for every 2° of glenohumeral abduction there must be approximately 1° of associated scapular motion to achieve 180° of arm elevation. If the scapulothoracic joint is not functioning

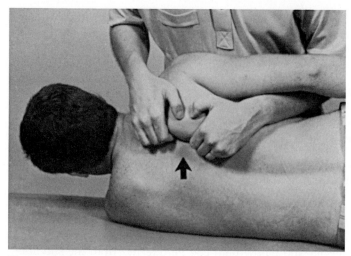

Figure 13–14. Scapula mobilization by distraction of the vertebral border of the scapula and lateral glide.

properly, the athlete may be able to attain only 100° to 120° of passive abduction, and active abduction may be even more limited.

The scapulothoracic joint should be evaluated for spasm in the rhomboids, latissimus dorsi, upper and lower trapezius, subscapularis, teres minor, infraspinatus, and supraspinatus muscles. These areas should also be assessed for active trigger points, as discussed by Travell and Simons.[97] The activation of trigger points in these muscles may refer pain to the middle deltoid and elbow and, in severe cases, down the arm. In addition, the clinician may find that the vertebral scapular border cannot be distracted off the thoracic cage; this results not only in increased pain for the athlete but also in an increase in muscle spasm.

Before decreased glenohumeral motion can be treated, scapulothoracic motion must be restored. This is usually accomplished by reducing the muscle spasm with moist heat, ultrasound, soft-tissue mobilization, trigger point release, and scapular mobilization (Figs. 13–14 and 13–15). In severe cases, the spray-and-stretch technique of Travell and Simons,[97] which uses Fluori-Methane spray to desensitize the trigger points, may be indicated. Trigger point injection may also be considered.[97] As trigger points are diminished, the athlete should report a

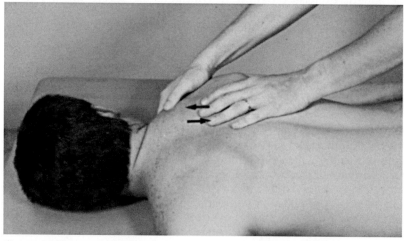

Figure 13–15. Scapula mobilization by superior and inferior scapula glides.

decrease in shoulder pain, neck stiffness, and referred pain, with an associated increase in glenohumeral abduction.

ROTATOR CUFF LESIONS

The rotator cuff can become injured through a variety of mechanisms. Most commonly, the cuff can become frayed and can progress to a full-thickness tear after repetitive wear, and it gradually degenerates. However, in young athletes, the cuff most commonly exhibits partial tearing or fraying, with symptoms of tendinitis. Andrews and Meister[3] have classified rotator cuff lesions into categories based on the pathomechanics (Table 13–3). We will briefly discuss a few of these categories as they pertain to the athlete with a shoulder injury. First, the athlete involved in overhead sports (i.e., thrower, swimmer) is prone to capsular laxity, which contributes to the clinical syndrome referred to as posterior impingement. In addition, such athletes are susceptible to undersurface cuff tearing (tensile overload) and occasionally to compressive cuff disease. In contrast, athletes involved in contact sports such as football, lacrosse, or hockey are more likely to sustain a traumatic cuff tear because of the athlete's arm being forcefully abducted or violently pulled away from the body. Full-thickness tears of the rotator cuff are unusual in young athletes.

Impingement Syndrome

The term "impingement syndrome" was popularized by Neer in 1972.[74] He emphasized that both the supraspinatus insertion to the greater tubercle and the bicipital groove lie anterior to the coracoacromial arch with the shoulder in the neutral position and that with forward flexion of the shoulder, these structures must pass beneath the coracoacromial arch, providing the opportunity for impingement.[68] He introduced the concept of a continuum in the impingement syndrome from chronic bursitis to partial or complete tears of the supraspinatus tendon, which may extend to involve ruptures of other parts of the rotator cuff.[68]

Impingement of the rotator cuff may occur in some athletes such as baseball players, quarterbacks, swimmers, and others whose activities involve repetitive use of the arm at and above 90° of shoulder abduction. Matsen and Arntz[68] have defined impingement as the encroachment of the acromion, coracoacromial ligament, coracoid process, or acromioclavicular joint on the rotator cuff mechanism that passes beneath them as the glenohumeral joint is moved, particularly in flexion and internal rotation. Impingement usually involves the supraspinatus tendon. When the supraspinatus muscle assists in stabilizing the head of the humerus within the glenoid, the greater tubercle cannot butt against the coracoacromial arch (Fig. 13–16).[88] Whether impingement is the primary event causing rotator cuff tendinitis or whether rotator cuff impingement occurs secondary to rotator cuff disease is undetermined.[88] In all likelihood both mechanisms of injury can occur.

There is approximately 5 to 10 mm of space between the humeral head and the undersurface of the acromial arch at 90° of shoulder abduction (depending

Table 13–3. Rotator Cuff Pathologic Classification

Primary compressive cuff disease (impingement)
Primary posterior impingement syndrome
Primary tensile overload
Traumatic overload
Secondary compressive cuff disease, primary instability
Secondary tensile failure, primary instability
Full-thickness cuff failure

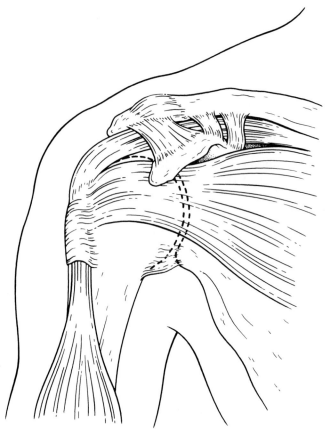

Figure 13–16. Anatomy relative to the impingement syndrome. The supraspinatus tendon is seen passing beneath the coracoacromial arch. (Redrawn from Matsen, F.A., III, and Arntz, C.T. [1990]: Subacromial impingement. *In*: Rockwood, C.A., Jr., and Matsen, F.A., III [eds.]: The Shoulder. Philadelphia, W.B. Saunders, p. 624.)

on anatomy). Thus, whenever the arm is elevated, some degree of rotator cuff impingement may occur.[88] The shoulder is most vulnerable to impingement when the arm is at 90° of abduction and the scapula has not rotated sufficiently upward to free the rotator cuff of the overhanging acromion and coracoacromial ligament. Impingement of the glenohumeral joint can occur with horizontal adduction of the arm, which causes impingement against the coracoid process. Forward flexion with internal rotation of the humerus also jams the greater tubercle under the acromion, the coracoacromial ligament, and, at times, the coracoid process.[88] If the arm is raised in external rotation, however, the greater tubercle is turned away from the acromial arch, and the arm can be elevated without impingement.

Impingement syndrome is perpetuated by the cumulative effect of many passages of the rotator cuff beneath the coracoacromial arch. This results in irritation of the supraspinatus and, possibly, the infraspinatus tendon, as well as in enlargement of the subacromial bursa, which can become fibrotic, thus further decreasing an already compromised space. Furthermore, with time and progression of wearing and attrition, microtears and partial-thickness rotator cuff tears may result. If these continue, secondary bony changes (osteophytes) can occur under the acromial arch, propagating full-thickness rotator cuff tears.

The etiology of the impingement syndrome is usually multifocal, and the supraspinatus tendon is the most likely structure to be involved. Several factors have been proposed that can contribute to the impingement syndrome. Tendon avascularity has long been thought to contribute to impingement. Lindblom,[62] in 1939, first reported avascularity of the rotator cuff at the supraspinatus attachment to the greater tubercle, describing this as the "critical zone"[25] in which many lesions occur. However, from their work, Moseley and Goldie[70] concluded that the critical zone is no more avascular than is the rest of the cuff. Finally, Iannotti and coworkers,[48] using laser Doppler technology, have reported substantial blood flow in the critical zone of the rotator cuff.

Although it now appears that the rotator cuff is not a completely avascular structure, Rathbun and Macnab[86] and Sigholm and associates[93] have proposed two mechanisms that may compromise supraspinatus blood flow. Rathbun and Macnab[86] have noted that shoulder adduction places the supraspinatus under tension and "wrings out" its vessels, resulting in tissue necrosis. Sigholm and colleagues[93] demonstrated that active forward flexion increases subacromial pressure to a level sufficient to reduce tendon microcirculation substantially.[68] However, in interpreting these findings, Matsen and Arntz pointed out that "since the shoulder is frequently moved, it is unclear whether either of these mechanisms could produce ischemia of sufficient duration to cause tendon damage."[68] Brewer[20] has reported that the blood supply to the critical zone diminishes with age. The relationship among cuff vascularity, impingement, and rotator cuff lesions is still speculative, and more research is needed. However, it appears that the critical zone is an area of hypovascularity and is prone to impingement and thus to tendon damage; this is especially true in the aging patient with shoulder injury.

The shape of the acromion has been studied in individuals with impingement syndrome.[13, 74] It appears that rotator cuff lesions are more likely to occur if a hooked acromion is present,[13, 72] but it cannot be determined whether the acromial shape is caused by or results from a cuff tear.[68] Figure 13–17 illustrates the three types of acromial shapes.

Finally, a weakened cuff mechanism can predispose an athlete to rotator cuff impingement. The rotator cuff functions to stabilize the shoulder against the actions of the deltoid and pectoralis major muscles. In the presence of a weakened cuff mechanism, contraction of the deltoid causes upward displacement of the humeral head so that it squeezes the remaining cuff against the coracoacromial arch (Fig. 13–18).[65] Other factors that can result in rotator cuff impingement include the following[68]: degenerative spurs, chronic bursal thickening, rotator cuff thickening related to chronic calcium deposits, tightness of the posterior shoulder capsule, and capsular laxity.

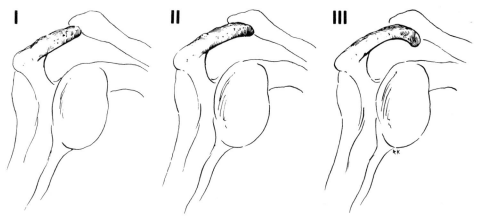

Figure 13–17. Biglianni et al.[13] have identified three different shapes of the acromion: type I—smooth; type II—curved; and type III—hooked. (From Jobe, C. M. [1990]: Gross Anatomy of the Shoulder. *In*: Rockwood, C.A., Jr., and Matsen, F.A. (eds.): The Shoulder. Philadelphia, W.B. Saunders, p. 45.)

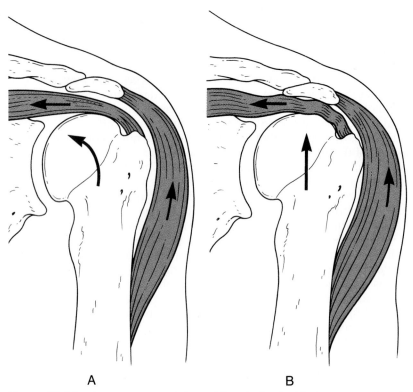

A   B

Figure 13–18. The supraspinatus helps stabilize the head of the humerus against the upward pull of the deltoid. *A*, Subacromial impingement is prevented by normal cuff function. *B*, Deep surface tearing of the supraspinatus weakens the ability of the cuff to hold the humeral head down, resulting in impingement of the tendon against the acromion. (Redrawn from Matsen, F.A., III, and Arntz, C.T. [1990]: Subacromial impingement. *In*: Rockwood, C.A., Jr., and Matsen, F.A., III [eds.]: The Shoulder. Philadelphia, W.B. Saunders, p. 624.)

Neer[74] has described three progressive stages of the impingement syndrome (Fig. 13–19). Stage I is a reversible lesion usually seen in individuals under 25 years of age; these patients present with an aching type of discomfort in the shoulder. This stage usually involves only inflammation of the supraspinatus tendon and long head of the biceps brachii. Stage II is generally seen in individuals 24 to 40 years of age and involves fibrotic changes of the supraspinatus tendon and subacromial bursa. Again, an aching type of pain is present, which may increase at night, and there may be an inability to perform the movement that results in the impingement syndrome. This stage sometimes responds to conservative treatment, but it may require surgical intervention. Stage III seldom occurs in those under the age of 40. In this stage, the individual has a long history of shoulder pain, and frequently there is osteophyte formation, a partial-thickness or eventually a full-thickness rotator cuff tear,[39] and an obvious wasting of the supraspinatus and infraspinatus muscles. This stage usually does not respond well to conservative treatment.

Rotator cuff impingement is a self-perpetuating process. Matsen and Arntz[68] have noted the following: (1) muscle or cuff tendon weakness causes impingement from loss of humeral head stabilization function leading to tendon damage, disuse atrophy, and additional cuff weakness (Fig. 13–20); (2) bursal thickening causes impingement from subacromial crowding, producing thickening of the bursa; and (3) posterior capsular tightness can lead to impingement, disuse, and stiffness, because the tight capsule forces the humeral head to rise up against the acromion. Numerous factors, structural and functional, contribute to im-

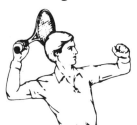

Stage I: Edema and hemorrhage

Typical age: <25 years
Differential diagnosis: Subluxation;
A/C arthritis
Clinical course: Reversible
Treatment: Conservative

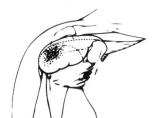

Stage II: Fibrosis and tendinitis

Typical age: 25–40 years
Differential diagnosis: Frozen shoulder; calcium

Clinical course: Recurrent pain with activity

Treatment: Consider bursectomy;
C/A ligament division

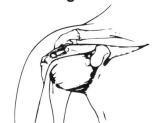

Stage III: Bone spurs and tendon rupture

Typical age: >40
Differential diagnosis: Cervical radiculitis;
Neoplasm
Clinical course: Progressive disability

Treatment: Anterior acromioplasty;
rotator cuff repair

Figure 13–19. Neer's three-stage classification of impingement syndrome. A/C, acromioclavicular joint; C/A, coracoacromial. (Reprinted with permission from Neer CS (1983). Impingement lesions. Clin Orthop Rel Res 173:70.)

pingement,[101] especially in young athletes. Additionally, if the capsule is especially lax and if the dynamic stabilizers are not sufficient, the humeral head may displace anterosuperiorly, leading to impingement complaints.

The goal in treating athletes with an impingement syndrome, either nonoperatively or surgically, is to reduce the compression and friction between the rotator cuff and subacromial space. Several factors[66, 68] are necessary to minimize the compression, including (1) shape of the coracoacromial arch, which allows passage of the adjacent cuff mechanism; (2) normal undersurface of the acromioclavicular joint; (3) normal bursa; (4) normal function of the humeral head stabilizers (rotator cuff); (5) normal capsular laxity; (6) smooth upper surface of the cuff mechanism; and (7) normal function of the scapular stabilizers. The primary complication of the impingement syndrome is a rotator cuff tear. If the impingement syndrome is diagnosed in its early stages, the prognosis is encouraging. In an acute impingement syndrome, time, rest from noxious stimuli, nonsteroidal anti-inflammatory drugs, modalities such as cold, heat, and electrical stimulation, and a general shoulder rehabilitation program of flexibility and PRE (as outlined at the end of this chapter) are indicated.

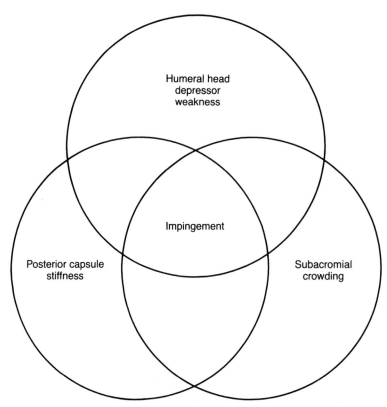

Figure 13–20. Normal shoulder tendon function depends on normal function of the humeral head depressors, normal capsular laxity, and adequate subacromial space. Some effects of impingement (e.g., weakness of the humeral head depressors, stiffness of the posterior capsule, and crowding of the subacromial space with thickened bursa) may further intensify impingement, producing a self-perpetuating process. (Modified from Matsen, F.A., III, and Arntz, C.T. [1990]: Subacromial impingement. *In*: Rockwood, C.A., Jr., and Matsen, F.A., III [eds.]: The Shoulder. Philadelphia, W.B. Saunders, p. 624.)

On evaluation, active range of motion may be limited with an empty or muscular guarding end feel as a result of pain. This may be caused by posterior capsule stiffness. In such cases moist heat, ultrasound, joint mobilization, and a general shoulder flexibility program with emphasis on supine internal and external rotation and horizontal adduction are appropriate. Most young throwers will exhibit a functional loss of internal rotation and, therefore, tightness of the posterior capsule. It is important to stretch the posterior capsule and normalize the degree of internal rotation. Table 13–4 outlines the protocol for nonoperative treatment of the impingement syndrome.

Injection of the subacromial space with lidocaine in an athlete with impingement syndrome decreases pain. Steroid injections into the tendons of the rotator cuff and biceps tendon may produce tendon atrophy or reduce the ability of a damaged tendon to repair itself.[68] Kennedy and Willis[57] have found a degenerative effect in the rabbit Achilles tendon after steroid injection. They concluded that physiologic doses of local steroids injected directly *into* a normal tendon weaken it significantly for up to 14 days postinjection. This weakness was attributed to cellular necrosis. When developing a rehabilitation program, the clinician must be aware of the potential effects of steroid injection.

Surgical intervention for patients with grade III impingement syndromes or for those who do not respond to nonoperative care consists of subacromial decompression, referred to as an acromioplasty. The goal in performing a subacromial decompression is to relieve the mechanical impingement and to prevent wear at the critical areas of the rotator cuff. Subacromial decompression consists of resection of the anteroinferior acromial undersurface to increase the space between the undersurface of the acromion and the rotator cuff/humeral head. Often, partial or complete resection of the coracoacromial ligament is also performed to further increase the available space. An acromioplasty may be performed in conjunction with a rotator cuff débridement or repair.

Surgical correction of the impingement syndrome can be done by arthroscopy or arthrotomy techniques. It is recommended that for an open subacromial

---

Table 13–4. Rehabilitation Protocol for Nonoperative Impingement Syndrome

I. **Phase I: Maximal Protection Acute Phase**
  Goals
  • Relieve pain and swelling
  • Decrease inflammation
  • Retard muscle atrophy
  • Maintain or increase flexibility
  1. Active rest: Eliminate any activity that causes an increase in symptoms
  2. Range-of-motion exercises
    (a) Pendulum exercises
    (b) Active-assisted range of motion—limited symptom-free available range
      • Rope-and-pulley exercises in flexion
      • L-bar exercises in flexion and neutral external rotation
  3. Joint mobilizations (grades I and II)
    (a) Inferior and posterior glides in scapular plane
  4. Modalities: Cryotherapy, transcutaneous electrical nerve stimulation, high-voltage galvanic stimulation
  5. Strengthening exercises
    (a) Isometrics (submaximal)
      • External rotation
      • Internal rotation
      • Biceps
      • Deltoid (anterior, middle, posterior)
  6. Patient education: Regarding activity, pathology, and avoiding overhead activity, reaching, and lifting
  Guidelines for progression
  • Decreases in pain or symptoms
  • Range of motion increased
  • Painful arc in abduction only
  • Muscular function improved
II. **Phase II: Motion Phase (Subacute Phase)**
  Goals
  • Re-establish nonpainful range of motion
  • Normalize arthrokinematics of shoulder complex
  • Retard muscular atrophy without exacerbation
  1. Range-of-motion exercises
    (a) Rope-and-pulley exercises in flexion and abduction (symptom-free motion)
    (b) L-bar exercises in flexion, abduction (symptom-free motion)
      • External rotation at 45° abduction, progress to 90° abduction
      • Internal rotation at 45° abduction, progress to 90° abduction
  2. Joint mobilizations (grades II, III, and IV)
    (a) Inferior, anterior, and posterior glides
    (b) Combined glides as required
  3. Modalities: Cryotherapy, ultrasound, phonophoresis
  4. Strengthening exercises
    (a) Continue isometric exercises
    (b) Initiate scapulothoracic strengthening exercises
  5. Initiate neuromuscular control exercises
  Guidelines for progression
  Begin to incorporate intermediate strengthening exercises as
  • Pain or symptoms decrease
  • Active-assisted range of motion normalizes
  • Muscular strength improves

Table continued on following page

Table 13–4. Rehabilitation Protocol for Nonoperative Impingement Syndrome *Continued*

III. **Phase III: Intermediate Strengthening Phase**
    Goals
- Normalized range of motion
- Perform symptom-free normal activities
- Improve muscular performance
1. Range-of-motion exercises
    (a) Aggressive L-bar active-assisted range of motion in all planes
    (b) Continue self-capsular stretching (anterior-posterior)
2. Strengthening exercises
    (a) Initiate isotonic dumbbell program:
      - Side-lying neutral internal and external rotation
      - Prone extension and horizontal abduction
      - Standing flexion to 90°; abduction to 90°; supraspinatus exercise
      - Initiate serratus exercises (wall push-ups)
      - Initiate tubing progression in slight abduction for internal and external rotation
3. Initiate arm ergometer for endurance
    Guidelines for progression
- Full nonpainful range of motion
- No pain or tenderness
- 70% of contralateral strength

    Goals
- Increase strength and endurance
- Increase power
- Increase neuromuscular control
1. Isokinetic test in internal-external rotation in modified neutral position and abduction-adduction
2. Initiate Throwers' Ten Exercise Program (Appendix C)
3. Isokinetics
    (a) Velocity spectrum exercises from 180°/sec to 300°/sec
    (b) Progress from modified neutral to 90/90 position as tolerated

---

decompression, a technique that does not compromise the deltoid attachments be employed, rather than separating the deltoid from its insertion during the surgical procedure. This approach results in less morbidity and allows for early postoperative motion, with almost no need for postoperative immobilization.[68] If the deltoid is detached from the acromion and distal clavicle, the rehabilitation program should proceed more slowly to allow for deltoid healing.

Modalities can be used initially after surgery to help control pain and inflammation, with the concurrent initiation of early range-of-motion exercises. In the early stages the athlete may complain of joint crepitus and a painful arc or catching points; these should be worked through as tolerated by the athlete. The crepitus and painful arc should subside in 7 to 10 days after initiation of exercises. We expect a patient to be restored to full passive range of motion or active-assisted range of motion in 2 to 3 weeks after arthroscopic decompression. As active range of motion is restored, a PRE program can be initiated. The protocol outlined in Table 13–5 presents the general postoperative course for an arthroscopic subacromial decompression. Coracoacromial ligament resection has no effect on the course of the rehabilitation. If a rotator cuff repair is performed in conjunction with the acromioplasty, a rotator cuff repair rehabilitation protocol should be followed.

Recently, posterior impingement has been described in the literature by Walch and colleagues.[100] Andrews and Carson[4] originally identified the lesion in the overhead thrower. This cuff lesion develops when the arm is abducted and externally rotated, such as in the cocking phase of throwing. During this movement, the humeral head tends to glide anteriorly (especially when the anterior capsule is hypermobile). As this motion occurs, the supraspinatus and infraspinatus impinge (or produce friction) on the posterosuperior edge of the glenoid

Table 13–5. Rehabilitation Protocol After Arthroscopic Subacromial Decompression

I. **Phase I: Motion Phase**
 Goals
  • Re-establish nonpainful range of motion
  • Retard muscular atrophy
  • Decrease pain and inflammation
 1. Range-of-motion exercises
   (a) Pendulum exercises
   (b) Rope-and-pulley exercises
   (c) L-bar exercises
    • Flexion-extension
    • Abduction-adduction
    • External-internal rotation (begin at 0° abduction, progress to 45° abduction, then to 90° abduction)
    • Self-stretches (capsular stretches)
 2. Strengthening exercises
   (a) Isometrics
   (b) May initiate tubing for external-internal rotation at 0° abduction in late phase
 3. Decrease pain and inflammation: Ice, nonsteroidal anti-inflammatory drugs, modalities
II. **Phase II: Intermediate Phase**
 Criteria to progress to phase II
  • Full range of motion
  • Minimal pain and tenderness
  • "Good" manual muscle test of internal rotation, external rotation, and flexion
 Goals
  • Regain and improve muscular strength
  • Normalize arthrokinematics
  • Improve neuromuscular control of shoulder complex
 1. Initiate isotonic program with dumbbells
   (a) Shoulder musculature
   (b) Scapulothoracic musculature
 2. Normalize arthrokinematics of shoulder complex
   (a) Joint mobilization
   (b) Control L-bar range of motion
 3. Initiate neuromuscular control exercises
 4. Initiate trunk exercises
 5. Initiate upper extremity endurance exercises
 6. Continue use of modalities; ice, as needed
III. **Phase III: Dynamic Strengthening Phase**
 Criteria to progress to phase III
  • Full, nonpainful range of motion
  • No pain or tenderness
  • Strength 70% compared to contralateral side
 Goals
  • Improve strength, power, and endurance
  • Improve neuromuscular control
  • Prepare athlete to begin to throw
 Emphasis of phase III
  • High-speed, high-energy strengthening exercises
  • Eccentric exercises
  • Diagonal patterns
 1. Exercises
   (a) Continue dumbbell strengthening (supraspinatus, deltoid)
   (b) Initiate tubing exercises in the 90/90 position for external and internal rotation (slow/fast speeds)
   (c) Continue tubing exercises for scapulothoracic musculature
   (d) Continue tubing exercises for biceps
   (e) Initiate plyometrics for rotator cuff
   (f) Initiate diagonal proprioceptive neuromuscular facilitation
   (g) Initiate isokinetics
   (h) Continue exercises for endurance and neuromuscular control

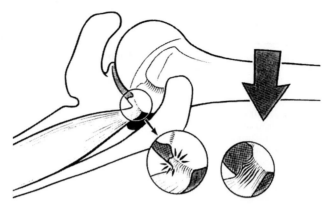

Figure 13–21. Posterior shoulder impingement. This occurs when the arm is abducted and externally rotated; the supraspinatus and infraspinatus muscles impinge (rub) on the posterosuperior rim of the glenoid cavity, leading to fraying of the cuff or labrum. (From Walch, G., Boileau, P., Noel, E., Donell, T. [1992]: Impingement of the deep surface of the supraspinatus tendon on the glenoid rim. J. Shoulder Elbow Surg., 1:239–245.

rim, resulting in an undersurface tearing of the rotator cuff and fraying of the posterosuperior glenoid labrum (Fig. 13–21). The nonoperative treatment for this type of lesion is to emphasize dynamic stabilization of the glenohumeral joint. If the nonoperative treatment is unsuccessful, surgery may be necessary. Most commonly, an arthroscopic débridement of the undersurface of the rotator cuff and the glenoid labrum is performed. After surgery, a thorough rehabilitation program emphasizing dynamic stabilization drills and normalization of motion is imperative.

Rotator Cuff Tears

The primary function of the rotator cuff is to provide dynamic stabilization and steer the humeral head. It appears that the cuff is well designed to bear tension and resist upward displacement of the humerus.[24, 25] The cuff balances the major forces applied by the prime mover muscles during motions such as flexion and abduction.[67]

The role of the rotator cuff in shoulder movements has long been, and still remains, somewhat controversial. Poppen and Walker[83, 84] have reported that the pull of the supraspinatus is fairly constant throughout the range of motion and actually exceeds that of the deltoid until 60° of shoulder abduction has been reached. Norkin and Levangie[77] have found that EMG activity of the deltoid in abduction shows a gradual increase in activity, peaking at 90° of humeral abduction and not plateauing until 180° has been reached. Colachis and coworkers[26, 27] used selective nerve blocks and noted that the supraspinatus and infraspinatus provide 45% of abduction and 90% of external rotation strength. Additionally, Howell and colleagues[46] measured the torque produced by the supraspinatus and deltoid in the forward flexion and elevation planes. They found that the supraspinatus and deltoid muscles are responsible equally for producing torque about the shoulder joint in functional planes of motions. Currently, it appears that both the deltoid and the supraspinatus contribute to abduction throughout the full range of motion. Active abduction is possible with loss of the deltoid or supraspinatus, with a corresponding loss in power.[26, 27]

The etiology of rotator cuff tears can be attributed to one or a combination of

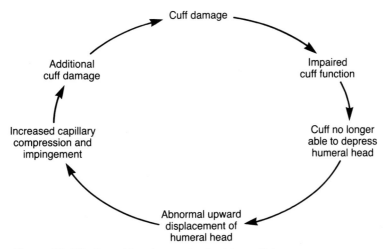

Figure 13–22. Potential pathogenesis of rotator cuff damage.

the following: repetitive microtrauma, disuse, overuse tendinitis, anatomic factors, and attrition. Neer[75] has reported that acute cuff tears occurring as a result of trauma account for approximately 3% to 8% of all tears. It has been postulated that rotator cuff tears result after the commonly diagnosed "cuff tendinitis" and that rotator cuff tears may actually represent failure of the rotator cuff fibers. This may explain why individuals with this injury usually recover with time and conservative treatment.[67] Matsen and Arntz have suggested the following explanation for perpetuation of rotator cuff failure[67]:

> The traumatic and degenerative theories of cuff tendon failure can be synthesized into a unified view of pathogenesis. Let us assume that the normal cuff starts out well vascularized and with a full complement of fibers. Through its life it is subjected to various adverse factors such as traction, contusion, impingement, inflammation, injections, and age-related degeneration. Each of these factors places fibers of the cuff tendons at risk. Even though laboratory studies show that normal tendon does not fail before failure of the musculotendinous junction or the tendon bone junction, in the clinical situation the cuff tendon ruptures both at its insertion to bone and in its mid-substance. With the application of loads (whether repetitive or abrupt, compressive, or tensile), each fiber fails when the applied load exceeds its strength. Fibers may fail a few at a time or in mass. Because these fibers are under load even with the arm at rest, they retract after their rupture. Each instance of fiber failure has at least three adverse effects: (1) it increases the load on the neighboring fibers (fewer fibers to share the load); (2) it detaches muscle fibers from bone (diminishing the force that the cuff muscles can deliver); and (3) it risks the vascular elements in close proximity by distorting their anatomy (a particularly important factor owing to the fact that the cuff tendons contain the anastomoses between the osseous and muscular vessels). Thus, the initially well-vascularized cuff tendon becomes progressively less vascular with succeeding injuries. Although some tendons, such as the Achilles tendon, have a remarkable propensity to heal after rupture, cuff ruptures communicate with joint and bursal fluid, which removes any hematoma that could contribute to cuff healing. Even if the tendon could heal with scar, scar tissue lacks the normal resilience of tendon and is, therefore, under increased risk for failure with subsequent loading (minor or major). These events weaken the substance of the cuff, impair its function, and render the cuff weaker, more prone to additional failure with less load, and less able to heal.

Figure 13–22 illustrates the vicious cycle of cuff degeneration that occurs if the problem is left untreated, regardless of the etiologic factors involved in cuff damage.

Arthroscopy has allowed investigators to examine rotator cuff lesions and make the following observations:

1. Failure of the musculotendinous cuff is almost always peripheral, near the attachment of the cuff to the greater tuberosity, and it nearly always begins in the supraspinatus part of the cuff near the biceps tendon.[68]
2. Partial-thickness tears appear to be two to three times as common as full-thickness lesions.[75, 108]
3. Often partial tears occur on the joint side and not on the bursal side.[37, 108]
4. Rotator cuff tears often begin deep and extend outward, therefore challenging the concept of subacromial impingement as the primary cause of defects.[32, 67, 107]
5. Full-thickness cuff tears appear to occur in tendons that are weakened by some combination of age, repeated small episodes of trauma, steroid injections, subacromial impingement, hypovascularity of the tendon, major injury, and previous partial tearing.[67]

Athletes presenting with rotator cuff tendinitis generally respond favorably to a well-designed rehabilitation program. The involved shoulder is usually stiff, especially in the posterior capsule, with appreciable glenohumeral crepitus. The stiffness limits one or a combination of the following motions: forward flexion, internal and external rotation, and horizontal adduction. The emphasis of the program is to correct any asymmetric capsular tightness. The athlete may also have difficulty reaching behind the back, because this movement elongates the musculotendinous unit and compresses it as it is pulled under the coracoacromial arch with internal rotation.[17] Modalities (such as moist heat, iontophoresis, and ultrasound), mobilization, and stretching exercises for the posterior capsule are indicated. Rest from the noxious stimuli and use of nonsteroidal anti-inflammatory drugs are also appropriate. Initiation of a general shoulder flexibility program and a rotator cuff PRE program, as outlined at the end of this chapter, are necessary to prevent progressive cuff degradation. The PRE program should concentrate on the posterior rotator cuff muscles, because these muscles are responsible for humeral head depression and contract eccentrically to slow the arm down during the deceleration phase of throwing.

Return to throwing should not begin until the entire rehabilitation program has been completed. The patient must exhibit specific criteria prior to initiating a throwing program. The criteria used by the authors include full nonpainful range of motion, satisfactory muscular strength, satisfactory clinical examination, and appropriate progression through the rehabilitation program. Once these criteria have been satisfied, an interval throwing program (see Appendix D) may be initiated. The athlete should continue with a program that includes strengthening and flexibility exercise after the throwing program has been initiated.

Patients who do not respond to nonoperative care may require surgical intervention. An acromioplasty is commonly performed in conjunction with a rotator cuff repair. Rotator cuff tears seen and treated arthroscopically are most often incomplete tears that are noted on the undersurface of the muscle. Larger lesions may require an open procedure to repair. There are numerous surgical techniques to repair a full-thickness rotator cuff tear. The "deltoid-splitting" procedure is recommended to decrease morbidity and promote early range of motion. Tables 13–6 to 13–8 outline rehabilitation program protocols for arthroscopic débridement and open rotator cuff repair, using the deltoid-splitting or arthroscopy-assisted surgical procedure. These protocols can easily be adapted to other rotator cuff procedures, if necessary. The rehabilitation approach we take is based on the size of the tear and tissue quality; hence, in Tables 13–6 to 13–8, three different protocols, based on the size of the tear, are illustrated. An abduction pillow (Fig. 13–23) can be used after rotator cuff repair to alleviate stress on the cuff repair, because the adducted position may cause undue early stress on the repair, especially in large to massive tears. Lesion size and extent of repair determine whether an abduction pillow will be used and the duration of use. In most cases, an abduction pillow or splint is not used after rotator cuff repair (except in large tears). Use of the pillow can range from 2 to 5 weeks. Immediately after the repair, passive range-of-motion exercises should be performed to minimize the patient's chances of developing adhesive capsulitis or a stiff shoulder. Active-assisted range of motion may be initiated once the physician feels that the repair has healed adequately. As active range of motion is restored, a PRE program should be initiated with a focus on posterior cuff and scapular stabilizer muscle strengthening. Postoperative rehabilitation depends on the extent of the cuff lesion, the tissue quality, and the procedure used to carry out the repair.

Anterior Instability

Shoulder instability is a common clinical problem, with anterior instability occurring most frequently. The anatomy of the glenohumeral joint predisposes the shoulder to instability. The glenoid cavity is relatively small and shallow, and the capsule tends to be loose in young, athletic individuals. These factors combine to make the shoulder susceptible to dislocations anteriorly.[21, 50, 85, 89] Anterior glenohumeral instability can be divided into acute traumatic dislocation and recurrent dislocation or subluxation. Most acute anterior dislocations occur with the arm abducted to 90°, extended, and externally rotated. This can occur when an athlete is attempting an arm tackle in football or when an abnormal force is applied to an arm that is executing a throw. The dislocated shoulder is characterized by a flattened deltoid contour, inability to move the arm, and severe pain. With this injury the head of the humerus is forced out of its articulation, past the glenoid labrum and then upward, to rest under the coracoid process.[5]

The dislocated shoulder is usually readily detectable, but the subluxing shoulder can be more subtle and may be overlooked. Anterior subluxation of the

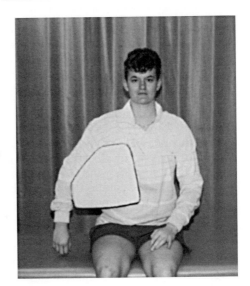

Figure 13–23. The use of an abduction pillow after rotator cuff repair can help alleviate stress placed on the repair.

Table 13–6. Rehabilitation Protocol After Type I Rotator Cuff Repair (Deltoid-Splitting Procedure): Small Tear (<1 cm)

I. **Phase I: Protective Phase (Weeks 0–6)**
  Goals
  - Achieve gradual return to full range of motion
  - Increase shoulder strength
  - Decrease pain
  A. Weeks 0–3
    1. Sling for comfort (1–2 weeks)
    2. Pendulum exercises
    3. Active-assisted range-of-motion exercises with L bar
    4. Rope-and-pulley exercises for flexion *only*
    5. Elbow range of motion and hand gripping
    6. Isometrics (submaximal, subpainful isometrics)
      - Abductors
      - External rotators
      - Internal rotators
      - Elbow flexors
      - Shoulder flexors
    7. Pain control modalities (ice, high-voltage galvanic stimulation)
    Note: Range-of-motion exercises are employed in a nonpainful range; gently and gradually increase motion to tolerance.
  B. Weeks 3–6
    1. Progress all exercises (continue all exercises listed above)
    2. Active-assisted range-of-motion exercises external-internal rotation (shoulder at 45° abduction)
    3. Surgical tubing external-internal rotation (arm at side)
    4. Initiate humeral head stabilization exercises
II. **Phase II: Intermediate Phase (Weeks 7–12)**
  Goals
  - Achieve full, nonpainful range of motion
  - Improve strength and power
  - Increase functional activities; decrease residual pain
  A. Weeks 7–10
    1. Active-assisted range-of-motion exercises with L bar
      - Flexion to 170–180°
      - External-internal rotation performed at 90° shoulder abduction—external rotation to 75–90°; internal rotation to 75–85°
      - External rotation exercises performed at 0° abduction
    2. Strengthening exercises for shoulder
      - Exercise tubing external-internal rotation, arm at side
      - Isotonic dumbbell exercises for deltoid, supraspinatus, elbow flexors, and scapulae muscles
    3. Initiate upper body ergometer for endurance
  B. Weeks 10–12
    1. Continue all exercises listed above
    2. Initiate isokinetic strengthening (scapular plane)
    3. Initiate side-lying external-internal rotation exercises (dumbbell)
    4. Initiate neuromuscular control exercises for scapulae

glenohumeral joint may develop without a history of trauma and is common in throwers. The subluxing shoulder is often referred to as the "dead arm syndrome," because it is characterized by a loss in shoulder strength and power. Rowe and Zarins[90] have reported that in 60 instances of dead arm syndrome, 26 patients were aware of shoulder subluxation, and 32 patients were not aware of its occurrence. Clinically, the athlete presents with soreness over the anterior aspect of the shoulder and reports a reproduction of the signs and symptoms in the cocking or acceleration phase of the throwing act. Athletes may also report a loss in shoulder strength and power and a feeling of clicking or sliding within the shoulder.

Several mechanisms of injury can explain the insidious onset of anterior instability. One of the most prevalent views is that in the cocking phase of throwing, external rotation places repeated stress on the anterior capsule and results in capsule attenuation and, ultimately, in anterior instability.

Table 13–6. Rehabilitation Protocol After Type I Rotator Cuff Repair (Deltoid-Splitting Procedure): Small Tear (<1 cm) *Continued*

III. **Phase III: Advanced Strengthening Phase (Weeks 13–21)**
  Goals
  • Maintain full, nonpainful range of motion
  • Improve strength of shoulder complex
  • Improve neuromuscular control
  • Gradually return to functional activities
  A. Weeks 13–18
    1. Active stretching program for the shoulder (active-assisted range of motion with L bar in flexion, external-internal rotation)
    2. Self-capsular stretches
    3. Aggressive strengthening program (isotonic program)
      • Shoulder flexion
      • Shoulder abduction
      • Supraspinatus
      • External-internal rotation
      • Elbow flexors and extensors
      • Scapulae muscles
    4. Isokinetic test at week 14 (modified neutral position)
      • External-internal rotation at 180°/sec and 300°/sec
    5. General conditioning program
  B. Weeks 18–21
    1. Continue all exercises listed above
    2. Initiate interval training program for sport
IV. **Phase IV: Return-to-Activity Phase (Weeks 21–26)**
  Goal
  • Gradually return to recreational and sports activities
    1. Isokinetic test (modified neutral position)
    2. Continue to comply with interval training program
    3. Continue Throwers' Ten Exercise Program (Appendix C) for strengthening and flexibility

---

Weakness of the scapula stabilizers is also believed to contribute to anterior instability.[54] The function of the scapula rotators (e.g., trapezius, rhomboids, serratus anterior) is to place the glenoid in the optimal position for the activities being performed. The rotator cuff seeks to stabilize the humeral head, and the glenohumeral ligament, particularly the inferior aspect, provides a static restraint at the margins of the joint.[54] Damage to the static restraints (gradual attenuation) results in instability, causing asynchronous firing of the scapula rotators and rotator cuff muscles. Greater stress is placed on the rotator cuff muscles in an attempt to stabilize the humeral head, producing rotator cuff damage and leading to rotator cuff impingement (described earlier). Thus, Jobe and associates[54] have reported that impingement problems are secondary to the primary lesion, glenohumeral instability.

Shoulder instability can be associated with an anterior glenoid labrum tear as the humeral head slips past the anterior aspect of the labrum and then reduces itself. A small portion of the anterior labrum may be torn, especially with recurrent episodes of instability. Additionally, Hill-Sachs and Bankart lesions (Fig. 13–24) are common with anterior instability, and their presence can be used to confirm this diagnosis. Bankart lesions result from an avulsion of the capsule and labrum from the glenoid rim and occur as the result of a traumatic glenohumeral joint dislocation. Individuals who have sustained a subluxation generally do not sustain a Bankart lesion. A Hill-Sachs lesion is a bony injury involving the posterolateral aspect of the humeral head as it strikes the rim of the glenoid at the time of dislocation.[89] Therefore, greater forces are required to dislocate a shoulder than to sublux it, and greater tissue damage results.

Whether the injury is a subluxation or a dislocation, nonoperative treatment is often attempted first. The success of nonoperative care is variable.[6, 7, 39, 44] Athletes who have dislocated their shoulders and thus have sustained Bankart lesions are less likely to return to unrestricted sports participation than are

---

Table 13–7. Rehabilitation Protocol After Type II Rotator Cuff Repair (Deltoid-Splitting Procedure): Medium to Large Tear (1 to 5 cm)

I. **Phase I: Protective Phase (Weeks 0–6)**
Goals
  • Achieve gradual increase in range of motion
  • Increase shoulder strength
  • Decrease pain and inflammation
  A. Weeks 0–3
    1. Brace or sling (as determined by physician)
    2. Pendulum exercises
    3. Active-assisted range-of-motion exercises with L bar
      • Flexion to 125°
      • External-internal rotation (shoulder at 40° abduction) to 30°
    4. Passive range of motion to tolerance
    5. Rope-and-pulley exercises in flexion
    6. Elbow range of motion
    7. Hand-gripping exercises
    8. Submaximal isometrics for flexors, abductors, external-internal rotation, and elbow flexors
    9. Ice and pain modalities
  B. Weeks 3–6
    1. Discontinue brace or sling
    2. Continue all exercises listed above
    3. Active-assisted range-of-motion exercises
      • Flexion to 145°
      • External-internal rotation performed at 65° abduction through range to tolerance
II. **Phase II: Intermediate Phase (Weeks 7–14)**
Goals
  • Achieve full, nonpainful range of motion (week 10)
  • Gradually increase strength
  • Decrease pain
  A. Weeks 7–10
    1. Active-assisted range-of-motion exercises with L bar
      • Flexion to 160°
      • External-internal rotation performed at 90° shoulder abduction to tolerance (greater than 45°)
    2. Strengthening exercises
      • Exercise tubing external-internal rotation, arm at side
      • Initiate humeral head stabilization exercises
      • Initiate dumbbell strengthening exercises for deltoid, supraspinatus, elbow flexion and extension, and scapulae muscles
  B. Weeks 10–14 (full range of motion desired by weeks 10–12)
    1. Continue all exercises listed above
    2. Initiate isokinetic strengthening (scapular plane)
    3. Initiate side-lying external-internal rotation exercises (dumbbell)
    4. Initiate neuromuscular control exercises for scapulae
    Note: If the athlete is unable to elevate the arm without the shoulder and scapula "hiking" (scapulothoracic substitution) before initiating isotonics, maintain the athlete on humeral head stabilization exercises.

---

individuals who have not sustained Bankart lesions. Rehabilitation should initially concentrate on decreasing the acute inflammation and pain and then gradually on restoring full shoulder motion. After normal motion is restored, an aggressive shoulder flexibility program is contraindicated because of the attenuation of the tissues. A strengthening program for the rotator cuff should be implemented, with a focus on the rotator cuff muscles and scapula stabilizers.[22]

If nonoperative treatment fails, several operative procedures can be used to restore function of the shoulder complex. These procedures attempt to restore static restraints or to compensate for the insufficiency in static structures with a dynamic (muscle transfer) procedure. The most commonly used dynamic repair procedure is the Bristow procedure. The Bristow procedure involves transfer of the coracoid process, with its tendon attachments through the subscapularis muscle, to the neck of the glenoid. The coracoid process is held to the glenoid with a screw, producing a bony block to deter anterior subluxation of the

Table 13–7. Rehabilitation Protocol After Type II Rotator Cuff Repair (Deltoid-Splitting Procedure): Medium to Large Tear (1 to 5 cm) *Continued*

III. **Phase III: Advanced Strengthening Phase (Weeks 15–26)**
   Goals
   - Maintain full, nonpainful range of motion
   - Improve strength of shoulder complex
   - Improve neuromuscular control
   - Gradually return to functional activities
   A. Weeks 15–20
   1. Continue active-assisted range-of-motion exercise with L bar in shoulder flexion, external-internal rotation
   2. Self-capsular stretches
   3. Aggressive strengthening program (isotonic program)
      - Shoulder flexion
      - Shoulder abduction to 90°
      - Supraspinatus
      - External-internal rotation
      - Elbow flexors and extensors
      - Scapulae muscles
   4. General conditioning program
   B. Weeks 21–26
   1. Continue all exercises listed above
   2. Isokinetic test (modified neutral position) for external-internal rotation at 180°/sec and 300°/sec
   3. Initiate interval training program for sport
IV. **Phase IV: Return-to-Activity Phase (Weeks 24–28)**
   Goal
   - Gradually return to sports activities
   1. Continue all strengthening exercises
   2. Continue all flexibility exercises
   3. Continue progression on interval training program

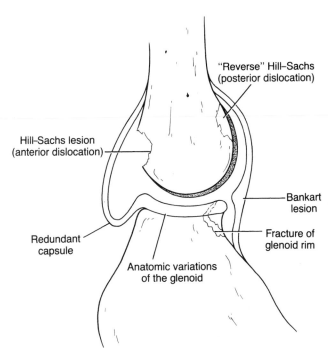

Figure 13–24. Anatomic lesions produced from shoulder insta-bility. (From Rowe, C.R. [1988]: The Shoulder. New York, Churchill Livingstone, p. 177.)

Table 13–8. Rehabilitation Protocol After Type III Rotator Cuff Repair (Deltoid-Splitting Procedure): Large to Massive Tear (>5 cm)

I. **Phase I: Protection Phase (Weeks 0–8)**
   A. Weeks 0–4
      1. Brace or sling (as determined by physician)
      2. Pendulum exercises
      3. Passive range of motion to tolerance
         • Flexion
         • External-internal rotation (shoulder at 45° abduction)
      4. Elbow range of motion
      5. Hand-gripping exercises
      6. Continuous passive motion
      7. Submaximal isometrics for abductors, external-internal rotation, elbow flexors
      8. Ice and pain modalities
      9. Gentle active-assisted range of motion with L bar at week 2
   B. Weeks 4–8
      1. Discontinue brace or sling
      2. Active-assisted range of motion with L bar in
         • Flexion to 100°
         • External-internal rotation to 40°, with shoulder at 45° abduction
      3. Continue pain modalities
II. **Phase II: Intermediate Phase (Weeks 8–14)**
   Goals
      • Achieve full range of motion (week 12)
      • Gradually increase strength
      • Decrease pain
   A. Weeks 8–10
      1. Active-assisted range-of-motion exercises with L-bar
         • Flexion to tolerance
         • External-internal rotation to tolerance with shoulder at 90° abduction
      2. Initiate isotonic strengthening
         • Deltoid to 90°
         • External-internal rotation in side-lying
         • Supraspinatus
         • Biceps and triceps
         • Scapulae muscles
   B. Weeks 10–14
      1. Full range of motion desired by weeks 12–14
      2. Continue all exercises listed above
      3. Initiate neuromuscular control exercises
      Note: If the athlete is unable to elevate the arm without the shoulder "hiking" (scapulothoracic substitution) before initiating isotonics, maintain the athlete on humeral head stabilization exercises.

humeral head when the arm is abducted and externally rotated. It has been previously stated that one of the major drawbacks to the Bristow procedure is the limitation imposed on external rotation that results in loss of approximately 10° in external rotation.[18] We recommend obtaining 90° of external rotation at 90° of abduction after this procedure. In addition, a concern of this procedure is migration of the screw used to fixate the conjoint tendon. Previously popular procedures such as the Putti-Platt and the Magnuson-Stack procedures are not as strongly advocated today because of the significant loss of external rotation[1, 28, 71] and because they are not an anatomic repair.

The most common techniques to repair the static restraints include the Bankart and the capsular shift (capsulorrhaphy) procedures, which address the glenohumeral ligament as the cause of instability. If the lesion is due to a traumatic injury, a Bankart lesion is probably present. If a Bankart lesion is present, an anatomic Bankart repair technique may be chosen, because it corrects not only the attenuated capsule but also the Bankart lesion. The Bankart repair can be performed either open or arthroscopically, and the procedure may require repairing the capsule to bone or repairing the capsulolabral complex. If the capsule is determined to be excessively redundant, then a capsular shift or a capsular

Table 13–8. Rehabilitation Protocol After Type III Rotator Cuff Repair (Deltoid-Splitting Procedure): Large to Massive Tear (>5 cm) *Continued*

III. **Phase III: Advanced Strengthening Phase (Weeks 15–26)**

   Goals
   - Maintain full, nonpainful range of motion
   - Improve strength of shoulder complex
   - Improve neuromuscular control
   - Gradually return to functional activities

   A. Weeks 15–20
   1. Continue active-assisted range-of-motion exercise with L bar in flexion, and external-internal rotation
   2. Self-capsular stretches
   3. Aggressive strengthening program (isotonic program)
      - Shoulder flexion
      - Shoulder abduction to 90°
      - Supraspinatus strengthening
      - External-internal rotation
      - Elbow flexors and extensors
      - Scapulae muscles
   4. General conditioning program

   B. Weeks 21–26
   1. Continue all exercises listed above
   2. Isokinetic test (modified neutral position) for external-internal rotation at 180°/sec and 300°/sec
   3. Initiate interval training program for sport

IV. **Phase IV: Return-to-Activity Phase (Weeks 24–28)**

   Goals
   - Gradually return to sports activities
   - Continue all strengthening exercises
   - Continue all flexibility exercises
   - Continue progression on interval training program

---

tensioning procedure may be performed concomitantly with the Bankart repair. There are numerous methods of fixation with a Bankart repair, including sutures, biodegradable tacks, suture anchors, and less preferably, metal tacks.

The capsulorrhaphy, or capsular shift procedure, is performed when instability is the result of an excessively loose capsule. Usually this procedure is performed on shoulders that exhibit atraumatic instability that may be multidirectional and in athletes who exhibit instability in the anteroinferior direction. The surgical technique involves taking the capsule off the bone (either on the humeral or on the glenoid side) and shifting the capsule in a superior direction. Essentially, this tightens the entire shoulder capsule. The position of the arm while applying tension to the capsule is very important, especially in overhead athletes (those who engage in repetitive overhead activities), because it partially determines the ability to regain external rotation range of motion postoperatively. The tendency is to overtighten the capsule to prevent recurrent instability, which results in a functional loss of external rotation and great difficulty in regaining motion.

Treatment after repair for anterior instability is essentially similar for both a static and a dynamic repair. Larger differences in treatment occur between arthroscopic and open stabilization procedures. In general, open procedures progress much more rapidly than do arthroscopic procedures. Table 13–9 outlines a rehabilitation protocol for athletes undergoing a Bristow repair; Table 13–10 outlines a rehabilitation protocol after a capsular shift procedure; and Tables 13–11 and 13–12 describe the rehabilitation after either open or arthroscopic Bankart procedures.

In some athletes who exhibit recurrent anterior instability and who are not required to abduct and externally rotate their arms above shoulder height, a shoulder brace may be used. Numerous devices are available, and these are designed to restrict combined abduction and external rotation. The Shoulder

---

Table 13–9. Rehabilitation Protocol After Bristow Procedure

I. **Phase I: Immediate Postoperative Phase (Days 1–5)**
  1. Range-of-motion exercises
    (a) Wrist flexion-extension
    (b) Elbow flexion-extension
    (c) Putty exercises for hand gripping
    (d) Initiate shoulder range of motion exercises (perform to tolerance)
      • Circumduction
      • Pendulum
      • Rope-and-pulley exercises in flexion-extension and abduction-adduction
      • L-bar exercises in flexion, abduction, internal and external rotation
  2. Strengthening exercises
    • Isometrics in flexion, extension, abduction, and internal-external rotation

II. **Phase II: Motion Phase (Weeks 2–6)**
  Goals
    • Increase range of motion
    • Improve strength and endurance
    • Decrease pain and inflammation
  A. Week 2
    1. Range-of-motion exercises
      (a) L-bar active-assisted exercises
        • External rotation at 45° abduction to tolerance
        • Internal rotation at 45° abduction to full range of motion
        • Shoulder flexion-extension
        • Shoulder abduction-adduction
      (b) Pendulum exercises
      (c) Rope-and-pulley exercises
    2. Initiate joint mobilization
    3. Strengthening exercises
      (a) Isometric internal-external rotation and abduction
      (b) Initiate isotonics for elbow in flexion-extension
      (c) Initiate isotonics for shoulder in abduction and flexion
      (d) Initiate isotonics for scapulothoracic musculature
  B. Week 4
    1. Range-of-motion exercises
      (a) Progress to tolerance on all exercises
        • External rotation at 90° abduction to tolerance
        • Internal rotation at 90° abduction to full range of motion
        • Continue all other range-of-motion exercises
    2. Strengthening exercises
      (a) Multiple-angle isometrics, 0° progressing to 45° abduction, flexion, internal and external rotation
      (b) Initiate shoulder isotonics for shoulder musculature in
        • Side-lying external rotation
        • Side-lying internal rotation
        • Abduction
        • Flexion
    3. Joint mobilization

III. **Phase III: Intermediate Phase (Weeks 6–10)**
  Goals
    • Regain and improve muscular strength
    • Normalize arthrokinematics
    • Improve neuromuscular control of shoulder complex
    • Normalize range of motion
  1. Continue isotonic strengthening
    (a) Flexion
    (b) Abduction
    (c) Internal rotation
    (d) External rotation
    (e) Supraspinatus
    (f) Extension
    (g) Shoulder shrugs
  2. Initiate surgical tubing exercises at 0° abduction in external-internal rotation
  3. Normalize arthrokinematics of shoulder complex
    (a) Continue joint mobilization
    (b) Improve neuromuscular control of shoulder complex
    (c) Initiate proprioceptive neuromuscular facilitation

Table 13–9. Rehabilitation Protocol After Bristow Procedure *Continued*

IV. **Phase IV: Advanced Strengthening Phase**
    Criteria to progress to phase IV
- Full, nonpainful range of motion
- No palpable tenderness
- Continued progression of resistance exercises

    Goals
- Improve strength, power, and endurance
- Improve neuromuscular control
- Prepare athlete for activity
  1. Continue isotonic strengthening (progressive-resistance exercises)
  2. Continue surgical tubing exercises
  3. Emphasize proprioceptive neuromuscular facilitation
  4. Initiate isokinetics

V. **Phase V: Return-to-Activity Phase**
    Criteria to progress to phase V
- Full range of motion
- No pain or palpable tenderness
- Satisfactory clinical examination
- Satisfactory isokinetic test

    Goals
- Progressively return athlete to prior full functional level
- Maintain optimal strength and endurance level

    Follow-up
- Isokinetic test
- Monitor exercise maintenance program
- Continue isotonic exercises for shoulder in external-internal rotation, abduction, flexion, and horizontal adduction, biceps, and triceps

Subluxation Inhibitor* is custom-fitted and is made of low- and high-density polyethylene. The SAWA shoulder orthosis† is an off-the-shelf brace made of cotton and rubber, with Velcro straps to limit motion. The Sully Brace‡ is another off-the-shelf brace made of neoprene. These types of braces have proven beneficial in athletes such as interior linemen, hockey players, and soccer players but have been completely unsuccessful in athletes who have to throw or catch a ball.

Posterior Instability

Posterior dislocation or subluxation is not as common as anterior instability, but it does occur. Usually, posterior subluxation results from traumatic forces that injure the posterior capsule. This can occur in football linemen who use their hands during blocking or rushing; with the elbow locked in extension and the shoulder flexed, the arm can be forcefully pushed posteriorly. Posterior dislocation may occur because of a fall onto an extended arm. The diagnosis is frequently missed because physical findings are not as dramatic as with an anterior dislocation.

Again, nonoperative treatment should be attempted first, using a balanced strengthening program for the anterior and posterior rotator cuff musculature. Strengthening of the posterior rotator cuff should be accomplished without placing the shoulder into a subluxated or apprehensive position.[78] An aggressive shoulder flexibility regimen is contraindicated because of the attenuated tissues. Engle and Canner[33] have reported success with a rehabilitation program that emphasizes PNF exercise techniques centered around development of the posterior cuff muscles. Success of the nonoperative program depends greatly on the type of athlete and the sport. Athletes who use their arms in an extended position in front of their body are more susceptible to recurrent symptoms.

Surgical management of those athletes who do not respond to nonoperative

*Available from SSI, Physical Support Systems, Inc., Windham, New Hampshire
†Available from Brace International, Scottsdale, Arizona
‡Available from The Saunders Group, Chaska, Minnesota

Table 13–10. Accelerated Rehabilitation Protocol After Anterior Capsular Shift

I. Phase I: Protection Phase (Weeks 0–6)
   Goals
   - Allow healing of sutured capsule
   - Begin early protected range of motion
   - Retard muscular atrophy
   - Decrease pain and inflammation
   A. Weeks 0–2
      1. Precautions
         (a) Sleep in immobilizer for 4 weeks
         (b) No overhead activities for 4–6 weeks
         (c) Wean from immobilizer and into sling as soon as possible
      2. Exercises
         (a) Gripping exercises with putty
         (b) Elbow flexion-extension and pronation-supination
         (c) Pendulum exercises (nonweighted)
         (d) Rope-and-pulley active-assisted exercises
            • Shoulder flexon to 90°
            • Shoulder abduction to 60°
         (e) L-bar exercises
            • External rotation to 15–20° with arm abducted to 40°
            • Shoulder flexion-extension to tolerance
         (f) Active range of motion for cervical spine
         (g) Isometrics for shoulder flexors, extensors, external and internal rotators and abductors
   Criteria for hospital discharge
   - Shoulder range of motion (active-assisted range of motion): Flexion 90°, abduction 45°, external rotation 40°
   - Minimal pain and swelling
   - "Good" proximal and distal muscle power
   B. Weeks 2–4
   Goals
   - Gradually increase range of motion
   - Normalize arthrokinematics
   - Improve strength
   - Decrease pain and inflammation
      1. Range-of-motion exercises
         (a) L-bar active-assisted exercises
            • External rotation in 40° abduction, progress to 45° abduction
            • Internal rotation in 40° abduction, progress to 45° abduction
            • Shoulder flexion-extension to tolerance
            • Shoulder abduction to tolerance
            • Shoulder horizontal abduction/adduction
         (b) Rope-and-pulley exercises in flexion-extension
         Note: All exercises are performed to tolerance. Athlete takes the movement to the point of pain or resistance and holds. *Gentle* self-capsular stretches are also performed.
      2. Gentle joint mobilization to re-establish normal arthrokinematics to scapulothoracic, glenohumeral, and sternoclavicular joints
      3. Strengthening exercises
         (a) Isometrics
         (b) May initiate tubing for external-internal rotation at 0° abduction
      4. Conditioning program for trunk, lower extremities, and cardiovascular system
      5. Decrease pain and inflammation: Use ice, nonsteroidal anti-inflammatory drugs, modalities
   C. Week 5
      1. Active-assisted range of motion flexion to tolerance
      2. Internal-external rotation at 45° abduction to tolerance
      3. Initiate isotonic (light weights) strengthening
      4. Gentle joint mobilization (grade III)
   D. Week 6
      1. Active-assisted range of motion: Continue all stretching exercises
      2. Progress external-internal rotation to 90° abduction

Table 13–10. Accelerated Rehabilitation Protocol After Anterior Capsular Shift *Continued*

II. **Phase II: Intermediate Phase (Weeks 7–12)**

Goals
- Achieve full nonpainful range of motion at weeks 8–10
- Normalize arthrokinematics
- Increase strength
- Improve neuromuscular control

A. Weeks 7–10
1. Range-of-motion exercises
   (a) L-bar active-assisted exercises
   (b) Continue all exercises listed above
   (c) Gradually increase range of motion to full range of motion by weeks 8–10
   (d) Continue self-capsular stretches
   (e) Continue joint mobilization
2. Strengthening exercises
   (a) Initiate isotonic dumbbell program for
      - Side-lying external rotation
      - Side-lying internal rotation
      - Shoulder abduction
      - Supraspinatus
      - Latissimus dorsi
      - Rhomboids
      - Biceps curl
      - Triceps curl
      - Shoulder shrug
      - Push-up in chair (serratus anterior)
   (b) Continue tubing at 0° for external-internal rotation
3. Initiate neuromuscular control exercise for scapulothoracic joint

B. Weeks 10–12
1. Continue all exercises listed above
2. Initiate tubing exercises for rhomboids, latissimus dorsi, biceps, and triceps
3. Initiate aggressive stretching and joint mobilization, if needed

III. **Phase III: Dynamic Strengthening Phase (Advanced Strengthening Phase) (Weeks 12–20)**

Criteria to progress to phase III
- Full, nonpainful range of motion
- No pain or tenderness
- Strength 70% or better compared to contralateral side

Goals
- Improve strength, power, and endurance
- Improve neuromuscular control
- Prepare athlete to begin to throw

Emphasis of phase III
- High-speed, high-energy strengthening exercises
- Eccentric exercises
- Diagonal patterns

A. Weeks 12–17
1. Exercises
   (a) Begin Throwers' Ten Exercise Program (Appendix C)
      - Initiate tubing exercises in 90/90 position for internal and external rotation (perform slow- and fast-speed sets)
      - Tubing for rhomboids
      - Tubing for latissimus dorsi
      - Tubing for biceps
      - Tubing for diagonal patterns D2 extension
      - Tubing for diagonal patterns D2 flexion
      - Continue dumbbell exercises for supraspinatus and deltoid
      - Continue serratus anterior strengthening exercises, floor push-ups
2. Continue trunk and lower extremity strengthening exercises
3. Continue neuromuscular exercises
4. Continue self-capsular stretches

Table continued on following page

Table 13–10. Rehabilitation Protocol After Accelerated Anterior Capsular Shift *Continued*

 B. Weeks 17–20
  1. Continue all exercises listed above
  2. Initiate plyometrics for shoulder
   • External rotation at 90° abduction
   • Internal rotation at 90° abduction
   • D2 extension plyometrics
   • Biceps plyometrics
   • Serratus anterior plyometrics
IV. **Phase IV: Throwing Phase (Weeks 20–26)**
 Criteria to progress to phase IV
  • Full range of motion
  • No pain or tenderness
  • Isokinetic test that fulfills criteria to throw
  • Satisfactory clinical examination
 Goal
  • Progressively increase activities to prepare athlete for full functional return
  1. Exercise
   (a) Initiate Interval Throwing Program (Appendix D) at week 20
    • Interval Throwing Program phase II at week 24
   (b) Continue Throwers' Ten Exercise Program
   (c) Continue plyometric exercises
  Return to sports at 26–30 weeks

care is controversial. The results after surgical reconstruction for posterior instability have been disappointing.[42, 90] Surgical techniques include shifting of the posterior capsule (capsulorrhaphy), posterior Bankart repair, or posterior osteotomy to help prevent dislocation. The posterior capsule tends to be much thinner than the anterior capsule and is thus prone to stretch out, which may contribute to diminished surgical success.

Rehabilitation after posterior capsulorrhaphy advances more slowly when compared to rehabilitation after anterior capsulorrhaphy. The most significant differences from the anterior capsulorrhaphy rehabilitation program include (1) no forward flexion above 90° and no horizontal adduction for 4 weeks to avoid stress on the repaired capsule; (2) slower restoration of internal rotation—internal rotation in the 90/90 position should not begin until approximately 6 weeks after surgery; and (3) a slower return to functional or sports activities.

Multidirectional Instability

Athletes who exhibit atraumatic (congenital), multidirectional instability pose a difficult problem, not only to the clinician but also to the surgeon. These individuals typically have generalized ligamentous and capsular laxity.[109] Most commonly these athletes are swimmers, gymnasts, and occasionally overhead athletes. The most common treatment plan for these individuals is a thorough nonoperative strengthening program. Although most frequently the program is successful, it is not uncommon for the athlete to experience intermittent symptoms.

Nonoperative treatment focuses on dynamic stabilization, proprioception, and neuromuscular control exercises. Rehabilitation techniques such as rhythmic stabilization, cocontractions, proprioceptive training, and motor control drills are the hallmark of a well-structured program. The program should attempt to balance the posterior and anterior musculature in an attempt to control and stabilize the glenohumeral joint. In patients with atraumatic instability it is critical to improve scapular muscle strength through an aggressive rehabilitation program.

Table 13–11. Rehabilitation Protocol After Open Anterior Capsulolabral (Bankart) Reconstruction

I. Phase I: Immediate Motion Phase
 A. Weeks 0–2
  1. Sling for comfort (1 week)
  2. Immobilization brace for 4 weeks (sleeping only)
  3. Gentle active-assisted range-of-motion exercises with L bar
   • Flexion to tolerance (0–120°)
   • External rotation at 20° abduction to tolerance (maximum 15–20°)
   • Internal rotation at 20° abduction to tolerance (maximum 45°)
  4. Rope-and-pulley exercises
  5. Elbow and hand range of motion
  6. Isometrics: External-internal rotation, abduction, biceps
  7. Squeeze ball exercises
  8. Elbow flexion-extension
  9. Ice
 B. Weeks 3–4
  1. Active-assisted range-of-motion exercises with L bar
   (a) Flexion to tolerance (maximum 120–140°)
   (b) External rotation at 45° abduction (acceptable 20–30°)
   (c) Internal rotation at 45° abduction (acceptable 45–60°)
  2. Initiate light isotonics for shoulder musculature in abduction, external-internal rotation and for supraspinatus and biceps
  3. Initiate scapular strengthening exercises; emphasize rhomboids, trapezius, serratus anterior
 C. Weeks 5–6
  1. Progress all range-of-motion exercises with active-assisted range of motion L bar
   • Flexion (maximum 160°)
   • External-internal rotation at 90° abduction: external rotation to 45–60°; internal rotation to 65–95°
  2. Upper extremity ergometer at 90° abduction
  3. Diagonal patterns, manual resistance
  4. Progress all strengthening exercises
II. Phase II: Intermediate Phase (Weeks 8–14)
 A. Weeks 8–10
  1. Progress to full range of motion
   • Flexion to 180°
   • External rotation in 90°
   • Internal rotation in 85°
  2. Isokinetic strengthening exercises (neutral position)
  3. Continue all strengthening exercises
  4. Initiate scapular strengthening exercises
 B. Weeks 10–14
  1. Continue all flexibility exercises, self-capsular stretches
  2. Throwers' Ten Exercise Program (Appendix C)
  3. Upper body ergometer, 90° abduction
  4. Initiate diagonal pattern (manual resistance)
III. Phase III: Advanced Phase (Months 4–6)
  1. Continue all flexibility exercises
   • External rotation stretch
   • Internal rotation stretch
   • Flexion stretch
   • Self-capsular stretches
  2. Continue Throwers' Ten Exercise Program
  3. Isokinetics external-internal rotation (90/90 position)
  4. Isokinetics test
  5. Plyometric exercises
  6. Initiate interval training program with physician approval
IV. Phase IV: Return-to-Activity Phase (Months 6–9)
  1. Continue all strengthening exercises—Throwers' Ten Exercise Program
  2. Continue all stretching exercises

Table 13–12. Rehabilitation Protocol After Arthroscopic Anterior Capsulolabral (Bankart) Reconstruction

I. **Phase I: Restricted Motion—Maximal Protection Phase**
  A. Weeks 0–2
    1. Sling for comfort (2 weeks)
    2. Immobilization brace for 4 weeks (sleeping only)
    3. Gentle active-assisted range of motion with L bar
      • Forward flexion to 60°
      • External rotation at 20° abduction (maximal motion 0°)
      • Internal rotation at 20° abduction (maximal motion 45°)
      Note: The athlete should not abduct and externally rotate shoulder during the first 4 weeks.
    4. Elbow and hand range of motion
    5. Isometrics: submaximal subpainful contraction—external and internal rotation, abduction of biceps with arm at side (0° abduction)
    6. Squeeze ball
    7. Ice, modalities to shoulder to control pain
  B. Weeks 3–4
    1. Discontinue use of sling
    2. Continue use of immobilization for sleep
    3. Continue gentle active-assisted range of motion with L bar
      • Flexion at 90°
      • External rotation at 20° abduction (maximal motion 15°)
      • Internal rotation at 20° abduction (maximal motion 65°)
    4. Initiate *light-weight* isotonic shoulder exercises for internal and external rotation, abduction, supraspinatus, biceps, triceps
    5. Initiate *light-weight* isotonic scapular strengthening in retraction, protraction, elevation, and depression
    6. Initiate upper body ergometer exercises at 70° abduction
II. **Phase II: Moderate Protection Phase (Weeks 7–14)**
  A. Weeks 7–9
    1. Progress all range-of-motion exercises
      • Flexion (0–180°)
      • External rotation at 90° abduction (maximal motion 75°)
      • Internal rotation at 90° abduction (maximal motion 85°)
    2. Continue isotonic strengthening program
    3. Initiate diagonal strengthening program
    4. Continue all scapular strengthening
    5. Initiate isokinetic exercises (neutral position)
    6. Initiate exercise tubing external-internal rotation (at 0° abduction)
  B. Weeks 10–14
  Goal
    • Achieve full range of motion by weeks 12–14
    1. Continue and progress all exercises listed above
    2. Initiate manual resistance exercise programs
III. **Phase III: Minimal Protection Phase (Weeks 15–21)**
  A. Weeks 15–18
    1. Continue all flexibility exercises and capsular stretches to maintain full range of motion
    2. Initiate Throwers' Ten Exercise Program (Appendix C)
    3. Initiate *light* swimming
    4. Initiate exercises in the 90° position
  B. Weeks 18–24
    1. Continue flexibility exercises
    2. Begin Interval Throwing Program (Appendix D) when
      • Full nonpainful range of motion is achieved
      • Strength is 90% of contralateral side
      • Pain or tenderness is absent
      • Clinical exam is satisfactory
    3. Continue Throwers' Ten Exercise Program
    4. Initiate plyometric exercise program
IV. **Phase IV: Advanced Strengthening Phase (Weeks 22–26)**
    1. Aggressive strengthening program for shoulder and scapular musculature
    2. Continue Throwers' Ten Exercise Program
    3. Continue plyometric program
    4. Progress to phase II of Interval Throwing Program
V. **Phase V: Return-to-activity Phase (Months 7–9)**
    1. Continue all strengthening exercises
    2. Continue all stretching exercises
    3. Begin unrestricted throwing

If nonsurgical treatment fails and the athlete is unable to participate in sports, surgical intervention may be indicated. Bigliani[12] has suggested that an inferior capsular shift may correct redundancy on all three sides: anterior, posterior, and inferior.

Glenoid Labrum Lesions

In recent years, increasing attention has been paid to the glenoid labrum. Glenoid labrum lesions are extremely common in athletes and can be classified as either atraumatic or traumatic lesions. Traumatic injuries to the glenoid capsulolabral complex are known to occur with glenohumeral dislocations or subluxations. With this mechanism of injury, a wide spectrum of glenoid labral injuries may occur, including a detachment of the labrum from the glenoid, a frank tear, or a combination of these lesions. Additionally, the labrum can be injured because of repetitive stresses during the throwing motion. Andrews and colleagues[2, 4] have described a tear of the superior aspect of the glenoid labrum at the origin of the biceps tendon. The authors theorized that this lesion may be due to repetitive forceful contraction of the biceps brachii during the follow-through phase of throwing.

Recently Snyder and associates[94] have described an anterosuperior labral complex lesion. This superior labrum, anterior, and posterior (SLAP) lesion begins posteriorly and extends anteriorly and involves the "anchor" of the long head of the biceps brachii to the labrum. Numerous mechanisms may produce this lesion. A labral tear may result from a fall onto an outstretched arm, from forceful muscular contraction of the biceps, or from repetitive strenuous overhead sport movements. Snyder and colleagues[94] have classified the SLAP lesions into four types (Fig. 13–25). In the type I lesion, the superior labrum is markedly frayed, but the attachments of the labrum and biceps tendon remain intact. The

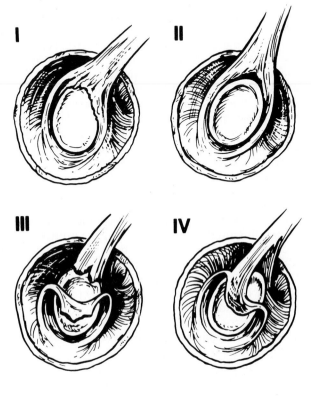

Figure 13–25. Classification of superior labrum, anterior and posterior lesions according to Snyder et al.[94] (From Zuckerman, J.D. [1993]: Glenoid labrum lesions. *In*: Andrews, J.R., and Wilk, K.E. [eds.]: The Athlete's Shoulder. New York, Churchill Livingstone, p. 232.)

type II lesion is similar in appearance to the type I lesion, except that the attachment of the superior labrum is compromised, resulting in instability of the labrum-biceps complex. The type III lesion consists of a bucket-handle tear of the labrum, which can displace into the joint. Type IV lesions are similar to type III lesions, except that the labral tear extends into the biceps tendon, allowing it to sublux into the joint.

Specific treatment recommendations are based on the type of labral lesion present. In type I lesions, the frayed labral tissue should be débrided back to the intact labrum. Type II lesions are usually treated with débridement, and the superior glenoid labrum should be reattached to the superior glenoid with an absorbable tack or with a similar surgical technique. In type III lesions the bucket-handle tear is excised, and in type IV lesions the tear is excised or tenodesed. The rehabilitation program must be designed differently for the débrided labral lesion compared to the reattached labral lesion. The patient with the reattached labrum requires a period of restricted motion in the immediate postsurgical period to allow adequate tissue healing. We emphasize no active contraction of the biceps for 6 to 8 weeks and no active forward flexion past 90° for 6 weeks. Conversely, in patients who have undergone labrum débridement, motion and strengthening may progress much more rapidly, and rehabilitation is based on signs and symptoms.

Acromioclavicular Separation

Injuries involving the acromioclavicular joint can occur insidiously from activities requiring repetitive overhead activity. Acute injuries occur either from direct trauma, in which the athlete falls on the tip of the shoulder and depresses the acromion process inferiorly, or from a fall on the outstretched arm, in which the forces are transmitted superiorly through the acromion process. The extent of acromioclavicular sprain or separation depends on whether the coracoclavicular ligaments are traumatized or the main stabilizing acromioclavicular ligaments are damaged. Rockwood[84] has identified six types of acromioclavicular joint sprains (Fig. 13–26). In the type I sprain the acromioclavicular ligament is injured. Type II injuries involve injury to the acromioclavicular ligament and a sprain of the coracoclavicular ligament. Type III injuries involve disruption of the acromioclavicular and coracoclavicular ligaments and some detachment of the deltoid and upper trapezius muscles from the distal clavicle. Type IV injuries are similar to type III injuries, except that in type IV acromioclavicular joint sprains, the clavicle displaces posteriorly through the trapezius muscle, and the deltoid and trapezius are detached. In type V injuries there is significant displacement of the clavicle by 100% to 300%. Type VI injuries involve the distal clavicle displacing inferiorly under the acromion. Somewhat similar classifications have been offered by other authors.[73]

Treatment for grade I and grade II injuries is nonoperative, but grade III injury treatment is still controversial. Many physicians elect to treat grade III injuries nonoperatively and believe that athletes do better with nonoperative management,[54, 76] whereas others believe the joint needs to be stabilized surgically. Depending on the extent of damage, a number of surgical measures are available including (1) stabilization of the clavicle to the coracoid process with a screw; (2) transarticular fixation of the acromioclavicular joint with pins after reduction; (3) resection of the outer end of the clavicle; and (4) transposition of the coracoacromial ligament to the top of the acromioclavicular joint. Biomechanical studies[36] have indicated that the superior acromioclavicular ligament is the most important for stabilizing the acromioclavicular joint for normal daily activities. The conoid ligament is the most important for supporting the joint against significant injury.

Rehabilitation following first- and second-degree acromioclavicular separa-

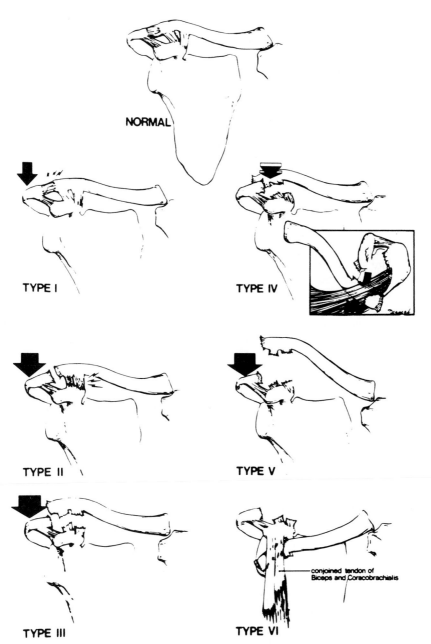

Figure 13–26. Rockwood classification of acromioclavicular joint sprains. (From Rockwood, C.A., and Young, D.C. [1990]: Disorders of the acromioclavicular joint. *In*: Rockwood, C.A., and Matsen, F.A. (eds.): The Shoulder. Philadelphia, W.B. Saunders, pp. 413–468.)

tions consists of progressing motion as tolerated and beginning a PRE program when active range of motion is equal bilaterally. Modalities may be used in the early stages of healing to help decrease inflammation and pain. Third-degree separations treated nonoperatively usually require 2 to 4 weeks of immobilization, with a gradual progression of motion and strengthening exercises after immobilization. Pendulum exercises, elbow range-of-motion exercises, isometrics in all planes, and rope-and-pulley exercises for shoulder flexion and abduction can be initiated as tolerated after immobilization. Precautions in rehabilitation after a surgical repair of the acromioclavicular joint are similar to those after conservative care of grade III injuries, including limitation of abduction and flexion to 90° for approximately 3 to 4 weeks. Pendulum and isometric exercises in all planes are encouraged in the initial stages of postsurgical rehabilitation. Range of motion is progressed to 90° in all planes as tolerated after 4 weeks. Rehabilitation should concentrate on strengthening the rotator cuff and scapula stabilizers and on restoring neuromuscular control and arthrokinematics, not unlike rehabilitation after other shoulder injuries.

SUMMARY

The mobility of the shoulder joint is acquired at the expense of stability. Shoulder injuries can be induced acutely through traumatic injuries, or they may arise with an insidious onset as a result of repetitive stresses over time. Overuse injuries to the shoulder are common in athletes whose endeavors require repetitive overhead activities, particularly throwers and swimmers. Most shoulder injuries occur during the late cocking, acceleration, and deceleration phases of throwing. The most common shoulder injuries include rotator cuff tendinitis or partial tears, compressive cuff disease, posterior impingement syndrome, and shoulder instability (most commonly anterior).

Rehabilitation of these injuries should concentrate on developing dynamic joint stability. Additionally, those athletes who are susceptible to shoulder pathology should be placed on an off-season shoulder flexibility and rotator cuff strengthening program to help prevent shoulder problems. They should continue this stretching and strengthening program two or three times weekly during the season. Preventive and postinjury exercises should also attempt to strengthen the rotator cuff muscles to dynamically stabilize the glenohumeral joint and the scapular stabilizers that help orient the glenoid fossa with the humeral head to maintain stability. Weakness in the scapula stabilizers can predispose the athlete to a variety of shoulder pathologies.

After shoulder surgery or injury, emphasis should be placed on addressing the inflammation process and restoring motion. After initiation of a rotator cuff strengthening program, PNF techniques may be implemented to help restore neuromuscular control. In the late phases of rehabilitation, eccentric, isokinetic, and plyometric exercises may be initiated. In the advanced strengthening phase, the goals of the program are to initiate sport-specific types of training for the shoulder joint complex.

The goals of shoulder rehabilitation are to prevent injuries through off-season and in-season conditioning programs addressing flexibility, rotator cuff strength, scapular stability, and neuromuscular control of the shoulder girdle. The program should be progressive and systematic, using the principles of periodization.

THERAPEUTIC SHOULDER EXERCISE PROGRAM
Range-of-Motion Exercises

Circumduction Pendulum Swings. The athlete leans over the table, supporting the body with the uninvolved arm and allowing the involved arm to hang

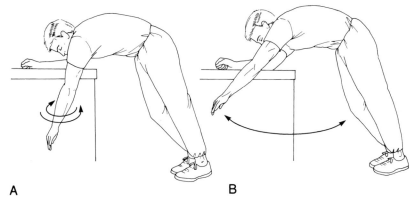

Figure 13–27. *A* and *B*, Circumduction pendulum swings.

straight down in a relaxed position. The athlete gently swings the arm in circles clockwise and counterclockwise (Fig. 13–27*A*), in a pendulum motion forward and backward (Fig. 13–27*B*) and side to side, repeating one set of 10 repetitions each and progressing to five sets of 10 repetitions each, as tolerated.

Rope-and-Pulley Exercises. The overhead rope and pulley should be positioned in a doorway. The athlete sits in a chair with the back against the door, directly underneath the pulley.

Active-Assisted Flexion. With the elbow straight and the back of the hand facing upward, the athlete raises the involved arm to the front of the body as high as possible (Fig. 13–28*A*), assisting as needed by pulling with the uninvolved arm and holding for 5 seconds. The arm is lowered slowly, using the uninvolved arm to control lowering as needed. The athlete repeats one set of 10 repetitions, progressing to five sets of 10 repetitions as tolerated.

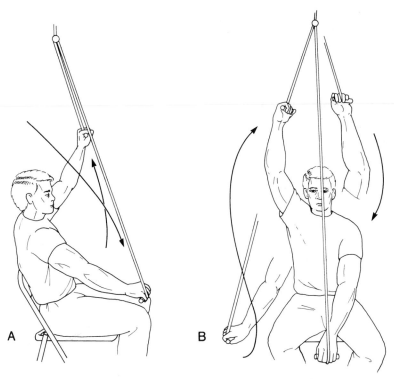

Figure 13–28. *A*, Active-assisted flexion. *B*, Active-assisted abduction.

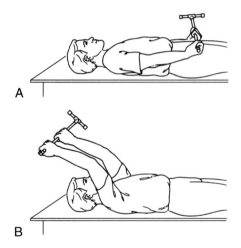

A

B

Figure 13–29. *A* and *B*, Supine flexion. (Redrawn from Wilk, K.E., Andrews, J.R., Arrigo, C.A., et al. [1997]: Preventive and Rehabilitative Exercises for the Shoulder and Elbow, 5th ed. Birmingham, Alabama, American Sports Medicine Institute.)

Active-Assisted Abduction. With the elbow straight and the hand rotated outward as far as possible, the athlete raises the involved arm to the side of the body as high as possible (Fig. 13–28*B*), assisting as needed by pulling with the uninvolved arm and holding for 5 seconds. The arm is lowered slowly using the uninvolved arm to control lowering as needed. The athlete repeats one set of 10 repetitions, progressing to five sets of 10 repetitions as tolerated.

Supine Flexion. The athlete lies on the back, grips the bar in both hands with the palms up and arms straight (Fig. 13–29*A*), raises both arms overhead as far as possible (Fig. 13–29*B*), and holds for 5 seconds before returning to the starting position. This is repeated 10 to 15 times. This may be performed with the thumb up as an alternate method, particularly if impingement syndrome is present.

Supine Abduction. The athlete lies on the back with the involved arm at the side of the body, straightens the involved arm, and rotates the hand outward as far as possible. Then the athlete slides the arm along the table, bed, or floor, moving the arm away from the side as far as possible and using a T bar to help push it up (Fig. 13–30*A* and *B*). This position is held for 5 seconds before returning to the starting position, and the exercise is repeated 10 to 15 times.

SUPINE EXTERNAL ROTATION

External Rotation (0° Abduction). The athlete lies on the back with the involved arm against the body and the elbow bent at 90° (Fig. 13–31*A*). Gripping the T-bar handle with the uninvolved arm, the athlete pushes the involved shoulder into external rotation with the T bar (Fig. 13–31*B*). This position is held for 5 seconds before returning to the starting position, and the exercise is repeated. A towel should be placed under the arm to stretch in the scapular plane.

Exercise Progression. Shoulder external rotation can be progressed by per-

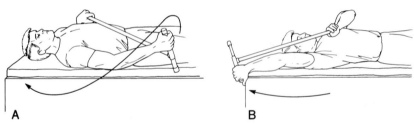

A

B

Figure 13–30. *A* and *B*, Supine abduction.

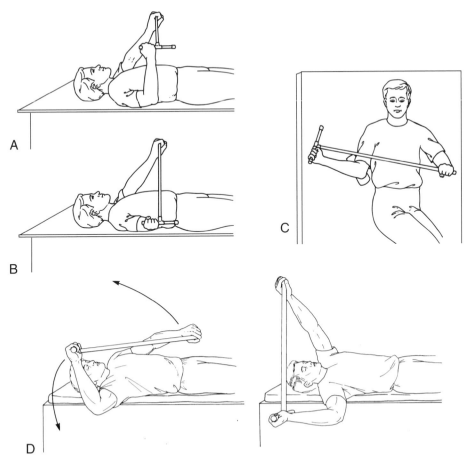

Figure 13–31. *A* and *B*, External rotation. *C* and *D*, Exercise progression. (*A* to *C* redrawn from Wilk, K.E., Andrews, J.R., Arrigo, C.A., et al. [1997]: Preventive and Rehabilitative Exercises for the Shoulder and Elbow, 5th ed. Birmingham, Alabama, American Sports Medicine Institute.)

forming this exercise at 45° (Fig. 13–31*C*) and 90° (Fig. 13–31*D*) degrees of shoulder abduction.

Standing External Rotation. With the involved arm overhead, the athlete holds a towel behind the neck and holds the other end of the towel with the uninvolved arm and pulls down (Fig. 13–32) As the left arm pulls in a downward direction, the right arm rotates externally. This position is held for 5 seconds before returning to the starting position, and the exercise is repeated 10 to 15 times.

Supine Internal Rotation. The athlete lies on the back with the involved arm out to the side of the body at 90° and the elbow bent at 90°. Gripping the T bar in the hand of the involved arm and keeping the elbow in a fixed position, the athlete uses the uninvolved arm to push the involved arm into internal rotation with the T bar (Fig. 13–33). This position is held for 5 seconds before returning to the starting position, and the exercise is repeated 10 to 15 times.

Standing Internal Rotation. The athlete's involved arm is behind the back holding a T bar or a towel (Fig. 13–34). The uninvolved arm is overhead, pulling the bar or towel upward. This action will further rotate the shoulder inward, internally rotating the involved arm. This position is held for 5 seconds before returning to the starting position, and the exercise is repeated 10 to 15 times.

Horizontal Abduction-Adduction. The athlete lies on the back and holds the T bar in front with the thumbs up (Fig. 13–35*A*). Keeping the arms straight, the athlete takes the arms as far as possible to one side of the body (Fig. 13–35*B*),

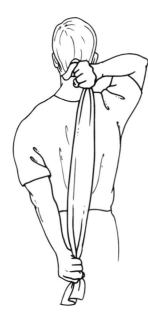

Figure 13–32. Standing external rotation. (Redrawn from Wilk, K.E., Andrews, J.R., Arrigo, C.A., et al. [1997]: Preventive and Rehabilitative Exercises for the Shoulder and Elbow, 5th ed. Birmingham, Alabama, American Sports Medicine Institute.)

holds for 5 seconds, and then take the arms as far as possible to the other side (Fig. 13–35C). Someone stabilizes the scapula on the affected side by holding the lateral border. This position is held for 5 seconds before returning to the starting position, and the exercise is repeated 10 to 15 times.

Posterior Capsular Stretch. The athlete grasps the elbow of the involved arm with the opposite hand and pulls the arm across the front of the chest (Fig. 13–36), holding for 5 seconds. The athlete then relaxes and repeats the exercise 10 to 15 times.

Inferior Capsular Stretch. The athlete holds the involved arm overhead with the elbow bent (Fig. 13–37A) and, using the uninvolved arm, stretches the arm farther overhead (Fig. 13–37B) until a stretching sensation is felt. This position is held for 5 seconds, and the exercise is repeated 10 to 15 times.

Anterior Capsular Stretch. The athlete stands in a doorway with the elbow straight and the shoulder abducted to 90° and externally rotated. With pressure

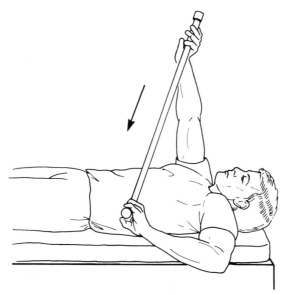

Figure 13–33. Supine internal rotation.

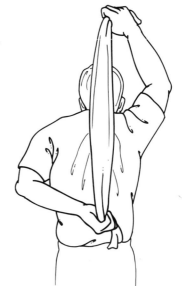

Figure 13–34. Standing internal rotation. (Redrawn from Wilk, K.E., Andrews, J.R., Arrigo, C.A., et al. [1997]: Preventive and Rehabilitative Exercises for the Shoulder and Elbow, 5th ed. Birmingham, Alabama, American Sports Medicine Institute.)

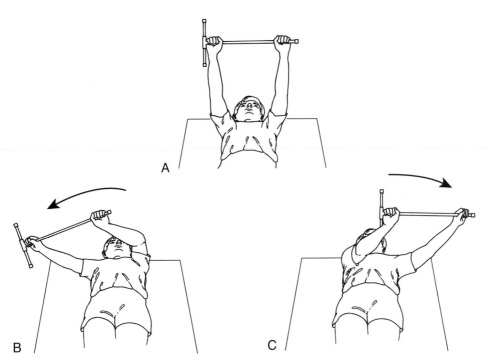

Figure 13–35. A to C, Horizontal abduction and adduction. (Redrawn from Wilk, K.E., Andrews, J.R., Arrigo, C.A., et al. [1997]: Preventive and Rehabilitative Exercises for the Shoulder and Elbow, 5th ed. Birmingham, Alabama, American Sports Medicine Institute.)

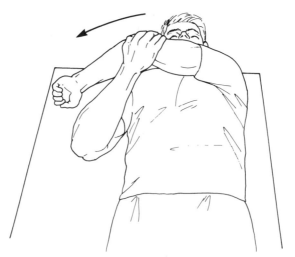

Figure 13–36. Posterior capsular stretch.

on the arm, the arm is forced back in order to stretch the front of the shoulder (Fig. 13–38). This position is held for 5 seconds, and the exercise is repeated 10 to 15 times.

Strengthening Exercises

ISOMETRICS

Flexion. The athlete stands facing out of a doorway, placing the involved arm in front (Fig. 13–39). The forearm and hand are placed on the door frame, and the athlete pushes as if to raise the arm overhead. The position is held at a submaximal force for 8 seconds, and the exercise is repeated.

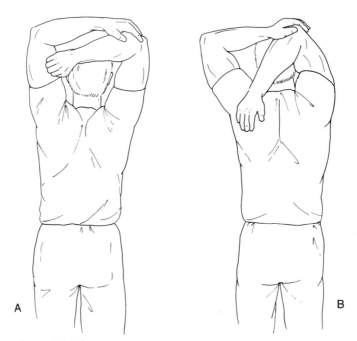

A   B

Figure 13–37. *A* and *B*, Inferior capsular stretch.

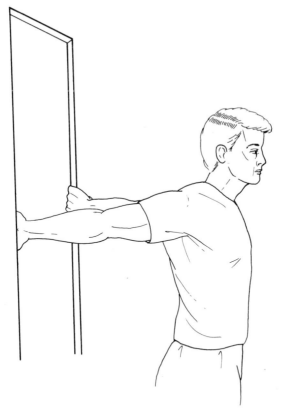

Figure 13–38. Anterior capsular stretch.

Figure 13–39. Flexion. (Redrawn from Wilk, K.E., Andrews, J.R., Arrigo, C.A., et al. [1997]: Preventive and Rehabilitative Exercises for the Shoulder and Elbow, 5th ed. Birmingham, Alabama, American Sports Medicine Institute.)

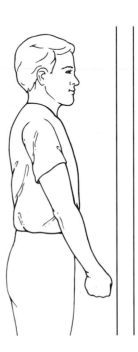

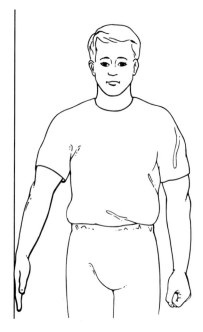

Figure 13–40. Abduction. (Redrawn from Wilk, K.E., Andrews, J.R., Arrigo, C.A., et al. [1997]: Preventive and Rehabilitative Exercises for the Shoulder and Elbow, 5th ed. Birmingham, Alabama, American Sports Medicine Institute.)

Abduction. The athlete stands against a wall or in a doorway with the involved arm at the side (Fig. 13–40) and presses back the forearm into the surface, keeping the arm at the side with the elbow straight. The position is held at a submaximal force for 8 seconds, and the exercise is repeated.

Extension. The athlete stands in a doorway in front of the door frame, places the involved arm slightly behind the body (Fig. 13–41), and pushes backward into the door frame. The position is held at a submaximal force for 8 seconds, and the exercise is repeated.

External Rotation. The athlete stands against a wall or in a doorway with the arm at the side and the elbow bent to 90° (Fig. 13–42) and presses the back of

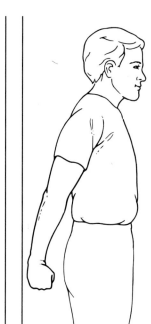

Figure 13–41. Extension. (Redrawn from Wilk, K.E., Andrews, J.R., Arrigo, C.A., et al. [1997]: Preventive and Rehabilitative Exercises for the Shoulder and Elbow, 5th ed. Birmingham, Alabama, American Sports Medicine Institute.)

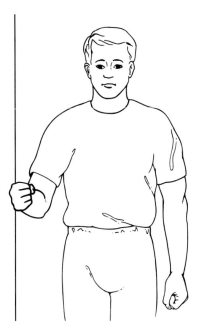

Figure 13–42. External rotation. (Redrawn from Wilk, K.E., Andrews, J.R., Arrigo, C.A., et al. [1997]: Preventive and Rehabilitative Exercises for the Shoulder and Elbow, 5th ed. Birmingham, Alabama, American Sports Medicine Institute.)

the forearm into the surface. The position is held at a submaximal force for 8 seconds, and the exercise is repeated.

Internal Rotation. The athlete stands against a wall or in a doorway with the arm at the side and the elbow bent to 90° (Fig. 13–43) and presses the front of the forearm into the surface. The position is held at a submaximal force for 8 seconds, and the exercise is repeated.

Elbow Flexion. The athlete uses the uninvolved arm to hold the involved elbow at angles of 45°, 90°, and 135° (Fig. 13–44) and flexes the elbow into the uninvolved hand, keeping the elbow still. The position is held at a submaximal force for 8 seconds, and the exercise is repeated.

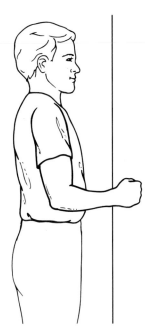

Figure 13–43. Internal rotation. (Redrawn from Wilk, K.E., Andrews, J.R., Arrigo, C.A., et al. [1997]: Preventive and Rehabilitative Exercises for the Shoulder and Elbow, 5th ed. Birmingham, Alabama, American Sports Medicine Institute.)

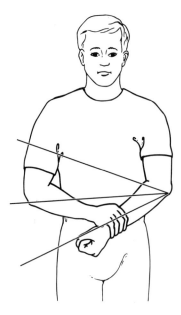

Figure 13–44. Elbow flexion. (Redrawn from Wilk, K.E., Andrews, J.R., Arrigo, C.A., et al. [1997]: Preventive and Rehabilitative Exercises for the Shoulder and Elbow, 5th ed. Birmingham, Alabama, American Sports Medicine Institute.)

ISOTONICS

Shoulder Flexion. The athlete stands with the elbow straight and the palm of the hand against the side, raises the involved arm out to the front of the body with the thumb up, and continues overhead as high as possible (Fig. 13–45). This position is held for 2 seconds, and the arm is slowly lowered.

Shoulder Abduction. The athlete stands with the elbow straight and the hand rotated outward as far as possible and raises the involved arm to the side of body as high as possible (Fig. 13–46). This position is held for 2 seconds, and the arm is slowly lowered.

Supraspinatus Strengthening ("Empty Can" Position). The athlete stands with the elbow straight and the hand rotated inward as far as possible and

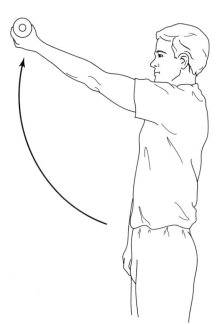

Figure 13–45. Shoulder flexion.

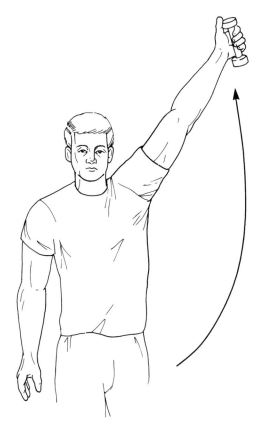

Figure 13-46. Shoulder abduction.

raises the arm to be parallel to the floor at a 30° angle to the body (Fig. 13–47). This position is held for 2 seconds, and the arm is slowly lowered.

Supraspinatus, Rotator Cuff, and Deltoid Strengthening ("Full Can" Position). The athlete stands with the elbow extended and the thumb up and raises the arm to shoulder level at a 30° angle in front of the body (Fig. 13–48). The arm should not go above shoulder level. This position is held for 2 seconds, and the arm is slowly lowered.

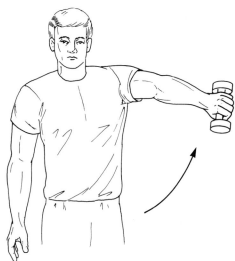

Figure 13-47. Supraspinatus strengthening ("empty can" position).

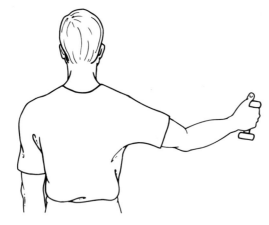

Figure 13–48. Strengthening, rotator cuff, and deltoid strengthening ("full can" position). (Redrawn from Wilk, K.E., Andrews, J.R., Arrigo, C.A., et al. [1997]: Preventive and Rehabilitative Exercises for the Shoulder and Elbow, 5th ed. Birmingham, Alabama, American Sports Medicine Institute.)

Prone Horizontal Abduction. The athlete lies on the table on the stomach, with the involved arm hanging straight to the floor. With the hand rotated outward as far as possible, the arm is raised out to the side, parallel to the floor (Fig. 13–49). This position is held for 2 seconds, and the arm is slowly lowered.

Prone Horizontal Abduction (100°). The athlete lies on the table on the stomach, with the involved arm hanging straight to the floor. With the hand rotated outward as far as possible and the shoulder at approximately 100° of abduction, the arm is raised out to the side, parallel to the floor (Fig. 13–50). This position is held for 2 seconds, and the arm is slowly lowered.

Shoulder Extension. The athlete lies on the table on the stomach, with the involved arm hanging straight to the floor. With the hand rotated outward as far as possible, the arm is raised straight back into extension as far as possible (Fig. 13–51). When lifting the arm straight back, the athlete continues to rotate the extremity externally as far as possible through the entire range of motion. This position is held for 2 seconds, and the arm is slowly lowered.

Side-lying External Rotation. The athlete lies on the uninvolved side, with the involved arm at the side of the body and the elbow bent at 90°. Keeping the elbow of the involved arm fixed to the side, the arm is rotated into external rotation (Fig. 13–52). This position is held for 2 seconds, and the arm is slowly lowered.

Side-lying Internal Rotation. The athlete lies on the involved side with the involved arm at the side of the body and the elbow bent at 90°. Keeping the elbow of the involved arm fixed to the side, the arm is rotated into internal

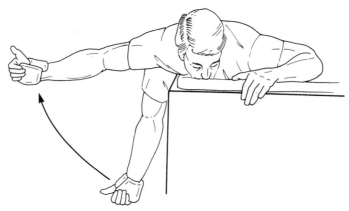

Figure 13–49. Prone horizontal abduction.

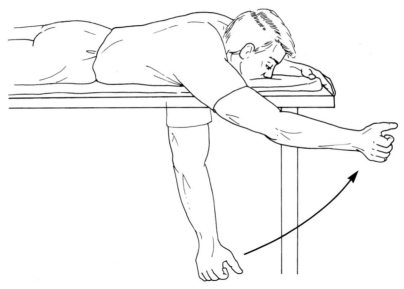

Figure 13–50. Prone horizontal abduction (100°).

rotation (Fig. 13–53). This position is held for 2 seconds, and the arm is slowly lowered.

Shoulder Shrug. The athlete stands with the arms by the side, lifts the shoulders up to the ears, holds for 2 seconds (Fig. 13–54A), pulls the shoulders back, and pinches the shoulder blades together (Fig. 13–54B). This position is held for 2 seconds, the shoulders are relaxed, and the exercise is repeated.

Biceps Curl. The athlete supports the involved arm with the opposite hand and bends the elbow to full flexion. This position is held for 2 seconds, and the arm is then extended completely (Fig. 13–55).

French Curl (Triceps). The athlete raises the involved arm overhead, providing support at the elbow with the opposite hand, and straightens the arm overhead (Fig. 13–56). This position is held for 2 seconds, and the arm is then slowly lowered.

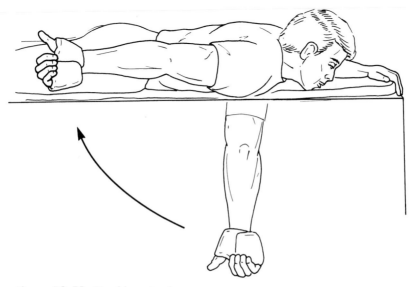

Figure 13–51. Shoulder extension.

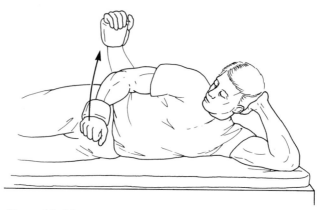

Figure 13–52. Side-lying external rotation.

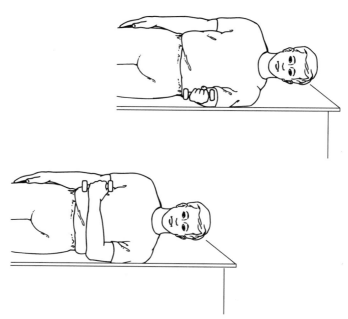

Figure 13–53. Side-lying internal rotation. (Redrawn from Wilk, K.E., Andrews, J.R., Arrigo, C.A., et al. [1997]: Preventive and Rehabilitative Exercises for the Shoulder and Elbow, 5th ed. Birmingham, Alabama, American Sports Medicine Institute.)

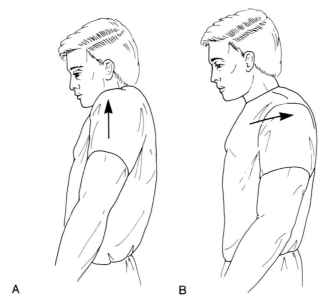

Figure 13–54. *A* and *B*, Shoulder shrugs.

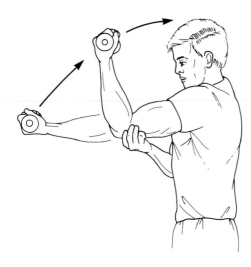

Figure 13–55. Biceps curl.

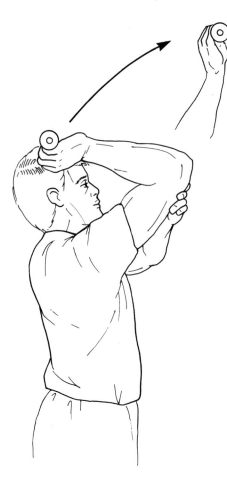

Figure 13–56. French curl (triceps).

Progressive Push-up. The athlete starts with a push-up into the wall, gradually progressing to the tabletop (Fig. 13–57) and then to the floor, as tolerated.

Punch. The athlete lies on the back, holding a medicine ball or dumbbell, and punches the arm up toward the ceiling, allowing the shoulder blade to lift off the table (Fig. 13–58). The position is held for 2 seconds, the arm is slowly returned to the starting position, and the exercise is repeated.

Seated Rowing. The athlete sits in a chair facing a wall to which tubing has been affixed at shoulder level (Fig. 13–59A). The athlete brings the arm out to 90°, holds the tubing with palms down, pulls the elbows back, and squeezes the shoulder blades together (Fig. 13–59B). The position is held for 2 seconds, the arm is returned to starting position, and the exercise is repeated.

Advanced Strengthening Exercises

External Rotation at 0° Abduction. Standing with the elbow fixed at the side, the elbow at 90° of flexion, and the involved arm across the front of the body, the athlete grips the tubing handle (the other end of the tubing is fixed) (Fig. 13–60A) and pulls out with the arm while keeping the elbow at the side (Fig. 13–60B). The tubing is returned slowly in a controlled manner.

Internal Rotation at 0° Abduction. Standing, with the elbow at the side fixed at 90° and the shoulder rotated out, the athlete grips the tubing handle (the other end of the tubing is fixed) (Fig. 13–61A) and pulls the arm across the body,

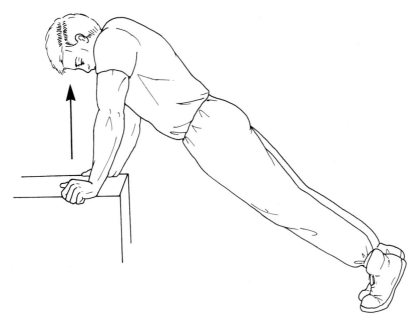

Figure 13–57. Progressive push-up.

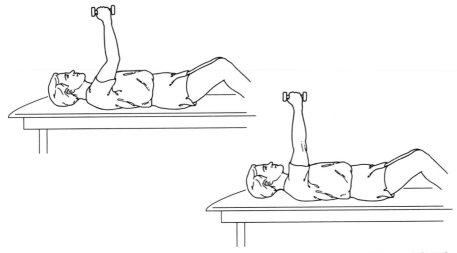

Figure 13–58. Punches. (Redrawn from Wilk, K.E., Andrews, J.R., Arrigo, C.A., et al. [1997]: Preventive and Rehabilitative Exercises for the Shoulder and Elbow, 5th ed. Birmingham, Alabama, American Sports Medicine Institute.)

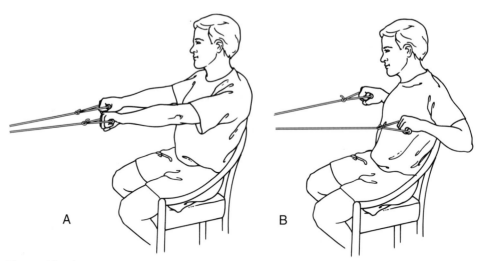

Figure 13–59. *A* and *B*, Seated rowing. (Redrawn from Wilk, K.E., Andrews, J.R., Arrigo, C.A., et al. [1997]: Preventive and Rehabilitative Exercises for the Shoulder and Elbow, 5th ed. Birmingham, Alabama, American Sports Medicine Institute.)

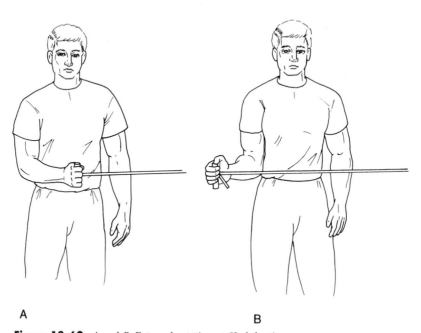

Figure 13–60. *A* and *B*, External rotation at 0° abduction.

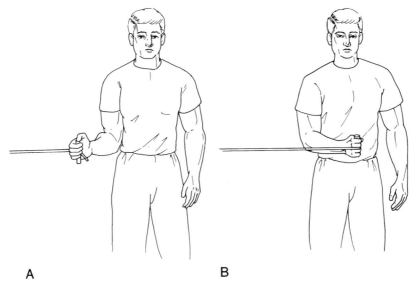

Figure 13–61. *A* and *B,* Internal rotation at 0° abduction.

keeping the elbow at the side (Fig. 13–61*B).* The tubing is returned slowly and in a controlled manner.

External Rotation at 90° Abduction—Slow. The athlete stands with the shoulder abducted 90° and the elbow flexed 90° and grips the tubing handle (the other end of the tubing is fixed straight ahead) (Fig. 13–62A and B). Keeping the shoulder abducted, the athlete rotates the shoulder back (keeping the elbow at 90°), slowly returns to the starting position, pauses, and repeats the exercise.

External Rotation at 90° Abduction—Fast. This exercise is the same as the previous one except that the athlete externally rotates the shoulder quickly, keeping the elbow at 90°. The tubing and hand are returned to the starting position quickly and in a controlled manner.

Internal Rotation at 90° Abduction—Slow. The athlete stands with the shoulder abducted to 90° and externally rotated to 90° and the elbow flexed to 90°

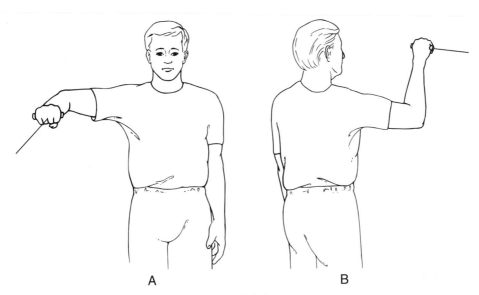

Figure 13–62. *A* and *B,* External rotation at 90° abduction.

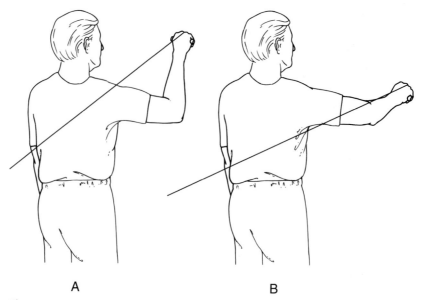

Figure 13–63. *A* and *B*, Internal rotation at 90° abduction.

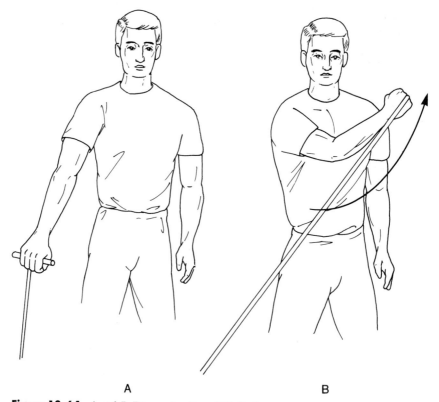

Figure 13–64. *A* and *B*, Diagonal pattern (D1) flexion.

and grips the tubing handle (the other end of the tubing is fixed straight ahead) (Fig. 13–63*A* and *B*). Keeping the shoulder abducted, the athlete rotates the shoulder back (keeping the elbow at 90°), slowly returns to the starting position, pauses, and repeats.

Internal Rotation at 90° Abduction—Fast. This exercise is the same as the previous one except that the athlete internally rotates the shoulder quickly, keeping the elbow at 90°. The tubing and hand are returned to the starting position quickly and in a controlled manner.

Diagonal Pattern (D1) Flexion. The athlete grips the tubing handle in the hand of the involved arm. The athlete begins with the arm out 45° from the side and the palm facing backward (Fig. 13–64*A*). After turning the palm forward, the athlete proceeds to flex the elbow and brings the arm up and over the uninvolved shoulder (Fig. 13–64*B*), then turns the palm down and reverses to take the arm to the starting position. The exercise should be performed in a controlled manner.

Diagonal Pattern (D2) Flexion. The athlete's involved hand grips the tubing handle across the body and against the opposite thigh (Fig. 13–65*A*). Starting with the palm down, the athlete rotates the palm up to begin, proceeds to flex

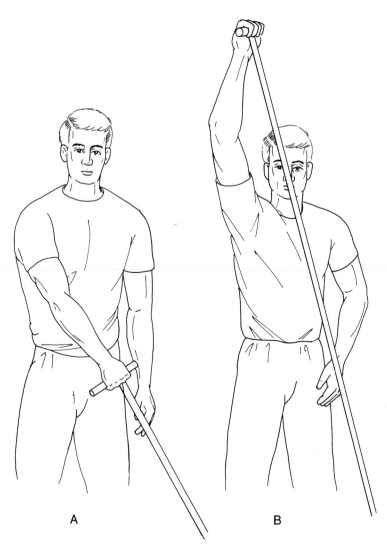

A   B

Figure 13–65. *A* and *B*, Diagonal pattern (D2) flexion.

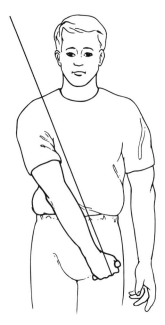

Figure 13–66. Diagonal pattern (D2) extension. (Redrawn from Wilk, K.E., Andrews, J.R., Arrigo, C.A., et al. [1997]: Preventive and Rehabilitative Exercises for the Shoulder and Elbow, 5th ed. Birmingham, Alabama, American Sports Medicine Institute.)

the elbow, and brings the arm up and over the involved shoulder with the palm facing inward (Fig. 13–65B). The palm is turned down, and the movement is reversed to take the arm to the starting position. The exercise should be performed in a controlled manner.

Diagonal Pattern (D2) Extension. The athlete grips the tubing handle overhead and out to the side with the involved hand and pulls the tubing down and across the body to the opposite side of the leg (Fig. 13–66), leading with the thumb during the motion.

References

1. Ahmadain, A.M. (1987): The Magnuson-Stack operation for recurrent anterior dislocation of the shoulder. J. Bone Joint Surg. [Br.], 69:111–114.
2. Andrews, J.R., and Carson, W.G. (1984): The arthroscopic treatment of glenoid labrum tears in the throwing athlete. Orthop. Trans., 8:44–49.
3. Andrews, J.R., and Meister K. (1993): Classification and treatment of rotator cuff injuries in the overhead athlete. J. Orthop. Sports Phys. Ther., 18:413–421.
4. Andrews, J.R., Carson, W.G., and McLeod, W.D. (1985): Glenoid labrum tears related to the long head of the biceps. Am. J. Sports Med., 13:337–341.
5. Arnheim, D. (1985): Modern Principles of Athletic Training. St. Louis, C.V. Mosby.
6. Aronen, J.G. (1986): Anterior shoulder dislocation in sports. Sports Med., 3:224–234.
7. Aronen, J.G., and Regan, K. (1984): Decreasing the incidence of recurrence of first-time anterior shoulder dislocations with rehabilitation. Am. J. Sports Med., 12:283–291.
8. Basmajian, J.V. (1963): The surgical anatomy and function of the arm-trunk mechanism. Surg. Clin. North Am., 43:1475–1479.
9. Bechtol, C. (1980): Biomechanics of the shoulder. Clin. Orthop., 146:37–41.
10. Berger, R.A. (1982): Applied Exercise Physiology. Philadelphia, Lea & Febiger, p. 267.
11. Reference deleted.
12. Bigliani, L.U. (1990): Multidirectional instability. Advances on the Knee and Shoulder. Cincinnati Sports Medicine, Cincinnati, OH.
13. Bigliani, L.U., Morrison, D., and April, E.W. (1986): The morphology of the acromion and its relationship to rotator cuff tears. Orthop. Trans., 10:228.
14. Blackburn, T.A. (1987): Throwing injuries to the shoulder. *In:* Donatelli, R. (ed.): Physical Therapy of the Shoulder. New York, Churchill Livingstone.
15. Blackburn, T.A., McLeod, W. D., White, B. W., and Wofford, L. (1990): EMG analysis of posterior rotator cuff exercises. Athl. Train., 25:40–45.
16. Bland, J. (1977): The painful shoulder. Semin. Arthritis Rheumatol., 7:21–47.
17. Boissonnault, W.G., and Janos, S.C. (1989): Dysfunction, evaluation, and treatment of the

shoulder. *In:* Donatelli, R., and Wooden, M.J. (eds.): Orthopaedic Physical Therapy. New York, Churchill Livingstone.

18. Braly, G., and Tullos, H.S. (1985): A modification of the Bristow procedure for recurrent anterior shoulder dislocation and subluxation. Am. J. Sports Med., 13:81–86.
19. Bratatz, J.H., and Gogia, P.P. (1987): The mechanics of pitching. J. Orthop. Sports Phys. Ther., 9:56–69.
20. Brewer, B.J. (1979): Aging of the rotator cuff. Am. J. Sports Med., 7:102–110.
21. Caillet, R. (1966): Shoulder Pain. Philadelphia, F.A. Davis.
22. Cain, P.R., Mutschler, T.A., Fu, F.A., et al. (1987): Anterior stability of the glenohumeral joint: A dynamic model. Am. J. Sports Med., 15:144–148.
23. Chu, D. (1989): Plyometric exercises with a medicine ball. Livermore, CA, Bittersweet Publishing Co.
24. Clark, J.C., Harryman, D.T. (1992): Tendons, ligaments, and capsule of the rotator cuff. J. Bone Joint Surg. [Am.], 74:713–719.
25. Codman, E.A. (1934): Rupture of the supraspinatus tendon and other lesions in or about the subacromial bursa. *In:* Codman, E.A. (ed.): The Shoulder. Boston, Thomas Todd.
26. Colachis, S.C., and Strohm, B.R. (1971): The effect of suprascapular and axillary nerve blocks and muscle force in the upper extremity. Arch. Phys. Med. Rehabil., 52:22–29.
27. Colachis, S.C., Strohm, B.R., and Brechner, V.L. (1969): Effects of axillary nerve block on muscle force in the upper extremity. Arch. Phys. Med. Rehabil., 50:647–654.
28. Collins, K.A., Capito, C., and Cross, M. (1986): The use of the Putti-Platt procedure in the treatment of recurrent anterior dislocation. Am. J. Sports Med., 14:380–382.
29. Davies, G.J., and Gould, J.A. (1985): Orthopaedic and Sports Physical Therapy. St. Louis, C.V. Mosby.
30. DeDuca, C.J., and Forrest, W.J. (1973): Force analysis of individual muscles acting simultaneously on the shoulder joint during isometric abduction. J. Biomech., 6:385–393.
31. Dempster, W.T. (1965): Mechanisms of shoulder movement. Arch. Phys. Med. Rehabil., 46A:49.
32. DePalma, A.F. (1973): Surgery of the Shoulder, 2nd ed. Philadelphia, J.B. Lippincott.
33. Engle, R.P., and Canner, G.C. (1989): Posterior shoulder instability approach to rehabilitation. J. Orthop. Sports Phys. Ther., 10:488–494.
34. Flatow, E.L., Soslowsky, L.J., Ticker, J.B., et al (1994): Excursion of the rotator cuff under the acromion: Patterns of subacromial contact. Am. J. Sports Med., 22:779–788.
35. Fleisig, G.S., Dillman, C.J., and Andrews, J.R.: Biomechanics of the shoulder during throwing. *In:* Andrews, J.R., and Wilk, K.E. (eds.): The Athlete's Shoulder. New York, Churchill Livingstone, pp. 355–368.
36. Fukuda, K., Craig, E.V., and An, K. (1986): Biomechanical study of the ligamentous system of the acromioclavicular joint. J. Bone Joint Surg. [Am.], 68:434–440.
37. Fukuda, H., Mikasa, M., Ogawa, K., et al. (1983): The partial-thickness tear of the rotator cuff. Orthop. Trans., 55:137.
38. Gambetta, V., and Odgers, S. (1991): The Complete Guide to Medicine Ball Training. Sarasota, FL, Optimum Sports Training.
39. Garth, W.P., Allman, F.L., and Armstrong, W.S. (1987): Occult anterior subluxations of the shoulder in noncontact sports. Am. J. Sports Med., 15:579–585.
40. Glousman, R., Jobe, F., Tibone, J., et al. (1988): Dynamic electromyographic analysis of the throwing shoulder with glenohumeral instability. J. Bone Joint Surg. [Am.], 70:220–226.
41. Hawkins, R., and Kennedy, J. (1980): Impingement syndrome in athletes. Am. J. Sports Med., 8:151–158.
42. Hawkins, R.J., Kippert, G., and Johnston, G. (1984): Recurrent posterior instability (subluxation) of the shoulder. J. Bone Joint Surg. [Am.], 66:169–174.
43. Hollingshead, W.H. (1958): Anatomy for Surgeons, Vol III. The Back and Limbs. New York, Hoeber & Harper.
44. Hovelius, L. (1987): Anterior dislocation of the shoulder in teen-agers and young adults. J. Bone Joint Surg. [Am.], 69:393–399.
45. Howell, S.M., Galinet, S.J. (1989): The glenoid labral socket: A constrained articular surface. Clin. Orthop., 243:122–129.
46. Howell, S.M., Imobersteg, A.M., Segar, D.H., and Marone, P.J. (1986): Clarification of the role of the supraspinatus muscle in shoulder function. J. Bone Joint Surg. [Am.], 68:398–404.
47. Hughston, J.C. (1985): Functional anatomy of the shoulder. *In:* Zarins, B., Andrews, J.R., and Carson, W.G. (eds.): Injuries to the Throwing Arm. Philadelphia, W.B. Saunders.
48. Iannotti, J.P., Swiontkowski, M., Esterhafi, J., and Boulas, H.F. (1989): Intraoperative assessment of rotator cuff vascularity using laser Doppler flowmetry (abstr.). Presented at the 1989 Meeting of the American Academy of Orthopaedic Surgeons, Las Vegas.
49. Inman, V., and Saunders, J.B. (1946): Observations of the function of the clavicle. Calif. Med., 65:158–166.
50. Inman, V., Saunders, M., and Abbott, L. (1944): Observations of the function of the shoulder joint. J. Bone Joint Surg. [Am.], 26:1–30.
51. Jobe, F.W., and Jobe, C.M. (1983): Painful athletic injuries of the shoulder. Clin. Orthop., 173:117–124.
52. Jobe, F.W., and Moynes, D.R. (1982): Delineation of diagnostic criteria and a rehabilitation program for rotator cuff injuries. Am. J. Sports Med., 10:336–339.

53. Jobe, F.W., Moynes, D.R., and Tibone, J.E. (1984): An EMG analysis of the shoulder in pitching: A second report. Am. J. Sports Med., 12:218–220.

54. Jobe, F.W., Tibone, J.E., Jobe, C.M., and Kvitne, R.S. Jr., (1990): The shoulder in sports. *In:* Rockwood, C.A., and Matsen, F.A., III (eds.): The Shoulder. Philadelphia, W.B. Saunders.

55. Jobe, F.W., Tibone, J.E., Perry, J., et al. (1983): An EMG analysis of the shoulder in throwing and pitching: A preliminary report. Am. J. Sports Med., 11:3–5.

56. Kelly, B.T., Kadrmas, W.R., and Speer, K.P. (1996): The manual muscle examination for rotator cuff strength. An electromyographic investigation. Am. J. Sports Med., 24B:581–588.

57. Kennedy, J.C., and Willis, R.B. (1976): The effects of local steroid injections on tendons: A biomechanical and microscopic correlative study. Am. J. Sports Med., 4:11–21.

58. Kent, B. (1971): Functional anatomy of the shoulder complex: A review. Phys. Ther., 51:867–887.

59. Kessel, L., and Watson, M. (1977): The painful arc syndrome. J. Bone Joint Surg. [Br.], 59:166–172.

60. Kuland, D. (1982): The Injured Athlete. Philadelphia, J.B. Lippincott.

61. Lilleby, H. (1984): Shoulder arthroscopy. Acta Orthop. Scand., 55:561–566.

62. Lindblom, K. (1939): On pathogenesis of ruptures of the tendon aponeurosis of the shoulder joint. Acta Radiol., 20:563–577.

63. Lucas, D.B. (1973): Biomechanics of the shoulder joint. Arch. Surg., 107:425–432.

64. MacConnail, M., and Basmajian, J. (1969): Muscles and Movement: A Basis for Human Kinesiology. Baltimore, Williams & Wilkins.

65. Malanga, G.A., Jenp Y.N., Growney E.C., and An K.N. (1996): EMG analysis of shoulder positioning in testing and strengthening the supraspinatus. Med. Sci. Sports Exerc., 28:661–664.

66. Matsen, F.A., III (1980): Compartmental Syndromes. San Francisco, Grune & Stratton.

67. Matsen, F.A., III and Arntz, C.T. (1990): Rotator cuff tendon failure. *In:* Rockwood, C.A., Jr., and Matsen, F.A., III (eds.): The Shoulder, Vol II. Philadelphia, W.B. Saunders, pp. 647–677.

68. Matsen, F.A., III, and Arntz, C.T. (1990): Subacromial impingement. *In:* Rockwood, C.A., Jr., and Matsen, F.A. III (eds.): The Shoulder, Vol II. Philadelphia, W.B. Saunders, pp. 623–646.

69. McLeod, W.D. (1985): The pitching mechanism. *In:* Zarins, B., Andrews, J.R., and Carson, W.G. (eds.): Injuries to the Throwing Arm. Philadelphia, W.B. Saunders, pp. 22–29.

70. McLeod, W.D., and Andrews, J.R. (1986): Mechanisms of shoulder injuries. Phys. Ther., 66:1901–1904.

71. Miller, L.S., Donahue, J.R., Good, R.P., and Staerk, A.J. (1984): The Magnuson-Stack procedure for treatment of recurrent glenohumeral dislocations. Am. J. Sports Med., 12:133–137.

72. Morrison, D.S., and Bigliani, L.U. (1987): The clinical significance of variation in acromial morphology. Presented at the Third Open Meeting of the American Shoulder and Elbow Surgeons, San Francisco.

73. Moseley, H.F., and Goldie, I. (1963): The arterial pattern of rotator cuff of the shoulder. J. Bone Joint Surg. [Br.], 45:780–789.

74. Neer, C.S. (1972): Anterior acromioplasty for the chronic impingement syndrome in the shoulder: A preliminary report. J. Bone Joint Surg. [Am.], 54:41–50.

75. Neer, C.S. (1983): Impingement syndrome. Clin. Orthop., 173:70–77.

76. Neviaser, R.J. (1987): Injuries to the clavicle and acromioclavicular joint. Orthop. Clin. North Am., 18:433–438.

77. Norkin, C., and Levangie, P. (1983): Joint Structure and Function: A Comprehensive Analysis. Philadelphia, F.A. Davis.

78. Norwood, L.A. (1985): Posterior shoulder instability. *In:* Zarins, B., Andrews, J.R., and Carson, W.G. (eds.): Injuries to the Throwing Arm. Philadelphia, W.B. Saunders, pp. 153–159.

79. O'Brien, S.J., Neves, M.C., and Arnoczky, S.J. (1990): The anatomy and histology of the inferior glenohumeral ligament complex of the shoulder. Am. J. Sports Med., 18:449–456.

80. Pappas, A.M., Zawacki, R.M., and Sullivan, T.J. (1985): Biomechanics of baseball pitching: A preliminary report. Am. J. Sports Med., 13:216–222.

81. Perry, J., and Glousman, R.E.(1990): Biomechanics of throwing. *In:* Nicholas, J.A., and Hershman, E.B. (eds.): The Upper Extremity in Sports Medicine. St. Louis, C.V. Mosby, pp. 727–751.

82. Podromos, C.C., Perry, J.A., and Schiller, J.A. (1990):Histological studies of the glenoid labrum from fetal life to old age. J. Bone Joint Surg. [Am.], 72:1344–1352.

83. Poppen, N.K., and Walker, P.S. (1976): Normal and abnormal motion of the shoulder. J. Bone Joint Surg. [Am.], 58:195–201.

84. Poppen, N., and Walker, P. (1978): Forces at the glenohumeral joint in adduction. Clin. Orthop., 135:165–170.

85. Protzman, R.R. (1980): Anterior instability of the shoulder. J. Bone Joint Surg. [Am.], 62:909–918.

86. Rathbun, J.B., and Macnab, I. (1970): The microvascular pattern of the rotator cuff. J. Bone Joint Surg. [Br.], 52:540–553.

87. Rockwood, C.A., and Young, D.C. (1990): Disorders of the acromioclavicular joint. *In:* Rockwood, C.A., and Matsen, F.A. (eds.): The Shoulder. Philadelphia, W.B. Saunders, pp. 413–468.

88. Rowe, C.R. (1988): Tendinitis, bursitis, impingement, "snapping scapula" and calcific tendinitis. *In:* Rowe, C.R. (ed.): The Shoulder. New York, Churchill Livingstone, pp. 105–129.

89. Rowe, C.R. (1988): The Shoulder. New York, Churchill Livingstone.

90. Rowe, C., and Zarins, B. (1981): Recurrent transient subluxation of the shoulder. J. Bone Joint Surg. [Am.], 63:863–871.

91. Saha, A. (1961): Theory of Shoulder Mechanism: Descriptive and Applied. Springfield, IL, Charles C Thomas.

92. Sarrafian, S. (1983): Gross and functional anatomy of the shoulder. Clin. Orthop., 173:11–19.
93. Sigholm, G., Styf, J., Korner, L., and Herberts, P. (1988): Pressure recording in the subacromial bursa. J. Orthop. Res., 6:123–128.
94. Snyder, S.J., Karzel R.P., DelPizzo, W., et al (1990): SLAP lesions of the shoulder. Arthroscopy, 6:274–276.
95. Steindler, A. (1955): Kinesiology of the human body. Springfield, IL, Charles C Thomas.
96. Townsend, H., Jobe, F.W., Pink, M., et al. (1992): EMG analysis of the glenohumeral muscles during a baseball rehabilitation program. Am. J. Sports Med., 19:264–269.
97. Travell, J.G., and Simons, D.G. (1983): Myofascial Pain and Dysfunction: The Trigger Point Manual. Baltimore, Williams & Wilkins.
98. Tullos, H.S., and King, J.W. (1973): Throwing mechanism in sports. Orthop. Clin. North Am., 4:709–721.
99. Turkel, S., Panio, M., Marshall, J., and Girgis, F. (1981): Stabilization mechanism preventing anterior dislocation of the glenohumeral joint. J. Bone Joint Surg. [Am.], 63:1208–1217.
100. Walch, G., Boileau, P., Noel, E., and Donell, T. (1992): Impingement of the deep surface of the supraspinatus tendon on the glenoid rim. J. Shoulder Elbow Surg., 1:239–245.
101. Walsh, D.A. (1989): Shoulder evaluation of the throwing athlete. Sports Med. Update, 4:24–527.
102. Wick, H.J., Dillman, C.J., Wisleder, D., et al (1991): A kinematic comparison between baseball pitching and football passing. Sports Med. Update, 6:13–16.
103. Wilk, K.E. (1996): Conditioning and Training Techniques. In: Hawkins, R.J., and Misamore, G.W. (eds.): Shoulder Injuries in the Athlete. New York, Churchill Livingstone, pp. 339–364.
104. Wilk, K.E., and Andrews, J.R. (1993): Rehabilitation following arthroscopic shoulder subacromial decompression. Orthopedics, 16:349–355.
105. Wilk, K.E., Andrews, J.R., Arrigo, C.A., et al. (1997): Preventive and Rehabilitative Exercises for the Shoulder and Elbow, 5th ed. Birmingham, AL, American Sports Medicine Institute.
106. Wilk, K.E., Voight, M., Keirns, M.A., et al. (1993): Stretch shortening drills for the upper extremity: Theory and clinical application. J. Orthop. Sports Phys. Ther., 17:225–239.
107. Wilson, C.F., and Duff, G.L. (1943): Pathologic study of degeneration and rupture of the supraspinatus tendon. Arch. Surg., 47:121–135.
108. Yamanaka, K., Fukuda, H., and Mikasa, M. (1987): Incomplete thickness tears of the rotator cuff. Clin. Orthop. 223:51–58.
109. Zarins, B., and Rowe, C.R. (1984): Current concepts in the diagnosis and treatment of shoulder instability in athletes. Med. Sci. Sports Exerc., 16:444–448.

Elbow Rehabilitation

Gary L. Harrelson, Ed.D., A.T.,C., and
Deidre Leaver-Dunn, M.Ed., A.T.,C.

Elbow injuries, whether induced by a direct blow or by overuse, are common in sports. The occurrence of elbow injuries in the throwing athlete has been well documented.[5, 14, 31, 38, 64, 80, 82] Because the etiology of many chronic elbow injuries has a strong biomechanical component, this aspect must be understood and addressed in the rehabilitation process. In addition, the clinician must have an appreciation of the effects of immobilization on the elbow. Regardless of the athlete's sport or the nature of the elbow injury, the rehabilitation program must include appropriate sport-specific activities and functional progressions.

BIOMECHANICS OF SPORTS AND ITS RELATIONSHIP TO ELBOW INJURIES

Both the act of throwing and the use of implements in sports can contribute to the development of elbow injuries. A basic understanding of the biomechanics of throwing and of the interaction between athlete and implement is necessary for understanding rehabilitation of injuries in these athletes. Clinicians must also be aware of the distinction between throwing injuries and injuries to throwers.[72] The term "throwing injuries of the elbow" refers to overuse syndromes that occur as a result of the repetitive stresses incurred by the structures about the elbow as a result of throwing over an extended period of time. Although the clinical manifestations may be acute at onset, the injuries are essentially the result of pathologic changes occurring at a subclinical level over varying periods of time. The term "injuries of the elbow in the throwing athlete" refers to generally acute, traumatic injuries that occur as a result of a single injury or episode and are not specific to the throwing act itself.

The Throwing Act

The throwing act has been described by many authors[13, 20, 18, 21, 22, 32, 44, 63, 67, 72, 73, 76, 84] (Fig. 14–1). Their analyses reveal that the elbow experiences distraction forces medially and compressive forces laterally. These forces place the elbow at greatest jeopardy for injury during the arm-cocking, acceleration, and deceleration phases of pitching.

Valgus torques, causing the elbow to undergo medial tension and lateral compression, are high during the arm-cocking phase.[16, 87] A strong varus torque

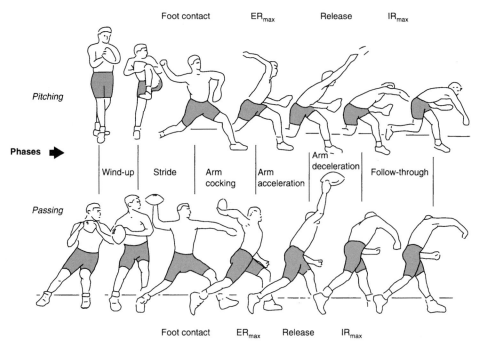

Figure 14–1. The six phases of throwing for baseball pitching *(top)* and football passing *(bottom)*: wind-up, stride, arm cocking, arm acceleration, arm deceleration, and follow-through. ER_{max}, maximum external rotation; IR_{max}, maximum internal rotation. (Reprinted by permission from G.S. Fleisig, et al., 1996, "Kinematic and Kinetic Comparison Between Baseball Pitching and Football Passing," Appl. Biomechanics, 12[2]:214, 216.)

is needed to counteract this valgus force. The ulnar collateral ligament (UCL) contributes to the production of a counteractive varus torque, but it is loaded near its maximum capacity during pitching and cannot withstand the valgus torque alone.[20, 18, 21, 87] Electromyographic studies have shown that the wrist flexor-pronator group, the triceps brachii and the anconeus, contribute dynamically to produce varus torque.[20, 18, 21, 87] In addition, the upper arm applies a medial force onto the forearm during arm cocking. This force serves to counteract the valgus torque and is greatest with fastball and curveball pitches.[18] Medial tension produces such injuries as spur formation with ulnar nerve compression, ulnar neuritis, medial epicondylitis, UCL sprains, flexor muscle strains, and Little Leaguer's elbow in the adolescent. Laterally, compression can result in radial head and capitellum hypertrophy, avascular necrosis, chip fractures, and osteochondritis dissecans in the young thrower.

During the short acceleration phase, extension velocity can approach 2300° per second,[19, 22, 87] with a maximum velocity of 2500° per second reported by Fleisig and Barrentine.[18] This rapid extension is possible because of reduced activity in the biceps brachii[87] and results primarily from centrifugal force generated by rotation of the upper trunk.[16, 18, 87] Centrifugal force and rapid elbow extension place distraction forces on the elbow joint that are counteracted by compression forces produced by muscular activity in the triceps brachii, wrist flexors and pronators, elbow flexors, and anconeus.[18, 87] The high rate of extension causes large shear forces to be imposed on the articular cartilage.[52] Valgus extension overload and Little Leaguer's elbow are also associated with the extension and resistance to valgus torque that occur with acceleration.

At the beginning of the deceleration phase the humerus has a relatively high rate of internal rotation, and the elbow is rapidly extending. After ball release, this extension causes humeral internal rotation to present itself as forearm pronation. Large forces, generated by eccentric contraction of the biceps brachii, brachialis, and brachioradialis, decelerate the rapidly moving forearm.[52, 87]

Rapid extension causes distraction forces about the elbow and shoulder joints. The ulnar and radial collateral ligaments stabilize the elbow. The UCL resists distraction, with assistance from compressive forces produced by the elbow extensors, wrist flexors and pronators, and wrist extensors.[87] Fastball and slider pitches result in the greatest compressive forces at the shoulder and elbow.[18] Activity by the elbow flexors also terminates elbow extension before impingement of the olecranon into the olecranon fossa.[18] If elbow extension is not decelerated, overextension injuries, common to the elbow, can occur; conversely, if elbow extension is decelerated too rapidly, the extremely high flexion forces required can overstress the biceps tendon.[2]

The curveball has the highest rate of elbow extension and, theoretically, is the most destructive pitch to the articular surfaces of the radial head and capitellum.[52] However, similarities demonstrated in the mechanics of curveball and fastball pitches may suggest that curveball pitches do not really lead to an increase in elbow injuries.[21, 71, 80]

Additionally, the kinematic differences at the elbow between a baseball pitch and a football pass have been investigated (see Fig. 14–1).[18, 19, 22] This research has shown that quarterbacks have shorter strides and stand more erect at ball release. During arm cocking, quarterbacks demonstrate greater elbow flexion and shoulder horizontal adduction. To decelerate the arm, pitchers generate greater compressive force at the elbow and greater compressive force and adduction torque at the shoulder. In summary, the two throws are similar but not identical, and pitchers produce higher joint angular velocities and higher limb velocities at the elbow and shoulder during delivery, with resultant greater ball velocities.[18, 21, 19, 22] The specific kinematic differences between baseball pitching and football passing are highlighted in Table 14–1.

As a result of the repetitive nature of throwing and the extreme forces produced, predictable osseous and muscular changes have been documented.[5, 31, 40, 44, 80] Medially, these changes are usually overuse injuries. The lateral side is prone to more serious damage such as radiocapitellar articular cartilage damage with subsequent degeneration.[52]

Implement-Forearm Interaction

Chronic elbow injuries are also common in athletes whose sport involves the use of implements such as clubs or racquets. The use of an implement with a small grip, with resultant excess activity of the wrist flexors and extensors, has been associated with the development of lateral and medial epicondylitis. As a component of their study of medial epicondylitis in golfers, Glazebrook and colleagues[29] investigated the effects of increased grip size on wrist flexor activity. Results of this investigation demonstrated no alteration in the activity of the common flexor muscles during the golf swing when a larger grip was used.[29]

The role of tennis racquet characteristics in the development of lateral epicondylitis has also been studied.[34] Hennig and colleagues[34] examined the relationship between racquet, shot, and athlete characteristics and the transfer of tennis racquet vibrations into the human forearm during the backhand stroke. These investigators found significantly greater vibration transfer with off-center impacts as well as with less proficient players. Larger racquet size and greater racquet resonance frequency were associated with lower vibration loads on the forearm. Greater acceleration of the forearm-racquet union necessitates greater dynamic control of wrist motion by the extensor group that may contribute to lateral epicondylitis. Giangarra and colleagues[28] have also reported that using a double-handed backhand stroke may contribute to the use of incorrect mechanics and enable impact forces to be transferred through the elbow.

Table 14–1. Kinematic Comparison Between Baseball Pitching and Football Passing

PARAMETER	PITCHING (n = 26)		PASSING (n = 26)	
	MEAN	SD	MEAN	SD
Instant of foot contact				
Stride length from ankle to ankle (% height)**	74	5	61	8
Shoulder abduction (°)	93	12	96	13
Shoulder horizontal adduction (°)**	−17	12	7	15
Shoulder external rotation*	67	24	90	33
Elbow flexion (°)**	98	18	77	12
Lead knee flexion (°)**	51	11	39	11
Arm-cocking phase				
Maximum pelvis angular velocity (°/sec)**	660	80	500	110
Maximum shoulder horizontal adduction (°)**	18	8	32	9
Maximum upper torso angular velocity (°/sec)**	1170	100	950	130
Maximum elbow flexion (°)**	100	13	113	10
Instant of maximum shoulder external rotation				
Maximum shoulder external rotation (°)*	173	10	164	12
Arm acceleration phase				
Maximum elbow extension velocity (°/sec)**	2340	300	1760	210
Average shoulder abduction during acceleration (°)**	93	9	108	8
Instant of ball release				
Ball velocity (m/s)**	35	3	21	2
Shoulder horizontal adduction (°)**	7	7	26	9
Elbow flexion (°)**	22	6	36	8
Trunk tilt forward (°)*	58	10	65	8
Trunk tilt sideways (°)**	124	9	116	5
Lead knee flexion (°)**	40	12	28	9
Arm deceleration phase				
Maximum shoulder internal rotation velocity (°/sec)**	7550	1360	4950	1080
Minimum elbow flexion (°)**	18	5	24	5
Average upper torso angular velocity (°/sec)**	470	160	310	110

From Fleisig, G.S., Escamilla, R.F., Andrews, J.R., et al. (1996): Kinematic and kinetic comparison between baseball pitching and football passing. J. Appl. Biomech., 12:207–224.
*$P < 0.01$ **$P < .001$
SD, standard deviation.

Upper Extremity Support of Body Weight

The elbow is subjected to increased forces in sports such as gymnastics in which the upper extremities are repetitively used to support body weight. These loads involve varus and valgus forces in addition to compression of the radiohumeral joint.[47] Forces about the elbow during the double-arm support phase of the back handspring have been shown to be similar to those seen during the baseball pitch.[47] Such loads can produce chronic lateral compartment injuries such as osteochondritis dissecans, as well as UCL sprains and other medial elbow injuries.

REHABILITATION PROGRAM

Traumatic injuries to the elbow usually require a period of immobilization or protected mobilization after injury. Range-of-motion and strengthening exercises should be started as quickly as possible, however, with wrist and hand exercises beginning during elbow immobilization. Conversely, overuse syndromes usually require no immobilization. A therapeutic exercise program, in combination with modalities such as ice, heat, ultrasound, and iontophoresis, may be initiated immediately with chronic lesions.

Postoperative rehabilitation, especially for those lesions treated arthroscopically, such as with débridement, loose body removal, or synovial resection, can be aggressive, with range-of-motion exercises beginning as early as the next postoperative day. Usually, the philosophy of instituting early range of motion can be followed regardless of whether an arthroscopy or arthrotomy is performed. The only exceptions are those procedures requiring a short period (usually 4 weeks) of soft-tissue healing such as repair of a torn flexor pronator origin.

In designing a rehabilitation program after elbow injury or surgery, it is important to keep the following three points in mind. (1) Re-establishing full elbow extension is a primary and critical goal during the initial phase of rehabilitation. (2) The concept of total arm strength should not be overlooked. The adage that proximal stability promotes distal mobility should be used to ensure adequate muscular performance and dynamic joint stability.[88] (3) During the throwing act, elbow extensors act concentrically and rapidly accelerate the arm during the acceleration phase, whereas the elbow flexors act eccentrically to decelerate the elbow and prevent elbow hyperextension or the potential pathologic abutting of the olecranon into its fossa during follow-through.[88] Each of these muscle groups should be trained according to the contraction it performs during the throwing activity.

The section on applications at the end of this chapter includes exercises that comprise a general rehabilitation program for postoperative and conservative treatment of elbow lesions. These exercises emphasize all planes of elbow motion and flexibility and are also appropriate for the rehabilitation of wrist injuries. The use of an adjustable weighted rod, such as the Press-Grip,* can be used to advance the athlete along a progressive-resistance exercise continuum (Fig. 14–2). This type of device is excellent for exercising pronation-supination and radial-ulnar deviation.

Guidelines for institution of any rehabilitative program are based on how quickly the athlete can advance while allowing the restraining structures time

---

*Available from L³ Enterprises, Ellenton, Florida

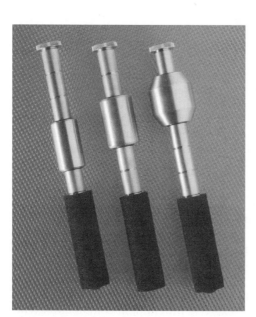

Figure 14–2. Use of an adjustable weighted rod, such as the Press-Grip, for elbow rehabilitation. (Photo courtesy of L³ Enterprises, Inc., Ellenton, Florida.)

to heal. Machines such as the Upper Body Ergometer (UBE)* can be used for endurance training as well as for the restoration of range of motion. Isokinetic exercises and inertial exercises† (Fig. 14–3) should be incorporated for proprioception, eccentric muscle contraction, and high-speed functional work.[1, 81]

Neuromuscular control exercises should be performed to enhance dynamic stability and proprioceptive skill. These exercises include proprioceptive neuromuscular facilitation (PNF) exercises such as rhythmic stabilizations and slow reversal holds, which can progress as tolerated to rapid diagonal movements.[88] Before returning to activity, the throwing athlete should participate in a high-speed program using surgical tubing, with a focus on functional patterns. Emphasis should be on the redevelopment of synergistic concentric and eccentric contraction patterns. Finally, the use of plyometrics has been reported to be extremely beneficial in rehabilitating athletes who perform overhead motions.[89] Plyometric exercise drills are performed for the entire upper extremity and body using plyoballs and a plyoback‡ (Figs. 14–4 and 14–5). These drills can be used to replicate the throwing motion, improve flexibility, or teach weight transferring and the use of the legs to accelerate the arm. A more complete description of the wide variety of plyometric exercises for the upper extremity has been provided by other authors[12, 25, 88, 89] and some upper extremity plyometric exercises can be found in Appendix A.

The throwing athlete should not neglect rehabilitation of the shoulder in conjunction with the elbow exercise program. Both joints are part of the total kinetic chain, and it would be remiss for one joint to be addressed without a concurrent rehabilitation program for the other. Rehabilitation, exercise progression, and restrictions for the most common injuries of the elbow are described next.

---

*Available from Cybex, Ronkonkoma, New York
†Available from E.M.A., Newnan, Georgia
‡Available from Functionally Integrated Technology, Dublan, California

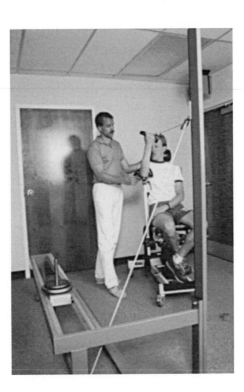

Figure 14–3. Inertia machine. This can be used in the later stages of elbow rehabilitation for proprioception, eccentric muscle contraction, and high-speed functional plane activity. (From Courson, R. [1989]: Rehabilitation of the thrower's elbow. Sports Med. Update, 4:7.)

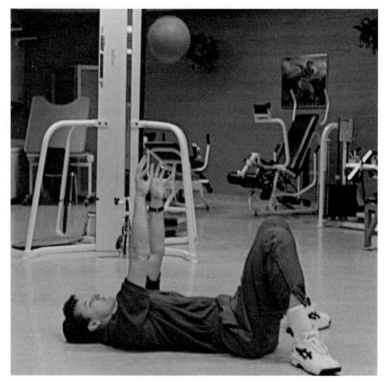

Figure 14–4. Supine plyometric chest press for elbow extensors using a medicine ball.

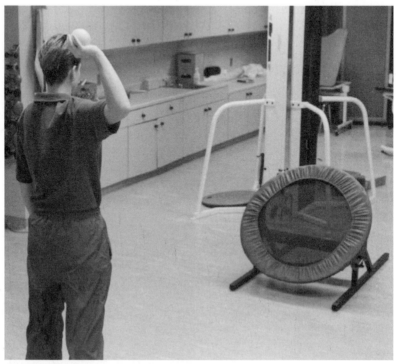

Figure 14–5. One-hand plyometric baseball throw with the arm in 90° of elbow flexion and 90° of shoulder abduction (90/90 position).

Common Elbow Injuries in Adults

EPICONDYLITIS

Lateral epicondylitis was first described in 1873 by Runge,[70] who noted this condition in the general population. The prevalence of lateral epicondylitis surged with the increase of participation in tennis, and hence the generic name of tennis elbow. Lateral epicondylitis is an overuse injury, usually involving the origin of the extensor carpi radialis brevis (ECRB) and, to a lesser degree, the extensor carpi radialis longus and anterior portion of the extensor communis.[48, 77]

Nirschl[55] has reported the development of fibroangiomatous hyperplasia in the involved tendon as a result of chronic repetitive trauma. Regan et al[67] recorded similar histologic abnormalities in a controlled study of patients with chronic lateral epicondylitis. These findings suggest that chronic epicondylitis (both lateral and medial) is a degenerative, rather than an inflammatory, condition.[67]

Although the precise site of pathology is not universal, Nirschl[55] has suggested that primarily the ECRB is involved. This hypothesis is supported by additional electromyographic studies.[28, 45] The ECRB is susceptible to increased stress when the wrist is flexed, with the ulna deviated, the elbow extended, and the forearm pronated, because the ECRB muscle must lengthen by 1.1 cm to allow full wrist flexion and pronation.[8] This is the same biomechanical principle as that of the tennis backhand, thus predisposing the tennis player to lateral epicondylar pain. This pain is usually reproduced as the racquet meets the ball. It is at the point of racquet to ball contact that the extensor muscles must contract to stabilize the wrist and hold the racquet. This results in repetitive muscle contraction, yielding chronic overload and causing lateral epicondylar pain. Giangarra and colleagues[28] have compared extensor muscle activity during single- and double-handed backhand strokes in elite tennis players. Results of this study showed no muscle activity differences between the two strokes, suggesting that poor mechanics is the primary contributor to the development of lateral epicondylitis. The relationship between flawed mechanics and lateral epicondylitis is further supported by the work of Kelley and associates.[45] This investigation demonstrated increased electromyographic activity of the wrist extensors and pronators during ball impact and early follow-through in symptomatic athletes who also exhibited a variety of errors in their single-handed backhand strokes.

Medial epicondylitis, which is less common, is generally associated with the golf address and swing and with the forehand, serve, or overhead strokes in tennis. This injury can also be seen in the throwing athlete as a result of valgus overload or overuse. The ratio of occurrence of lateral epicondylitis to medial epicondylitis is approximately 7:1.[48]

Ollivierre and colleagues[58] have identified the flexor carpi radialis–pronator teres interval as the most common site of pathology in chronic medial epicondylitis. Histologic studies in patients with chronic medial epicondylitis show collagen degeneration and angiofibroblastic tissue formation at the tendon origin.[58] Improper tennis[58] and golf mechanics[29, 58] cause excessive tension to be developed by the medial elbow musculature; when repeated over time, this overload results in the development of epicondylitis.

Individuals with epicondylitis usually complain of increased pain, on either the medial or lateral epicondyle. There is point tenderness over the involved epicondyle, and resisted wrist extension (lateral epicondylitis) or resisted wrist flexion (medial epicondylitis) exacerbates the symptoms, depending on the involved area. Grip strength can also decrease, and gripping action can refer pain to the symptomatic epicondyle.

Treatment of medial and lateral epicondylitis is similar. A rehabilitation program should be initiated before the symptoms and pain escalate, because the longer medial or lateral epicondylitis is symptomatic, the more difficult and prolonged the treatment.[48] Table 14–2 includes a sample epicondylitis treatment protocol.

With epicondylitis that is chronic or has passed the acute stage, the athlete with only mild pain or pain that does not increase may continue to play while undergoing treatment; however, if the activity exacerbates the symptoms, the athlete should stop the activity. Therapeutic exercises may worsen the symptoms for the first 7 to 10 days after initiation of the rehabilitation program, so the athlete should be instructed in the treatment of possible escalating symptoms. If the pain becomes severe, the exercises should be decreased or stopped. After 1 to 2 weeks with chronic lesions, the increase in symptoms should dissipate, and the athlete should notice a decrease in pain. Table 14–2 outlines a program for the rehabilitation of chronic and postacute epicondylitis. The interval tennis, golf, or throwing program (see Appendix D) can be used to return athletes to their sport, if applicable.

Relatively few cases (5% to 10%) of lateral epicondylitis require surgery.[9] A postoperative protocol can be found in Table 14–2. Nirschl[56] has reported that full power and flexibility in the extensor muscle mass returns at approximately 4 months postsurgery.

Table 14–2. Epicondylitis Treatment Protocol

I. Conservative treatment of acute epicondylitis
  A. Initial phase
    • Rest or active rest
    • Cock-up splint to decrease stress on the lateral epicondyle (remove the splint 3 or 4 times daily for elbow and wrist active range-of-motion exercises)
    • Cryotherapy
    • Electrical stimulation
    • Nonsteroidal anti-inflammatory drugs
    • Possible corticosteroid injection
  B. Intermediate phase
    • More aggressive range-of-motion exercises
    • Progressive-resistance exercise for wrist flexors, extensors, pronators, and supinators
    • Counterforce brace
II. Conservative treatment of chronic or postacute epicondylitis
  • Moist heat
  • Ultrasound
  • Ultrasound phonophoresis with 10% hydrocortisone cream
  • Iontophoresis
  • Wrist extensor and wrist flexor stretches
  • Progressive-resistance exercise for all muscle groups acting on the forearm and wrist
  • Counterforce brace
III. Postoperative rehabilitation for epicondylitis
  A. Initial phase
    1. Day of surgery
      • Posterior splint in neutral position and 90° elbow flexion
    2. Postoperative day 1
      • Gentle hand, wrist, elbow, and shoulder active range of motion in splint
    3. Postoperative days 7–10
      • Discontinue splint
      • Begin total body conditioning
  B. Intermediate phase
    1. Postoperative week 3
      • Goal: Full active range of motion of wrist and elbow
      • Begin elbow, wrist, and hand progressive-resistance exercise with counterforce brace, progressing to 2–3 lb
    2. Postoperative weeks 4–6
      • Eccentric training
      • Functional rehabilitation
  C. Advanced phase: postoperative month 2
    • Gradual return to sports participation
    • Interval program (see Appendix D)
    • Strength and flexibility maintenance program daily

Halle and associates[33] have compared the effectiveness of four treatment protocols, in association with a home program, for lateral epicondylitis: (1) ultrasound; (2) ultrasound with 10% hydrocortisone; (3) transcutaneous electrical nerve stimulation; and (4) subcutaneous steroid injection. It was determined that the four treatment protocols do not significantly differ in effectiveness. All are effective in decreasing pain and symptoms, but it should be noted that a home therapeutic exercise program is a common denominator in all four protocols.

Corticosteroid injection has been somewhat successful in treating epicondylitis symptoms. However, this is only a palliative measure if not performed in conjunction with a therapeutic exercise program to increase muscular strength and endurance. Iontophoresis is a favorable alternative to corticosteroid injection. The benefits of iontophoresis over injection include decreased systemic side effects, short-term administration, avoidance of further tissue damage from injection, and prevention of discomfort from needle insertion at an already tender area.[26] Current commercial iontophoresis units use a buffered electrode as a delivery mechanism (Fig. 14–6). The buffered electrode does not require lidocaine, and the amount of dexamethasone used is directly proportional to the electrode size and can range from 1.5 ml to 2.5 ml.

The use of counterforce bracing has long been advocated by many authors.[8, 9, 23, 37, 48, 55, 56, 57, 64] Froimson[23] and Ilfeld and Field[37] first reported the use of a counterforce brace for lateral epicondylitis. In 1966, Ilfeld and Field[37] described a tennis elbow brace designed to support the elbow between two lateral hinged metal stirrups that limited extension and rotation, somewhat different from the current proximal forearm band described by Froimson[23] (Fig. 14–7). The rationale behind the use of counterforce bracing for lateral epicondylitis is that the brace either decreases the amount of internally generated muscle contractile tension or alters and directs potentially abusive force overloads to less sensitive tissues, possibly to the brace itself.[32, 55] In patients whose symptoms are severe, the counterforce brace can be used during the therapeutic exercise program.

The counterforce brace is thought to exert its effect by gentle compression of musculotendinous areas, which partially decreases muscle expansion at the time of intrinsic muscle contraction or minimizes exaggerated tendon movement. A number of objective studies have supported the efficacy of counterforce bracing.[32, 77, 78, 86] Glazebrook and colleagues[29] analyzed wrist flexor muscle activity in golfers with and without medial epicondylitis after the application of a counterforce brace. Results of this investigation showed no decreases in muscle activity in either group with the braced condition and suggest that the symptomatic

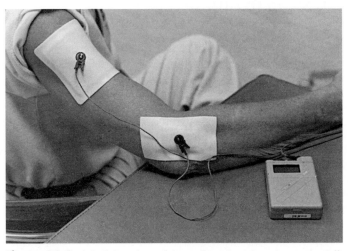

Figure 14–6. Administration of iontophoresis using a commercially available unit with a buffered electrode.

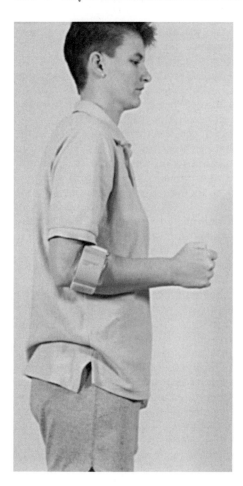

Figure 14–7. Counterforce brace for tennis elbow. The brace either decreases the quantity of internally generated muscle contraction tension or alters and directs potentially abusive force overloads to less sensitive tissues and probably to the brace itself.

relief associated with counterforce braces is due to a mechanism other than decreased activity in the involved muscle-tendon complex.

VALGUS EXTENSION OVERLOAD

The repetitive nature of throwing results in muscular and osseous hypertrophy around the elbow.[44] This bony hypertrophy is usually located on the olecranon process, primarily posteromedially, and results in a bony block and loss of elbow extension. Valgus stress plus forced extension is the major pathologic mechanism that produces scarring, fibrous tissue deposition in the olecranon fossa, and osteophyte formation on the tip or posteromedial aspect of the olecranon process.[2, 79, 83] Traditionally, emphasis was placed on osteophyte formation on the posterior olecranon tip as a result of extension overload.[2, 46, 90] True symptomatic lesions, however, are caused by the posteromedial osteophyte as it abuts into the medial margin of the olecranon fossa.[4, 46] This impingement can result in osteochondrosis in this area.

Athletes suffering from valgus extension overload usually have already developed secondary soft-tissue contractures as a result of fibrous tissue deposition in the olecranon fossa, olecranon osteophyte formation, loose bodies, or radial head hypertrophy. King and colleagues[46] have reported that 50% of all professional baseball pitchers have elbow flexion contracture, and approximately 30% have cubitus valgus deformity as a result of repetitive throwing. Although a flexion deformity is usually present, it does not appear to alter pitching performance.[2] This is probably due to the elbow's stopping short of full extension during the pitching act.[19]

These athletes complain of elbow pain that is accentuated with throwing, as well as joint catching, locking, crepitus, and loss of elbow range of motion, particularly extension. The elbow end feel is hard, painful, and unyielding when tested, clinical features that are generally associated with a mechanical block.

Conservative treatment is indicated for athletes with mild valgus extension overload. Surgery is indicated for patients in whom pain persists and exercise increases symptoms. Postoperative rehabilitation can begin the day following arthroscopic or arthrotomy excision of loose bodies and osteophytes. If an arthrotomy is performed for removal of the osteophytes, the goal is restoration of full elbow extension in 7 to 10 days postoperatively and gradual return of flexion. The same exercises are indicated as for an arthroscopic procedure. Protocols for rehabilitation with conservative and surgical treatment of valgus extension overload are presented in Table 14–3. Additionally, the importance of training the athlete to control the rapid elbow extension that occurs during the acceleration and deceleration phases of throwing and to dynamically stabilize the elbow against the valgus strain has been reported.[88] Specifically, the biceps brachii, brachioradialis, and brachialis contract eccentrically to control the rapid rate of elbow extension and the abutting of the olecranon within the medial aspect of the fossa.[88]

ULNAR NERVE LESIONS

The ulnar nerve is highly susceptible to the valgus forces encountered in throwing, which produce traction on the medial aspect of the elbow. The ulnar nerve can be injured by direct trauma, repetitive traction caused by ligament laxity, compression secondary to muscular hypertrophy, recurrent subluxation or dislocation of the nerve out of the ulnar groove, or fixation of the nerve in the cubital tunnel by adhesions. All of these etiologies can be aggravated by repetitive throwing. Although protected in the proximal and distal cubital tunnel by muscle mass, the ulnar nerve is relatively unprotected and is vulnerable to compressive forces.[82] The floor of the cubital tunnel is formed by the UCL. The arcuate ligament, which forms the roof of the cubital tunnel, is taut at 90° of flexion and can compress the ulnar nerve as elbow flexion increases.[82, 85] Furthermore, any deficiency in the anterior bundle of the UCL that allows the elbow to open in valgus places undue stress on the ulnar nerve and sometimes may lead to tardy ulnar nerve palsy.[23, 27]

Typically, once ulnar nerve lesions become symptomatic, surgical intervention may often be necessary. Some athletes respond to conservative care including rest, cryotherapy, nonsteroidal anti-inflammatory drugs, and changes in pitching biomechanics. Surgical procedures usually transpose the nerve anteriorly. The nerve may be repositioned in the forearm musculature, but extensive scarring and compression have been observed with this procedure.[7, 49] In addition, throwing athletes tend to have a hypertrophied forearm flexor mass that may compress the nerve during contraction.[7] Some surgeons elect to reflect the flexor mass and resect the medial epicondyle before anterior transposition.[24, 54] Subcutaneous transposition of the ulnar nerve has been advocated to avoid muscular compression of the nerve.[3, 15, 66, 69] More commonly, fasciodermal slings are used to subcutaneously transpose the nerve anteriorly.[3, 15] Excellent results with this technique have been reported by Rettig and Ebben.[68] The protocol outlined in Table 14–4 can be used as a guideline for rehabilitation after subcutaneous transposition of the ulnar nerve using fascial slings.

LOSS OF RANGE OF MOTION

Loss of elbow range of motion is a common complication, particularly in athletes who have suffered an elbow dislocation, radial head or olecranon

---

Table 14–3. Postoperative Rehabilitation After Elbow Arthroscopy (Posterior Compartment or Valgus Extension Overload)

I. Phase I: Immediate Motion Phase

Goals
- Improve or regain full range of motion
- Decrease pain or inflammation
- Retard muscular atrophy

A. Days 1–4
- Range of motion to tolerance (extension-flexion and supination-pronation). Often full elbow extension is not possible because of pain
- Gentle overpressure into extension
- Wrist flexion-extension stretches
- Gripping exercises with putty
- Isometrics, wrist extension-flexion
- Isometrics, elbow extension-flexion
- Compression dressing, ice 4–5 times daily

B. Days 5–10
- Range-of-motion exercises to tolerance (at least 20°–90°)
- Overpressure into extension
- Joint mobilization to re-establish range of motion
- Wrist flexion-extension stretches
- Continue isometrics
- Continue use of ice and compression to control swelling

C. Days 11–14
- Range-of-motion exercises to tolerance (at least 10°–100°)
- Overpressure into extension (3–4 times daily)
- Continue joint mobilization techniques
- Initiate light dumbbell program (progressive-resistance exercise for biceps, triceps, wrist flexors, extensors, supinators and pronators)
- Continue use of ice postexercise

II. Phase II: Intermediate Phase

Goals
- Improve strength, power, and endurance
- Increase range of motion
- Initiate functional activities

A. Weeks 2–4
- Full range-of-motion exercises (4–5 times daily)
- Overpressure into elbow extension
- Continue progressive-resistance exercise program for elbow and wrist musculature
- Initiate shoulder program (external rotation and rotator cuff)
- Continue joint mobilization
- Continue ice postexercise

B. Weeks 4–7
- Continue all exercises listed above
- Initiate light upper body program
- Continue use of ice postactivity

III. Phase III: Advanced Strengthening Program

Goals
- Improve strength, power, and endurance
- Gradual return to functional activities

Criteria to enter phase III
- Full nonpainful range of motion
- Strength 75% or more of contralateral side
- No pain or tenderness

A. Weeks 8–12
- Continue progressive-resistance exercise program for elbow and wrist
- Continue shoulder program
- Continue stretching for elbow and shoulder
- Initiate interval throwing program and gradually return to sports activities

---

From Wilk, K.E., Arrigo, C.A., Andrews, J.R., and Azar, F.M. (1996): Rehabilitation following elbow surgery in the throwing athlete. Operative Tech. Sports Med., 4:114–132.

Table 14–4. Postoperative Rehabilitation After Ulnar Nerve Transposition

I. **Phase I: Immediate Postoperative Phase (Week 0–1)**
   Goals
   - Allow soft-tissue healing of relocated nerve
   - Decrease pain and inflammation
   - Retard muscular atrophy
   A. Week 1
      1. Posterior splint at 90° elbow flexion with wrist free for motion (use sling for comfort)
      2. Compression dressing
      3. Exercises such as gripping exercises, wrist range of motion, shoulder isometrics
   B. Week 2
      1. Remove posterior splint for exercise and bathing
      2. Progress elbow range of motion (passive range of motion, 15°–120°)
      3. Initiate elbow and wrist isometrics
      4. Continue shoulder isometrics

II. **Phase II: Intermediate Phase (Weeks 3–7)**
   Goals
   - Restore full pain-free range of motion
   - Improve strength, power, and endurance of upper extremity musculature
   - Gradually increase functional demands
   A. Week 3
      1. Discontinue posterior splint
      2. Progress elbow range of motion, emphasize full extension
      3. Initiate flexibility exercise for wrist extension-flexion, forearm supination-pronation, and elbow extension-flexion
      4. Initiate strengthening exercises for wrist extension-flexion, forearm supination-pronation, elbow extensors and flexors, and a shoulder program
   B. Week 6
      1. Continue all exercises listed above
      2. Initiate light sport activities

III. **Phase III: Advanced Strengthening Phase (Weeks 8–12)**
   Goals
   - Increase strength, power, and endurance
   - Gradually initiate sports activities
   A. Week 8
      1. Initiate eccentric exercise program
      2. Initiate plyometric exercise drills
      3. Continue shoulder and elbow strengthening and flexibility exercises
      4. Initiate interval throwing program

IV. **Phase IV: Return to Activity Phase (Weeks 12–16)**
   Goal
   - Gradually return to sports activities
   A. Week 12
      1. Return to competitive throwing
      2. Continue Throwers' Ten exercise program

From Wilk, K.E., Arrigo, C.A., Andrews, J.R., and Azar F.M. (1996). Rehabilitation following elbow surgery in the throwing athlete. Operative Tech. Sports Med., 4:114–132.

fracture, osteochondritis, or osteochondritis dissecans. With any injury, the elbow will respond to the pain and effusion by flexing. Thus, over time, the periarticular tissue and joint capsule become shortened and fibrotic, with a resultant loss in range of motion.[88] Because the elbow is susceptible to flexion contractures, initiation of early range of motion, even in a limited range, is an important deterrent. Immobilization for longer than 2 weeks after injury or surgery can affect the long-term outcome.[53] Re-establishment of full elbow extension is a primary and critical goal during the initial phases of elbow rehabilitation after injury or surgery to the elbow.[88] Wilk et al[88] allude to several factors that may contribute and predispose an athlete to developing an elbow flexion contracture: (1) the intimate congruency of the elbow complex, especially of the humeroulnar joint; (2) the tightness of the elbow joint capsule; and (3) the tendency of the anterior capsule to scar and become adhesive. General guidelines for increasing

Table 14–5. Guidelines for Increasing Elbow Range of Motion

Avoid strong passive loading of the joint.
Perform range-of-motion exercises at end ranges many times daily, once allowed by physiologic healing restraints.
Perform exercises only in the range of normal synergy.
Rest in a comfortable position to prolong the period of stretch stimulus.
Perform low-load, prolonged stretching to minimize joint trauma.

elbow range of motion can be found in Table 14–5. Additional information on range of motion and flexibility is contained in Chapter 6.

High-intensity, short-duration stretching is contraindicated for any elbow with limited range of motion. This can stimulate ossification, potentially resulting in traumatic myositis ossificans, additional loss of motion, and increased pain, which translate into poor outcomes.[35, 66] Rather, joint mobilization of the humeroulnar and radioulnar joint and low-load, long-duration stretching is advocated. Low-load, long-duration stretching can be accomplished through the application of a dynamic splint (Fig. 14–8) or by using techniques similar to the one described by Wilk and colleagues (Fig. 14–9).[88]

Flexion contractures are best treated in the subacute stage with modalities in combination with a therapeutic exercise program. The use of moist heat and ultrasound prior to, or in conjunction with, range-of-motion exercises may stimulate vasodilation and increase collagen elasticity, thereby allowing greater elongation with less associated structural damage. The athlete can perform range-of-motion exercises while immersing the elbow in a warm whirlpool, combining the heating effects with the buoyancy of the water.

Also, the UBE is an excellent range-of-motion tool. The seat and arm attachments can be adjusted to accommodate an athlete with a range-of-motion deficit, and it may be used for passive, active-assisted, or active range of motion. Exercise with the UBE increases local temperature and blood flow around the joint and stimulates synovial fluid disbursement. When appropriate, soft-tissue and joint mobilization techniques may be beneficial.

Use of a dynamic splint (see Chap. 6), which applies a prolonged, low-

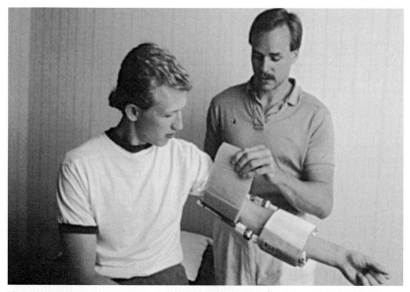

Figure 14–8. Elbow dynamic splint. This can provide a low-force, long-duration stretch for an elbow with loss of range of motion. (From Courson, R. [1989]: Rehabilitation of the thrower's elbow. Sports Med. Update, 4:6.)

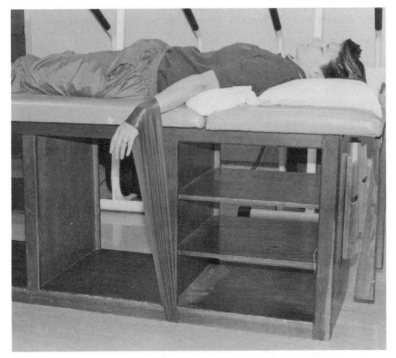

Figure 14-9. Low-load, long-duration stretch as described by Wilk et al.[88]

intensity force, has met with success in treating loss of elbow range of motion without the risk of traumatizing the joint by forceful and vigorous stretching (see Fig. 14–8).[35] To obtain the best results, the dynamic splint is generally advocated for use at night while the athlete is sleeping, but it may be worn during the day. Usually, the athlete who can achieve extension from 0° to 10° is fully functional and does not notice the loss of elbow extension.[2, 6, 46]

If conservative treatment fails, an arthroscopic arthrolysis may be necessary. Rehabilitation after arthroscopic arthrolysis is aggressive in order to restore full range of motion, particularly extension. However, care must be taken not to be too aggressive and inflame the joint, which would result in further pain and reflex splinting. Table 14–6 outlines a rehabilitation protocol for postarthroscopic arthrolysis.

ULNAR AND RADIAL COLLATERAL LIGAMENT SPRAINS

Injuries involving the UCL and radial collateral ligament most often result from overuse, a direct blow, or an elbow dislocation. Damage to the UCL occurs most frequently, particularly in throwers. The medial distraction forces associated with throwing contribute to the gradual attenuation of the UCL, which predisposes the elbow to further degeneration (Fig. 14–10). In addition, Glousman and colleagues[30] have identified asynchronous elbow and forearm muscle activity during pitching in throwers with UCL insufficiency. Such altered function may predispose the elbow to further injury.

The UCL is formed by three distinct bands: anterior, posterior, and transverse (Fig. 14–11). The primary stabilizer to valgus stress is the anterior oblique part of the UCL.[73] This band is taut throughout the full elbow range of motion. Conversely, the posterior band is taut with flexion and lax with extension, with the transverse band contributing little to medial stability.[73, 82] Sectioning of the posterior fibers of the UCL does not result in valgus instability, but resection of

Table 14–6. Elbow Rehabilitation After Arthroscopic Arthrolysis

I. **Phase I: Immediate Motion Phase**
   Goals
   - Improve range of motion
   - Re-establish full passive extension
   - Retard muscular atrophy
   - Decrease pain or inflammation
   A. Days 1–3
   - Range of motion to tolerance (elbow extension-flexion) (2 sets of 10 hourly)
   - Overpressure into extension (at least 10°)
   - Joint mobilization
   - Gripping exercises with putty
   - Isometrics for wrist and elbow
   - Compression, ice hourly
   B. Days 4–9
   - Range of motion extension-flexion (at least 5°–120°)
   - Overpressure into extension—5-lb weight, elbow in full extension (4–5 times daily)
   - Joint mobilization
   - Continue isometrics and gripping exercises
   - Continue use of ice
   C. Days 10–14
   - Full passive range of motion
   - Range-of-motion exercises, 2 sets of 10 hourly
   - Stretch into extension
   - Continue isometrics
II. **Phase II: Motion Maintenance Phase**
   Goals
   - Maintain full range of motion
   - Gradually improve strength
   - Decrease pain or inflammation
   A. Weeks 2–4
   - Range-of-motion exercise (4–5 times daily)
   - Overpressure into extension 00 stretch for 2 min (3–4 times daily)
   - Initiate progressive-resistance exercise program (light dumbbells)—elbow extension-flexion, wrist extension-flexion
   - Continue use of ice postexercise
   B. Weeks 4–7
   - Continue all exercises listed above
   - Initiate interval sports program

From Wilk, K.E., Arrigo, C.A., Andrews, J.R., and Azar, F.M. (1996). Rehabilitation following elbow surgery in the throwing athlete. Operative Tech. Sports Med., 4:114–132.

the anterior oblique UCL fibers alone does.[82] Also, resection of the radial head contributes to medial instability, even if the anterior oblique UCL fibers remain intact.[82]

With acute valgus instability, direct repair of the anterior portion of the UCL using the ligament itself is an appropriate option. However, at surgery, the ligament is often found to be attenuated and is sacrificed. Thus, primary repair of the UCL is difficult, if not contraindicated. In such cases other connective tissues may be transferred to compensate for the insufficiency, or a reconstruction may be attempted using a tendon graft from the palmaris longus, plantaris, or long toe extensor. Jobe and colleagues[41] have described reconstruction of the UCL with autogenous tendon grafts to allow the athlete to return to the previous level of throwing. With this technique, 10 out of 16 throwing athletes successfully returned to their previous level of throwing ability.[41] Schwab and associates[73] have also reported good results using a procedure for osteotomy of the medial epicondyle with transfer to a proximal and anterior position on the humerus in the reconstruction of chronically lax UCL; however, this technique has had no widespread use for throwers.

Recent advances in arthroscopy have resulted in the development of arthroscopic techniques for the elbow. Although these methods are less invasive,

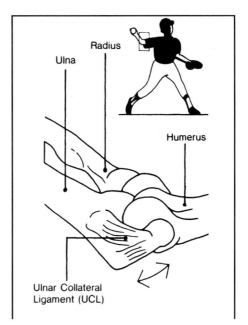

Figure 14–10. Because of the distractive forces that occur medially during the pitching act, the ulnar collateral ligament can be injured from acute or subacute trauma. (From Schemmel, S.P., and Andrews, J.R. [1988]: Acute and chronic ulnar collateral ligament injuries in the throwing athlete. Sports Med. Update, 3:10.)

adequate visualization of the entire anterior portion of the UCL may not be possible through the arthroscope.[17, 50] Use of posterior approaches also necessitates great care in avoiding the ulnar nerve.[17] A medial approach is recommended by Lindenfeld[41] because of its distance from crucial neurovascular structures. Arthroscopic stress views to determine or verify medial laxity have been advocated by Andrews et al.[3]

Rehabilitation after reconstruction of the UCL varies depending on the type of surgery performed, the method of transposition of the ulnar nerve, and the extent of injury within the elbow joint.[88] Seto and colleagues[74] described a rehabilitation program after UCL reconstruction using a palmaris longus tendon graft and transposition of the ulnar nerve within the flexor muscle mass. The rehabilitation program outlined in Table 14–7 is based on the surgical technique described by Andrews and colleagues,[4] which uses an autogenous graft such as the palmaris longus tendon or plantaris tendon to reconstruct the anterior bundle of the UCL along with subcutaneous transposition of the ulnar nerve using fascial slings.

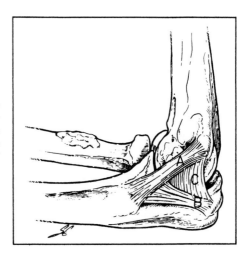

Figure 14–11. Medial aspect of the elbow illustrating the three bundles of fibers that comprise the ulnar collateral ligament. *A*, Anterior. *B*, Transverse. *C*, Posterior. (From Medich, G.F. [1989]: Little League elbow. Sports Med. Update, 4:15.)

572 ◆ Gary L. Harrelson and Deidre Leaver-Dunn

Table 14–7. Postoperative Rehabilitation After Chronic Ulnar Collateral Ligament Reconstruction Using Autogenous Graft

I. **Phase I: Immediate Postoperative Phase (Weeks 0–3)**
   Goals
   - Protect healing tissue
   - Decrease pain or inflammation
   - Retard muscular atrophy
   A. Postoperative week 1
      1. Posterior splint at 90° elbow flexion
      2. Wrist active range of motion extension-flexion
      3. Elbow compression dressing (2–3 days)
      4. Exercises such as gripping exercises, wrist range of motion, shoulder isometrics (except shoulder external rotation), biceps isometrics
      5. Cryotherapy
   B. Postoperative week 2
      1. Apply functional brace, 30°–100° (Fig. 14–12)
      2. Initiate wrist isometrics
      3. Initiate elbow flexion-extension isometrics
      4. Continue all exercises listed above
   C. Postoperative week 3
      1. Advance brace 15°–110° (gradually increase range of motion by 5° extension and 10° flexion per week)

II. **Phase II: Intermediate Phase (Weeks 4–8)**
   Goals
   - Gradually increase range of motion
   - Promote healing of repaired tissue
   - Regain and improve muscular strength
   A. Week 4
      1. Functional brace set (10°–120°)
      2. Begin light resistance exercises for arm (1 lb wrist curls, extensions, pronation-supination, elbow extension-flexion)
      3. Progress shoulder program, emphasize rotator cuff strengthening (avoid external rotation until week 6)
   B. Week 6
      1. Functional brace set (0°–130°); active range of motion 0°–145° (without brace)
      2. Progress elbow strengthening exercises
      3. Initiate shoulder external rotation strengthening
      4. Progress shoulder program

III. **Phase III: Advanced Strengthening Phase (Weeks 9–13)**
   Goals
   - Increase strength, power, and endurance
   - Maintain full elbow range of motion
   - Gradually initiate sports activities
   A. Week 9
      1. Initiate eccentric elbow flexion-extension
      2. Continue isotonic program—forearm and wrist
      3. Continue shoulder program—Throwers' Ten exercise program
      4. Initiate manual resistance diagonal patterns
      5. Initiate plyometric exercise program
   B. Week 11
      1. Continue all exercises listed above
      2. May begin light sports activities (i.e., golf, swimming)

IV. **Phase IV: Return to Activity Phase (Weeks 14–26)**
   Goals
   - Continue to increase strength, power, and endurance of upper extremity musculature
   - Gradually return to sports activities
   A. Week 14
      1. Initiate interval throwing program (Phase I)
      2. Continue strengthening program
      3. Emphasize elbow and wrist strengthening and flexibility exercises
   B. Weeks 22–26
      1. Return to competitive throwing

From Wilk, K.E., Arrigo, C.A., Andrews, J.R., and Azar, F.M. (1996). Rehabilitation following elbow surgery in the throwing athlete. Operative Tech. Sports Med., 4:114–132.

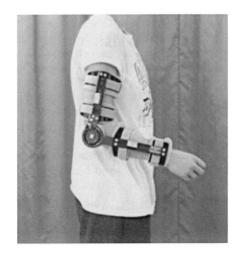

Figure 14-12. Hinged brace for limitation of range of motion with ulnar collateral ligament repairs.

Conservative management of attenuated UCL lesions is an option. This, however, may be only a palliative measure for those athletes who continue to throw and stress the elbow medially.

Athletes returning to contact and collision sports after acute first- or second-degree UCL sprains should have the elbow taped or should wear an orthosis that prevents the last 15° to 30° of extension and protects the elbow from valgus forces. Stress radiography has demonstrated increased medial stability with application of a functional elbow brace after UCL injury.[62]

CONTUSIONS AND STRAINS

Most elbow contusions occur to its bony prominences, the medial and lateral epicondyles and the olecranon process. These injuries, depending on their severity, can result in a transitory loss of flexion, extension, or both. Initial treatment includes cryotherapy and electrical stimulation to decrease effusion and pain and active or active-assisted range of motion. On the second or third day postinjury, the athlete can progress with an elbow exercise program as tolerated and return to practice as early as the next day postinjury, with the area protected for contact sports. A throwing athlete with this injury should return gradually to throwing by accelerating the interval throwing program (see Appendix D).

DISLOCATIONS

Most elbow dislocations result from hyperextension associated with a fall on an outstretched arm. Johansson[43] reported elbow dislocations caused by violent hyperextension and abduction forces that resulted in ruptures of the anterior oblique ligament and anterior joint capsule. Posterior and posterolateral dislocations are most common. Osborne and Cotterill[59] have maintained that the ligaments are the sole factors that prevent posterior dislocations while the elbow is in extension.

Most often, elbow dislocations are treated conservatively. After reduction, the use of an arm sling and a posterior splint at approximately 90° of flexion for 6 weeks have traditionally been the accepted modes of treatment. Prolonged immobilization, however, is accompanied by detrimental effects such as flexion contracture. The rationale for the use of prolonged immobilization is the prevention of a recurrent dislocation; this is rare, even when early mobilization is initiated.[43, 53, 73] Mehlhoff et al[53] retrospectively examined the long-term effects of early mobilization on elbow dislocations. Results of the investigation found that prolonged immobilization after injury is strongly associated with an unsatisfactory result. The longer the immobilization, the larger the flexion contracture and the more severe the pain. From these data the authors recommended that immobilization not exceed 2 weeks after an elbow dislocation.[53] This report is consistent with other findings that have promoted early elbow mobilization after dislocation.[43, 65] Protzman[65] has noted no recurrence of dislocations in 27 patients treated with active range of motion less than 5 days postreduction. Even if some instability still exists, immobilization should never exceed 3 to 4 weeks.[53]

Rehabilitation of the elbow after dislocation can proceed according to the protocol outlined in Table 14–8. Soft-tissue mobilization, PNF patterns, and joint mobilization techniques may be incorporated according to the athlete's needs. A functional brace should be worn for return to activity. These orthoses have been shown to increase medial support in the unstable elbow.[62]

Elbow Injuries in Adolescents

Although adolescent pitchers subject the elbow to the same stresses as do adult pitchers, the manifestation of lesions differs because of the degree of skeletal maturity. In adolescent baseball players the elbow is the most frequent area of complaint. Most of the osseous changes seen in the adolescent as a result of the pitching act are manifested at the radiohumeral joint.[83] The two most common injuries in the adolescent pitcher are osteochondritis dissecans and Little Leaguer's elbow.

OSTEOCHONDRITIS DISSECANS

Osteochondritis dissecans is a lesion to the bone and articular cartilage that commonly occurs on the anterolateral surface of the capitellum (Fig. 14–13).[40] The condition results from repeated lateral compression of the radiocapitellar joint that can injure the articular cartilage, creating loose bodies.[57, 82] Although it

---

Table 14–8. Elbow Dislocation Treatment Protocol

I. **Phase I: Initial Phase (Postinjury Days 1–10)**
   - Note: No passive range of motion
   - Posterior splint at 90° flexion
   - Gripping exercises
   - Wrist active range of motion in all planes
   - Exercise out of splint after 3–4 days
   - Elbow active range of motion in all planes
   - Multiple-angle flexion isometrics
   - Multiple-angle extension isometrics

II. **Phase II: Intermediate Phase (Postinjury Days 10–14)**
   - Discontinue posterior splint
   - Hinged brace with motion from 15°–90°
   - Wrist flexor stretch
   - Wrist extensor stretch
   - Wrist curls
   - Reverse wrist curls
   - Neutral wrist curls
   - Pronation
   - Supination
   - Biceps curls
   - French curls

III. **Phase III: Advanced Phase (Postinjury Weeks 2–6)**
   - Progressive-resistance exercises for previous wrist and elbow exercises
   - Sport-specific activities
   - Functional progressions
   - Interval throwing program (see Appendix D)
   - Daily strength and flexibility maintenance program

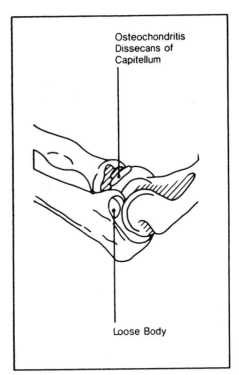

Figure 14–13. Osteochondritis dissecans of the capitellum. (From Medich, G.F. [1989]: Little League elbow. Sports Med. Update, 4:16.)

is most often seen in throwers, osteochondritis dissecans has been reported in adolescent table tennis players[63] and motorcross riders.[39] Osteochondritis dissecans is considered the leading cause of permanent elbow disability in the young pitching athlete.[2, 38, 79] Andrews[2] has reported that this group usually has the most severe flexion contractures and obtains the least benefit from surgery. Unlike lesions occurring to the medial side of the elbow, lateral lesions can result in permanent elbow damage and often shorten or terminate a throwing athlete's career.[83]

The exact cause of osteochondritis dissecans is unknown. It is believed, however, that repeated traumatic impact of the radial head into the capitellum during the cocking and acceleration phases of throwing can result in a circulatory disturbance at the radiocapitellar joint. Primary changes occur to the bone and secondary changes to the cartilage.[60] Instead of presenting as loose body formation, as in the mature thrower, osteochondritis dissecans is seen as aseptic necrosis of the radial head in the adolescent. This can also result in the progressive formation of loose bodies, overgrowth of the radial head, and early arthritic changes.

Osteochondritis dissecans represents a major threat to the elbow joint, and it is important that it be diagnosed early. The athlete complains of anterolateral elbow tenderness along with decreased pronation and supination, suggesting radiocapitellar incongruity or radial head fracture.[82] The most common finding is a loss of full elbow extension. It is not unusual for the athlete to lack as much as 20° of extension.[11, 79, 91]

Initial conservative treatment consists of avoiding noxious stimuli and using modalities for the relief of pain and inflammation. The athlete may begin an elbow exercise program, as tolerated. An overly aggressive approach with osteochondritis dissecans, however, can result in progressive loss of motion. If avascular changes are noted on the lateral side of the elbow in the young thrower, abstinence from throwing should be maintained until revascularization of the affected area has occurred.

Most authors recommend surgical removal of symptomatic loose bodies and avoidance of other surgical procedures, unless there are changes that could compromise the architectural support of the capitellum.[61, 75, 91] Prognosis of osteochondritis dissecans after simple loose body removal is good if diagnosis is made early and no degenerative changes are associated. There is slow recovery to normal function, however, and some limitation of full extension is likely to remain. Tivnon and colleagues[79] have reported an average elbow range of motion preoperatively of 30° to 134°, yielding an average arc of motion of 104°. Follow-up average range of motion was 11° to 136°, with an average arc of 125° of motion. Others have reported a similar response of range of motion after surgery.[11] Therefore, if range of motion is to be re-established or increased after loose body extraction in this condition, early mobilization is paramount.

Degenerative changes of the radiocapitellar joint have a poor prognosis for the athlete returning to pitching.[38] Although the osteophytes and loose bodies can be removed surgically, ankylosis may remain in the young athlete, who is then unable to throw.[36] Singer and Roy[75] reported that of five gymnasts treated for osteochondritis dissecans, four could not return to full workout without recurring symptoms in a 3-year follow-up period.

LITTLE LEAGUER'S ELBOW

Brogdon and Crow[10] coined the term Little Leaguer's elbow to describe an avulsion of the ossification center of the medial epicondyle caused by the pitching act in the adolescent athlete.[36] Since the initial description, several pathologic conditions have been included under this term, including strain of the flexor muscles, ulnar neuropathy, and osteochondritis dissecans.

Forces associated with this condition injure the epiphyseal plate because this is the weakest link in the adolescent kinetic chain. The injury is associated with repetitive throwing and results from the medial traction forces experienced during the acceleration phase. Hypertrophy of the medial epicondyle develops as a physiologic response to throwing. A widened growth line or displacement of the epicondyle is evidence of a fracture (Fig. 14–14).

The adolescent athlete suffering from Little Leaguer's elbow most commonly presents with a history of progressive medial elbow pain over a few weeks, which worsens with pitching and is relieved by rest. Additional signs and symptoms include limitation of complete extension, tenderness over the medial epicondyle, and pain with passive extension of the wrist and fingers. Radiographic changes include accelerated growth and separation and fragmentation

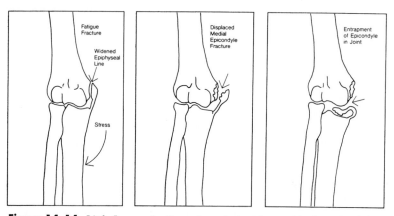

Figure 14–14. Little Leaguer's elbow characterized by a widening growth line and eventual epicondyle displacement. (From Medich, G.F. [1989]: Little League elbow. Sports Med. Update, 4:17.)

of the medial epicondylar epiphysis. Less commonly, the athlete may present with dramatic symptoms, including the report of a popping sensation followed by medial elbow pain, the inability to throw because of pain, and swelling accompanied by medial ecchymosis.

Prevention remains the best treatment for Little Leaguer's elbow. It is important that coaches and parents be educated about proper warm-up, conditioning, and off-season training of the adolescent pitcher. Also, the throwing of curveballs and other breaking pitches by pitchers in the 9- to 14-year age group should be prohibited, because this stress considerably increases the force on wrist flexion and pronation.[13, 61] Pitchers should be taught proper pitching mechanics, and a pitching maximum should be established. Currently, Little League International pitching rules advise six innings per week, with 3 days of rest between pitching turns.[51] However, there are no rules or recommendations that govern the amount of practice pitching.

Treatment in the early stages of Little Leaguer's elbow includes rest from noxious stimuli, application of ice, and possibly immobilization. If radiographic findings reveal capitellum osteochondritis dissecans, it is recommended that the player stop pitching for the remainder of the baseball season.

After initial conservative treatment, if the athlete returns to throwing and there is any recurrence of symptoms, there should be complete abstinence from throwing until the next season. A medial epicondylar fracture that is displaced by more than 1 cm may occur in a small percentage of athletes. These injuries should be opened and fixed internally with a screw. With open and internal fixation, the elbow is immobilized for approximately 3 to 4 weeks, and the athlete should not engage in any throwing activity until the following season. Also, in later stages sometimes, surgery may be indicated if loose bodies are present. Criteria for return to competition include no pain, normal elbow range of motion, and no weakness in muscle strength or endurance in all planes of wrist and elbow range of motion. The return to throwing should be gradual and should follow the Little League interval throwing program (see Appendix D). Fortunately, most elbow injuries in the adolescent thrower are adequately treated by rest and cause no permanent disability.

SUMMARY

Elbow injuries, particularly in throwers, are a common complaint. Most elbow injuries are a result of subacute trauma over a period of time. The nature of the pitching act, which results in medial distraction and lateral compressive forces, causes predictable connective-tissue and osseous changes. Some injuries seen in adult throwers result from cumulative microtrauma associated with the volatile action of throwing. Most elbow lesions caused by overuse usually respond well to avoidance of noxious stimuli, the use of modalities, nonsteroidal anti-inflammatory drugs, and a low-weight, high-repetition rehabilitation regimen.

Although adolescent throwers subject themselves to the same mechanical elbow stresses as do adult throwers, the injuries are different because of the maturation process and can be more debilitating. If these injuries are detected early they can be managed with no debilitating effects; but if the athlete continues to throw and the injuries are left untreated, permanent disability can ensue.

Initial treatment of elbow injuries after conservative management or surgery is concerned with decreasing the athlete's pain and inflammation and with restoring normal joint arthrokinematics. As pain decreases and healing restraints allow, range-of-motion exercises can be increased, and a progressive-resistance exercise regimen can be implemented. Later stages of rehabilitation should concentrate on the athletes' performing exercises in functional planes at functional speeds to ready them for return to their sport. This return to competition should be preceded by an interval throwing program or by an interval program

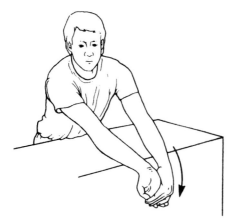

Figure 14–15. Wrist flexor stretch. (From Wilk, K.E., Andrews, J.R., Arrigo, C.A., et al. [1997]: Preventive and Rehabilitative Exercises for the Shoulder and Elbow. Birmingham, Alabama, American Sports Medicine Institute.)

that is applicable for the individual athlete and allows for gradual return to participation.

APPLICATION

(All elbow exercises in this section [except for ulnar and radial deviation] are from Wilk, K.E., Andrews, J.R., Arrigo, C.A., et al. [1997]: Preventive and Rehabilitative Exercises for the Shoulder and Elbow. Birmingham, Alabama, American Sports Medicine Institute.)

Soft-Tissue and Range-of-Motion Techniques

Deep Friction Massage. Deep transverse friction massage is applied across the area of the elbow that is sore for 5 minutes, several times daily.

Grip. The athlete uses a grip apparatus (e.g., putty, small rubber ball) frequently throughout the day.

Stretch Flexors. The athlete straightens the elbow completely and, with the palm facing up, grasps the middle of the hand and thumb (Fig. 14–15). The wrist is pulled down as far as possible, held for a count of 10, and released. The exercise is repeated 5 to 10 times before and after each exercise session.

Stretch Extensors. The athlete straightens the elbow completely and, with the palm facing down, grasps the back of the hand and pulls the wrist down as

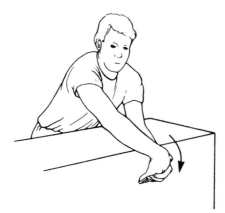

Figure 14–16. Wrist extensor stretch. (From Wilk, K.E., Andrews, J.R., Arrigo, C.A., et al. [1997]: Preventive and Rehabilitative Exercises for the Shoulder and Elbow, 5th ed. Birmingham, Alabama, American Sports Medicine Institute.)

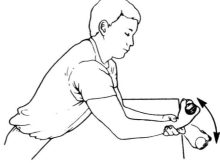

Figure 14–17. Wrist curls. (From Wilk, K.E., Andrews, J.R., Arrigo, C.A., et al. [1997]: Preventive and Rehabilitative Exercises for the Shoulder and Elbow, 5th ed. Birmingham, Alabama, American Sports Medicine Institute.)

far as possible (Fig. 14–16). This is held for a count of 10 and released and repeated 5 to 10 times before and after each exercise session.

Progressive-Resistance Exercises (PRE)

Each PRE session is started with three sets of 10 repetitions (or 30 times) without weight, progressing to five sets of 10 repetitions (or 50 times) as tolerated. When the athlete can easily perform five sets of 10 repetitions, he or she may begin adding weight. Each PRE session begins with three sets of 10 repetitions with a 1-pound weight, progressing to five sets of 10, as tolerated over the next 2 to 3 days. When the athlete can easily perform five sets of 10 repetitions with a 1-pound weight, he or she may begin to progress the weight in the same manner.

Wrist Curls. The forearm should be supported on a table with the hand off the edge; the palm should face upward. Using a weight, the athlete lowers the hand as far as possible and then curls the wrist up as high as possible (Fig. 14–17), holding for a count of 2.

Reverse Wrist Curls. The forearm should be supported on a table with the hand off the edge; the palm should face downward. Using a weight, the athlete lowers the hand as far as possible and then curls the wrist up as high as possible (Fig. 14–18), holding for a count of 2.

Radial Deviation. Standing with the arm by the side, the athlete holds an adjustable rod or hammer as depicted (Fig. 14–19), radially deviating the wrist, keeping the elbow straight, and holding for a count of 2.

Ulnar Deviation. Standing with the arm by the side, the athlete holds an

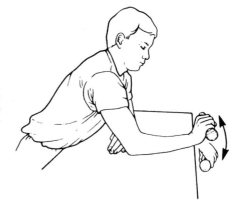

Figure 14–18. Reverse wrist curls. (From Wilk, K.E., Andrews, J.R., Arrigo, C.A., et al. [1997]: Preventive and Rehabilitative Exercises for the Shoulder and Elbow, 5th ed. Birmingham, Alabama, American Sports Medicine Institute.)

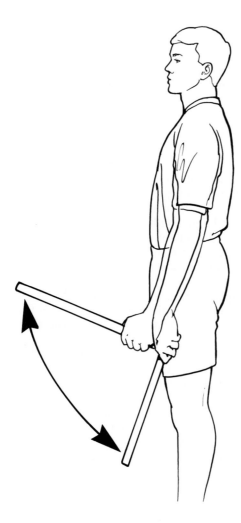

Figure 14–19. Radial deviation.

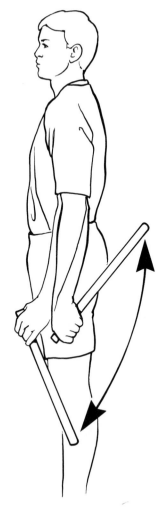

Figure 14–20. Ulnar deviation.

adjustable rod or hammer as depicted (Fig. 14–20), ulnarly deviating the wrist, keeping the elbow straight, and holding for a count of 2.

Pronation. The forearm should be supported on a table with the wrist in the neutral position (Fig. 14–21*A*). Using a hammer or adjustable rod, the athlete rolls the wrist and brings the hammer or rod into pronation as far as possible (Fig. 14–21*B*), holding for a count of 2, and then raising back to starting position.

Supination. The forearm should be supported on the table with the wrist in the neutral position (Fig. 14–22*A*). Using a hammer or adjustable rod, the athlete rolls the wrist and brings the hammer or rod into full supination (Fig. 14–22*B*), holding for a count of 2 and raising back to the starting position.

Broomstick Curl-Up. A 1- to 2-foot broom handle with a 4- to 5-foot cord attached in the middle is used, with a 1- to 5-pound weight tied in the center.

Extensors. The athlete grips the stick on each side of the rope with the palms down (Fig. 14–23*A*). The cord is curled up by turning the stick toward the athlete (the cord is on the side of the stick away from the athlete). Once the weight is pulled to the top, the weight is lowered by unwinding the stick, rotating it away from the athlete. This is repeated 3 to 5 times.

Flexors. This is the same as the exercise for the extensors, but the palms are facing upward (Fig. 14–23*B*).

Biceps Curl. The athlete supports the arm on the opposite hand, bends the elbow to full flexion, and then straightens the arm completely (Fig. 14–24).

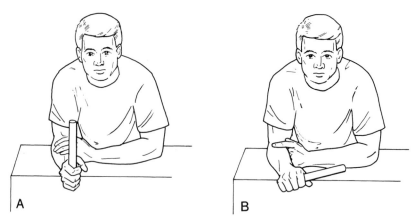

Figure 14–21. *A* and *B*, Pronation. (Modified from Wilk, K.E., Andrews, J.R., Arrigo, C.A., et al. [1997]: Preventive and Rehabilitative Exercises for the Shoulder and Elbow, 5th ed. Birmingham, Alabama, American Sports Medicine Institute.)

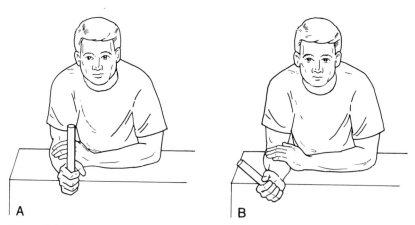

Figure 14–22. *A* and *B*, Supination. (Modified from Wilk, K.E., Andrews, J.R., Arrigo, C.A., et al. [1997]: Preventive and Rehabilitative Exercises for the Shoulder and Elbow, 5th ed. Birmingham, Alabama, American Sports Medicine Institute.)

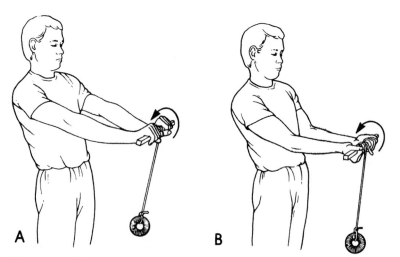

Figure 14–23. Broomstick curl-ups. *A*, For flexors. *B*, For extensors. (From Wilk, K.E., Andrews, J.R., Arrigo, C.A., et al. [1997]: Preventive and Rehabilitative Exercises for the Shoulder and Elbow, 5th ed. Birmingham, Alabama, American Sports Medicine Institute.)

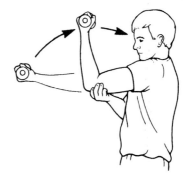

Figure 14–24. Biceps curl. (From Wilk, K.E., Andrews, J.R., Arrigo, C.A., et al. [1997]: Preventive and Rehabilitative Exercises for the Shoulder and Elbow, 5th ed. Birmingham, Alabama, American Sports Medicine Institute.)

French Curl. The athlete raises the arm overhead, using the opposite hand to support the elbow (Fig. 14–25). The elbow is straightened over the head, holding for a count of 2.

Eccentric Elbow Program

Flexion. The athlete places the arm on the table, holding it straight with the hand facing up and off the table. Tubing is placed around the hand, with the opposite end tied tightly to the table leg (Fig. 14–26A). With the palm up, the opposite hand assists the wrist to a flexed position, and the athlete works to starting position within a count of 5 (Fig. 14–26B), repeating three to five sets of 10 repetitions.

Extension. The athlete places the arm on the table, holding it straight with the hand facing down and off the table. The tubing is placed around the hand, with the opposite end tied tightly to the table leg (Fig. 14–27A). The opposite hand is used to assist the wrist to an extended position, and the athlete works back to starting position within a count of 5 (Fig. 14–27B), repeating three to five sets of 10 repetitions.

Pronation. The athlete places the arm straight on the table with the thumb up, holding the hammer (with the tubing secure around the top of the hammer and the opposite end of the tubing tied to the table leg nearest the involved arm) (Fig. 14–28A). The hammer is assisted with the opposite hand pushing the hammer and palm down, slowly returning to neutral within a count of 5 (Fig. 14–28B). This is repeated for 3 to 5 sets of 10 repetitions.

Figure 14–25. French curl. (From Wilk, K.E., Andrews, J.R., Arrigo, C.A., et al. [1997]: Preventive and Rehabilitative Exercises for the Shoulder and Elbow, 5th ed. Birmingham, Alabama, American Sports Medicine Institute.)

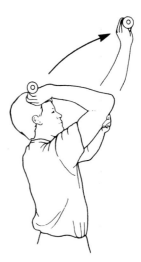

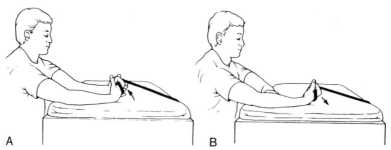

Figure 14–26. *A* and *B*, Eccentric wrist flexion. (From Wilk, K.E., Andrews, J.R., Arrigo, C.A., et al. [1997]: Preventive and Rehabilitative Exercises for the Shoulder and Elbow, 5th ed. Birmingham, Alabama, American Sports Medicine Institute.)

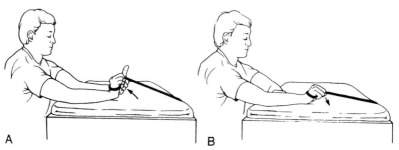

Figure 14–27. *A* and *B*, Eccentric wrist extension. (From Wilk, K.E., Andrews, J.R., Arrigo, C.A., et al. [1997]: Preventive and Rehabilitative Exercises for the Shoulder and Elbow, 5th ed. Birmingham, Alabama, American Sports Medicine Institute.)

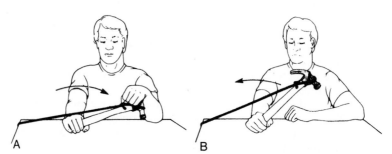

Figure 14–28. *A* and *B*, Eccentric pronation. (From Wilk, K.E., Andrews, J.R., Arrigo, C.A., et al. [1997]: Preventive and Rehabilitative Exercises for the Shoulder and Elbow, 5th ed. Birmingham, Alabama, American Sports Medicine Institute.)

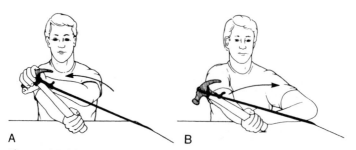

Figure 14–29. *A* and *B*, Eccentric supination. (From Wilk, K.E., Andrews, J.R., Arrigo, C.A., et al. [1997]: Preventive and Rehabilitative Exercises for the Shoulder and Elbow, 5th ed. Birmingham, Alabama, American Sports Medicine Institute.)

Supination. The athlete places the arm straight on the table with the thumb up, holding the hammer (with the tubing secure around the top of the hammer and the opposite end of the tubing tied to the table leg opposite the involved arm). The hammer is pushed down with the opposite hand, turning the involved hand palm up (Fig. 14–29A) and slowly returning to neutral position within a count of 5 (Fig. 14–29B). This is repeated three to five times.

References

1. Albert M.S., Hillegass, E., and Spiegel, P. (1994): Muscle torque changes caused by inertial exercise training. J. Orthop. Sports Phys. Ther., 20:254–261.
2. Andrews, J.R. (1985): Bony injuries about the elbow in the throwing athlete. In: Stauffer, E.S. (ed.): Instructional Course Lectures, Vol. 36. St. Louis, C.V. Mosby, pp. 323–331.
3. Andrews, J.R., and Wilson, F. (1985): Valgus extension overload in the pitching elbow. In: Zarins, B., Andrews, J.R., and Carson, W.G. (eds.): Injuries to the Throwing Athlete. Philadelphia, W.B. Saunders, pp. 250–257.
4. Andrews, J.R., Joyce, M., Jelsma R., et al. (1996): Open surgical procedures for injuries to the elbow in throwers. Operative Tech. Sports Med., 4:109–113.
5. Barnes, W.G., and Tullos, H.S. (1978): An analysis of 100 symptomatic baseball players. Am. J. Sports Med., 6:62–67.
6. Bennett, G.E. (1941): Shoulder and elbow lesions of the professional baseball pitcher. JAMA, 117:510–514.
7. Berkely, M.E., Bennett, J.B., and Woods, G.W. (1985): Surgical management of acute and chronic elbow problems. In: Zarins, B., Andrews, J.R., and Carson, W.G. (eds.): Injuries to the Throwing Arm. Philadelphia, W.B. Saunders, pp. 235–249.
8. Bernhang, A.M., Dehner, W., and Fogerry, C. (1974): Tennis elbow: A biomechanical approach. J. Sports Med., 2:235–258.
9. Boyd, C.A., and McLeod, A.L. (1973): Tennis elbow. J. Bone Joint Surg. [Am.], 55:1183–1187.
10. Brogdon, B.S., and Crow, M.D. (1960): Little Leaguer's elbow. Am. J. Roentgenol., 85:671–677.
11. Brown, R., Blazina, M.E., Kerlan, R.K., et al. (1974): Osteochondritis of the capitellum. J. Sports Med., 2:27–46.
12. Chu, D. (1992). Jumping into plyometrics. Champaign, IL, Human Kinetics Publishers.
13. DeHaven, K.E., and Evarts, C.M. (1973): Throwing injuries of the elbow in athletes. Orthop. Clin. North Am., 4:801–808.
14. Del Pizzo, W., Jobe, F.W., and Norwood, L. (1977): Ulnar nerve entrapment syndrome in baseball players. Am. J. Sports Med., 5:182–185.
15. Eaton, R.G., Crowe, J.F., and Parkes, J.C. (1980): Anterior transposition of the ulnar nerve using a non-compressing fasciodermal sling. J. Bone Joint Surg. [Am.], 62:820–825.
16. Feltner, M.E. (1989): Three dimensional interactions in a two-segment kinetic chain. Part II: Application to the throwing arm in baseball pitching. Int. J. Sport Biomech., 5:420–450.
17. Field, L.D., Callaway, G.H., O'Brien, S.J., and Altchek, D.W. (1995): Arthroscopic assessment of the medial collateral ligament complex of the elbow. Am. J. Sports Med., 23:396–400.
18. Fleisig, G.S., and Barrentine, S.W. (1995): Biomechanical aspects of the elbow in sports. Sports Med. Arthrosc. Rev., 3:149–159.
19. Fleisig, G.S., and Escamilla, R.F. (1996). Biomechanics of the elbow in the throwing athlete. Operative Tech. Sports Med., 4:62–68.
20. Fleisig, G.S., Andrews, J.R., Dillman, C.J., and Escamilla, R.F. (1995): Kinetics of baseball pitching with implications about injury mechanisms. Am. J. Sports Med., 23:233–239.
21. Fleisig, G.S., Barrentine, S.W., Escamilla, R.F., and Andrews, J.R. (1996): Biomechanics of overhand throwing with implications for injuries. Sports Med., 6:421–437.
22. Fleisig, G.S., Escamilla, R.F., Andrews, J.R., et al. (1996). Kinematic and kinetic comparison between baseball pitching and football passing. J. Appl. Biomech., 12: 207–224.
23. Froimson, A.I. (1971): Treatment of tennis elbow with forearm support. J. Bone Joint Surg. [Am.], 53:183–184.
24. Froimson, A.I., and Zahrawi, F. (1980): Treatment of compression neuropathy of the ulnar nerve at the elbow by epicondylectomy and neurolysis. J. Hand Surg., 5:391–396.
25. Gambetta, V., and Odgers, S. (1991). The Complete Guide to Medicine Ball Training. Sarasota, FL, Optimum Sports Training.
26. Garver, A.A. (1989): Iontophoresis Protocol: Tennis Elbow. Iomed, Salt Lake City.
27. Gay, J.R., and Love, J.G. (1947): Diagnosis and treatment of tardy paralysis of the ulnar nerve. J. Bone Joint Surg. [Am.], 29:1087–1095.
28. Giangarra, C.E., Conroy, B., Jobe F.W., et al. (1993): Electromyographic and cinematographic analysis of elbow function in tennis players using single- and double-handed backhand strokes. Am. J. Sports Med., 21:394–399.
29. Glazebrook, M.A., Curwin, S., Islam, M.N., et al. (1994): Medial epicondylitis: An electromyographic analysis and an investigation of intervention strategies. Am. J. Sports Med., 22:674–679.

30. Glousman, R.E., Barron, J., Jobe, F.W., et al. (1992): An electromyographic analysis of the elbow in normal and injured pitchers with medial collateral ligament insufficiency. Am. J. Sports Med., 20:311–317.
31. Grana, W.A. (1980): Pitchers elbow in adolescents. Am. J. Sports Med., 8:333–336.
32. Groppel, J.L., and Nirschl, R.P. (1986): A mechanical and electromyographical analysis of the effects of various joint counterforce braces on the tennis player. Am. J. Sports Med., 14:195–200.
33. Halle, J.S., Franklin, R.J., and Karalfa, B.L. (1986): Comparison of four treatment approaches for lateral epicondylitis of the elbow. J. Orthop. Sports Phys. Ther., 8:62–68.
34. Hennig, E.M., Rosenbaum, D., and Milani, T.L. (1992): Transfer of tennis racquet vibrations onto the human forearm. Med. Sci. Sports Exerc., 24:1134–1140.
35. Hepburn, G.R., and Crivelli, R.J. (1984): Use of elbow Dynasplint for reduction of elbow flexion contractures: A case study. J. Orthop. Sports Phys. Ther., 5:269–274.
36. Hunter, S.C. (1985): Little Leaguer's elbow. In: Zarins, B., Andrews, J.R., and Carson, W.G. (eds.): Injuries to the Throwing Arm. Philadelphia, W.B. Saunders, pp. 228–234.
37. Ilfeld, F.W., and Field, S.M. (1966): Treatment of tennis elbow. JAMA, 195:111–114.
38. Indelicato, P.A., Jobe, F.W., Kerlan, R.K., et al. (1979): Correctable elbow lesions in professional baseball players: A review of 25 cases. Am. J. Sports Med., 7:72–75.
39. Inoue, G. (1991): Bilateral osteochondritis dissecans of the elbow treated with Herbert screw fixation. Br. J. Sports Med., 25:142–144.
40. Jobe, F.W., and Nuber, G. (1986): Throwing injuries of the elbow. Clin. Sports Med., 5:621–636.
41. Jobe, F.W., Stark, H., and Lombardo, S.J. (1986): Reconstruction of the ulnar collateral ligament in athletes. J. Bone Joint Surg. [Am.], 68:1158–1163.
42. Jobe, F.W., Moynes, D.R., Tibone, J.E., and Perry, J. (1984): An EMG analysis of the shoulder in pitching: A special report. Am. J. Sports Med., 12:218–220.
43. Johansson, O. (1962): Capsular and ligament injuries of the elbow joint: A clinical and arthrographic study. Acta Chir. Scand. Suppl., 287:5–71.
44. Jones, H.H., Priest, J.D., Hayes, W.C., et al. (1977): Humeral hypertrophy in response to exercise. J. Bone Joint Surg. [Am.], 59:204–209.
45. Kelley, J.D., Lombardo, S.J., Pink, M., et al. (1994): Electromyographic and cinematographic analysis of elbow function in tennis players with lateral epicondylitis. Am. J. Sports Med., 22:359–363.
46. King, J.W., Brelsford, H.J., and Tullos, H.S. (1969): Analysis of the pitching arm of the professional baseball pitcher. Clin. Orthop., 67:116–122.
47. Koh, T.J., Grabiner, M.D., and Weiker, G.G. (1992): Technique and ground reaction forces in the back handspring. Am. J. Sports Med., 20:61–66.
48. Leach, R.E., and Miller, J.K. (1987): Lateral and medial epicondylitis of the elbow. Clin. Sports Med., 6:259–272.
49. Levy, D.M., and Apfelberg, D.B. (1972): Results of anterior transposition for ulnar neuropathy at the elbow. Am. J. Surg., 123:304–308.
50. Lindenfeld, T.N. (1990): Medial approach in elbow arthroscopy. Am. J. Sports Med., 18:413–417.
51. Little League International. (1996): 1996 Youth Baseball Handbook. Williamsport, PA, Little League International.
52. McLeod, W.D. (1985): The pitching mechanism. In: Zarins, B., Andrews, J.R., and Carson, W.G. (eds.): Injuries to the Throwing Arm. Philadelphia, W.B. Saunders, pp. 22–29.
53. Melhoff, T.L., Noble, P.C., Bennett, J.B., and Tullos, H.S. (1988): Simple dislocation of the elbow in the adult. J. Bone Joint Surg. [Am.], 70:244–249.
54. Neblett, C., and Ehini, G. (1970): Medial epicondylectomy for ulnar palsy. J. Neurosurg., 32:55–60.
55. Nirschl, R.P. (1973): Tennis elbow. Orthop. Clin. North Am., 4:787–799.
56. Nirschl, R.P. (1975): The etiology and treatment of tennis elbow. Am. J. Sports Med., 2:308–323.
57. Nirschl, R.P. (1986): Soft-tissue injuries about the elbow. Clin. Sports Med., 5:637–653.
58. Ollivierre, C.O., Nirschl, R.P., and Pettrone, F.A. (1995): Resection and repair for medial tennis elbow: A prospective analysis. Am. J. Sports Med., 23:214–221.
59. Osborne, G., and Cotterill, P. (1966): Recurrent dislocation of the elbow. J. Bone Joint Surg. [Br.], 48:340–346.
60. Pappas, A.M. (1981): Osteochondrosis dissecans. Clin. Orthop., 158:59–69.
61. Pappas, A.M. (1982): Elbow problems associated with baseball during childhood and adolescence. Clin. Orthop., 164:30–41.
62. Pincivero, D.M., Rijke, A.M., Heinrichs, K., and Perrin, D.H. (1994): The effects of a functional elbow brace on medial joint stability: A case study. J. Athl. Train., 29:232–234, 237.
63. Pintore, E., and Maffulli, N. (1991): Osteochondritis dissecans of the lateral humeral epicondyle in a table tennis player. Med. Sci. Sports Exerc., 23:889–891.
64. Priest, J.D. (1976): Tennis elbow: The syndrome and a study of average players. Minn. Med., June:367–371.
65. Protzman, R.R. (1978): Dislocation of the elbow joint. J. Bone Joint Surg. [Am.], 60:539–541.
66. Raney, R.B., and Brasher, H.R. (1971): Shands' Handbook of Orthopaedic Surgery. St. Louis, C.V. Mosby, pp. 429–431.
67. Regan, W., Wold, L.E., Coonrad, R., and Morrey, B.F. (1992): Microscopic histopathology of chronic refractory lateral epicondylitis. Am. J. Sports Med., 20:746–749.
68. Rettig, A.C. and Ebben, J.R. (1993): Anterior subcutaneous transfer of the ulnar nerve in the athlete. Am. J. Sports Med., 21:836–840.

69. Richmond, J.C., and Southmayd, W.W. (1982): Superficial anterior transposition of the ulnar nerve at the elbow for ulnar neuritis. Clin. Orthop., 164:42–44.

70. Runge, F. (1873): Zur Genese und Behandlung des Schreibekrampfes. Berl. Klin. Wochenschr., 21:245–248.

71. Sakuri, S., Ikegami, Y., Okamoto, A., et al. (1993): A three-dimensional cinematographic analysis of upper limb movement during fastball and curveball baseball pitches. J. Appl. Biomech., 9:47–65.

72. Schemmel, S.P., and Andrews, J.R. (1988): Acute and chronic ulnar collateral ligament injuries in the throwing athlete. Sports Med. Update, 3:10–11.

73. Schwab, G.H., Bennett, J.B., Woods, G.W., and Tullos, H.S. (1980): Biomechanics of elbow instability: The role of the medial collateral ligament. Clin. Orthop., 146:42–52.

74. Seto, J.L., Brewster, C.E., Randall, C.C., et al. (1991). Rehabilitation following ulnar collateral ligament reconstruction of athletes. J. Orthop. Sports Phys. Ther., 14:100–105.

75. Singer, K.M., and Roy, S.P. (1984): Osteochondrosis of the humeral capitellum. Am. J. Sports Med., 12:351–360.

76. Sisto, D.J., Jobe, F.W., Moynes, D.R., and Antonelli, D.J. (1987): An electromyographic analysis of the elbow in pitching. Am. J. Sports Med., 15:260–263.

77. Snyder-Mackler, L., and Epler, M. (1989): Effect of standard and Aircast tennis elbow bands on integrated electromyography of forearm extensor musculature proximal to the bands. Am. J. Sports Med., 17:278–281.

78. Stonecipher, D.R., and Catlin, P.A. (1984): The effect of a forearm strap on wrist extensor strength. J. Orthop. Sports Phys. Ther., 6:184–189.

79. Tivnon, M.C., Anzel, S.H., and Waugh, T.R. (1976): Surgical management of osteochondritis dissecans of the capitellum. Am. J. Sports Med., 4:121–128.

80. Torg, J.S., Pollack, H., and Sweterlitsch, P. (1972): The effect of competitive pitching on the shoulders and elbows in preadolescent baseball players. Pediatrics, 49:267–271.

81. Tracy, J.E., Obuchi, S., and Johnson, B. (1995): Kinematic and electromyographic analysis of elbow flexion during inertial exercise. J. Athl. Train., 30:254–258.

82. Tullos, H.S., and Bryan, W.J. (1985): Examination of the throwing elbow. In: Zarins, B., Andrews, J.R., and Carson, W.G. (eds.): Injuries to the Throwing Athlete. Philadelphia, W.B. Saunders, pp. 201–210.

83. Tullos, H.S., and King, J.W. (1972): Lesion of the pitching arm in adolescents. JAMA, 220:264–271.

84. Tullos, H.S., and King, J.W. (1973): Throwing mechanism in sports. Orthop. Clin. North Am., 4:709–721.

85. Vanderpool, D.W., Chalmers, J., Lamb, D.W., and Winston, T.B. (1968): Peripheral compression lesion of the ulnar nerve. J. Bone Joint Surg. [Br.], 50:792–803.

86. Wadsworth, C.T., Nielson, D.H., Burns, L.T., et al. (1989): Effect of the counterforce armband on wrist extension and grip strength and pain in subjects with tennis elbow. J. Orthop. Sports Phys. Ther., 11:192–197.

87. Werner, S.L., Fleisig, G.S., Dillman, C.J., and Andrews, J.R. (1993): Biomechanics of the elbow during baseball pitching. J. Orthop. Sports Phys. Ther., 17:274–278.

88. Wilk, K.E., Arrigo, C.A., Andrews, J.R., and Azar, F.M. (1996). Rehabilitation following elbow surgery in the throwing athletes. Operative Tech. Sports Med., 4:114–132.

89. Wilk, K.E., Voight, M., Keirns, M.J. (1993). Plyometrics for the upper extremities: Theory and clinical application. J. Orthop. Sports Phys. Ther., 17:225–239.

90. Wilson, F.D., Andrews, J.R., and McCluskey, G. (1983): Valgus extension overload in the pitching elbow. Am. J. Sports Med., 11:83–87.

91. Woodward, A.H., and Bianco, A.J. (1975): Osteochondritis dissecans of the elbow. Clin. Orthop., 110:35–41.

Chapter 15

Rehabilitation of Wrist and Hand Injuries

Tim L. Uhl, M.S., P.T., A.T.,C., Sejal Shah, O.T.R./L., and Joe Gieck, Ed.D., A.T.,C., P.T.

The purpose of this chapter is to provide a commonsense approach to treating athletes with injuries to their wrists, hands, and fingers. These injuries are often minimized and not given the full attention they deserve because athletes are often able to continue participation after minimal care. However, these injuries, if left untreated, can result in permanent disability.[13] As with any other sport injury, the primary goal is to return the athlete to full participation as soon as possible without risking further injury or permanent disability.[23] The primary emphasis of this chapter will be management of common wrist, hand, and finger injuries to minimize time to return to participation and prevent permanent disability or deformity.

The chapter briefly discusses common mechanisms of injury, pathology of the involved structures, and clinical assessment of the injury. Commonsense management of the injury is presented with regard to protective splinting, taping, and initiation of rehabilitation. A summary of splinting procedures for each injury can be found in Table 15–1. Exercises are described to help the athlete return to participation and maximize return of full function of the injured structure.

COMMON INJURIES: MECHANISMS AND MANAGEMENT

Mallet Finger

Mallet injury occurs frequently in sports in which balls are being caught, especially football, basketball, baseball, and softball.[31] The distal phalanx is impacted by a ball or some other object, forcing flexion or hyperextension of the distal phalanx while the extensor mechanism is active.[1, 33] The mallet finger deformity is readily observed, and the athlete is unable to actively extend the distal phalanx. McCue[23] classifies this injury into five types (Table 15–2).

The treatment of a mallet finger depends on the type of injury the distal interphalangeal joint (DIP) and extensor mechanism have sustained. The first three types may be treated conservatively by splinting the DIP joint in full extension.[31] This may be achieved through a variety of splinting techniques, including commercially available stack splints and dorsal or volar aluminum or thermoplastic splints (Fig. 15–1).[51]

Treatment of types IV and V injuries generally involves surgery. With appro-

Table 15–1. Splinting Summary

INJURY	JOINT POSITION	CONSTANT SPLINTING	COMPETITION SPLINTING	BEGIN MOTION AT
Mallet finger	Extension DIP	9 wk	Add 3 wk	9 wk
DIP and PIP dislocations	30° flexion	3 wk	Add 3 wk	3 wk
Jersey finger and FDP repair	MCP in 70° flexion; PIP and DIP in extension	3 wk	Add 3 wk	3 wk
Boutonnière deformity	PIP in extension; DIP and MCP free	6–8 wk	Add 6–8 wk	6–8 wk
Pseudoboutonnière deformity	30° flexion	5 wk	Add 3 wk	3 wk
Metacarpal fracture	MCP, 30°	3–6 wk	Add 3–4 wk	3 wk
UCL sprain of thumb	Thumb spica cast	3 wk	Add 3–6 wk	3 wk
Bennett's fracture	Thumb spica cast	6 wk	Add 6 wk	4 wk
Scaphoid fracture	Thumb spica cast	9 wk	Until season is over	Once snuffbox is painless
Hamate fracture	Padding	Symptomatically		
Wrist sprain and ganglion cyst	Cock-up splint	3–7 days	As needed	3–7 days
de Quervain's tenosynovitis	Thumb spica cast	3–6 wk	As needed	3–6 wk as symptoms allow
Carpal tunnel syndrome	10° wrist extension	4–6 wk	As needed	1–2 wk as symptoms allow

DIP, Distal interphalangeal; MCP, metacarpophalangeal; PIP, proximal interphalangeal; UCL, ulnar collateral ligament.

priate protective splinting, the athlete may return to participation as pain allows.[31]

The DIP joint must be immobilized for 9 weeks.[29] Management of initial swelling can be accomplished with the use of a wrapping such as Coban wrap, ice, and elevation. A dorsal aluminum or thermoplastic splint has advantages for those athletes who handle the ball and need more tactile control because the fingertip is kept free while the DIP joint still has three-point fixation.[30] Care should be taken that the DIP joint is not splinted into hyperextension because such may cause an impairment of blood supply to the joint, resulting in a skin slough over the DIP joint.[28] The splint and skin must be kept dry to prevent maceration. The clinician must educate the athlete about ensuring skin integrity. The athlete should be instructed to remove the splint regularly to clean and dry the area under the splint. On initial removal of the splint, the athlete must be supervised and instructed to keep the DIP in full extension. If any flexion occurs at any time during the immobilization phase, the 9-week immobilization period

Table 15–2. Classification of Mallet Finger

TYPE	INJURY
I	Tendon stretch
II	Tendon rupture
III	Tendon rupture with avulsion of distal phalanx
IV	Distal phalanx fracture involving the articular surface
V	Epiphyseal fracture

Data from McCue, F.C. (1982): The elbow, wrist, and hand. *In* Kulund, D.N. (ed.): The Injured Athlete. Philadelphia, J.B. Lippincott, pp. 295–329.

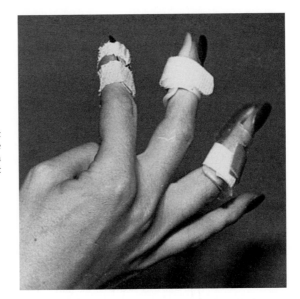

Figure 15-1. Three types of mallet finger splints: a dorsal splint on the index finger, a thermoplastic splint on the middle finger, and a stack splint on the ring finger.

starts again from that day. The athlete should be allowed to return to play with the splint at the physician's discretion.[24] After the initial 9 weeks of continuous splinting, the athlete is advised to continue wearing the splint during athletic activities for 6 to 8 more weeks.[31]

Rehabilitation of mallet finger is initiated after the 9 weeks of immobilization. Active range-of-motion exercises are initiated at this time to establish normal range of motion. Passive DIP flexion may be initiated if there is a significant loss in active flexion that does not seem to be returning with the active exercises after 2 weeks. The athlete may begin strengthening exercises as long as there is no loss of DIP extension and range of motion is improving. Refer to specific exercises in the rehabilitation section later in this chapter.

DIP Joint Fracture and Dislocations

Fractures of the DIP are commonly caused by direct crushing injuries, and the fractures are not usually displaced.[41] Crepitus and point tenderness in the distal phalanx are classic signs of a fracture. Along with the fracture, the digit may have a subungual hematoma. Radiographs must be obtained to confirm presence of a fracture, but it is not generally necessary to acquire radiographs immediately. With all finger injuries in which there is ecchymosis and edema as a result of trauma, ligamentous instability, or painful passive compression of the finger, radiographs must be obtained.

Acute management of a nondisplaced fracture requires a compressive dressing and placement of the DIP joint in an extension gutter splint. Edema control may be achieved via elastic wrap (e.g., Coban wrap or digi sleeve) (Fig. 15–2). The subungual hematoma can be drained in a sterile environment to reduce pain and pressure. Healing of the fracture usually takes 3 to 4 weeks. If the fracture is displaced and there is disruption of the nail and nailbed, surgery may be necessary.[41]

Rehabilitation to regain motion is initiated after clinical and radiographic healing of the fracture has occurred, generally in 3 to 4 weeks. At this point, a progression of active motion for 2 weeks is begun, followed by pain-free passive range of motion. The patient advances to resistance exercises as tolerated over

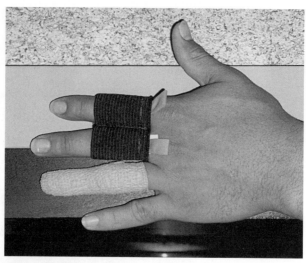

Figure 15–2. Coban wrap for swelling on the ring finger and a double digi sleeve on the index and middle fingers.

the next 3 to 4 weeks. Even with an aggressive rehabilitation program, complete re-establishment of full range of motion of the DIP joint is rare when there is a fracture through the joint.

DIP joint dislocations are rare but can occur from hyperextension or from a lateral force. Dorsal dislocation of the distal phalanx on the middle phalanx is the most common. Volar dislocation occurs less frequently. These dislocations are reducible at the time of injury and are generally stable. However, consideration must be given to the collateral ligaments and volar plate, and these structures must be carefully checked when an obvious dislocation is not present, such as in DIP sprains.[21] Assessment of collateral ligaments is performed with slight flexion of the distal phalanx. The volar plate is assessed by gently hyperextending the distal phalanx on the middle phalanx. If the dislocation is open, care should be taken to prevent infection of the wound.[42] These injuries require surgical débridement to prevent infection of the bone and joint and need surgical repair of the soft tissues damaged.[56]

Postreduction splinting of the DIP dislocations in 30° of flexion for 3 weeks is recommended, along with buddy taping to the adjacent finger to prevent collateral ligament damage (Fig. 15–3). Functional splinting of the DIP joint at 30° is recommended for sprains to decrease stress on the volar plate and to prevent the collateral ligaments from healing in a shortened position. This promotes function during and after the immobilization period.[21]

Management of DIP sprains or dislocations consists of continuous immobilization of the DIP joint in the appropriate position for 3 weeks, leaving the PIP and metacarpophalangeal (MCP) joints free. Active range-of-motion exercises are initiated at 3 weeks postinjury, but continued use of splinting for an additional 3 weeks is recommended. The splint is usually worn for practice and games through the remainder of the competitive season. The same progression of exercises as for fractures is followed for sprains. In most cases, athletes may return to play immediately with a protective splint as soon as they are comfortable.

Jersey Finger (Flexor Digitorum Profundus Rupture)

An athlete may sustain this injury when attempting to grasp an opponent or the opponent's jersey while the opponent is breaking away. The distal phalanx

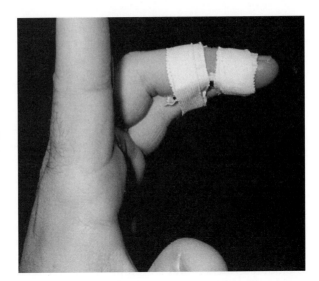

Figure 15–3. Buddy taping of fingers with a 30°-distal interphalangeal splint.

is forcibly extended while the flexor digitorum profundus is active during grasping. This may cause an avulsion of the flexor digitorum profundus at the insertion of the distal phalanx.[5, 25, 49] The injury can occur at any finger, but it most commonly involves the ring finger.[25, 26]

Examination of this injury requires isolating the function of the flexor tendons. The flexor profundus is isolated by blocking proximal interphalangeal (PIP) joint motion while actively flexing the DIP joint. The flexor digitorum superficialis is isolated by blocking all other fingers into extension and allowing PIP flexion of the injured finger (Fig. 15–4). Inability to isolate and actively flex the DIP joint should raise suspicion of flexor profundus injury.[31, 49] Palpating for the retracted tendon along its path is important in identifying the level of retraction. Jersey finger is classified by Leddy and Packer[25] into three types by level of retraction (Table 15–3).

Management of this injury is dependent on the level of disability from the injury, the athlete's participation level, the point in the season, the athlete's team

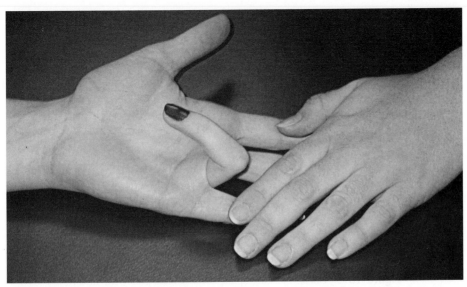

Figure 15–4. Isolation muscle test for flexor digitorum superficialis of the ring finger.

Table 15–3. Classification of Jersey Finger

TYPE	AMOUNT OF RETRACTION	TIME TO REPAIR
I	Retracted to palm	7 days
II	Retracted to PIP joint	10 days
III	Avulsion of distal phalanx	2 wk

Data from Leddy, J.P., and Packer, J.W. (1977): Avulsion of the profundus tendon insertion in athletes. J. Hand Surg., 2:66–69.

position and future sports career plans, and the philosophy of the treating physician. In general, acute repair within 2 weeks is recommended for best return; however, there is a possibility of rerupturing the tendon.[33]

The pre- and postsurgical rehabilitation program consists of edema control, athlete education with regard to precautions, and appropriate splinting position. A modified Klienert and Duran postoperative rehabilitation protocol is described in Table 15–4 for the repair of a torn flexor digitorum profundus (Fig. 15–5).[8, 20]

Boutonnière Injuries

The mechanism of these types of injuries is a direct blow on the dorsum of the PIP joint or forced flexion of the PIP joint while the extensor mechanism is actively extending the joint (e.g., opening the hand to catch a pass and being struck on the dorsum of the hand at the same time). Anatomically, the central slip of the extensor mechanism is ruptured at the base of the middle phalanx.[43] In acute cases, it is difficult to differentiate a PIP joint sprain from a boutonnière injury. In both cases, the athlete can present with swelling, pain, and inability to actively extend the PIP joint. A digital block performed by a physician can block the inhibiting effect of the pain and assist in detection of a ruptured extensor mechanism by the inability to actively extend the PIP joint.[3]

If a boutonnière injury goes untreated or is treated as a PIP joint sprain by splinting the finger in slight flexion, a boutonnière deformity can occur. This presents as a flexion deformity of the PIP joint with a hyperextension deformity

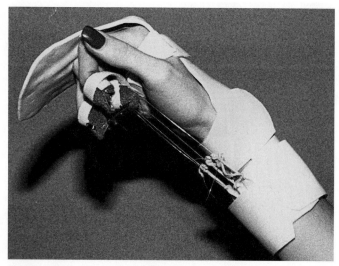

Figure 15–5. Dorsal blocking splint via a palmar pulley for flexor tendon repairs.

Table 15–4. Postoperative Rehabilitation Protocol After Flexor Tendon Repair

I. Days 1–3
  A. Bulky postoperative dressing removed
  B. Fabrication of dorsal blocking splint with inclusion of all digits with a palmar pulley bar: (see Fig. 15–5)
   • Wrist in 20–30° of flexion
   • MCP joints in 60–70° of flexion
   • PIP and DIP joints in full extension
   • Dynamic traction via palmar pulley with night resting strap
  C. Exercise program
   1. Perform active extension of IP joints to the hood of the splint, 10 repetitions every hour without traction through the palmar pulley
   2. Perform passive flexion of the digits, full fist and isolated MCP, PIP, and DIP joint flexion, 10 repetitions 4–6 times a day in splint
   3. Release dynamic traction at night with night strap
   4. Begin scar-tissue massage the day after stitches removed and wound healed; may use wrapping to control edema
II. Weeks 4–6
  A. Continue splinting with modifying wrist into neutral position
  B. Exercise program
   1. Begin place-and-hold exercises
   2. Begin gentle active flexion exercises as directed by physician
III. Week 6
  A. Discontinue splint
  B. If extension contracture exists, begin dynamic splinting
  C. Exercise program
   1. Begin tendon gliding exercises
   2. Begin light activities of daily living
   3. Continue PROM, scar massage
   4. Begin active wrist flexion and extension
   5. Begin making composite fist and flex wrist, then extend wrist and fingers
   6. Begin electrical stimulation on flexor superficialis and profundus, if needed to facilitate finger flexion
IV. Weeks 6–8
  A. Exercise program
   1. Begin joint-blocking exercises
   2. Begin light putty strengthening exercises
   3. Return to play
V. Week 12
  A. Begin return to normal activities of the sport and the usual training activities that would involve the injured finger

DIP, Distal interphalangeal; IP, interphalangeal; MCP, metacarpophalangeal; PIP, proximal interphalangeal; PROM, passive range of motion.

of the MCP and DIP joints. This deformity can occur as a result of the swelling, which laterally displaces and shortens the ruptured extensor mechanism. The unopposed action of the flexor digitorum superficialis along with the displaced extensor mechanism results in the boutonnière deformity.[45]

Appropriate acute treatment for disruption of the extensor mechanism is to splint the PIP joint in extension while allowing DIP flexion. Continuous splinting is recommended for 6 to 8 weeks, and participation in sports is allowed.[34] During this period of immobilization, the athlete is encouraged to perform active and passive range of motion of the DIP and MCP joints to prevent joint contracture and assist in healing of the extensor mechanism.[49] Active range-of-motion exercises for the PIP are begun after the initial immobilization period. Splinting should continue until full pain-free motion is restored.[35] Passive flexion of the PIP joint can begin 2 weeks after initiating active range-of-motion exercises. Caution should be taken to maintain active extension of the PIP joint while progressing PIP joint flexion. If a loss of active extension develops, passive

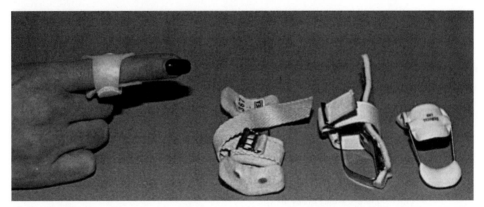

Figure 15–6. Splints for boutonnière deformities. *From left to right:* custom-made proximal interphalangeal extension splint on index finger, safety pin splint, Joint Jack splint, and wire foam splint for severe flexion contractures.

exercises should be discontinued and intermittent splinting restarted.[56] Strengthening exercises may commence once active extension is ensured.

If the athlete delays presentation and has a soft endfeel flexion contracture at the PIP joint, there are a variety of splinting techniques that can be used to treat the contracture. If no contracture is present, a custom-made thermoplastic PIP joint extension splint should be fabricated. If there is a contracture of the PIP joint less than 25°, a prefabricated safety pin splint or Joint Jack splint may be used. If contracture is greater than 25°, a prefabricated wire foam splint or a short dorsal outrigger PIP joint extension splint is recommended (Fig. 15–6). All splints will provide low-load progressive extension stretch to PIP joint volar soft tissue.[48]

If there is a solid flexion contracture and the athlete has active PIP joint flexion, serial casting is recommended until a soft endfeel is achieved. At this point, the athlete should switch back to static or dynamic extension splinting until the PIP joint reaches full extension. The PIP joint is held continuously in full extension for 3 more weeks, and the same active range-of-motion exercises as for acute injuries are then started.[48] Only those cases that do not respond to splinting are considered for surgery. This option is rarely used, because results are less predictable than with conservative management.[37]

PIP Joint Sprains and Dislocations

PIP joint sprains and dislocations are very common, so much so that they are often overlooked and undertreated. The mechanism of injury varies and is generally poorly reported by the athlete other than "I jammed my finger." Like the DIP joint dislocations, many times PIP joint dislocations are reduced on the field by the coach, athletic trainer, physician, or athlete. The player is then allowed to return to the game with buddy taping.[32] The problem with reducing the joint on the field is that the athlete may not have a simple dislocation but rather may have a fracture or other soft-tissue injury such as a volar plate injury. Sotereanos et al[51] advise delaying reduction until a radiographic evaluation can be performed. If reduction of the dislocation is performed on the field, follow-up radiographs are required. It is important for the athlete to receive follow-up splinting so that a painful, stiff, or deformed finger does not develop 2 to 3 months later. This condition, which can develop without appropriate follow-up, has been termed "coach's finger."[34]

Anatomically, the collateral ligaments of the PIP joint are under the greatest tension when the joint is in full extension and at maximum flexion; therefore, examination of joint stability must be performed with the PIP joint in extension and flexion.[19] Treatment of collateral ligament sprains is successful with simple PIP joint splinting at 30° of flexion or buddy taping while the athlete continues sports participation. Continued use of the splint or taping during off-field activities for 3 weeks is critical to prevent small aggravations to the injured joint that can prolong recovery. Without this simple but appropriate care, these sprains can manifest through the entire season. Active exercises are begun at 3 weeks, and continued splinting or taping is recommended for another 3 weeks during sports participation.

Of the three types of PIP dislocations, the most common is the dorsal dislocation, with the other two types being volar and lateral dislocations. The dislocated PIP joint is typically treated with closed reduction. However, surgical intervention may be necessary depending on the joint's stability postreduction or on the clinician's inability to reduce the dislocation.

Dorsal dislocations involve dislocation of the middle phalanx dorsally, frequently causing the volar plate to be torn from the insertion of the middle phalanx. Lateral dislocation damages the collateral ligaments and volar plate. Volar dislocation may cause an avulsion of the central slip of the extensor mechanism.[32] Once reduction is performed, the finger is immobilized with a dorsal extension blocking gutter with the PIP joint in 25° to 30° of flexion for 2 to 3 weeks.[48] Edema should be controlled with 1-inch Coban wrap. After the initial immobilization period, protected active range-of-motion exercises are begun. The athlete is instructed not to extend the PIP joint beyond the limits of the splint for 2 weeks to protect the volar plate and prevent hyperextension. After the protected phase, the athlete is instructed to progress to full active range-of-motion exercises. Strengthening exercises are initiated at 6 to 8 weeks postinjury. Protective splinting is continued during athletic events until complete, pain-free motion is achieved.

Pseudoboutonnière Deformity

Pseudoboutonnière deformity occurs after a PIP joint injury involving the volar plate.[36] Its presentation is very similar to that of a boutonnière deformity, with flexion deformity of the PIP joint. The slight difference occurs in the DIP joint, in which a boutonnière deformity presents in hyperextension, but a pseudoboutonnière deformity allows normal motion.[46]

If the patient has flexion contractures of less than 45°, dynamic or static extension splinting can be done as in a boutonnière deformity. Active range-of-motion exercises are initiated during splinting to facilitate active flexion and extension. Splints should be removed to perform exercises four times a day.[32]

If there is a flexion contracture of greater than 45°, surgical intervention is usually necessary. Postoperatively, the PIP joint is splinted in full extension, with the DIP joint free, for 3 weeks. Active and passive range-of-motion exercises of the MCP and DIP joints are performed during this period. At 3 weeks postoperatively, PIP active range-of-motion exercises are begun as with a boutonnière injury. At 6 to 8 weeks, strengthening exercises are commenced for the PIP joint.[32]

Metacarpal Fractures

Metacarpal fractures may be the result of direct trauma, indirect compression, or rotational trauma.[16, 40] Metacarpal fractures generally present with focal area of point tenderness and swelling within the hand. Careful inspection of rotation is done by having the athlete attempt to make a flat fist (a fist with MCP and PIP flexion and DIP extension) and observing whether all fingers point to the same point. Radiographs are always necessary to confirm type, location, and angulation of fracture.

Stabilization of a metacarpal fracture is dependent on the location, angulation, and rotation of the fracture. Fractures involving the third or fourth metacarpal are inherently more stable than those involving the second or fifth metacarpal. This is due to the presence of soft tissue, ligaments, and interosseous muscle surrounding the middle metacarpals. Most commonly, fractures of the metacarpal head, neck, and shaft are immobilized with the wrist extended to 15° to 20° and with the involved and adjacent MCP joints flexed to 65° to 70°.[48] This position allows the MCP collateral ligaments to help stabilize the fracture and assists in preventing shortening of the fracture.[18] Stabilizing the fracture without bulky immobilization is critical to allowing the return of normal range of motion of the uninvolved joints, promoting healing, and maximizing function.[58]

A variety of splinting and bracing techniques are available for metacarpal fractures, depending on the location, type, and stability of the fracture and the preference of the treating physician. An ulnar or radial gutter cast or a custom-made thermoplastic splint can be used. The thermoplastic splints have the advantage of being remolded as needed for changes in swelling. A stable shaft fracture may be protected during healing with a well-molded splint that holds all four fingers' metacarpals together as one, while allowing full finger motion. A prefabricated Galveston brace, a three-point fixation device, is available for treatment of metacarpal shaft fractures.[6]

Whatever form of stabilization is chosen, sports participation is another important consideration. The recent rule change in football that now allows sports participation with a cast that is covered with a ½-inch closed-cell foam has enabled early return of athletes to participation. This early return places added responsibility on the sports medicine team to ensure that the fracture is adequately stabilized, protected, and maintained in correct alignment during the healing process.

Rehabilitation of these metacarpal fractures managed by closed reduction includes active motion of the joints not splinted during the initial immobilization that usually lasts 3 to 6 weeks.[48] Edema should be managed using ice, elevation, and compressive dressing during and after the splinting phase to facilitate motion and reduce adhesions. Gentle active motion of immobilized joints can be initiated as early as 3 weeks if tolerated by the athlete and if radiographs show appropriate healing. Passive motion may be initiated after clinical healing, at approximately 6 weeks.[48, 59] At 8 weeks, light progressive strengthening may be initiated for the wrist, hand, and fingers.

Bennett's Fracture

Bennett's fracture is a small intra-articular fracture at the carpometacarpal joint of the thumb resulting from axial compression.[37] This small fragment is generally treated with closed reduction and percutaneous pin fixation.[37, 44] A thumb spica cast or splint is applied and worn for 3 to 4 weeks continuously. At approximately 4 weeks the intra-articular pin is removed and active motion of the thumb and wrist is begun. After 6 to 8 weeks the remaining pins are removed and rehabilitation is progressed to passive and resistance exercises.[30]

An athlete who does not regularly handle the ball may return to play as early as 2 to 3 weeks after injury if pins are in place and a protective cast is used. If the fracture is treated with rigid internal fixation, the player may return earlier, with protective splinting.[44] Protective splinting is continued during competition until full strength and pain-free range of motion are re-established.[37]

Ulnar Collateral Ligament Injury of the Thumb

The "gamekeeper's thumb," as this injury is also commonly called, arises from a hyperabduction or hyperextension of the thumb or a combination of the two and is seen commonly in skiers who fall on a ski pole or football players and wrestlers who are attempting to grab their opponents.[21, 22] Injury to the ulnar collateral ligament (UCL) proper, accessory UCL, adductor pollicis, and volar plate and avulsion of the first proximal phalanx (Stener's lesion) are possible with this mechanism of injury.

The athlete with a thumb UCL injury presents with pain and swelling in the web space or on the ulnar side of the MCP joint of the thumb.[35] Examination of the UCL requires stressing the ligament in full extension to asses accessory UCL function and in flexion to asses UCL status properly.[2, 35] Hyperextension laxity of the MCP would indicate volar plate involvement. Stress films are indicated for documenting abduction instability and identifying bony involvement.[37]

UCL sprains are generally treated with a thumb spica splint or cast with the thumb in slight adduction, approximately 40° from the palm, continuously for 3 weeks (Figs. 15–7 and 15–8). As healing progresses, active range-of-motion exercises can be initiated after the immobilization period. Protective splinting is recommended for at least another 3 weeks or until pain subsides and full range of motion and strength are regained.[27, 37]

Surgical treatment of these injuries is indicated for acute injuries with gross clinical instability, injuries that cannot be reduced because of bone or soft-tissue obstruction, injuries with significant articular surface fragment, bony displacement, or a rotation fracture fragment. Surgical management of UCL chronic instability is determined by the athlete's pain, instability, and loss of pinch strength.[35]

Scaphoid Fracture

Of all the carpal bones, the scaphoid is the bone most commonly fractured. The usual mechanism of injury is falling on an outstretched hand with the wrist in extension.[54] Scaphoid fractures should be suspected in any athlete presenting with tenderness over the anatomic snuffbox, palmar side of the scaphoid, or radial side of the wrist. Diagnostic radiographic series should include antero-

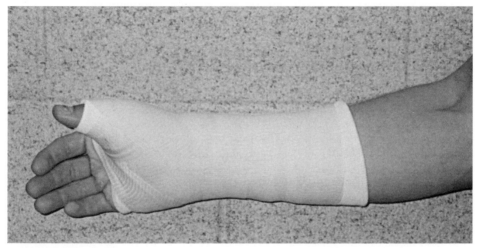

Figure 15–7. Thumb spica cast.

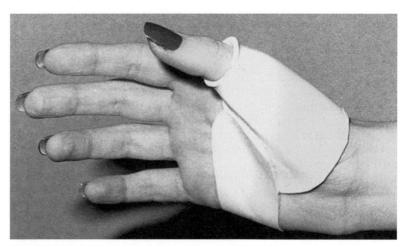

Figure 15–8. Thumb spica thermoplastic splint.

posterior, lateral, right and left oblique, and clenched-fist views in maximal radial and ulnar deviation.

Conservative treatment of all scaphoid fractures is critical because of the precarious blood supply. The scaphoid's proximal pole is primarily supplied by a single artery arising from the dorsal branch of the radial artery. Therefore, a large number of scaphoid fractures proceed to nonunion or avascular necrosis.[15] Thirty percent of mid-third fractures and approximately 100% of proximal fractures develop avascular necrosis.

Scaphoid fractures can be broken down by anatomic distribution, with 20% being proximal, 70% being middle, and 10% being distal fractures.[47] An indication that a scaphoid fracture will proceed to nonunion or avascular necrosis is that (1) the fracture has delayed presentation, (2) the fracture is in the proximal third, or (3) the fragment is displaced.[7]

The management of all athletes who present with scaphoid tenderness should consist of a radiographic series and at least 2 weeks in a short-arm thumb spica cast followed by re-examination and radiographs. If the radiographs are negative but the athlete remains symptomatic, a bone scan should be ordered to evaluate the status of the scaphoid. Continuous casting for 3 to 4 months, with radiographs and refitting of a cast every 3 to 4 weeks, is a standard treatment for scaphoid fractures advocated by McCue.[37] Nonunion of scaphoid fracture after 6 months of conservative treatment requires surgical intervention.[37]

The decision to bivalve a cast for hygienic reasons depends on the compliance of the athlete and the preference of the sports medicine staff. Removing the cast for showering and wearing one cast for practice and another for activities of daily living can have a negative impact during the early healing period. After union of the scaphoid fracture, active range-of-motion exercises are initiated to restore normal motion of the thumb and wrist. Resistance exercises are initiated gradually as tolerated.

Hamate Fracture

The classic scenario leading to a hamate hook fracture is the golf swing that takes a large divot, in which the club shaft is levered against the hypothenar area, shearing off the hook of the hamate. This fracture can also occur in other sports in which racquets or bats are held.[60]

Diagnosis is made by point tenderness over the hook of the hamate and is confirmed by a carpal tunnel view radiograph. Treatment is generally symptomatic, with management of pain with standard acute injury measures such as ice, compression, elevation, and rest. A pad can be fabricated to protect the area and relieve pressure. However, if the injury is very symptomatic, early surgical excision of the fractured fragment is common, usually allowing return to full participation in 4 to 6 weeks.[52] Typically, postoperative active range-of-motion exercises for the wrist and hand are performed as soon as comfort allows. Protective splinting or padding is needed for sports participation for at least 1 to 2 months to alleviate pain from pressure over the fracture site.[38]

Ganglion Cysts

Ganglion cysts generally arise because of overuse of the musculotendinous structures around the wrist and are most common on the radial side, on either the volar or the dorsal surface. The ganglion cyst arises from the synovial lining of the tendon sheath or from the joint.[4] The athlete will complain of wrist pain with motion, and the wrist is tender on palpation. The conservative treatment of choice is rest, nonsteroidal anti-inflammatory medications, and a wrist cock-up splint. Aspiration and surgical intervention are alternative treatments if conservative methods fail.[37]

Wrist Sprains and Tendonitis

Wrist sprains commonly occur when the wrist is forced into hyperextension. The athlete generally presents with tenderness over the dorsum of the wrist, with pain and limitation of wrist motion.

Tendonitis is generally due to an overuse of the forearm or wrist musculature. This is commonly seen in racquet sports or in heavy weight-lifting activities. Placing the wrist and hand in unusual positions or in extremes of motion and loading the tissue can predispose the athlete to tendonitis or wrist sprains.

Treatment of both these problems is similar. The use of a wrist splint for a few days to allow the injured tissues to rest is very beneficial. Ice and anti-inflammatory medication are commonly prescribed.[50] On reduction of initial symptoms, active range-of-motion exercises are initiated within pain-free ranges. The athlete can progress to strengthening exercises within 1 to 2 weeks after active range-of-motion exercises are begun.

de Quervain's Tenosynovitis

de Quervain's tenosynovitis involves the irritation of the tendon and its covering sheath of the first dorsal extensor compartment encompassing the extensor pollicis brevis and abductor pollicis longus. It is usually caused by overuse and may occur from a direct blow to the first dorsal compartment. It is seen most often in players of racquet sports and also in gymnasts and golfers.[26, 55, 57] The athlete presents with pain on the radial side of the wrist localized over the radial styloid area. A positive Finkelstein test indicates a strong possibility of de Quervain's tenosynovitis. The test is performed by the athlete's flexing the thumb into the palm and making a full fist; the wrist is then forcefully and passively deviated ulnarly by the clinician. The test is positive if the athlete feels excruciating pain over the radial styloid area.[12]

The injury is treated conservatively first, with splinting with a short-arm thumb spica splint to rest the area. The wrist is placed in approximately 15° of extension, the thumb in 40° of abduction and 10° flexion, with the IP joint free, for 6 weeks.[48] Nonsteroidal anti-inflammatory medications are usually prescribed, and therapeutic modalities are used to decrease pain and inflammation. Active range-of-motion exercises of the wrist and thumb, within pain limits, are initiated two times a day after immobilization.[57] If symptoms do not decrease, steroid injections may be considered. If symptoms persists, surgery may be necessary to release the tendon sheath.[40] Postoperative treatment is initiated at 1 week with active and passive exercises of the thumb and wrist. Scar management is initiated 2 weeks postoperatively, and usually in 3 to 4 weeks, return to normal activities is allowed.

Trigger Finger

Trigger finger is the thickening of the tendon sheath, with the tendon forming a nodular or hourglass shape. This results in decrease in smooth gliding through the A1 pulley located on the palmar aspect of the MCP joint, causing triggering or, in advanced cases, causing the digit to lock in flexion or extension. It is caused by repetitive injury to the tendon sheath via repetitive gripping activities and direct pressure at the MCP joint.[11] The finger has point tenderness at the A1 pulley with full passive range of motion of the involved digit.

Conservative treatment includes splinting the MCP joint at 0° of extension of the involved fingers, with the PIP and DIP joints free (Fig. 15–9). The athlete performs active range-of-motion exercises including tendon excursions and tendon gliding exercises with the splint on, with 20 repetitions every 2 hours.[10] Corticosteroid injections to decrease the inflammation and promote smooth gliding of the tendon have been used.[14]

Unsuccessful conservative treatment may require surgery to release the A1 pulley. Postoperative rehabilitation includes the following: (1) Focus on edema control and initiation of active and passive range-of-motion exercises in the first 2 weeks; (2) Begin scar management and continue range-of-motion exercises after removal of stitches at approximately 2 weeks; (3) Progress to hand strengthening as tolerated at approximately 4 to 6 weeks.

Carpal Tunnel Syndrome

Carpal tunnel syndrome is the compression of the median nerve in the carpal tunnel. The carpal tunnel houses nine tendons and the median nerve, enclosed by a concave arch of the carpal bones and the flexor retinaculum, also called the transverse carpal ligament.[53] Inflammation in the tunnel causes pressure on the median nerve, leading to symptoms of numbness and tingling in the median

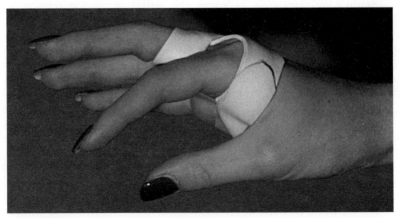

Figure 15–9. Trigger-finger splint holding the metacarpophalangeal joint at 0°.

nerve distribution, thumb, and index and middle fingers. The athlete may report night numbness and pain that can progress to weakness and dropping of objects. Carpal tunnel syndrome may develop from any sport or activity that requires repetitive wrist flexion and extension or after a wrist fracture.[37] Two tests to assist in identification of carpal tunnel syndrome are Phalen's maneuver and Tinel's sign. To perform Phalen's maneuver, the athlete flexes both wrists and places them with the dorsa of both hands touching. If numbness is reported within 60 seconds of holding the test position, the test is positive. Tinel's sign is positive when the carpal tunnel is tapped and the athlete reports tingling in the median nerve distribution.[39] Electromyography and nerve conduction velocity tests are commonly performed to assist in confirming the diagnosis of carpal tunnel syndrome.[17]

Conservative treatment consists of splinting to take pressure off the median nerve with the wrist placed in a neutral position to 10° of extension, with digits free to allow full motion. The splint should be worn during athletic activities and at night. The athlete is instructed in tendon gliding exercise to continue tendon excursion through the carpal tunnel along with wrist active range-of-motion exercises to prevent stiffness at the wrist. Nonsteroidal anti-inflammatory drugs together with compliant splint wearing should facilitate a decrease in symptoms.[51] If the athlete does not respond with conservative splinting, steroidal injections may be given.[37]

A carpal tunnel release may be required if there is no response to conservative treatment. Postoperative rehabilitation of an open carpal tunnel release begins at 2 weeks when the postoperative splint is removed along with stitches. Edema is controlled via Tubi-Grip and use of modalities as necessary. Scar management is initiated with scar massage and a silicone sheet application to the scar once the wound is healed, for remodeling of the scar. Active and passive range-of-motion exercises for the wrist and digits, along with light grip-strengthening exercises, are also begun. Desensitization activities are started if hypersensitivity exists at the incision site. At approximately 4 to 6 weeks after surgery, wrist-strengthening exercises can begin. The athlete may return to participation as soon as the athletic activities can be performed without pain. The athlete's full strength is generally expected to return by 3 to 4 months postoperatively.[51]

REHABILITATIVE EXERCISES

Active Motion Exercises for the Digits

The individual active range-of-motion exercises for the fingers will be described below and can be used for all injuries when they are cleared for active range-of-motion exercises. After each description of the exercise, recommendations for indications are given. Each exercise should be performed within the pain tolerance of the injured athlete. Sets and repetitions are dependent on the clinician's preference; generally one to two sets of 5 to 12 repetitions four to six times a day are used with these active exercises. The injured athlete is educated in all appropriate exercises. After demonstrating the proper techniques with the exercises, the athlete is encouraged to take responsibility for performing the exercises several times a day independently. Performing these exercises in a warm whirlpool is an excellent way to loosen stiff joints, as long as swelling is not a concern. Soft-tissue massage is commonly prescribed to loosen a stiff joint or facilitate scar mobility.

The use of thin silicone sheets such as Topigel over a completely healed incision site for several hours a day also assists in scar management.

Finger Abduction and Adduction. The athlete should spread the fingers apart and together. This will facilitate a decrease in edema along with working the intrinsic musculature of the hand. This is recommended for all wrist and hand injuries.

Opposition. The athlete should touch every fingertip with the thumb starting with the index finger and progressing by sliding the thumb down the small finger into the palm of the hand to facilitate full flexion of the thumb. This exercise is recommended for Bennett's fracture, UCL injuries of the thumb, wrist fractures, distal radius and ulna fractures, and de Quervain's tenosynovitis.

MCP Flexion with IP Flexion and Extension. The athlete should flex the MCP joint to 90°, then alternately flex and extend the IP joints into full flexion and full extension to facilitate the interossei and lumbricals (Fig. 15–10).[9] This exercise is recommended for all PIP joint injuries and any injuries that result in lack of extension at the PIP.

Tendon Gliding Exercises or Stage Fisting. This exercise involves the digits' making various types of fists in a progression starting with full extension, followed by a tabletop (intrinsic-plus) position, a flat fist, a full fist without thumb, and finally a hook (intrinsic-minus) position (Fig. 15–11). These exercises are designed to facilitate the gliding of the flexor digitorum superficialis (FDS) and flexor digitorum profundus (FDP) tendons through the carpal tunnel. This exercise is recommended for all wrist and hand injuries.

Isolated Tendon Excursions or Joint-Blocking Exercises. These exercises are designed to isolate the FDS, FDP, and flexor profundus longus (FPL) tendons to increase active range of motion of a specific joint. To perform these exercises, the athlete should hold the MCP joints of all fingers in extension. To isolate the FDS, the athlete should hold the finger below the crease of the PIP joint, then flex and extend the PIP joint. For FDP tendon excursion, the athlete should hold the finger below the DIP joint crease, then flex and extend the DIP joint (Fig. 15–12). For the FPL, the athlete should hold the finger below the crease of the thumb IP joint, then flex and extend the IP joint. It is critical that joints are properly stabilized during these exercises to prevent substitution. This exercise is recommended for all finger injuries.

Extensor Digitorum Communis Exercise. The athlete should place all IP joints in flexion and the MCP joints in extension (intrinsic-minus position), then

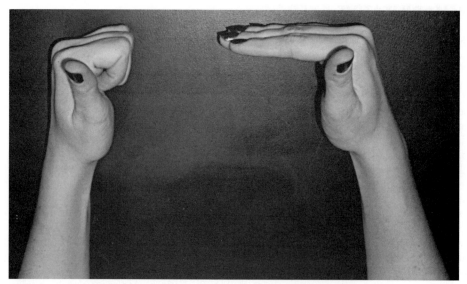

Figure 15–10. Strengthening exercise for interossei and lumbrical muscles. The starting position is with the metacarpophalangeal joint flexed to 90° and the interphalangeal (IP) joints in full extension *(right hand)*; the IP joints are then flexed *(left hand)*.

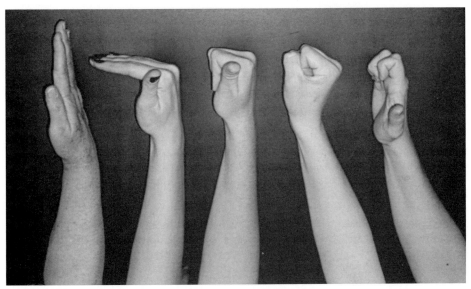

Figure 15–11. Tendon gliding exercises. *From left to right:* beginning position in full extension; a tabletop position (intrinsic-plus position); flat fist; full fist; and a hook position (intrinsic-minus position).

actively flex and extend the MCP joints. If needed, wrap the IP joints to keep them in flexion. This exercise prevents adhesions to the extensor digitorum communis tendons. This exercise is recommended for metacarpal fractures to decrease adhesions to the extensor digitorum communis tendons.

Passive Motion Exercises for the Digits

The goal of rehabilitation for digits is to obtain full flexion without losing extension. Passive range-of-motion exercises should be gentle and should not be performed if extension of the digit is being compromised. Passive exercises are

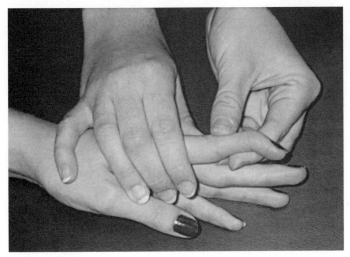

Figure 15–12. Joint blocking for distal interphalangeal joint flexion of the index finger.

often combined with the active exercises described above and are performed with gentle overpressure by either the athlete or the treating clinician. It is recommended that the athlete hold a stretch for 5 to 10 seconds and repeat this 5 to 10 times, four to six times a day. Pushing the joint beyond the pain threshold should be avoided, because this can cause an inflammatory reaction and can slow progression. These exercises are generally initiated after 2 weeks of active range-of-motion activities. Care should be taken not to overstretch the extensor hood with aggressive passive flexion exercises.

One special technique that can be used to help regain normal range of motion of the digits is successive induction. This technique is a combination of proprioceptive neuromuscular facilitation techniques. An example of successive induction is the procedure for gaining DIP flexion after immobilization: The athlete actively flexes the DIP through the available range of motion. The clinician then lightly resists active extension of the DIP for 3 to 5 seconds and immediately has the athlete attempt to flex the DIP joint. The finger is then held in the new range and the process is repeated four to six times. The advantage of this technique is that no forced passive flexion is placed on the extensor hood. The athlete can be instructed to perform this exercise two or three times a day.

Strengthening Exercises for the Digits

All active range-of-motion exercises described above can be used for strengthening exercises with the use of manual resistance or light resistive elastic bands. Isolation techniques such as joint blocking are very useful for strengthening weakened tissue (Fig. 15–13). Techniques are limited only by the imagination of the treating clinician.

Gripping exercises for strengthening the flexor tendons are common. Various devices can be used, from putty, soft rubber balls, and wet washcloths to resistive gripping devices. Progression should be guided by pain, maintenance of active extension, and healing restraints of the particular injury. Generally two to three sets of 10 to 25 repetitions are prescribed two to three times a day for all strengthening exercises.

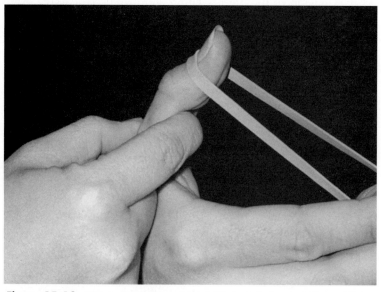

Figure 15–13. Metacarpophalangeal joint blocked during resistive extension with an elastic band.

Strengthening Exercises for the Wrist and Forearm

These are a group of exercises that facilitate active motion of the wrist and forearm and that can be used as strengthening exercise by the incorporation of weights or resistive elastic bands. These have also been called Super 7 exercises for the wrist. Stretching exercises are generally held for 10 to 15 seconds and repeated three to five times, in two sessions per day.

Strengthening exercises are usually performed two times a day for three sets of 10 repetitions at progressing weights from 1 to 5 pounds as tolerated.

1. Wrist flexion stretching with passive overpressure from the opposite hand (Fig. 15–14).
2. Wrist extension stretching with passive overpressure from the opposite hand (Fig. 15–15).
3. Wrist flexion, initiating the exercise with the wrist in maximal wrist extension and flexing through the available amount of flexion (Fig. 15–16).
4. Wrist extension, initiating the exercise with the wrist in maximal wrist flexion and extending through the available amount of extension (Fig. 15–17).
5. Radial deviation, initiating the exercise with the wrist in maximal ulnar deviation and moving through the available range into maximal radial deviation (Fig. 15–18).
6. Ulnar deviation, initiating the exercise with the wrist in maximal radial deviation and moving through the available range into maximal ulnar deviation (Fig. 15–19).

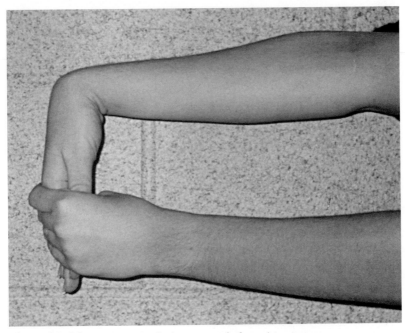

Figure 15–14. Passive wrist flexion to stretch the wrist extensors.

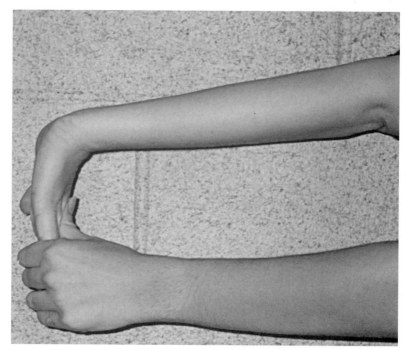

Figure 15–15. Passive wrist extension to stretch the wrist flexors.

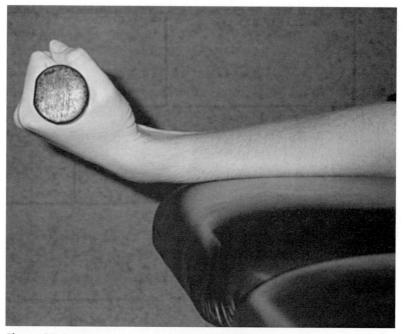

Figure 15–16. Resistive wrist flexion to strengthen the wrist flexors.

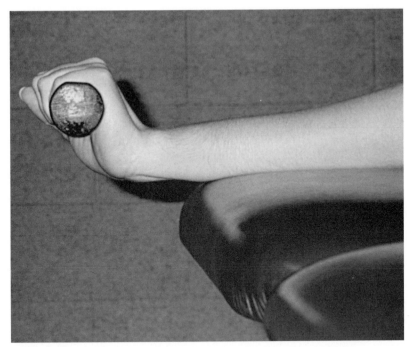

Figure 15–17. Resistive wrist extension to strengthen the wrist extensors.

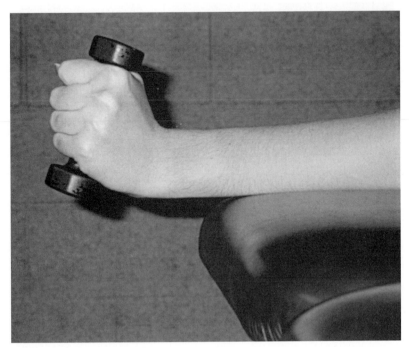

Figure 15–18. Resistive radial deviation.

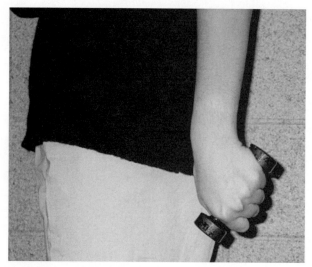

Figure 15–19. Resistive ulnar deviation.

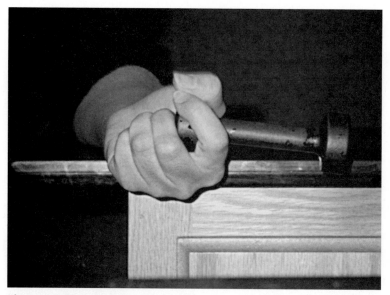

Figure 15–20. Resistive supination.

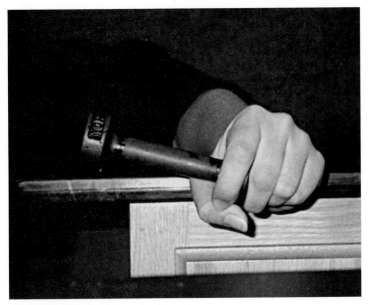

Figure 15–21. Resistive pronation.

7. Pronation and supination, performed with the wrist beginning in neutral rotation and then maximally supinating the wrist and forearm (Figs. 15–20 and 15–21). The direction is then reversed into maximal pronation.

Protective Splinting

Athletes in high school and college sports can now return to participation in sports activities with a cast on their upper extremities as long as it is covered with 1/2-inch closed-cell foam. This, along with the use of silicone rubber splints

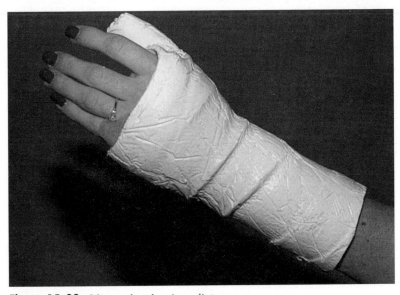

Figure 15–22. Silicone thumb spica splint.

(Fig. 15–22), has allowed athletes to return to competition earlier. This rule change has placed added responsibility on the sports medicine team that is caring for the injured athlete to ensure that the injury is diagnosed and splinted properly so that the athlete is not placed at further risk of injury.

References

1. Abouna, J.M., and Brown, H. (1968): The treatment of mallet finger. The results in a series of 148 consecutive cases and a review of the literature. Br. J. Surg., 55:653–667.
2. Adams, B.D., and Muller, D.L. (1996): Assessment of thumb positioning in the treatment of ulnar collateral ligament injuries. A laboratory study. Am. J. Sports Med., 24:672–675.
3. Burton, R.I., and Eaton, R.G. (1973): Common hand injuries in the athlete. Orthop. Clin. North Am., 4:809–838.
4. Bush, D.C. (1995): Soft-tissue tumors of the hand. In: Hunter, J.M., Macken, E.J., and Callhan, A.B. (eds.): Rehabilitation of the Hand: Surgery and Therapy. St. Louis, Mosby-Year Book Inc., pp. 1017–1033.
5. Carroll, R.E., and Match, R.M. (1970): Avulsion of the profundus tendon insertion. J. Trauma, 10:1109.
6. Colditz, J.C. (1995): Functional fracture bracing. In: Hunter, J.M., Macken, E.J., and Callhan, A.B. (eds.): Rehabilitation of the Hand: Surgery and Therapy. St. Louis, Mosby-Year Book Inc., pp. 395–406.
7. Cooney, W.P., Linscheid, R.L., and Dobyns, J.H. (1996): Fracture and dislocation of the wrist. In: Rockwood, C.A., Green, D.P., and Bucholz, R.W. (eds.): Fracture in Adults. Philadelphia, Lippincott-Raven, pp. 745–867.
8. Duran, R., and Houser, R. (1975): Controlled passive motion following flexor tendon repair in zone 2 and 3. In: AAOS Symposium on Tendon Surgery in the Hand. St. Louis, C.V. Mosby.
9. Evans, R.B. (1995): An update on extensor tendon management. In: Hunter, J.M., Macken, E.J., and Callhan, A.B. (eds.): Rehabilitation of the Hand: Surgery and Therapy. St. Louis, Mosby-Year Book Inc., pp. 565–606.
10. Evans, R.B., Hunter, J.M., and Burkhalter, W.E. (1988): Conservative management of the trigger finger: A new approach. J. Hand Ther., 1:59–68.
11. Fahey, J.J., and Bollinger, J.A. (1954): Trigger finger in adults and children. J. Bone Joint Surg. [Am.], 36:1200–1218.
12. Finkelstein, H. (1930): Stenosing tendovaginitis at the radial styloid process. J. Bone Joint Surg., 12:509–540.
13. Foreman, S, and Gieck, J.H. (1992): Rehabilitative management of injuries to the hand. Clin. Sports Med., 11:239–252.
14. Freiberg, A., Mulholland, R.S., and Levine, R. (1989): Nonoperative treatment of trigger fingers and thumbs. J. Hand Surg., 14A:553–558.
15. Gelberman, R.H., Panagis, J.S., Taleisnk, J., and Baumgaertner, M. (1983): The arterial anatomy of the human carpus. Part I. The extraosseous vascularity. J. Hand Surg., 8:367–375.
16. Hastings, H. (1992): Management of extraarticular fractures of the phalanges and metacarpals. In: Strickland, J.W., and Rettig, A.C. (eds.): Hand Injuries in Athletes. Philadelphia, W.B. Saunders, pp. 129–153.
17. Hunter, J.M., Lance, B.D., and Fedus, L.M. (1995): Major neuropathies of the upper extremity: the median nerve. In: Hunter, J.M., Macken, E.J., and Callhan, A.B. (eds.): Rehabilitation of the Hand: Surgery and Therapy. St. Louis, Mosby-Year Book Inc., pp. 905–916.
18. Jahss, S.A. (1938): Fractures of the metacarpals: a new method of reduction and immobilization. J. Bone Joint Surg., 20:178–186.
19. Kapandji, I.A. (1982): The physiology of joints. Vol I. Upper Limb. New York, Churchill Livingstone, pp. 1860–1891.
20. Kleinert, H.E., Kutz, J.E., and Cohen, M.J. (1975): Primary repair of zone 2 flexor tendon lacerations. AAOS symposium on tendon surgery in the hand. St. Louis, C.V. Mosby.
21. Kulund, D.N. (1982): The Injured Athlete. Philadelphia, J.B. Lippincott, pp. 295–329.
22. Lane, L.B. (1995): Acute ulnar collateral ligament rupture of the metacarpophalangeal joint of the thumb. In: Torg, J.S., and Shepard, R.J. (eds.): Current Therapy in Sports Medicine. St. Louis, C.V. Mosby, pp. 151–161.
23. Leadbeter, W.B., Buckwalter, J.A., and Gordon, S.L. (1990): Sport-Induced Inflammation: Clinical and Basic Science Concepts. Park Ridge, IL, American Academy of Orthopaedic Surgeons.
24. Leddy, J.F., and Dennis, T.R. (1992): Tendon injuries. In: Stricklan, J.W., and Rettig, A.C. (eds.): Hand Injuries in Athletes. Philadelphia, W.B. Saunders, pp. 175–207.
25. Leddy, J.P., and Packer, J.W. (1977): Avulsion of the profundus tendon insertion in athletes. J. Hand Surg., 2:66–69.
26. Manske, P.R., and Lesker, P.A. (1978): Avulsion of the ring finger digitorum profundus tendon: An experimental study. Hand, 10:52–55.
27. Mayer, V.A., and McCue, F.C. (1995): Rehabilitation and protection of the hand and wrist. In:

Nicholas, J.A., and Hershman, E.B. (eds.): The Upper Extremity in Sports Medicine, 2nd ed. St. Louis, Mosby-Year Book Inc., pp. 591–634.

28. McCue, F.C. (1982): The elbow, wrist, and hand. *In:* Kulund, D.N. (ed.): The Injured Athlete. Philadelphia, J.B. Lippincott, pp. 295–329.

29. McCue, F.C., and Bruce, J.F. (1994): Hand and wrist. *In:* DeLee, J.C., and Drez, D., Jr. (eds.): Orthopaedic Sports Medicine Principles and Practice, Vol I. Philadelphia, W.B. Saunders, pp. 913–944.

30. McCue, F.C., and Cabrera, J.N. (1992): Common athletic digital joint injuries of the hand. *In:* Strickland, J.W., and Rettig, A.C. (eds.): Hand Injuries in Athletes. Philadelphia, W.B. Saunders, pp. 49–94.

31. McCue, F.C., and Garroway, R.Y. (1985): Sport injuries to the hand and wrist. *In:* Schneider, R.C. (ed.): Sport Injuries: Mechanism, Prevention, and Treatment. Baltimore, Williams & Wilkins, pp. 743–764.

32. McCue, F.C., and Redler, M.R. (1990): Coach's finger. *In:* Torg, J.S., Welsh, P.R., and Shepard, R.J. (eds.): Current Therapy in Sports Medicine. Toronto, B.C. Decker Inc., pp. 438–443.

33. McCue, F.C., and Wooten, S.L. (1986): Closed tendon injuries of the hand in athletics. Clin. Sports Med., 5:741–755.

34. McCue, F.C., Andrew, J.R., and Hakala, M. (1974): The coach's finger. Am. J. Sports Med., 2:270–275.

35. McCue, F.C., Hakala, M.H., Andrews, J.R., and Gieck, J.H. (1974): Ulnar collateral ligament injuries of the thumb in athletes. J. Sports Med., 2:70–80.

36. McCue, F.C., Honner, R., and Gieck, J.H., et al. (1975): A pseudo-boutonniere deformity. Hand, 7:166–170.

37. McCue, F.C., Hussamy, O.D., and Gieck, J.H. (1996): Hand and wrist injuries. *In:* Zachazewski, J.E., Magee, D.J., and Quillen, W.S. (eds.): Athletic Injuries and Rehabilitation, Philadelphia, W.B. Saunders, pp. 585–597.

38. Melone, C.P. (1990): Fracture of the wrist. *In:* Nicholas, J.A., and Hershman, E.B. (eds.): The Upper Extremity in Sports Medicine. St. Louis, C.V. Mosby, pp. 419–456.

39. Phalen, G.S. (1972): The carpal tunnel syndrome: Clinical evaluation of 598 hands. Clin. Orthop., 83:29–40.

40. Posner, M.A. (1990): Hand injuries. *In:* Nicholas, J.A., and Hershman, E.B. (eds.): The Upper Extremity in Sports Medicine. St. Louis, C.V. Mosby, pp. 495–594.

41. Redler, M. (1989): Phalangeal and metacarpal fractures. Sport Injury Management, 2(1):53–58, 1989.

42. Redler, M. (1989): Dislocation of the interphalangeal joints and metacarpophalangeal joints. Sport Injury Management, 2(1):59–66.

43. Rettig, A.C. (1992): Closed tendon injuries of the hand and wrist in the athlete. Clin. Sports Med., 11:77–99.

44. Rettig, A.C., and Rowdon, G.A. (1995): Metacarpal fractures. *In:* Torg, J.S., and Shepard, R.J. (eds.): Current Therapy in Sports Medicine. St. Louis, C.V. Mosby, pp. 152–156.

45. Rosenthal, E.A. (1995): The extensor tendons: Anatomy and management. *In:* Hunter, J.M., Macken, E.J., and Callhan, A.B. (eds.): Rehabilitation of the Hand: Surgery and Therapy. St. Louis, Mosby-Year Book Inc., pp. 519–564.

46. Ruby, L.K. (1980): Common hand injuries in the athlete. Orthop. Clin. North Am., 11:819–839.

47. Russe, O. (1960): Fracture of the carpal navicular: Diagnosis, non-operative and operative treatment. J. Bone Joint Surg. [Am.], 42:759–768.

48. Sadler, J.A., and Koepfer, J.M. (1992): Rehabilitation and the splinting of the injured hand. *In:* Strickland, J.W., and Rettig, A.C. (eds.): Hand Injuries in Athletes. Philadelphia, W.B. Saunders, pp. 235–276.

49. Schneider, L.H. (1990): Tendon injuries of the hand. *In:* Nicholas, J.A., and Hershman, E.B. (eds.): The Upper Extremity in Sports Medicine. St. Louis, C.V. Mosby, pp. 595–618.

50. Shaw Wilgis, E.F., and Yates, A.Y. (1990): Wrist pain. *In:* Nicholas, J.A., and Hershman, E.B. (eds.): The Upper Extremity in Sports Medicine. St. Louis, C.V. Mosby, pp. 483–494.

51. Sotereanos, D.G., Levy, J.A., and Herndon, J.H. (1994): Hand and wrist injuries. *In:* Fu, F.H., and Stone, D.A. (eds.): Sport Injuries: Mechanisms, Prevention, Treatment. Baltimore, Williams & Wilkins, pp. 937–947.

52. Stark, H.H., Jobe, F.W., Boyes, J.H., and Ashworth, C.R. (1977): Fractures of the hook of the hamate in athletes. J. Bone Joint Surg. [Am.], 59:575–582.

53. Tubiana, R., Thomine, J.M., and Mackin, E. (1996): Functional anatomy. *In:* Examination of the Hand and Wrist. St Louis, Mosby-Year Book Inc., p. 12.

54. Weber, E.R., and Chao, E.Y. (1978): An experimental approach to the mechanism of scaphoid wrist fractures. J. Hand Surg., 3:142–148.

55. Weiker, G.G. (1992): Hand and wrist problems in the gymnast. *In:* Culzer, J.E. (ed.): Clinical Sports Medicine: Injuries of the Hand and Wrist. Philadelphia, W.B. Saunders, pp. 189–202.

56. Wilson, R.L., and Hazen, J. (1995): Management of joint injuries and intraarticular fractures of the hand. *In:* Hunter, J.M., Macken, E.J., and Callhan, A.B. (eds.): Rehabilitation of the Hand: Surgery and Therapy. St. Louis, Mosby-Year Book Inc., pp. 377–394.

57. Wright, H.H., and Rettig, A.C. (1995): Management of common sports injuries. *In:* Hunter, J.M., Macken, E.J., and Callhan, A.B. (eds.): Rehabilitation of the Hand: Surgery and Therapy. St. Louis, Mosby-Year Book Inc., pp. 1809–1838.

58. Wright, S.C. (1990): Fracture and dislocation in the hand and wrist. *In:* Torg, J.S., Welsh, P.R., and Shepard, R.J. (eds.): Current Therapy in Sports Medicine. Toronto, B.C. Decker Inc., pp. 443–446.

59. Wright, T.A. (1968): Early mobilization in fractures of the metacarpals and phalanges. Can. J. Surg., 11:491–498.

60. Zemmel, N.P., and Stark, H.H. (1986): Fractures and dislocations of the carpal bones. Clin. Sports Med., 5:709–724.

Chapter 16

Aquatic Rehabilitation

Cheryl S. Fuller, M.S., A.T.,C.

Hydrotherapy, or the utilization of water as a therapeutic modality, dates back many centuries. Throughout history water has been used to treat a wide variety of diseases. In the fifth century B.C. the Greeks began to use baths for the treatment of physical ailments. Hippocrates (c. 460 to 375 B.C.) used hot and cold baths to treat diseases including muscle spasms, rheumatism, and paralysis.[6] The Romans, noted for their architectural and construction skills, built large public bathhouses for rest, recreation, and exercise.[7] The ruins of these elaborate baths are still visible today.

During the Middle Ages, bathhouses became a source of disease, and bathing for therapeutic as well as for hygienic purposes declined.[15] It was not until the nineteenth century that there seemed to be a resurgence in the use of water as a therapeutic medium. Spas built near natural springs emerged in Europe, and the medical discipline of hydrotherapy became accepted as a treatment for a variety of conditions.

The use of hydrotherapy in the United States began in the 1920s.[6] At this time, exercise in water was used for the physical rehabilitation of polio patients and injured war veterans.[14] Today hydrotherapy is a widely accepted therapeutic modality, used for various injuries and disabilities. Although hydrotherapy has been used for centuries, recently there has been a dramatic increase in the ways that the medical community is using water to attain rehabilitation goals. However, the term hydrotherapy is so broad that for our purpose we will distinguish hydrotherapy from aquatic rehabilitation. Generally, hydrotherapy is the use of water as a therapeutic agent accompanied by active remedial exercises of a particular joint. Aquatic rehabilitation in sports medicine uses a much more aggressive approach. Not only is water used as a therapeutic agent for healing the injury, but the physical properties of water are used to maintain or achieve physical conditioning.

PHYSICAL PROPERTIES OF WATER

Aquatic rehabilitation is commonly used in sports medicine today. The use of water as a medium for exercise after an injury has proven to be a safe means of promoting range of motion, enhancing muscular strength and endurance, increasing cardiovascular endurance, and progressing weight-bearing and functional activities. A thorough understanding of the physical properties of water and the laws of physics that govern these properties is necessary for the practical application of aquatic rehabilitation in sports medicine.

Specific Gravity

The specific gravity or relative density of an object is the property that determines whether the object will sink or float in water. The specific gravity is actually the ratio of the weight of an object to the weight of an equal volume of water.

The specific gravity of water equals 1; therefore, if the specific gravity of an object is greater than 1, the object will sink, and if it is less than 1, the object will float.[4] The average specific gravity of the human body is 0.974; consequently, the body will float. However, each individual's specific gravity will vary because of differences in body composition. Lean body mass, which includes bone, muscle, connective tissue, and organs, has a relative density of 1.1, and fat mass has a density of 0.90.[7]

Buoyancy

Buoyancy and specific gravity are very closely related. Buoyancy is the upward force experienced by a body in a fluid. The Greek mathematician Archimedes (287 to 212 B.C.) discovered the physical principle of buoyancy.[9] Archimedes' principle states that when a body is wholly or partially immersed in a fluid at rest, the body experiences an upward thrust equal to the weight of the fluid displaced.[17] The force of buoyancy acts in a direction opposite that of the force of gravity and is responsible for the feeling of weightlessness in water. Buoyancy can assist, resist, or support movement through water. Movement toward the surface of the water will be assisted by the force of buoyancy, movement toward the bottom of the pool will be resisted by the force of buoyancy, and movement that is parallel to the surface of the water will be supported by the force of buoyancy.

Moment of Force

To determine the amount of assistance or resistance of a given movement in water, buoyancy must be examined as a moment of force. A moment of force is the turning effect of a force about an axis. The moment of buoyancy is represented by the equation $M = fd$, where M is the moment of buoyancy, f is the upward force of buoyancy, and d is the perpendicular distance from a vertical line through the axis of rotation to the center of buoyancy.[8] Figure 16–1 illustrates the result of the turning effect of buoyancy on the arm with shoulder abduction. As the limb moves closer to the surface of the water, the effect of buoyancy becomes greater because of the increased distance of the center of buoyancy of the limb to the axis of rotation (see Fig. 16–1A).[2] The moment of buoyancy may be modified by increasing or decreasing the length of the lever arm and also by using and placing flotation devices (see Fig. 16–1B and C).

Viscosity

Viscosity is a physical property of water that makes strengthening a benefit of aquatic rehabilitation. Viscosity is friction that occurs between molecules of a liquid and causes resistance to flow of the liquid. It provides resistance to movement as the molecules of water adhere to the surface of an object moving through it. Movement through water also creates resistance from pressure. There is positive pressure in front of a moving object that tends to impede its progress. This is known as the bow wave and accounts for about 10% of the resistance to

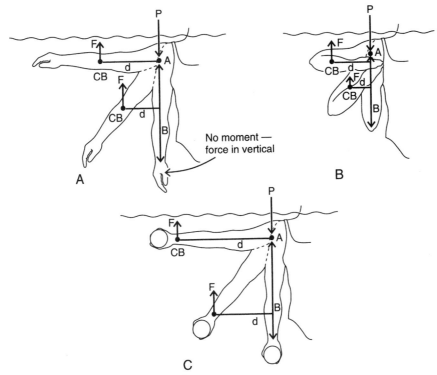

Figure 16–1. The turning effect of buoyancy on the arm. *A*, With arm extended (long lever). *B*, With elbow bent (short lever). *C*, Holding a float. P, pivot point; F, upward force of buoyancy; d, horizontal distance from the vertical (AB) to the center of buoyancy (CB). (From Bates, A., and Hanson, N. [1996]: Aquatic Exercise Therapy. Philadelphia, W.B. Saunders, p. 24.)

movement. The wake, which forms behind the moving object, is caused by water flowing into the area immediately to the rear of the object. This results in an area of low pressure behind the object that tends to hold the object back. This drag force produces the majority of resistance to movement.[8]

Movement Through Water

Movement through water may also be modified to alter the resistance desired for strengthening. The velocity of an object moving through water determines the amount of resistance produced. The drag force is proportional to the square of the velocity of movement. Therefore, the faster the movement, the greater the drag force and the resistance to movement.[4] Also, the frontal area of the object moving through the water is directly proportional to the drag force produced and may be used to alter resistance. The flow of the water is another factor that affects resistance.[2] Turbulent water flow increases the friction between molecules and therefore increases the resistance to movement. It is important to consider all of these factors and their effects on movement through water when one is designing aquatic exercises.

Hydrostatic Pressure

Pascal's law of hydrostatic pressure states that a fluid exerts a pressure equally on all surfaces of an immersed body at rest at any given depth.[2] Hydrostatic pressure increases with the depth and the density of the fluid. Water exerts a pressure of 22.4 mm Hg per foot of water depth.[4] At a depth of 5 feet, the hydrostatic pressure would equal 112 mm Hg, which substantially exceeds venous pressure. Because of this pressure, there is improved venous return, which prevents pooling of blood in the lower extremities. Therefore, aquatic rehabilitation may be used to control and possibly aid the resolution of edema in an injured body part.

PHYSIOLOGIC EFFECTS OF WATER IMMERSION

The physiologic effects of water immersion are well documented. There has been more research in hydrotherapy than most people realize. Much of the research was performed in Europe and reported in the European literature but was never translated and reported in the American literature. Then in the 1960s, when President John F. Kennedy came into office and wanted to put a man on the moon, aquatic research became vital in the United States because the weightless environment of water mimicked the weightless environment of space.[3] In order to study the effects of weightlessness for the space program, research on the physiologic effects of water immersion was funded by the federal government. Most of the research was performed by the National Aeronautics and Space Administration and was reported in the aerospace literature. This research deals with the physiologic effects of water immersion at rest on the circulatory, respiratory, musculoskeletal, renal, central and peripheral nervous, and endocrine systems.[1, 10, 11, 16] Unfortunately, there are very little correlative data in the aerospace literature and the medical literature.

Cardiovascular System

The physiologic effects of water immersion on the cardiovascular system are extensive. The reduced gravity, along with the hydrostatic pressure, shifts blood and fluid from the lower extremities and abdomen upward to the thorax. This shift of blood from the periphery to the central circulation is about 0.7 L. Of that 0.7 L, one third goes to the heart and two thirds goes to the pulmonary arterial circulation.[3] This increase in blood volume distends the heart and increases myocardial wall tension, which produces a greater contraction of the heart. The result is an increase in mean stroke volume of approximately 35%. There is also a corresponding drop in the heart rate by about 13 beats per minute, as well as a decrease in blood pressure. This occurs because of the increased cardiac filling time and the hemodynamic changes of blood volume and venous tone.[5] These changes correspond to an increase in cardiac output, which provides more oxygenated blood to the working muscles.

Musculoskeletal System

The physiologic effects of water immersion on the musculoskeletal system are particularly significant in sports medicine. The more efficient circulation of blood to working muscles enhances delivery of oxygen and removal of carbon dioxide and lactic acid, thus decreasing muscle soreness. The buoyancy of the water decreases the compressive forces on the joints of the spine and lower extremities, allowing the safe progression of weight-bearing activities.[12] This permits strengthening and conditioning without the potentially harmful effects of impact. Figure 16–2 illustrates the approximate percentage of weight bearing during

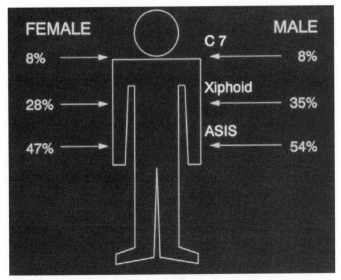

Figure 16–2. Approximate values for percentage weight bearing. ASIS, anterior superior iliac spine. (Data from Harrison, R.A. and Bulsfrode, S.J. [1987]: Percentage of weight-bearing during partial immersion in the hydrotherapy pool. Physiotherapy, 3:60–63.)

partial immersion in water according to Harrison.[12] By selecting gradually decreasing depths of water, weight-bearing forces may be increased in a controlled manner to provide progressive loading and to facilitate the transition to land-based activities.

Central and Peripheral Nervous Systems

Throughout history, relaxation and pain reduction have been the most noted effects of hydrotherapy. It is theorized that these effects result from a sensory overload generated by the buoyancy, hydrostatic pressure, viscosity, temperature, and turbulence of the water. These properties not only aid in relaxation and pain reduction but also provide more stimuli for kinesthetic awareness and proprioception. Water provides an ideal medium to enhance performance because it optimizes neuromuscular responses. The viscosity of the water provides a three-dimensional resistance environment that improves synchronization of motor unit contractions, facilitates maximal muscle unit contraction through the entire range of motion, and increases motor unit recruitment of all muscle fibers. This permits earlier functional activities that stimulate balance and coordination, which would otherwise go unstimulated until the later phases of rehabilitation.

THERAPEUTIC VALUE OF AQUATIC REHABILITATION

Aquatic rehabilitation is one of the most valuable, and certainly one of the most enjoyable, techniques used in sports medicine. Postinjury rehabilitation is a traumatic time for athletes. The emotional pain of inactivity is often more intense for an athlete than the injury itself. Aquatic rehabilitation allows an athlete to maintain physical conditioning while rehabilitating an injury. This speeds an athlete's return to play at preinjury conditioning levels. It also improves the psychologic and emotional outlook of an athlete during rehabilitation as well as after return to the sport.

Because of the physical properties of water and the physiologic changes that occur during exercise in water, aquatic rehabilitation offers many advantages over land-based rehabilitation after an injury. Buoyancy counteracts gravity and alleviates body weight and the compressive forces on the joints. Buoyancy and hydrostatic pressure provide support that allows for comfortable positioning and movement. This helps reduce pain and muscle spasm, making range-of-motion exercises more effective. Movement increases blood flow to the injured area, which aids the healing process.

The resistance of the water provides a safe and effective strengthening medium. Because of the viscosity of the water, resistance is encountered in all directions of movement. In the pool, resistance is easily modified by adjusting the lever arm, the speed of motion, and the turbulence of the water. The use of equipment may also serve to increase resistance for optimal strengthening. Water provides an accommodating resistance to exercise that makes aquatic rehabilitation safe for an injured athlete. As the speed of the activity or movement increases or decreases, so does the resistance to that movement. If pain is encountered, the resistance may be immediately reduced to within tolerance limits by slowing the activity.

Water is an ideal environment for endurance training or cardiovascular conditioning. Maintaining aerobic conditioning is vital for an injured athlete. Owing to the therapeutic nature of water, an athlete may exercise at a high intensity for a long duration without overstressing healing tissue. Cardiovascular conditioning in the water may begin immediately after an injury. The physiologic effects of buoyancy and hydrostatic pressure on the circulatory system place the heart in a training mode. As discussed earlier, the heart becomes a more efficient pump with immersion in water. The stroke volume increases, as does cardiac output, so even before an athlete begins to exercise, the heart is pumping more oxygen-rich blood throughout the body.

Athletic trainers and therapists probably use the pool most for the rehabilitation of injuries that limit weight bearing. The buoyancy of water negates the effects of gravity, reducing or eliminating the compressive forces experienced on land. The more submerged the body, the smaller the compressive forces acting on the body. After an injury, an athlete may perform rehabilitation exercises as well as functional sport activities in the deep water to prepare the injured area for weight bearing. As appropriate, the depth of water is decreased to progress weight bearing. Increasing the speed of a weight-bearing activity in shallow water will also provide progressive loading.[13]

AQUATIC REHABILITATION GUIDELINES

When designing an aquatic exercise program for athletic injuries, it is essential to follow the basic principles of sports rehabilitation. A complete and accurate diagnosis should be made by a physician. After the evaluation, aquatic rehabilitation may be initiated, with the emphasis placed on minimizing inflammation and preventing further damage to the injury. Each program should be designed by considering the injury, the athlete's sport and position, and the athlete's goals. Exercises are then initiated to recover full range of motion and stability of the involved joint. Endurance activities for maintaining or regaining an athlete's cardiovascular condition should be performed as soon as possible, providing adequate protection to the injury so that the healing tissue will not be overstressed. These activities may be performed in deep water with the aid of flotation devices if the injury prevents weight bearing. Isolated strengthening, weight bearing, and gait training are initiated next and progressed, as tolerated, within the healing restraints of the injury. The final phase of aquatic rehabilitation involves advanced cardiovascular conditioning in combination with complex movement patterns for balance, coordination, agility, power, and simulation of athletic skills.

Not only is aquatic rehabilitation efficient in maintaining or regaining athletic fitness, but because of the inherent properties of water, it also reduces injuries related to impact and overuse. For this reason, many athletic teams are using water not only for rehabilitating injured athletes but also for preseason conditioning and cross-training. Personnel involved in conditioning of athletes believe that aquatic exercise is an important adjunct to their land-based activities.

Increasing Range of Motion

Because of the support provided by buoyancy and hydrostatic pressure, water provides an optimal environment for range-of-motion and stretching exercises. The reduced-gravity environment relaxes the muscles and decreases protective spasms, which aids in reducing pain, allowing an athlete to achieve a greater range of motion. With proper positioning of the athlete, buoyancy may also help an athlete perform a range of motion that is not possible because of weakness.

Increasing Strength

Progressive resistance strengthening is easily achieved in the water (Figs. 16–3 to 16–8). Accommodating resistance is provided by the viscosity of the water. Exercises performed in the pool may be isometric, with the athlete attempting to stabilize against the movement of water. Dynamic exercises performed in the water may be isotonic or isokinetic and may produce a concentric or eccentric contraction. A concentric contraction involves the shortening of a muscle during contraction and usually occurs with the generation of force to move against a resistance. In water, this occurs when an athlete moves a body part against the

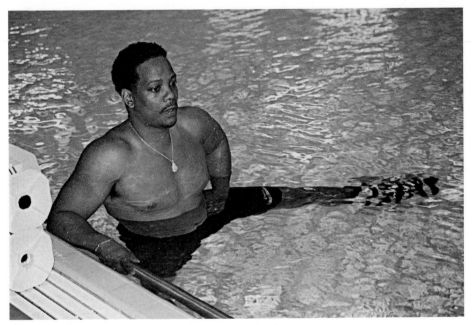

Figure 16–3. Hip abduction and adduction strengthening.

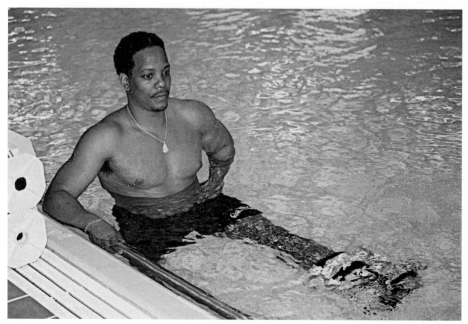

Figure 16–4. Hip flexion and extension strengthening with straight leg for increased lever arm resistance.

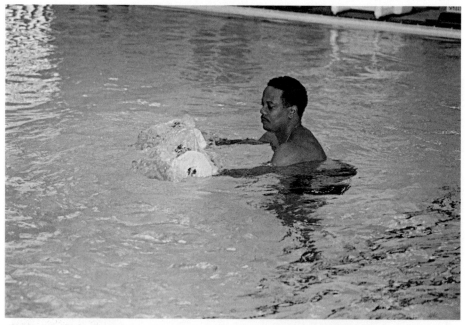

Figure 16–5. Wrist flexion and extension for range of motion and strengthening.

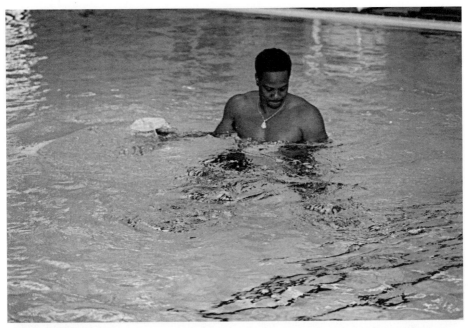

Figure 16–6. Shoulder internal and external rotation for range of motion and strengthening.

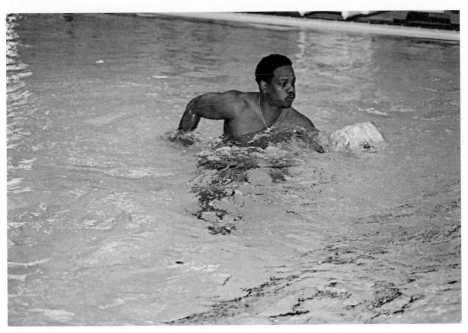

Figure 16–7. Shoulder and elbow flexion and extension strengthening.

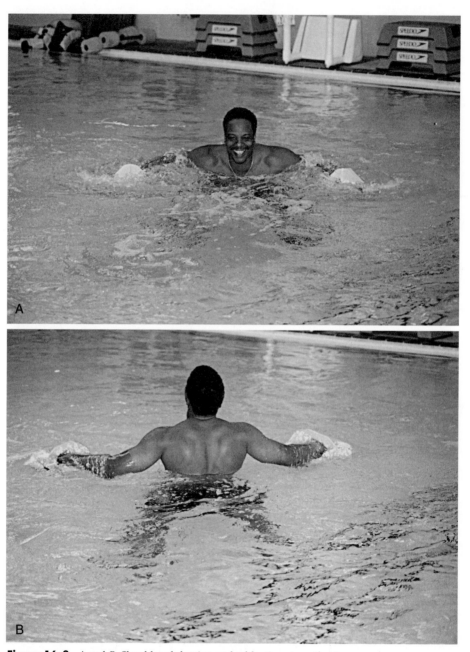

Figure 16–8. *A* and *B*, Shoulder abduction and adduction strengthening.

force of buoyancy or against the force generated by the viscosity of the water. An eccentric contraction involves the lengthening of the muscle during contraction and occurs during deceleration motions. In water, this occurs when an athlete controls the action of a body part moving with a force such as buoyancy. The resistance of these exercises may be progressed by changing the speed of movement or the length of the lever arm or by using equipment designed to increase the surface area or alter the buoyant force.

Increasing Cardiovascular Endurance

Many activities may be performed to increase cardiovascular endurance. Deep-water running is ideal for injured athletes because running is involved in the majority of sports and is a familiar exercise. Deep-water running consists of simulated running in the deep end of the pool with the aid of a flotation device that maintains the head above water (Fig. 16–9). The athlete may run the length of the pool or run in place if secured by a tether system. This activity eliminates all impact forces because no contact is made with the bottom of the pool. Swimming is also an excellent endurance activity but may not be the activity of choice because of a lack of skill. There are an infinite number of activities that may be used for cardiovascular conditioning in the water. Any skill that is familiar to the athlete and that involves repetitive motion of large muscle groups may be suitable as an exercise for endurance.

Functional Progression

The ultimate goal of aquatic rehabilitation in sports medicine is to return the athlete to competition as soon as possible at 100% of preinjury strength and conditioning levels. To achieve this, the focus must ultimately become the performance of functional or sport-specific activities (Figs. 16–10 to 16–13). Water

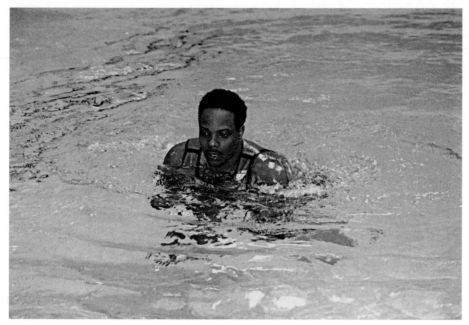

Figure 16–9. Deep water running with the aid of a flotation vest.

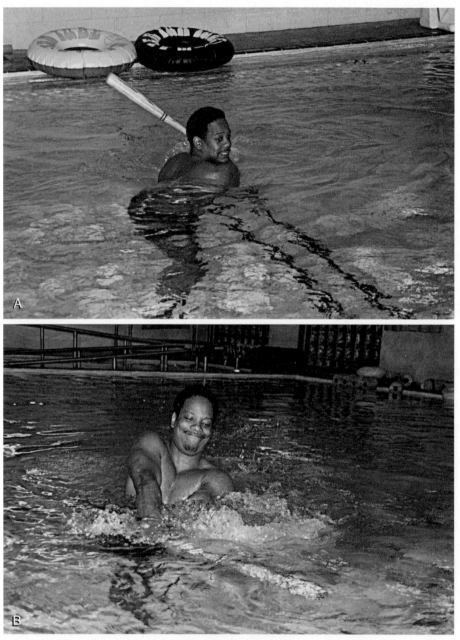

Figure 16–10. *A* and *B,* Functional activity simulation: baseball swing.

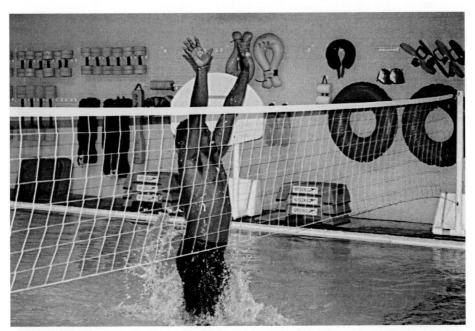

Figure 16–11. Functional activity simulation: volleyball blocking.

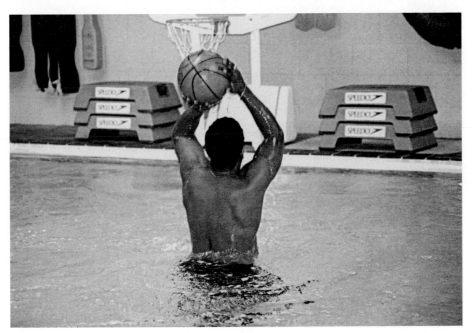

Figure 16–12. Functional activity simulation: basketball jump shot.

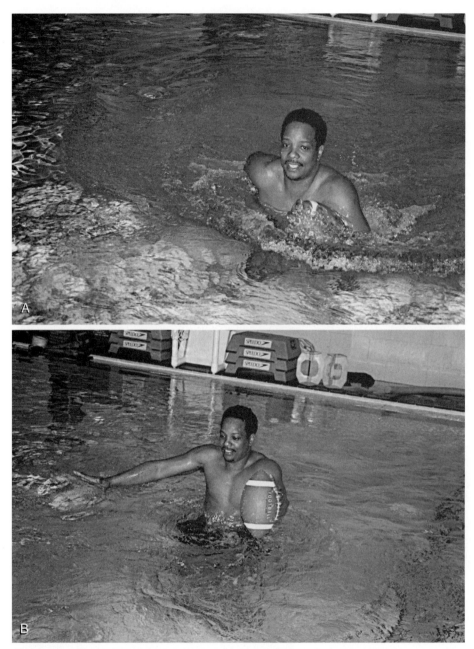

Figure 16–13. Functional activity simulation. *A*, Runningback. *B*, Quarterback.

is an ideal environment to initiate functional activities. The buoyancy of water may be used to decrease, and even eliminate, the compressive forces encountered with land exercise. This is especially important to those athletes with injuries that limit weight bearing. Range-of-motion, strength, and endurance activities performed in deep water are used to prepare the athlete for weight bearing. When the athlete has been cleared to begin weight bearing, gait training is performed in decreasing water depths to increase the loading of the joints and spine (Fig. 16–14). Weight bearing and closed-chain and sport-specific activities prepare the athlete for return to full unlimited activity. Table 16–1 outlines an example of aquatic progression after an anterior cruciate ligament reconstruction.

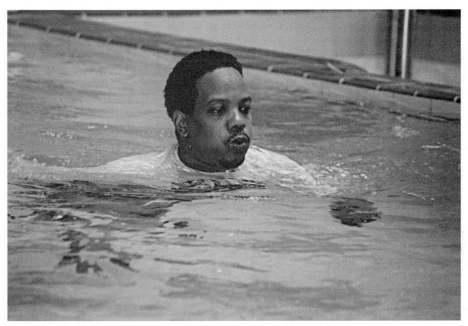

Figure 16–14. Running in water at neck level for 10% weight bearing.

Table 16–1. Aquatic Exercise Progression After Anterior Cruciate Ligament Reconstruction

I. **Phase I: Maximum Protection Phase**
  A. Weeks 2–6
    1. Gait training
      • Forward
      • Backward
      • Sideways
    2. Resistive exercises
      • Minisquats
      • Hip flexion and extension with knee flexion
      • Hip abduction and adduction
    3. Deep-well endurance activity
      • Bicycling
      • Scissor kick
      • Hip abduction and adduction
    4. Hamstring and gastrocnemius/soleus stretching
  B. Weeks 3–6
    1. Barbell minisquats
    2. Straight leg hip flexion and extension
    3. Addition of resistance exercise equipment
II. **Phase II: Controlled Ambulation Phase**
  A. Weeks 6–9
    1. Continue resistance exercises
    2. Side-lying cycling: forward and backward
    3. Lateral step-ups
    4. Cariocas
    5. Jogging: forward and backward
    6. Swimming with buoy
    7. Back-lying flutter kick
III. **Phase III: Moderate Protection Phase**
  A. Weeks 9–14
    1. Continue resistance exercises
    2. Kickboard lap swimming
    3. Resistance kickboard running
IV. **Phase IV: Light Activity Phase**
  A. Months 3–4
    1. 3 Months
      • Swimming
      • Vertical jumping
      • Resistance running with jets
      • Agility patterns
      • Diagonal cutting
    2. 3.5 Months
      • Kickboard laps with fins
      • Deep-well running with fins
      • Tethered shallow-water running

From Arrigo, C.A., Fuller, C.S., and Wilk, K.E., (1992): Aquatic rehabilitation following ACL-PTG reconstruction. Sports Med. Update, 7:22–27.

SUMMARY

Aquatic rehabilitation is a valuable tool in the management, progression, and successful rehabilitation of sports injuries. Exercising in water decreases the compressive forces of weight bearing, allowing earlier performance of functional activities during rehabilitation. The water provides an environment for effective range-of-motion exercises, strengthening, and cardiovascular conditioning, aimed at returning the athlete to his or her sport as soon as possible at preinjury conditioning levels. In addition, aquatic rehabilitation keeps the athlete motivated during rehabilitation by allowing sport-specific activities that enhance the athlete's successful return to competition.

References

1. Arborelius, M., Balldin, U.I., Lilla, B., et al. (1973): Regional lung function in man during immersion with the head above water. Aerosp. Med., 43:701–707.
2. Bates, A., and Hanson, N. (1996): Aquatic Exercise Therapy. Philadelphia, W.B. Saunders.
3. Becker, B.E. (1994): The biologic aspects of hydrotherapy. J. Back Musculoskel. Rehabil., 4:255–264.
4. Becker, B.E. (1997): Aquatic physics. In: Ruoti, R.G., Morris, D.M., and Cole, A.J. (eds.): Aquatic Rehabilitation. Philadelphia, J.B. Lippincott, pp. 15–23.
5. Bookspan, J. (1997): Physiologic effects of immersion at rest. In: Ruoti, R.G., Morris, D.M., and Cole, A.J. (eds.): Aquatic Rehabilitation. Philadelphia, J.B. Lippincott, pp. 25–37.
6. Campion, M.R. (1990): Adult Hydrotherapy: A Practical Approach. Oxford, England, Heinemann Medical Books, pp. 3–5, 39–40.
7. Cunningham, J. (1994): Historical review of aquatics and physical therapy. Orthop. Physical Therapy Clin. North Am., 2:83–93.
8. Davis, B., and Harrison, R.A. (1993): Hydrotherapy in Practice. New York, Random House.
9. Edlich, R.F., Towler, M.A., Goitz, R.J., et al. (1987): Bioengineering principles of hydrotherapy. J. Burn Care Rehabil., 8:579–584.
10. Gabrielsen, A., Johansen, L.B., and Norsk, P. (1993): Central cardiovascular pressures during graded water immersion in humans. Am. Phys. Soc., 75:581–585.
11. Haffor, A.S.A., Mohler, J.G., and Harrison, A.C. (1995): Effects of water immersion on cardiac output of lean and fat male subjects at rest and during exercise. Aviat. Space Environ. Med., 2:123–127.
12. Harrison, R.A., and Bulstrode, S.J. (1987): Percentage of weight-bearing during partial immersion in the hydrotherapy pool. Physiotherapy, 3:60–63.
13. Harrison, R.A., Hillman, M., and Bulstrode, S. (1992): Loading of the lower limb when walking partially immersed. Physiotherapy, 78:164–166.
14. Irion, J.M. (1997): Historical overview of aquatic rehabilitation. In: Ruoti, R.G., Morris, D.M., and Cole, A.J. (eds.): Aquatic Rehabilitation. Philadelphia, J.B. Lippincott, pp. 1–13.
15. Lowman, C. (1952): Therapeutic Use of Pools and Tanks. Philadelphia, W.B. Saunders.
16. Norsk, P., Drummer, C., Johansen, L.B., et al. (1993): Effect of water immersion on renal natriuretic peptide (urodilatin) excretion in humans. Am. Phys. Soc., 74:2881–2885.
17. Skinner, A.T., and Thomson, A. (1983): Duffield's Exercise in Water, 3rd ed. London, Bailliere Tindall.

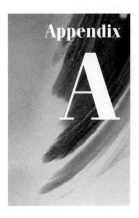
Upper Extremity Plyometrics*

Kevin E. Wilk, P.T.

Chest Pass (Fig. A–1). The athlete stands facing a plyoback. Using both hands to hold a 3-pound medicine ball against the chest, the athlete pushes the ball away from the chest into the plyoback. The athlete's arm should return to the starting position as he or she catches the ball rebounding off the plyoback.

Two-Hand Overhead Soccer Throw (Fig. A–2). The athlete stands or kneels facing a plyoback. Holding a 3- to 5-pound medicine ball in both hands, the athlete raises the ball overhead, then throws it into the plyoback. The athlete should catch the ball overhead as it rebounds from the plyoback.

Two-Hand Side-to-Side Throw (Fig. A–3). The athlete stands facing a plyoback holding a 3- to 5-pound medicine ball with both hands, positioned over one shoulder. The athlete throws the ball into the plyoback, then catches it with both hands over the opposite shoulder. The athlete continues alternating sides. This exercise can also be used to train the rotators of the hips and trunk by allowing the body to rotate slightly as the ball is caught.

Baseball Toss at 90/90 (Fig. A–4). The athlete stands facing a plyoback with the arm at a 90°-angle away from the body and the elbow bent to 90° (cocking position). Holding a 1-pound medicine ball, the athlete forcefully throws the ball into the plyoback, then catches it as it rebounds, maintaining the same position

---

*From Wilk, K.E., Andrews, J.R., Arrigo, C.A., et al. (1997). Preventive and Rehabilitative Exercises for the Shoulder and Elbow. Birmingham, Alabama, American Sports Medicine Institute, pp. 30–31.

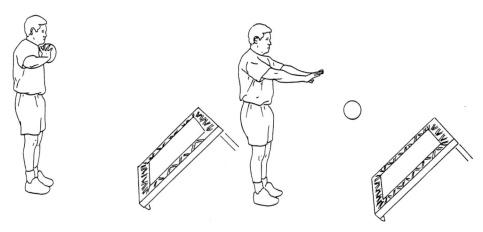

Figure A-1. Chest pass.

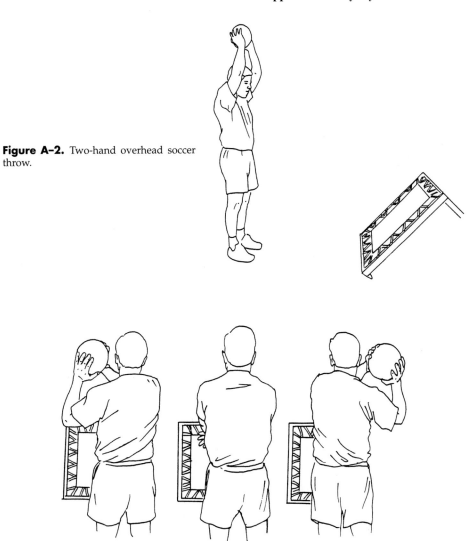

Figure A-2. Two-hand overhead soccer throw.

Figure A-3. Two-hand side-to-side throw.

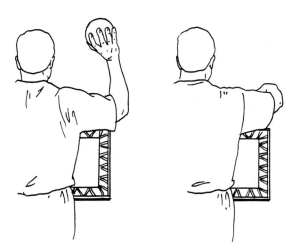

Figure A-4. Baseball toss at 90/90.

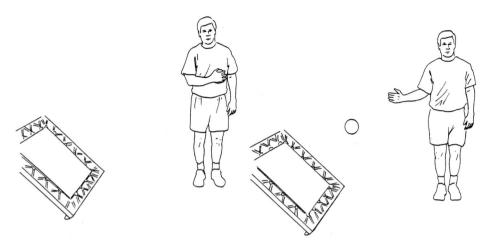

Figure A–5. Backhand external rotation at 0°.

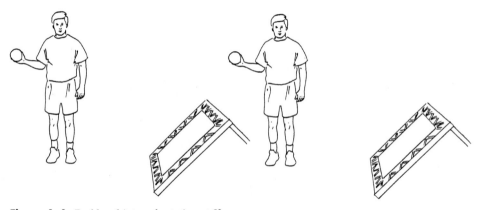

Figure A–6. Backhand internal rotation at 0°.

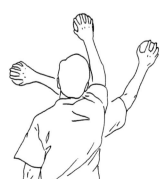

Figure A–7. Wall dribble.

of the arm and elbow. The exercise can also be used to train the legs and trunk to accelerate the arm by stepping out as the ball is thrown.

Backhand External Rotation at 0° (Fig. A–5). The athlete stands sideways with the involved side toward the plyoback and a 1- to 3-pound medicine ball in the involved hand. Keeping the upper arm against the body and the elbow bent to 90°, the athlete internally rotates the arm toward the chest, then forcefully externally rotates the arm, throwing the ball into the plyoback. The athlete should try catching the ball as it rebounds with the palm toward the body and upper arm close to the side.

Backhand Internal Rotation at 0° (Fig. A–6). The athlete stands sideways with the uninvolved side nearest the plyoback and a 1- to 3-pound medicine ball in the involved hand, keeping the upper arm of the involved side close to the body and the elbow bent to 90°. After the athlete externally rotates the arm, he or she forcefully throws the ball into the plyoback by internally rotating the arm. The athlete should catch the ball while maintaining the upper arm against the body.

Wall Dribbling (Fig. A–7). The athlete stands facing a wall, holding a 1- to 3-pound medicine ball slightly above shoulder level. The athlete should dribble the ball against the wall. This exercise can be progressed by dribbling the ball in an arch along the wall.

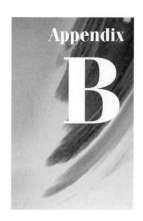

Knee and Leg Rehabilitation Exercises

Gary L. Harrelson, Ed.D., A.T.,C.

RANGE-OF-MOTION EXERCISES

Patella Mobilization. With the athlete's leg straight and thigh musculature relaxed, the athlete or clinician places the fingers of each hand on each side of the patella and gently mobilizes the patella side to side for 1 to 2 minutes. This is repeated, with mobilization of the patella up and down for 1 to 2 minutes.

Passive Knee Flexion. The athlete sits in a chair, pushes the lower leg on the involved side as far back as possible with the opposite leg (Fig. B–1), and holds for 10 seconds. To straighten, the athlete hooks the foot of the uninvolved leg

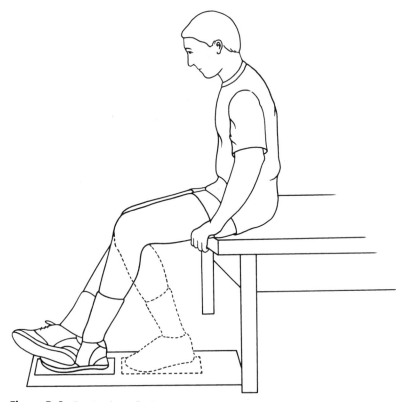

Figure B–1. Passive knee flexion.

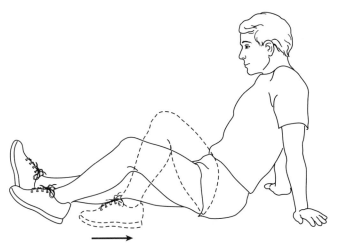

Figure B–2. Heel slide.

behind the involved leg's ankle and guides the involved knee straight without contracting the quadriceps.

Heel Slide. The athlete pulls the heel toward the buttocks, flexing the knee; holds for 5 seconds; straightens the leg by sliding the heel downward; and holds for 5 seconds (Fig. B–2). In later stages of rehabilitation the athlete may grasp the lower leg with both hands and pull the heel toward the buttocks. During straightening of the leg, pressure may be put on the leg above the patella to aid in regaining extension.

Active-Assisted Knee Flexion. The athlete sits in a chair and slides the lower leg on the involved side as far back as possible. Keeping the foot stationary, the athlete slides the hips forward (Fig. B–3), holds for 5 seconds, and relaxes.

Knee Flexion Pulley. The athlete, seated and with the pulley secured to the

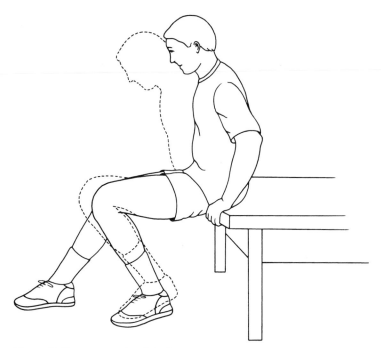

Figure B–3. Active-assisted flexion.

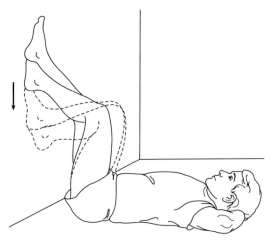

Figure B–4. Wall slide.

back of the chair, slides the involved foot as far back as possible. The handle on the pulley rope is grasped and pulled gently to bend the knee farther back.

Wall Slide. The athlete lies on the back with the involved foot on the wall (Fig. B–4). Using a towel between the wall and the foot, the athlete allows the foot to slide down the wall by bending the knee. The other leg is used to apply pressure downward.

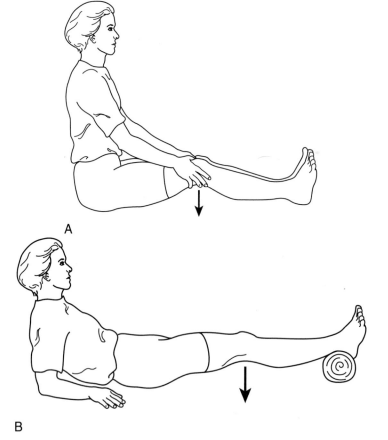

A

B

Figure B–5. *A,* Passive knee extension. *B,* Passive knee extension.

Passive Knee Extension. (1) The athlete straightens the involved leg by sliding the heel downward and uses the hands to apply pressure on the leg above the patella, trying to make the knee as straight as possible; holds for 10 seconds; relaxes; and repeats the exercise (Fig. B–5A). (2) The athlete places a towel roll under the heel and allows the involved leg to straighten with the assistance of gravity and gentle pressure from the hands (Fig. B–5B). (3) The athlete places a weight on the thigh above the knee.

ISOMETRIC EXERCISES

Quad Set. With the leg as straight as possible, the athlete tightens the front thigh muscles (quadriceps), trying to pull the patella superiorly; holds for 5 seconds, contracting the muscles as tightly as possible; completely relaxes the thigh; and rests for 2 seconds. This exercise may be performed standing, sitting, or lying down.

Multiple-Angle Isometrics. Seated, the athlete places the foot against the wall with the knee bent to 90° (Fig. B–6), gently pushes into the wall as if to kick out, holds for 10 seconds, and relaxes for 4 seconds. The exercise is repeated at 90°, 60°, and 30° of knee flexion.

Isometric Hip Adduction. The athlete places a rolled towel or pillow between the thighs (Fig. B–7), squeezes the legs together tightly, holds for 10 seconds, relaxes and rests for 4 seconds, and repeats.

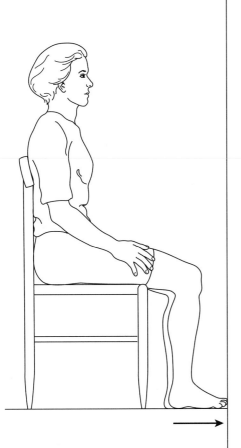

Figure B–6. Multiple-angle isometrics.

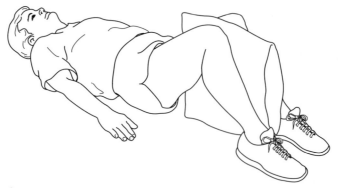

Figure B–7. Isometric hip adduction.

Cocontraction. The athlete tightens both the quadriceps and the hamstring muscles at the same time by "digging" the heel downward (Fig. B–8), holds for 5 seconds, contracts the muscles as tightly as possible, and then completely relaxes the thigh and rests for 4 seconds. This exercise may be performed sitting up, lying down, or seated in a chair. Cocontractions may be modified by performing each set with the knee bent at a different angle.

ISOTONIC EXERCISES

Straight Leg Raise. The athlete tightens the quadriceps as in a quad set, keeps the leg straight, lifts the heel off the table approximately 6 inches (Fig. B–9),

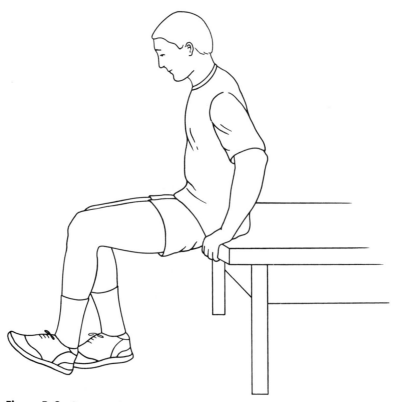

Figure B–8. Cocontraction.

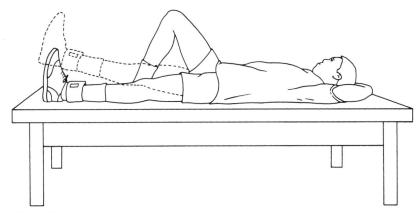

Figure B–9. Straight leg raise.

holds for 6 seconds, slowly lowers the leg, completely relaxes the thigh, and rests for 4 seconds.

Hip Adduction. The athlete lies on the side of the involved leg, places the opposite foot just in front of the involved knee, lifts the involved leg 6 inches up and away from the table (Fig. B–10), holds for 6 seconds, slowly lowers the leg, and relaxes, resting for 4 seconds.

Hip Abduction. The athlete lies on the side of the uninvolved leg, bending the leg at the knee for stability; straightens the top leg; lifts upward toward the ceiling without rotating the leg outward (Fig. B–11); holds for 6 seconds; slowly lowers the leg; and relaxes, resting for 4 seconds.

Hip Extension. The athlete lies prone on the table with the feet off the table edge; lifts the involved leg straight up about 6 inches, keeping the leg straight (Fig. B–12); holds for 6 seconds; slowly lowers to the resting position; and rests for 4 seconds. This exercise can also be performed in the standing position, with the athlete lying over the table edge at the waist.

Gluteal Extension. The athlete lies prone on the table, flexes the knee on the involved side to about 90°, lifts the involved leg straight up (Fig. B–13), holds for 6 seconds, slowly lowers the leg to the resting position, and rests for 4 seconds.

Hip Flexion. The athlete sits on the edge of a firm surface with the feet resting on the floor, lifts the knee toward the chest (Fig. B–14), holds for 6 seconds, slowly lowers the leg to the resting position, and rests for 4 seconds.

Terminal Knee Extension. A hard roll is placed under the involved knee, allowing the knee to bend approximately 30°. The athlete extends the leg slowly

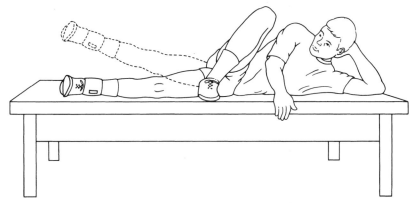

Figure B–10. Hip adduction.

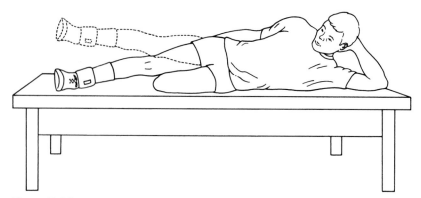

Figure B–11. Hip abduction.

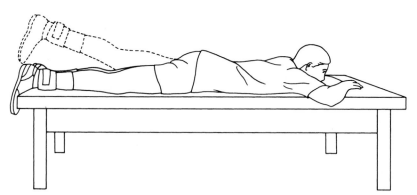

Figure B–12. Hip extension.

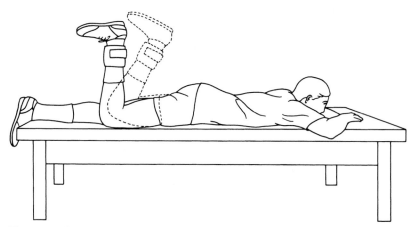

Figure B–13. Gluteal extension.

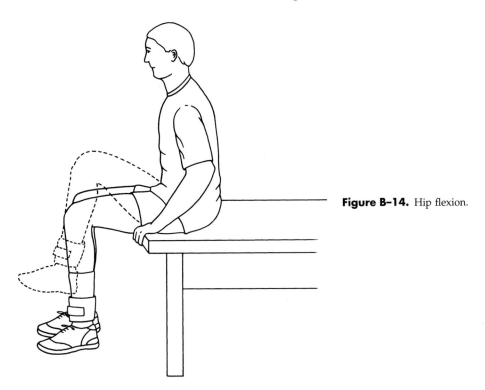

Figure B-14. Hip flexion.

until it is straight (Fig. B–15), pauses, slowly lowers the leg to the starting position, and rests for 4 seconds.

90°-to-45° Knee Extension. In a sitting position, the athlete extends the involved leg slowly to a 45° angle (Fig. B–16), holds for 6 seconds, slowly lowers the leg to the starting position, and rests for 4 seconds.

90°-to-0° Knee Extension. In a sitting position, the athlete extends the involved leg slowly until it is straight (Fig. B–17), holds for 6 seconds, slowly lowers the leg to the starting position, and rests for 4 seconds.

Static Weight Loading. Sitting on the edge of a chair, the athlete straightens the leg, with the foot resting on the floor; tightens the quadriceps as in a quad set, keeping the leg straight; raises the leg until it is parallel to the floor (Fig. B–18); and holds for 10 seconds. The athlete then lowers the leg to the floor, rests, and repeats the exercise, performing 10 repetitions. This is increased in 5-second intervals up to 1 minute. No weight is used until 1 minute is reached; the hold time is then reduced, progressing to 1 minute again.

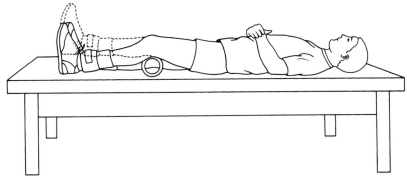

Figure B-15. Terminal knee extension.

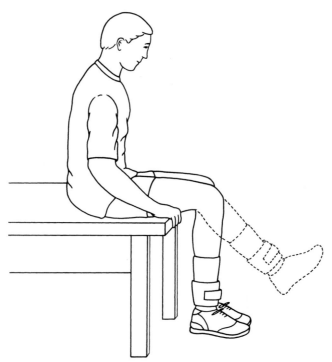

Figure B-16. Knee extension (90° to 45°).

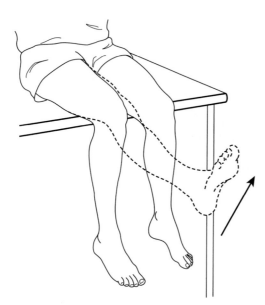

Figure B-17. Knee extension (90° to 0°).

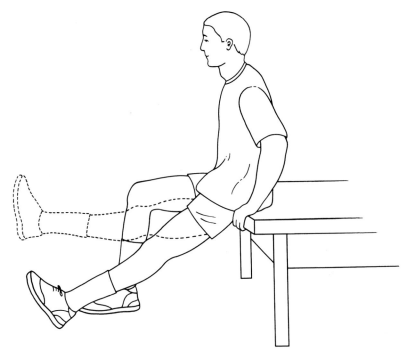

Figure B–18. Static weight loading.

Hip Internal Rotation. Seated, the athlete slowly lifts the foot to the outside, rotating the upper leg inward; holds for 6 seconds; slowly returns the foot to the starting position; and rests for 4 seconds (Fig. B–19). This exercise can be done with a weight wrapped around the lower leg or with rubber tubing wrapped around the lower leg with the other end of the tubing anchored to a fixed object.

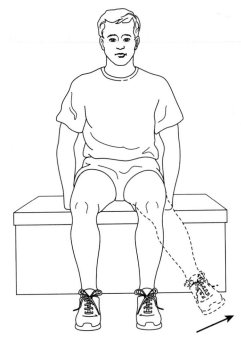

Figure B–19. Hip internal rotation.

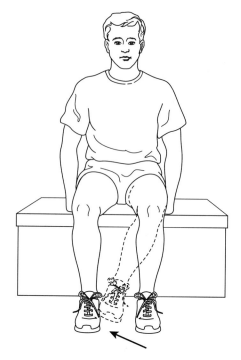

Figure B–20. Hip external rotation.

Hip External Rotation. Seated, the athlete slowly lifts the foot to the inside, rotating the upper leg outward; holds for 6 seconds; slowly returns the foot to the starting position; and rests for 4 seconds (Fig. B–20). This exercise can be done with a weight wrapped around the lower leg or with rubber tubing wrapped around the lower leg with the other end of the tubing anchored to a fixed object.

Prone Hamstring Curl. The athlete lies prone on the table with the feet off the table edge; bends the knee slowly, bringing the heel toward the buttocks (Fig. B–21); holds for 6 seconds; slowly lowers to starting position; and rests for 4 seconds.

Standing Hamstring Curl. The athlete stands straight with the thigh resting against a table or wall, raises the heel slowly toward the buttocks (Fig. B–22), holds for 6 seconds, slowly lowers the leg, and rests for 4 seconds.

Resisted Plantar Flexion. With the leg as straight as possible, the athlete loops a towel around the ball of the foot, holding the ends of the towel with both hands; and pushes the foot downward, providing resistance with the towel (Fig. B–23). After a pause, the athlete pulls the foot back as far as possible, stretching the Achilles tendon. A variation of this would be to use rubber tubing to provide the resistance.

Heel Raise. The athlete stands with the feet slightly pigeon-toed, using a wall

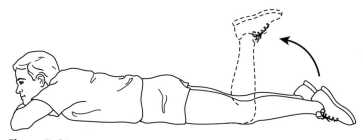

Figure B–21. Prone hamstring curl.

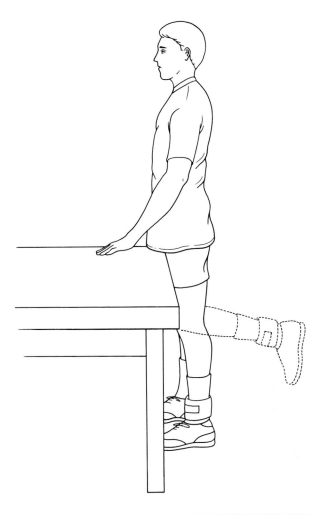

Figure B–22. Standing hamstring curl.

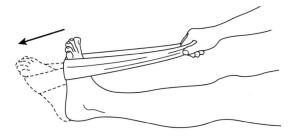

Figure B–23. Resisted plantar flexion.

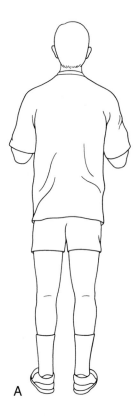 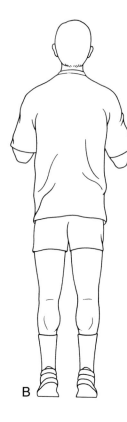

A

B

Figure B-24. *A* and *B*, Heel raise.

or table for balance (Fig. B–24*A*); pushes up on the toes and lifts the heels (Fig. B–24*B*); holds for 6 seconds; slowly lowers the heel; relaxes; and repeats the exercise.

Hip Abduction with Elastic Resistance. The athlete secures one end of an elastic band to a fixed object and the other end to the involved or uninvolved ankle. The athlete stands with the involved or uninvolved leg next to the fixed object; rapidly moves the leg away about 1 foot, keeping the knee straight (Fig. B–25); returns to the starting position; and repeats. *Note:* The elastic band may be attached to the involved or the uninvolved leg, depending on the goal of the exercise.

Hip Adduction with Elastic Resistance. The athlete secures one end of an

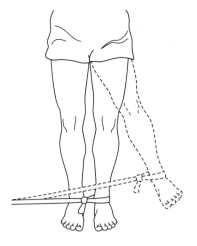

Figure B-25. Hip abduction with elastic resistance.

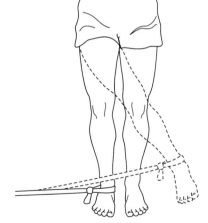

Figure B–26. Hip adduction with elastic resistance.

elastic band to a fixed object and the other end to the involved or uninvolved ankle. The athlete stands with the involved or uninvolved leg next to the fixed object; rapidly moves the leg away about 1 foot, keeping the knee straight (Fig. B–26); returns to the starting position; and repeats. *Note:* The elastic band may be attached to the involved or the uninvolved leg, depending on the goal of the exercise.

Hip Extension with Elastic Resistance. The athlete secures one end of an elastic band to a fixed object and the other end to the involved or uninvolved ankle. The athlete stands facing the fixed object; rapidly pulls the leg back until the toes are across the heel of the opposite foot, keeping the knee straight (Fig. B–27); returns to the starting position; and repeats. *Note:* The elastic band may be attached to the involved or the uninvolved leg, depending on the goal of the exercise.

Hip Flexion with Elastic Resistance. The athlete secures one end of an elastic band to a fixed object and the other end to the involved or uninvolved ankle. The athlete stands facing away from the fixed object. Keeping the knee straight, the athlete rapidly moves the leg forward until the heel is across the toes of the

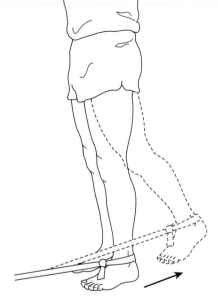

Figure B–27. Hip extension with elastic resistance.

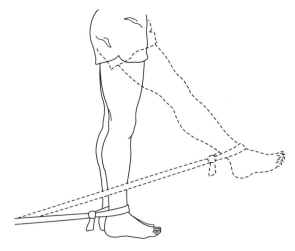

Figure B–28. Hip flexion with elastic resistance.

opposite foot (Fig. B–28); returns to the starting position; and repeats. *Note:* The elastic band may be attached to the involved or the uninvolved leg, depending on the goal of the exercise.

CLOSED-CHAIN EXERCISES

Mini Squats. The athlete stands with the feet shoulder-width apart and rotated outward slightly and, using a table for support, bends at the knees to

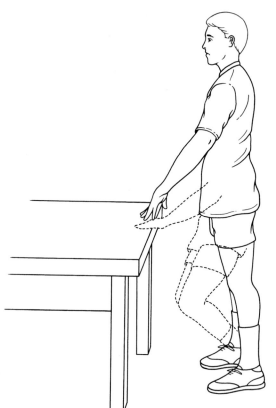

Figure B–29. Minisquats.

30°; holds for 4 seconds (Fig. B–29); slowly straightens to 15°; and repeats. This exercise can be progressed by using no support, with the back against the wall, and by using only the involved leg. It can be performed with tubing to provide resistance, with the athlete standing on the tubing and holding the tubing at waist level.

Forward Lunge. The athlete stands, lunges the involved or the uninvolved leg (depending on the goal of the exercise) forward approximately 2 to 3 feet, bending the hips and knees; pauses; returns to the starting position; and repeats (Fig. B–30). The athlete should *not* take the knee past the toes, and knee flexion may need to be limited, depending on the injury or surgical procedure.

Lunges with Elastic Resistance

1. Forward Lunge. While standing, the athlete lunges the involved or uninvolved leg (depending on the goal of the exercise) forward approximately 2 to 3 feet, bending at the hips and knees; pauses; returns to the starting position; and repeats (Fig. B–31*A*). The athlete should *not* take the knee past the toes, and knee flexion may need to be limited, depending on the injury or surgical procedure.

2. Sidestep Lunge. While standing, the athlete lunges the involved or uninvolved leg (depending on the goal of the exercise) to the side approximately 2 to 3 feet, bending at the hips and knees; pauses; returns to the starting position; and repeats (Fig. B–31*B*). The athlete should *not* take the knee past the toes, and knee flexion may need to be limited, depending on the injury or surgical procedure.

3. Cross-step Lunge: While standing, the athlete lunges the involved or uninvolved leg (depending on the goal of the exercise) across the body, bending at the hips and knees; pauses; returns to the starting position; and repeats (Fig. B–31*C*). The athlete should *not* take the knee past the toes, and knee

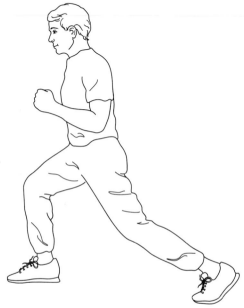

Figure B–30. Forward lunge.

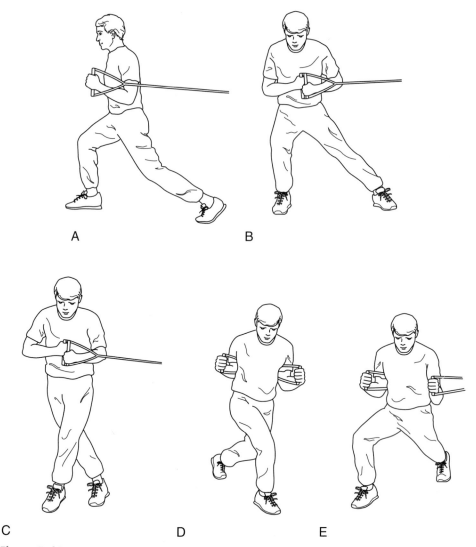

Figure B–31. Lunges with elastic resistance. *A*, Forward lunge. *B*, Sidestep lunge. *C*, Cross-step lunge. *D*, Diagonal cross-step lunge. *E*, Diagonal lunge.

flexion may need to be limited, depending on the injury or surgical procedure.

4. Diagonal Cross-step Lunge. While standing, the athlete lunges the involved or uninvolved leg (depending on the goal of the exercise) forward approximately 2 to 3 feet and across in front of the other leg, bending at the hips and knees; pauses; returns to the starting position; and repeats (Fig. B–31D). The athlete should *not* take the knee past the toes, and knee flexion may need to be limited, depending on the injury or surgical procedure.

5. Diagonal Lunge. While standing, the athlete lunges the involved or uninvolved leg (depending on the goal of the exercise) forward approximately 2 to 3 feet and out to the side, bending at the hips and knees; pauses; returns to the starting position; and

repeats (Fig. B–31*E*). The athlete should *not* take the knee past the toes, and knee flexion may need to be limited, depending on the injury or surgical procedure.

Lateral Step-ups. The athlete stands with the involved leg toward a step, places the foot on the step (Fig. B–32*A*), and lifts the body with the involved leg (Fig. B–32*B*). The exercise may be advanced to standing on the heel of the uninvolved leg and lifting the entire body with no push-off. The athlete begins with about a 4-inch step and gradually progresses to an 8-inch step, as tolerated. Resistance can be provided by having the athlete stand on rubber tubing with the involved leg, hold the tubing as high as possible, and perform the exercise as described above.

Closed-Chain Terminal Knee Extensions. The athlete stands with the feet shoulder-width apart and with tubing looped around the involved leg above the knee (the other end is looped around a fixed object) and performs the following exercises: (1) With the tubing pulling out from the side of the body, the athlete bends the knees to 30°, pauses, slowly straightens, and repeats the movement. (2) With the tubing pulling forward in front of the body, the athlete bends knees to 30°, pauses, slowly straightens, and repeats the movement.

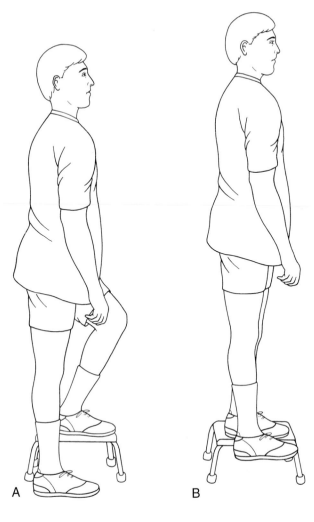

Figure B–32. *A* and *B*, Lateral step-ups.

A   B

Stationary Cycling. The seat height is adjusted so that the involved leg is almost straight when the ball of the foot is on the lower pedal (Fig. B–33). The tension should be set to allow minimum to moderate resistance.

Hamstring Stretch. (1) The athlete straightens the supported leg with the opposite leg to the side; slowly leans forward, keeping the toe pulled back and the knee straight until a stretch is felt in the hamstrings (Fig. B–34*A*); and holds for 10 seconds. This stretch is performed with the chin up and the back straight and with no bouncing. (2) The athlete lies on the back and bends the leg toward the chest until the knee is pointed upward; slowly straightens the leg until a stretch is felt in the hamstrings; holds for 10 seconds; and repeats (Fig. B–34*B*).

Quadriceps Stretch. The athlete holds on with one arm for balance, grasps the foot of the injured extremity with the hand, and brings the heel to the buttocks (Fig. B–35). While standing straight, the athlete slowly extends the leg while maintaining the hold on the foot, and holds for 10 seconds.

Hip Flexor Stretch. The athlete kneels on the involved leg and places the other leg out in front of the the body with the knee bent at 90° (Fig.B–36). Keeping the body upright, the athlete leans forward until a stretch is felt in the muscle on the front of the involved leg, holds for 10 seconds, returns to starting position, and repeats.

Achilles Stretch. The athlete stands and leans into a wall with the weight on the heels and the back knee straight (Fig. B–37). Keeping the feet pointed straight ahead, the athlete slowly leans forward until a stretch is felt in the calf, holds for 10 seconds, and repeats with each leg.

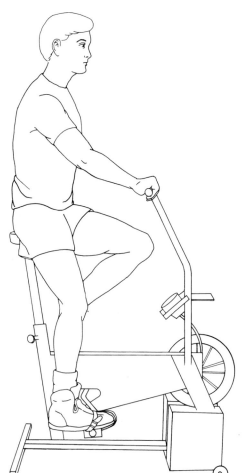

Figure B–33. Stationary cycling.

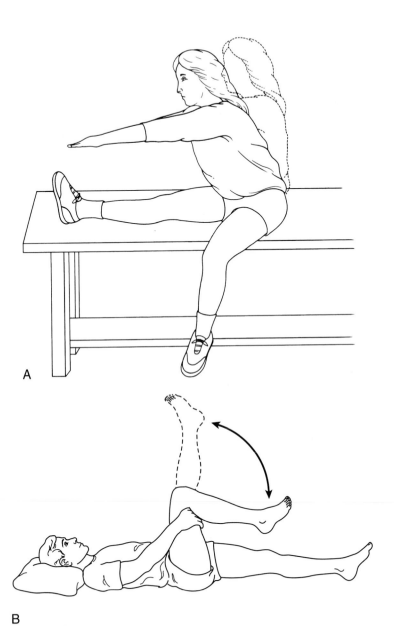

Figure B–34. *A* and *B,* Hamstring stretches.

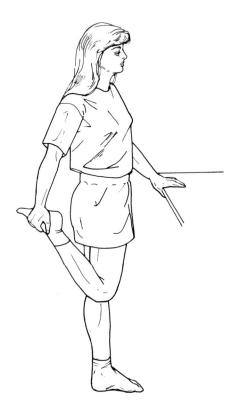

Figure B–35. Quadriceps stretch.

Figure B–36. Hip flexor stretch.

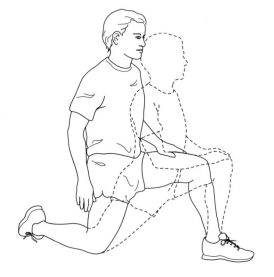

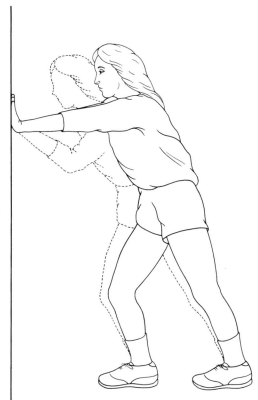

Figure B–37. Achilles stretch.

Soleus Stretch. The athlete stands and leans into a wall with the weight on the heels and the knees slightly bent and slowly leans forward until a stretch is felt in the calf (Fig. B–38), holds for 10 seconds, and repeats with each leg.

WEIGHT MACHINE EXERCISES

Multi-Hip Machine

The platform height should be adjusted so that the hip joint is aligned with the axis of the pivot arm. The leg pad should be adjusted to be just above the knee joint.

Hip Adduction. The involved leg is positioned with the hip at the axis of the pivot arm (Fig. B–39*A*). The athlete stands facing the weight. The pivot arm is positioned so that the leg pad rests against the inner part of the thigh as the involved leg is abducted away as far as possible. The athlete grasps the handles for stabilization, lifts the weight by moving the involved leg across in front of the uninvolved leg *without* twisting the body, pauses, lowers the weight to the starting position in a slow and controlled manner, and repeats.

Hip Flexion. The involved leg is positioned with the hip at the axis of the pivot arm (Fig. B–39*B*). The athlete stands facing the stabilizing arm, with the involved leg closest to the weight. The pivot arm is positioned so that the leg pad rests against the front of the thigh as the athlete is standing on both legs. The athlete grasps the handles for stabilization, lifts the weight by lifting the involved thigh until the thigh is level with the ground *without* arching the back, pauses, lowers the weight to the starting position in a slow and controlled manner, and repeats.

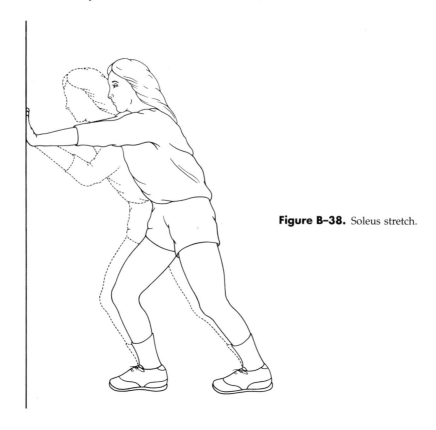

Figure B–38. Soleus stretch.

Hip Abduction. The involved leg is positioned with the hip at the axis of the pivot arm (Fig. B–39C). The athlete stands facing the weight. The pivot arm is positioned so that the leg pad rests against the outer part of the thigh as the athlete stands with the involved leg across the uninvolved leg. The athlete grasps the handles for stabilization, lifts the weight by moving the involved leg across and away from the body *without* twisting the body, pauses, lowers the weight to the starting position in a slow and controlled manner, and repeats.

Hip Extension. The involved leg is positioned with the hip at the axis of the pivot arm (Fig. B–39D). The athlete stands facing the stabilizing bars with the involved leg closest to the weight. The pivot arm is positioned so that the leg pad rests against the back of the thigh as the athlete's thigh is raised to parallel to the floor. The athlete grasps the handles for stabilization, lifts the weight by moving the involved thigh down as the knee is straightened *without* arching the back, pauses, lowers the weight to the starting position in a slow and rhythmic controlled manner, and repeats.

Standing Calf Raises. The shoulder pads are positioned so that the knees are slightly bent while the athlete is standing in the machine (Fig. B–40). The athlete places the ball of each foot of the footplate approximately shoulder-width apart, lifts the weight by raising upon the balls of the feet, lowers the weight slowly and rhythmically in a controlled manner as far as possible, and repeats.

Minisquats. The shoulder pads are positioned so that the knee can be flexed to the appropriate degrees of flexion for the injury (Fig. B–41). The feet are placed approximately shoulder-width apart. The athlete lifts the weight by straightening the knees, pauses, lowers the weight to the starting position in a slow and controlled manner, and repeats.

Leg Press. The plate is adjusted so that the athlete's knees are flexed to the appropriate degrees of flexion for the injury (Fig. B–42). The feet are placed shoulder-width apart. The athlete lifts the weight with both legs until the legs

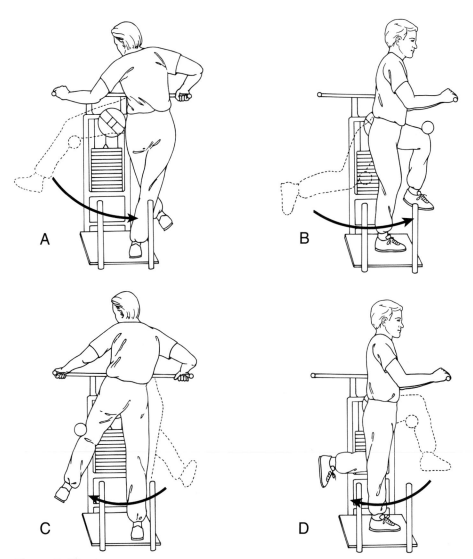

Figure B-39. Multi-hip machine. *A*, Hip adduction. *B*, Hip flexion. *C*, Hip abduction. *D*, Hip extension.

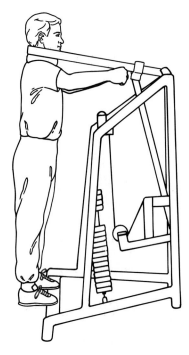

Figure B–40. Standing calf raises.

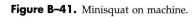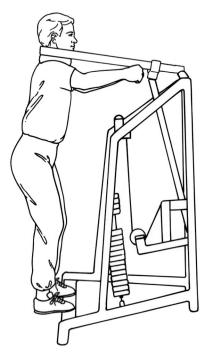

Figure B–41. Minisquat on machine.

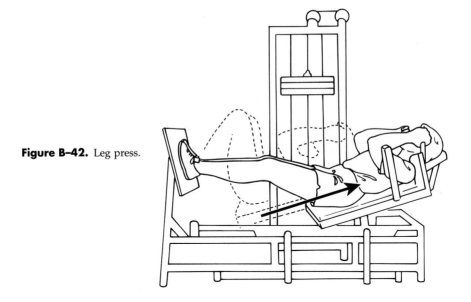

Figure B–42. Leg press.

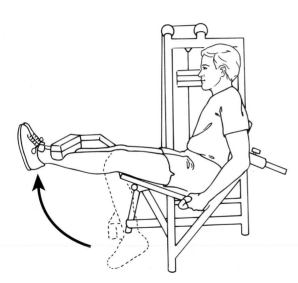

Figure B–43. Knee extension.

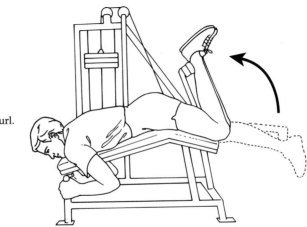

Figure B–44. Hamstring curl.

are almost straight, *without* locking the knees, pauses, lowers the weight to the starting position in a slow and controlled manner, and repeats.

Knee Extension. The seat is adjusted back so that the pad is flat against the athlete's back and the knees are aligned with the axis of the pivot arm (Fig. B–43). The leg pad is adjusted to just above the ankle, and the set range-of-motion limits are indicated. The athlete lifts the weight by straightening both knees, pauses, lowers the weight to the starting position in a slow and controlled manner, and repeats.

Hamstring Curl. The leg pad is adjusted to just above the Achilles tendon (Fig. B–44). The athlete lies on the bench with the knees on the surface of the pad and aligned with the axis of the pivot arm, lifts the weight by bending both knees, pauses, lowers the weight to the starting position in a slow and controlled manner, and repeats.

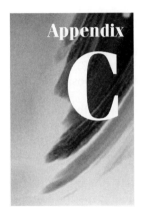

Appendix C

Throwers' Ten Exercise Program

Kevin E. Wilk, P.T.

The Throwers' Ten Exercise Program* is designed to exercise the major muscles necessary for throwing. The goal of the program is to be an organized and concise exercise program. In addition, all exercises included are specific to the thrower and are designed to improve strength, power, and endurance of the musculature of the shoulder complex.

Diagonal Pattern (D2) Extension. The athlete grips the tubing handle overhead and out to the side with the involved hand. The athlete pulls the tubing down and across the body to the opposite side of the leg (Fig. C–1A). During the motion, the athlete leads with the thumb.

*Modified from Wilk, K.E., Andrews, J.R., Arrigo, C.A., et al. (1997): Preventive and Rehabilitative Exercises for the Shoulder and Elbow, 5th ed. Birmingham, Alabama, American Sports Medicine Institute.

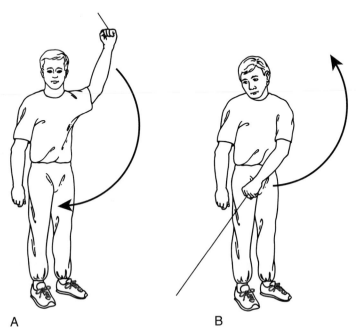

A   B

Figure C–1. Diagonal patterns. *A*, Extension. *B*, Flexion. (Redrawn from Wilk, K.E., Andrews, J.R., Arrigo, C.A., et al. [1997]: Preventive and Rehabilitative Exercises for the Shoulder and Elbow, 5th ed. Birmingham, Alabama, American Sports Medicine Institute.)

Diagonal Pattern (D2) Flexion. The athlete grips the tubing handle in the hand of the involved arm and brings the arm out 45° from the side, palm facing backward. After turning the palm forward, the athlete proceeds to flex the elbow and bring the arm up and over the uninvolved shoulder (Fig. C–1*B*). The palm is turned down and reversed to take the arm to the starting position. The exercise should be performed in a controlled manner.

External Rotation at 0° of Abduction. The athlete stands with the involved elbow fixed at the side, elbow at 90°, and the involved arm across the front of the body. The athlete grips the tubing handle (the other end of the tubing is fixed) and pulls out with the arm, keeping the elbow at the side (Fig. C–2*A*), and returns the tubing slowly and in a controlled manner.

Internal Rotation at 0° of Abduction. The athlete stands with the elbow at the side, fixed at 90°, and the shoulder rotated out. The athlete grips the tubing handle (the other end of the tubing is fixed) and pulls the arm across the body, keeping the elbow at the side (Fig. C–2*B*), and returns the tubing slowly and in a controlled manner.

External Rotation at 90° of Abduction. The athlete stands with the shoulder abducted to 90° and elbow flexed to 90°. The athlete grips the tubing handle (the other end is fixed straight ahead, slightly lower than the shoulder). Keeping the shoulder abducted, the athlete rotates the shoulder back, keeping the elbow at 90° (Fig. C–2*C*). Slow- and fast-speed sets should be performed with the tubing. The clinician will need to change the tubing resistance as appropriate.

Internal Rotation at 90° of Abduction. The athlete stands with the shoulder abducted to 90°, externally rotated to 90°, and the elbow bent to 90°. Keeping the shoulder abducted, the athlete rotates the shoulder forward, keeping the elbow bent at 90° (Fig. C–2*D*), and then returns the tubing and hand to the starting position. Slow- and fast-speed sets should be performed with the tubing. The clinician will need to change the tubing resistance as appropriate.

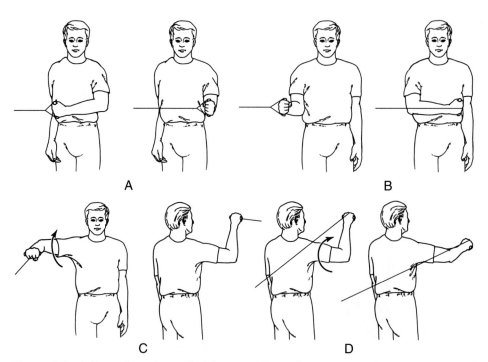

Figure C–2. *A*, External rotation at 0° abduction. *B*, Internal rotation at 0° abduction. *C*, External rotation at 90° abduction. *D*, Internal rotation at 90° abduction. (Redrawn from Wilk, K.E., Andrews, J.R., Arrigo, C.A., et al. [1997]: Preventive and Rehabilitative Exercises for the Shoulder and Elbow, 5th ed. Birmingham, Alabama, American Sports Medicine Institute.)

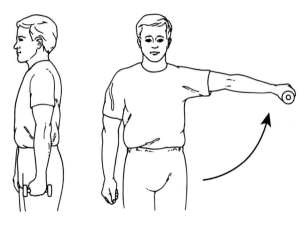

Figure C–3. Shoulder abduction to 90°. (Redrawn from Wilk, K.E., Andrews, J.R., Arrigo, C.A., et al. [1997]: Preventive and Rehabilitative Exercises for the Shoulder and Elbow, 5th ed. Birmingham, Alabama, American Sports Medicine Institute.)

Shoulder Abduction to 90°. The athlete stands with the arm at the side, the elbow straight, and the palm against the side and raises the arm to the side, palm down, until the arm reaches 90° (shoulder level) (Fig. C–3). The athlete holds the position for 2 seconds and lowers the arm slowly.

Scaption, Internal Rotation. The athlete stands with the elbow straight and thumb down and raises the arm to shoulder level at a 30° angle in front of body (Fig. C–4), not going above shoulder height. The athlete holds the position for 2 seconds and lowers the arm slowly.

Prone Horizontal Abduction (Neutral). The athlete lies on the table, face down, with the involved arm hanging straight to the floor and the palm facing down. The arm is raised out to the side, parallel to the floor (Fig. C–5A). The athlete holds the position for 2 seconds and lowers the arm slowly.

Prone Horizontal Abduction (Full External Rotation, 100° of Abduction). The athlete lies on the table, face down, with the involved arm hanging straight to the floor and the thumb rotated up (hitchhiker position). The arm is raised out to the side with the arm slightly in front of the shoulder, parallel to the floor (Fig. C–5B). The athlete holds the position for 2 seconds and lowers the arm slowly.

Press-ups. The athlete, seated on a chair or on a table, places both hands firmly on the sides of the chair or table, palm down and fingers pointed outward. The hands should be on a straight line with the shoulders. The athlete slowly pushes downward through the hands to elevate the body (Fig. C–6). The athlete holds the elevated position for 2 seconds and lowers the body.

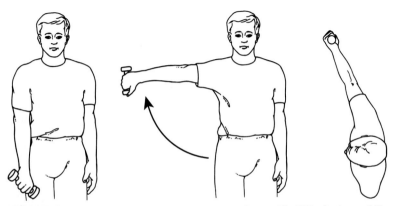

Figure C–4. Scaption internal rotation. (Redrawn from Wilk, K.E., Andrews, J.R., Arrigo, C.A., et al. [1997]: Preventive and Rehabilitative Exercises for the Shoulder and Elbow, 5th ed. Birmingham, Alabama, American Sports Medicine Institute.)

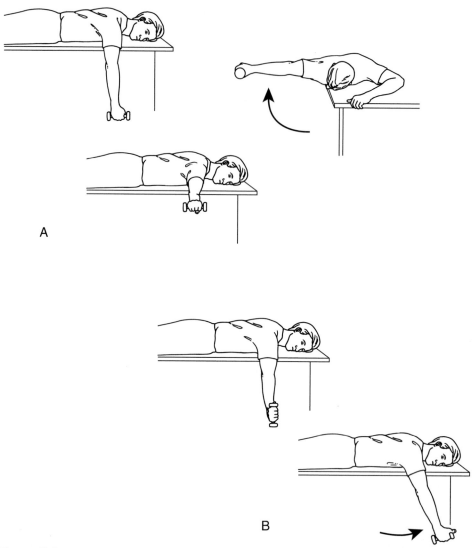

Figure C–5. Prone horizontal abduction. *A,* Neutral. *B,* Full external rotation, 100° abduction. (Redrawn from Wilk, K.E., Andrews, J.R., Arrigo, C.A., et al. [1997]: Preventive and Rehabilitative Exercises for the Shoulder and Elbow, 5th ed. Birmingham, Alabama, American Sports Medicine Institute.)

Prone Rowing. The athlete lies on the stomach with the involved arm hanging over the side of the table, a dumbbell in the hand, and the elbow straight. The athlete slowly raises the arm, bending the elbow, and bringing the dumbbell as high as possible (Fig. C–7). The athlete holds the position for 2 seconds and lowers the arm slowly.

Push-ups. The athlete starts in the down position with the arms in a comfortable position. The hands should be placed no more than shoulder-width apart. The athlete pushes up as high as possible, rolling the shoulders forward after the elbows are straight (Fig. C–8). The athlete can start with a push-up into the wall and can gradually progress to a table and eventually to the floor, as tolerable.

Elbow Flexion. With the arm against the side and the palm facing inward, the athlete bends the elbow upward, turning the palm up as he or she progresses (Fig. C–9A). The athlete holds the position for 2 seconds and lowers the elbow slowly.

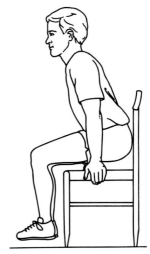

Figure C–6. Press-ups. (Redrawn from Wilk, K.E., Andrews, J.R., Arrigo, C.A., et al. [1997]: Preventive and Rehabilitative Exercises for the Shoulder and Elbow, 5th ed. Birmingham, Alabama, American Sports Medicine Institute.)

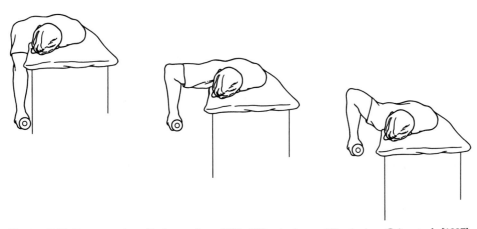

Figure C–7. Prone rowing. (Redrawn from Wilk, K.E., Andrews, J.R., Arrigo, C.A., et al. [1997]: Preventive and Rehabilitative Exercises for the Shoulder and Elbow, 5th ed. Birmingham, Alabama, American Sports Medicine Institute.)

Figure C–8. Push-ups. (Redrawn from Wilk, K.E., Andrews, J.R., Arrigo, C.A., et al. [1997]: Preventive and Rehabilitative Exercises for the Shoulder and Elbow, 5th ed. Birmingham, Alabama, American Sports Medicine Institute.)

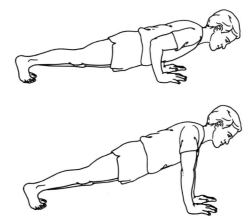

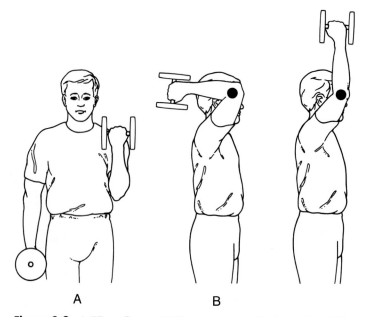

A   B

Figure C-9. *A*, Elbow flexion. *B*, Elbow extension. (Redrawn from Wilk, K.E., Andrews, J.R., Arrigo, C.A., et al. [1997]: Preventive and Rehabilitative Exercises for the Shoulder and Elbow, 5th ed. Birmingham, Alabama, American Sports Medicine Institute.)

Elbow Extension. The athlete raises the involved arm overhead, with the uninvolved hand providing support at the elbow. The arm is straightened overhead (Fig. C–9*B*). The athlete holds the position for 2 seconds and lowers the arm slowly.

Wrist Extension. Supporting the forearm and with the palm facing downward, the athlete raises a weight in the hand as far as possible (Fig. C–10*A*). The athlete holds the position for 2 seconds and lowers the arm slowly.

Wrist Flexion. Supporting the forearm and with the palm facing upward, the athlete lowers a weight in the hand as far as possible and then curls it up as high as possible (Fig. C–10*B*). The athlete holds the position for 2 seconds and lowers the arm slowly.

Supination. With the forearm supported on the table and the wrist in a neutral position, the athlete holds the position a weight or hammer and rolls the wrist, taking the palm up (Fig. C–10*C*). The athlete holds the position for 2 seconds, and the arm is returned to the starting position.

Pronation. The athlete supports the forearm on a table, with the wrist in a neutral position. Using a weight or hammer, the athlete rolls the wrist, taking the palm down (Fig. C–10*D*). The athlete holds the position for 2 seconds, and the arm is returned to the starting position.

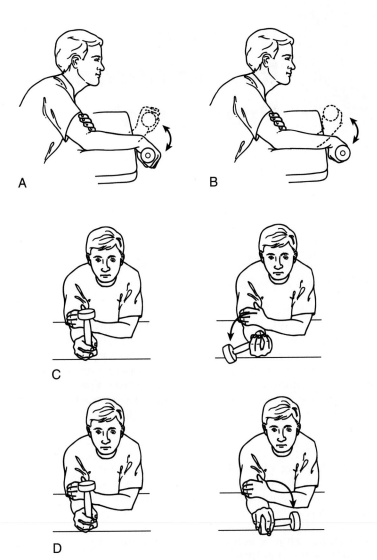

Figure C-10. *A*, Wrist extension. *B*, Wrist flexion. *C*, Wrist supination. *D*, Wrist pronation. (Redrawn from Wilk, K.E., Andrews, J.R., Arrigo, C.A., et al. [1997]: Preventive and Rehabilitative Exercises for the Shoulder and Elbow, 5th ed. Birmingham, Alabama, American Sports Medicine Institute.)

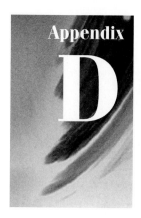

Appendix D

Interval Rehabilitation Programs*

Gary L. Harrelson, Ed.D., A.T.,C., and
Kevin E. Wilk, P.T.

INTERVAL THROWING PROGRAM FOR BASEBALL PLAYERS

The Interval Throwing Program (ITP) is designed to bring about a gradual return of motion, strength, and confidence to the throwing arm after injury or surgery by slowly progressing the athlete through graduated throwing distances. The ITP can be initiated after clearance by the athlete's physician for the resumption of throwing and is carried out under the supervision of the rehabilitation team (physician, athletic trainer, or physical therapist). The program is set up to minimize the chance of reinjury and emphasizes prethrowing warm-up and stretching. In the development of the ITP, the following factors are considered most important:

1. The act of throwing a baseball involves the transfer of energy from the feet, through the legs, pelvis, trunk, and out the shoulder through the elbow and hand. Therefore, any return to throwing after injury must include attention to the entire body.
2. The chance for reinjury is lessened by a graduated progression of interval throwing.
3. Proper warm-up is essential.
4. Most injuries occur as the result of fatigue.
5. Regard for proper throwing mechanics lessens the incidence of reinjury.
6. Baseline requirements for throwing include a pain-free range of motion of all joints involved in throwing and adequate muscle power and resistance to fatigue.

Because there is individual variability in all throwing athletes, there is no set timetable for completion of the ITP. Most athletes, by nature, are highly competi-

*The Interval Throwing Program, Parts I and II; The Little Leaguer Interval Training Program; The Interval Tennis Program; The Interval Racquetball Program; and The Interval Golf Program have been reprinted with permission from Wilk, K.E., Andrews, J.R., Arrigo, C.A. et al. (1997): Preventive and Rehabilitative Exercises for the Shoulder and Elbow, Birmingham, Alabama, American Sports Medicine Institute, p. 42; pp. 38–41; p. 43; p. 44.

tive individuals who wish to return to competition at the earliest possible time. Although this is a necessary characteristic in all athletes, the proper channeling of the athlete's energies into a rigidly controlled throwing program is essential to lessen the chance of reinjury during the rehabilitative period. The athlete may want to increase the intensity of the throwing program, but this can increase the incidence of reinjury and may greatly retard the rehabilitation process. It is recommended that the program be followed rigidly, because that is the safest route for returning to competition.

During the recovery process the athlete may experience soreness and a dull, diffuse, aching sensation in the muscles and tendons. If the athlete experiences sharp pain, particularly in the joint, all throwing activity should be stopped until this pain abates. Throwing should also be discontinued if the athlete's elbow or shoulder becomes swollen. Heat on the shoulder or elbow may help loosen up the joint prior to throwing. Ice alone is recommended after throwing or to treat swelling.

Weight Training

The athlete should supplement the ITP with a high-repetition, low-weight exercise program. The strengthening regimen should maintain a proper balance between the anterior and posterior musculature so that the shoulder is not predisposed to injury. Special emphasis must be given to the posterior rotator cuff musculature in any strengthening program. Weight training does not increase throwing velocity but increases the resistance of the arm to fatigue and injury. Weight training should be done the same day as throwing; however, it should be performed *after* throwing is completed. The day in between throwing should be used for flexibility exercises and recovery. A weight-training pattern or routine should be stressed at this point as a "maintenance program." This pattern can and should accompany the athlete into and throughout the season as a deterrent to further injury. It must be stressed that weight training is of no benefit unless accompanied by a sound flexibility program.

Individual Variability

The ITP is designed so that each level is achieved without pain or complication before the next level is started. This sets up a progression—a goal is achieved prior to advancement, instead of advancement according to a specific time frame. Thus, the ITP may be used for those with different levels of skills and abilities, from athletes in high school to professionals. The reasons for performing the ITP vary from person to person, so the length of time required to complete each step successfully also varies. For example, one athlete may wish to throw on alternate days, with or without using weights in between, and another athlete may have to throw every third or fourth day because of pain or swelling. Athletes should progress as their bodies dictate. Again, completion of the ITP steps is subject to individual variation. There is no fixed timetable in terms of days to completion.

Warm-up

Jogging increases blood flow to the muscles and joints, thus increasing their flexibility and decreasing the chance for reinjury. Because the length of the warm-up varies among individuals, the athlete should jog until a light sweat develops and then progress to the stretching phase.

Stretching

Throwing involves all muscles in the body, so all muscle groups should be stretched prior to throwing. This should be done in a systematic fashion, beginning with the legs and including the trunk, back, neck, and arms and continuing with capsular stretches and T-bar range-of-motion exercises.

Throwing Mechanics

A critical aspect of the ITP is maintenance of proper throwing mechanics throughout its advancement. The use of the crow-hop method simulates the throwing act, allowing emphasis on proper body mechanics. This method should be adopted from the onset of the ITP. Throwing flatfooted encourages improper body mechanics, placing increased stress on the throwing arm and thus predisposing the arm to reinjury. The pitching coach and sports biomechanist (if available) may be valuable allies to the rehabilitation team because of their knowledge of throwing mechanics.

The crow-hop method begins with a hop and then a skip and is followed by the throw. The velocity of the throw is determined by the distance—the ball should have enough momentum to travel only the designated distance. Again, emphasis should be placed on proper throwing mechanics when the athlete begins part II of the program (Throwing off the Mound) or returns to his or her playing position to decrease the chance of reinjury.

Throwing

Using the crow-hop method, the athlete should begin warm-up throws at a comfortable distance (approximately 30 to 45 feet; part I of the ITP) and then progress to the distance indicated for that phase (Fig. D–1). The objetive of each phase is for the athlete to be able to throw the ball the specified number of feet (45, 60, 90, 120, 150, or 180) without pain, 75 times at each distance. Athletes who can throw the ball 180 feet, 50 times, without pain are ready for part II of the ITP (Throwing off the Mound) or returning to their playing positions (step 14). At this point, full strength and confidence in the athlete's arm should be restored. It is important to stress the crow-hop method and proper mechanics with each throw. Just as advancement to this point has been gradual and progressive, the return to unrestricted throwing must follow the same principles. A pitcher should first throw only fastballs at 50% intensity, progressing to 75%,

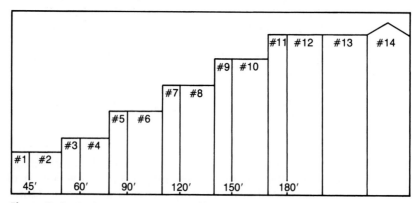

Figure D–1. Graduation of the Interval Throwing Program.

and finally to 100%. At this time the athlete may begin to throw more stressful pitches, such as breaking balls. The position player should simulate a game situation, again progressing from 50% to 75% to 100%.

Once again, if an athlete has increased pain, particularly at the joint, the intensity of the ITP should be reduced. Readvancement should be under the direction of the rehabilitation team members.

Batting

Depending on the type of injury, the time of return to batting should be determined by the physician. Stress placed on the arm and shoulder during the batting motion is very different from that during the throwing motion. Return to unrestricted use of a bat should also follow the same progressive guidelines as those for the throwing program. The athlete should begin with dry swings, progress to hitting off the tee, then hit a soft toss, and finally progress to live pitching.

Summary

By using the ITP in conjunction with a structured rehabilitation program, the athlete should be able to return to full competition, minimizing the chance of reinjury. The program and its progression should be modified to meet the specific needs of each individual athlete. A comprehensive program consisting of a maintenance strength and flexibility regimen, appropriate warm-up and cool-down procedures, proper pitching mechanics, and progressive throwing and batting will assist the baseball player in returning to competition safely.

I. Part I
  A. 45-foot phase
    1. Step 1
      (a) Warm-up throwing
      (b) 45 feet (25 throws)
      (c) Rest 15 minutes
      (d) Warm-up throwing
      (e) 45 feet (25 throws)
    2. Step 2
      (a) Warm-up throwing
      (b) 45 feet (25 throws)
      (c) Rest 10 minutes
      (d) Warm-up throwing
      (e) 45 feet (25 throws)
      (f) Rest 10 minutes
      (g) Warm-up throwing
      (h) 45 feet (25 throws)
  B. 60-foot phase
    1. Step 3
      (a) Warm-up throwing
      (b) 60 feet (25 throws)
      (c) Rest 15 minutes
      (d) Warm-up throwing
      (e) 60 feet (25 throws)
    2. Step 4
      (a) Warm-up throwing
      (b) 60 feet (25 throws)
      (c) Rest 10 minutes
      (d) Warm-up throwing

      (e) 60 feet (25 throws)
      (f) Rest 10 minutes
      (g) Warm-up throwing
      (h) 60 feet (25 throws)
  C. 90-foot phase
    1. Step 5
      (a) Warm-up throwing
      (b) 90 feet (25 throws)
      (c) Rest 15 minutes
      (d) Warm-up throwing
      (e) 90 feet (25 throws)
    2. Step 6
      (a) Warm-up throwing
      (b) 90 feet (25 throws)
      (c) Rest 10 minutes
      (d) Warm-up throwing
      (e) 90 feet (25 throws)
      (f) Rest 10 minutes
      (g) Warm-up throwing
      (h) 90 feet (25 throws)
  D. 120-foot phase
    1. Step 7
      (a) Warm-up throwing
      (b) 120 feet (25 throws)
      (c) Rest 15 minutes
      (d) Warm-up throwing
      (e) 120 feet (25 throws)

2. Step 8
   (a) Warm-up throwing
   (b) 120 feet (25 throws)
   (c) Rest 10 minutes
   (d) Warm-up throwing
   (e) 120 feet (25 throws)
   (f) Rest 10 minutes
   (g) Warm-up throwing
   (h) 120 feet (25 throws)
E. 150-foot phase
   1. Step 9
      (a) Warm-up throwing
      (b) 150 feet (25 throws)
      (c) Rest 15 minutes
      (d) Warm-up throwing
      (e) 150 feet (25 throws)
   2. Step 10
      (a) Warm-up throwing
      (b) 150 feet (25 throws)
      (c) Rest 10 minutes
      (d) Warm-up throwing
      (e) 150 feet (25 throws)
      (f) Rest 10 minutes
      (g) Warm-up throwing
      (h) 150 feet (25 throws)

F. 180-foot phase
   1. Step 11
      (a) Warm-up throwing
      (b) 180 feet (25 throws)
      (c) Rest 15 minutes
      (d) Warm-up throwing
      (e) 180 feet (25 throws)
   2. Step 12
      (a) Warm-up throwing
      (b) 180 feet (25 throws)
      (c) Rest 10 minutes
      (d) Warm-up throwing
      (e) 180 feet (25 throws)
      (f) Rest 10 minutes
      (g) Warm-up throwing
      (h) 180 feet (25 throws)
   3. Step 13
      (a) Warm-up throwing
      (b) 180 feet (25 throws)
      (c) Rest 10 minutes
      (d) Warm-up throwing
      (e) 180 feet (25 throws)
      (f) Rest 10 minutes
      (g) Warm-up throwing
      (h) 180 feet (50 throws)
   4. Step 14 Begin ITP off the mound or return to playing position

II. Part II: Throwing off the Mound
   All throwing off the mound should be done in the presence of the pitching coach to stress proper throwing mechanics. A speed gun can be used to aid in effort control.
   A. Stage one: fastball only
      1. Step 1
         (a) Interval throwing
         (b) 15 throws off mound, 50%
      2. Step 2
         (a) Interval throwing
         (b) 30 throws off mound, 50%
      3. Step 3
         (a) Interval throwing
         (b) 45 throws off mound, 50%
      4. Step 4
         (a) Interval throwing
         (b) 60 throws off mound, 50%
      5. Step 5
         (a) Interval throwing
         (b) 30 throws off mound, 50%
      6. Step 6
         (a) 30 throws off mound, 75%
         (b) 45 throws off mound, 50%
      7. Step 7
         (a) 45 throws off mound, 75%
         (b) 15 throws off mound, 50%
      8. Step 8
         (a) 60 throws off mound, 75%
   B. Stage two: fastball only

1. Step 9
   (a) 45 throws off mound, 75%
   (b) 15 throws in batting practice
2. Step 10
   (a) 45 throws off mound, 75%
   (b) 30 throws in batting practice
3. Step 11
   (a) 45 throws off mound, 75%
   (b) 45 throws in batting practice

C. Stage three
1. Step 12
   (a) 30 throws off mound, 75% warm-up
   (b) 15 throws off mound, 50% breaking balls
   (c) 45 to 60 throws in batting practice (fastball only)
2. Step 13
   (a) 30 throws off mound, 75%
   (b) 30 breaking balls, 75%
   (c) 30 throws in batting practice
3. Step 14
   (a) 30 throws off mound, 75%
   (b) 60 to 90 throws in batting practice, 25% breaking balls
4. Step 15
   (a) Simulated game—progressing by 15 throws per workout

NOTE
   (a) Use interval throwing to 120-foot phase as warm-up
   (b) All throwing off the mound should be done in the presence of a pitching coach to stress proper throwing mechanics
   (c) Use a speed gun to aid in effort control

LITTLE LEAGUER INTERVAL TRAINING PROGRAM

The Little Leaguer Interval Throwing Program parallels the ITP in returning the Little Leaguer to a graduated progression of throwing distances. Warm-up and stretching should be performed prior to throwing.

A. 30-foot phase
1. Step 1
   (a) Warm-up throwing
   (b) 30 feet (25 throws)
   (c) Rest 15 minutes
   (d) Warm-up throwing
   (e) 30 feet (25 throws)
2. Step 2
   (a) Warm-up throwing
   (b) 30 feet (25 throws)
   (c) Rest 10 minutes
   (d) Warm-up throwing
   (e) 30 feet (25 throws)
   (f) Rest 10 minutes
   (g) Warm-up throwing
   (h) 30 feet (25 throws)

B. 45-foot phase
1. Step 3
   (a) Warm-up throwing
   (b) 45 feet (25 throws)
   (c) Rest 15 minutes
   (d) Warm-up throwing
   (e) 45 feet (25 throws)

2. Step 4
   (a) Warm-up throwing
   (b) 45 feet (25 throws)
   (c) Rest 10 minutes
   (d) Warm-up throwing
   (e) 45 feet (25 throws)
   (f) Rest 10 minutes
   (g) Warm-up throwing
   (h) 45 feet (25 throws)

C. 60-foot phase
1. Step 5
   (a) Warm-up throwing
   (b) 60 feet (25 throws)
   (c) Rest 15 minutes
   (d) Warm-up throwing
   (e) 60 feet (25 throws)
2. Step 6
   (a) Warm-up throwing
   (b) 60 feet (25 throws)
   (c) Rest 10 minutes
   (d) Warm-up throwing
   (e) 60 feet (25 throws)

(f) Rest 10 minutes
(g) Warm-up throwing
(h) 60 feet (25 throws)
D. 90-foot phase
  1. Step 7
    (a) Warm-up throwing
    (b) 90 feet (25 throws)
    (c) Rest 15 minutes
    (d) Warm-up throwing
    (e) 90 feet (25 throws)

  2. Step 8
    (a) Warm-up throwing
    (b) 90 feet (25 throws)
    (c) Rest 10 minutes
    (d) Warm-up throwing
    (e) 90 feet (25 throws)
    (f) Rest 10 minutes
    (g) Warm-up throwing
    (h) 90 feet (25 throws)

INTERVAL TENNIS PROGRAM

The same principles should be followed with the interval tennis program as for the interval baseball program. Proper warm-up, stretching, and strengthening should be implemented throughout the entire interval tennis rehabilitation program. As the athletes begin the program they should remember that mechanics play an important role in their recovery.

WEEK	MONDAY	WEDNESDAY	FRIDAY
1	12 FH 8 BH 10-min rest 13 FH 7 BH	15 FH 8 BH 10-min rest 15 FH 7 BH	15 FH 10 BH 10-min rest 15 FH 10 BH
2	25 FH 15 BH 10-min rest 25 FH 15 BH	30 FH 20 BH 10-min rest 30 FH 20 BH	30 FH 25 BH 10-min rest 30 FH 15 BH 10 OH
3	30 FH 25 BH 10 OH 10-min rest 30 FH 25 BH 10 OH	30 FH 25 BH 15 OH 10-min rest 30 FH 25 BH 15 OH	30 FH 30 BH 15 OH 10-min rest 30 FH 15 OH 10-min rest 30 FH 30 BH 15 OH
4	30 FH 30 BH 10 OH 10-min rest Play 3 games 10 FH 10 BH 5 OH	30 FH 30 BH 10 OH 10-min rest Play set 10 FH 10 BH 5 OH	30 FH 30 BH 10 OH 10-min rest Play 1½ sets 10 FH 10 BH 3 OH

BH, Backhand ground strokes; FH, forehand ground strokes; OH, overhead shots.

INTERVAL RACQUETBALL PROGRAM

Warm-up. Jogging increases blood flow to the muscles and joints, thus increasing their flexibility and decreasing the chance of reinjury. Because the amount of warm-up will vary from person to person, the athlete should jog until developing a light sweat, then progress to the stretching phase.

Stretching. Because racquetball involves all muscles in the body, all muscle groups should be stretched prior to playing. This should be done in a systemic fashion beginning with the legs and including the trunk, back, neck, and arms. The athlete should continue with capsular stretches and T- or L-bar range-of-motion exercises.

WEEK	MONDAY	WEDNESDAY	FRIDAY
1	12 FH 8 BH 10-min rest 13 FH 7 BH	15 FH 8 BH 10-min rest 15 FH 7 BH	15 FH 10 BH 10-min rest 15 FH 10 BH
2	25 FH 15 BH 10-min rest 25 FH 15 BH	30 FH 20 BH 10-min rest 30 FH 20 BH	30 FH 25 BH 10-min rest 30 FH 15 BH 10 BH
3	30 FH 25 BH 10 OH 10-min rest 30 FH 25 BH 10 OH	30 FH 25 BH 15 OH 10-min rest 30 FH 25 BH 15 OH	30 FH 30 BH 15 OH 30 FH 15 OH 10-min rest 30 FH 30 BH 15 OH
4	30 FH 30 BH 10 OH 10-min rest Play 11-point game 10 FH 10 BH 5 OH	30 FH 30 BH 10 OH 10-min rest Play 21-point game 10 FH 10 BH 5 OH	30 FH 30 BH 10 OH 10-min rest Play 1½ games 10 FH 10 BH 3 OH

BH, Backhand shots; FH, forehand shots; OH, overhead shots.

INTERVAL GOLF PROGRAM

The same principles should be followed with the interval golf program as for the interval baseball program. Proper warm-up, stretching, and strengthening should be implemented throughout the entire interval golf rehabilitation program. As athletes begin the program, they should remember that mechanics play an important role in their recovery.

The athlete should perform flexibility exercises before hitting and use ice after hitting.

WEEK	MONDAY	WEDNESDAY	FRIDAY
1	10 putts 10 chips 5-min rest 15 chips	15 putts 15 chips 5-min rest 25 chips	20 putts 20 chips 5-min rest 20 putts 20 chips 5-min rest 10 chips 10 short irons
2	20 chips 10 short irons 5-min rest 10 short irons	20 chips 15 short irons 10-min rest 15 short irons 15 chips Putting	15 short irons 10 medium irons 10-min rest 20 short irons 15 chips
3	15 short irons 15 medium irons 10-min rest 5 long irons 15 short irons 15 medium irons 10-min rest 20 chips	15 short irons 10 medium irons 10 long irons 10-min rest 10 short irons 10 medium irons 5 long irons 5 wood	15 short irons 10 medium irons 10 long irons 10-min rest 10 short irons 10 medium irons 10 long irons 10 wood
4	15 short irons 10 medium irons 10 long irons 10 drives 15-min rest Repeat	Play 9 holes	Play 9 holes
5	Play 9 holes	Play 9 holes	Play 18 holes

Chips:
- pitching wedge
- short irons — W 9, 8
- medium irons — 7, 6, 5
- long irons — 4, 3, 2
- woods — 3, 5
- drives — driver

INTERVAL RUNNING PROGRAM

The athlete should always stretch completely before and after the workout and should use ice when necessary.

WEEK	RUN	WALK	RUN	WALK
1	¼ mile	¼ mile	¼ mile	¼ mile
2	¼ mile	¼ mile	½ mile	¼ mile
3	½ mile	¼ mile	½ mile	¼ mile
4	½ mile	¼ mile	¾ mile	¼ mile
5	¾ mile	¼ mile	¾ mile	¼ mile
6	¾ mile	¼ mile	1 mile	¼ mile
7	1 mile	¼ mile	1 mile	¼ mile

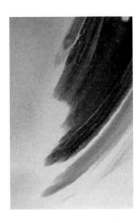

Index

Note: Page numbers in *italics* indicate figures; those followed by t indicate tables.

Abdominal sit-ups, for spondylolisthesis, 468, *468*
Abduction, of hip, isotonic, 641, *642*
    with elastic resistance, 648, *648*
    with multi-hip machine, 658, *659*
  of shoulder. See *Shoulder(s), abduction of.*
Absorption, of solutions, from joint space, 16–17
Acceleration, isokinetic exercises and, 252
Acceleration phase, of throwing, elbow in, 486–487, 555
  shoulder in, 486–487
Accommodating resistance, definition of, 220
Achilles tendon, rupture of, *284,* 284–285, 286t–287t
  stretching exercise for, 655, *657*
  tendinitis of, 285, 288–289
ACL. See *Anterior cruciate ligament (ACL).*
Acromioclavicular joint, arthrology of, 479–480
  glides of, anterior and posterior, technique for, 163–164, *165*
  separation of, 526, *527,* 528
  shoulder elevation and, 483
Acromioplasty, for rotator cuff tears, 510
Active exercise(s), 183–191
  concentric and eccentric contractions and, 183–184
  dynamic, 184
  inertial, 185–186, *188*
  isokinetic, 185, *187*
  isotonic, 185, *185, 186*
  plyometric, 186–191, *188–191*
Active tall kneeling, on Swiss ball, 474
Adduction, of hip, isometric, 639, *640*
  isotonic, 641, *641*
    with elastic resistance, 648–649, *649*
    with multi-hip machine, 657, *659*
  of shoulder, horizontal, 531–532, *533*
    strength of, isokinetic testing of, 239–240
Adolescents, elbow injuries in, 574–577
    Little Leaguer's elbow as, *576,* 576–577
    osteochondritis dissecans as, 574–576, *575*
Anatomic zero position, for goniometric measurements, 58, 59t

Ankle(s), 261, 295–313. See also *Lower extremity(ies).*
  goniometric measurements of, 75, 77, *78, 79,* 79–80
  injuries of, mechanisms of, 295, 296t
  inversion sprains of, 295, 297–305
    signs and symptoms of, 298t
    treatment and rehabilitation of, 297, *297,* 299, *299,* 300t–301t, *302–308,* 303–305
  joint mobilization techniques for, 170–171, *171, 172*
  peroneal tendon subluxation of, 309, 313, *313*
  proprioception training for, 198
  syndesmotic sprains of, 305–306, 309
    lateral ankle reconstructions for, postsurgical management of, 306, 306t, 309
    mechanism of injury of, 305, *309*
    postimmobilization fracture management and, 309, *310–313*
Annulus fibrosus, 428
Anterior cruciate ligament (ACL), 333–335, 334t, 335t
  functional testing of, 395–396
  reconstructive treatment of, 365–368
    allografts for, 367–368, 375–376
    autografts for, 367, 367t
    closed kinetic chain exercises following, 253
    closed kinetic chain isokinetic testing following, 232–233
  rehabilitation for, 365–376
    biofeedback in, 368, 374, *374, 375*
    electrical stimulation in, 368
    functional progression program for, 375, 376t
    progression in, time-frame for, 368
    protocols for, 368, 369t–373t
    strengthening exercises in, 375, *375,* 376t
  shear forces on, during stationary cycling, 351–352
Anterior tibialis tendinitis, 289
Anthropometric assessment, of lower extremity. See *Lower extremity(ies), anthropometric assessment of.*

Antishear devices, for knee, 394, *394*
Apophysitis, calcaneal, 314
Aquatic rehabilitation, 615–630
  guidelines for, 620–628
    in functional progression, 625, 626–629, 628, 630t
    in increasing cardiovascular endurance, 625, *625*
    in increasing range of motion, 621
    in increasing strength, 621, *621–624*, 625
  therapeutic value of, 619–620
  water and, 615–618
    buoyancy and, 616
    hydrostatic pressure and, 617–618
    moment of force and, 616, *617*
    movement through, 617
    specific gravity of, 616
    viscosity of, 616–617
  water immersion and, physiologic effects of, 618–619
    on cardiovascular system, 618
    on central and peripheral nervous systems, 619
    on musculoskeletal system, 618–619, *619*
Arm-cocking phase, of throwing, elbow in, 554–556
  shoulder in, 485–486
Arthrofibrosis, 21–25, *22, 24,* 24t
  phases of, 23, 24t
Arthrofibrotic loop, 23, 24f
Arthrokinematics, 261–267
  of interphalangeal joint, 266
  of metatarsophalangeal joint, *266,* 266–267
  of midtarsal joint, *265,* 265–266, *266*
  of subtalar joint, 262–265, *263,* 263t, *264*
  of talocrural joint, 261–262, *262,* 262t
  of tarsometatarsal joint, 266, *266*
  of tibiofibular joint, 261
Arthrometry, of knee, 390–393, *391,* 392t
Arthrotomy, quadriceps shutdown following, 19
Articular cartilage, immobilization and, 25–26
  of knee, rehabilitation for injuries of, 383
  remobilization and, 30
  response to injury and, 17, *17*
Articular receptors, proprioception and, 192, 193
Assistive devices, 149, *150–152*
Attentional focus, 4–5

Balance testing, 195, *196–199,* 197–199
  for isokinetic power evaluation, 224
Balance training, on minitrampoline, *306*
  on multiaxial wobble board, *305*
Bankart procedure, 516–517
  rehabilitation protocol following, 523t, 524t
BAPS (Biomechanical Ankle Platform System), *199, 200, 297, 362, 363*
Baseball pitching. See *Throwing.*
Baseball toss, 632, *633,* 635
Bennett's fractures, 598
Biceps curl, 542, *543,* 581, *583*
Bilateral comparison, in isokinetic testing, 229
Biodex Stability System, *196*
Biofeedback, 132–137, *134*
  application of, 134–136, *136*
  contraindications to, 136–137
  for anterior cruciate ligament injuries, 368, *374, 374, 375*

Biofeedback *(Continued)*
  indications for, 136
Biomechanical Ankle Platform System (BAPS), *199, 200, 297, 362, 363*
Bird dog exercise, for spondylolisthesis, 469, *470*
  on Swiss ball, *473*
Blix curve, 220
Blood pressure cuff, for biofeedback, 368, 374, *374, 375*
Bone(s), immobilization and, 27
  of foot, 261
  remobilization and, 30
Boundary conditions, for open and closed kinetic chain exercises, 179–180, 180t
Boutonnière injuries, 594–596, *596*
Bracing, counterforce, for epicondylitis, 563–564, *564*
  effect of, on proprioception, 199, 201
  functional, of knee, 388–390
  patellofemoral, 388
Bridging, on Swiss ball, *473*
Bristow procedure, 514, 516
  rehabilitation protocol following, 518t–519t
Broomstick curl-up exercise, for elbow, 581
Bubble inclinometer, 57, *58*
Buoyancy, 616
Bursitis, retrocalcaneal, 314, *315*

Calcaneal glides, lateral, *311*
  medial, *311*
Calcaneus, injuries of, 313–315, *315, 316*
Calf raises, standing, with multi-hip machine, 658, *660*
Capillary permeability, increased, following injury, 14
Capsular shift procedure, 516–517
  rehabilitation protocol following, 520t–522t
Capsular stretch(es), of shoulder, anterior, 532, 534, *535*
  inferior, 532, *534*
  posterior, 532, *534*
Capsulorrhaphy, 516–517
  rehabilitation protocol following, 520t–522t
Cardiovascular system, endurance of, aquatic rehabilitation to increase, 625, *625*
  water immersion and, effects of, 618
Care plans, developing, 49–50
Carpal tunnel syndrome, 602–603
Carpometacarpal joint, of thumb, Bennett's fracture of, 598
Cartilage, articular. See *Articular cartilage.*
Casting, for ulnar collateral ligament injuries of thumb, 599, *599*
Cell degeneration (death), 13–14
Cellular metabolism, cryotherapy effect on, 83
  therapeutic heat effects on, 93–94
Central nervous system, water immersion and, effects of, 619
Chest pass, 632, *632*
Chondrocyte transplantation, for osteochondritis, 383
Chondromalacia patellae, 385–386
Circulation, cryotherapy effect on, 84
  therapeutic heat effects on, 93
Circumduction pendulum swings, 528–529, *529*
Circumferential measurements, 46
Closed kinetic chain (CKC), 175

Closed kinetic chain exercise(s) (CKCE), 178–182, *179*, 180t, 251–252
for anterior cruciate ligament injuries, 368, 373t
for knee, 359–360, 360t, *361*
for knee and leg, 650–654, *650–658*, 657
Closed kinetic chain (CKC) pattern, 222
Closed kinetic chain (CKC) testing, functional performance on, open kinetic chain testing correlated with, 233
isokinetic, squat, for isokinetic power evaluation, 225–226
supine, for isokinetic power evaluation, 224, 225t
"Coach's finger," 596
Coban wrap, 591, *592*
Cocking phase, of throwing, elbow in, 554–556
shoulder in, 485–486
Cocontraction, 640, *640*
Cold, therapeutic. See *Cryotherapy.*
Cold packs, 88–90
commercial, 89–90, *90*
conventional, 88–89, *89*
Collagen, of fibrous connective tissue, 21, 22f
Collateral ligament(s), lateral, 337
medial, 336–337
immobilization and, 27
rehabilitation for injuries of, 376–377, 380t–382t
ulnar, injury of, of thumb, 599, *599, 600*
sprain of, 569–571, *571*, 572t, 573
Compartmental compression syndromes, of lower leg, 293–295, 294t, 295t
Competition, return to, following lower extremity injury, 326, *327*, 328
Compliance, with rehabilitation program, 7–8
Compression, 137–139, *138*
application of, 138
contraindications to, 139
indications for, 138–139
Compression forces, during stationary cycling, 352
Compression test, in low back pain evaluation, 443, *445*
Compressive load, about knee joint, during stationary cycling, 353–355, *354*
Concentric contractions, 183–184
Concentric dynamic strength assessment, eccentric assessment versus, 240
Connective tissue, periarticular, immobilization and, 20–25, *22, 24*, 24t
remobilization and, 31
stretching and, 146
Continuous passive motion (CPM), 27–29, *28*
Contract-relax technique, for proprioceptive neuromuscular facilitation, 154, *155*
Contralateral kicks, *307*
Contrast baths, 96
Contusion(s), of elbow, 573
of quadriceps, 411–415, *413–416*, 417
Coping strategies, 10
Coracromial arch, arthrology of, 481–482
Corticosteroid injections, for epicondylitis, 563
Counterforce bracing, for epicondylitis, 563–564, *564*
CPM (continuous passive movement), 27–29, *28*
Cranial shear test, in low back pain evaluation, 447, *447*
Crepitus, in shoulder, 497
Cross-step lunge, with elastic resistance, 650–651, *652*

Cruciate ligament. See *Anterior cruciate ligament (ACL); Posterior cruciate ligament (PCL).*
Crutch training, 206–208, *207–209*
Cryostretching, of hamstring, 406, 409, *410*
Cryotherapy, 82–92
cold packs for, 88–90, *89*, 89t, *90*
considerations for use of, 86–88, *87*
contraindications to, 88
excessive cooling using, 87–88
ice buckets or baths for, 91, *91*
ice massage for, 91–92, *92*
indications for, 88
physiologic effects of, 82–86
proprioception following, 198–199
Cuboid syndrome, 318–319, *319*
Curl-up exercise, broomstick, for elbow, 581
Curveballs, elbow injury due to, 556
Cutaneous receptions, proprioception and, 193
Cybex Reactor, 47, *48*
Cycling, stationary, 654, *654*
biomechanics of, 351–355, 352t, 353t, *354*
for ankle rehabilitation, *303*
Cyst(s), ganglion, 601

Daily adjustable progressive-resistance exercise (DAPRE), 203–204, 204t
de Quervain's tenosynovitis, 601–602
Dead bug exercise, for spondylolisthesis, 469, *469*
Deceleration, isokinetic exercises and, 252
Deceleration phase, of throwing, elbow in, 555–556
shoulder in, 487
Deep friction massage, of elbow, 578
Deep heating modalities, 98–105
physiologic effects of, 98
shortwave diathermy as, 98–99
ultrasound as, *100*, 100–105, 102t
Deep tendon reflexes, testing of, 442, 442t
DeLorme program, 202–203
Deltoid, "empty can" position for strengthening, 539, *540*
Derangements, lumbar, treatment for, 457–466, *460–463, 465*
Dermatomes, in low back pain evaluation, 442
Diagonal cross-step lunge, with elastic resistance, 651, *652*
Diagonal lunge, with elastic resistance, 651–652, *652*
Diagonal pattern throwing exercises, 663–664
extension, 663, *663*
flexion, *663*, 664
Diathermy, shortwave, 98–99
Digit(s). See *Finger(s); Thumb(s); Toe.*
DIP joint. See *Distal interphalangeal (DIP) joint.*
Direct current electrical stimulation, 130–132
application of, 121–132, *131*, 133t
for denervated muscle stimulation, 130
for iontophoresis, 130–132
Disc(s), intervertebral, 427, 428–429
pressure between, *429*, 429–430, *430*
prolapse of, 430t, 430–431
Discharge parameters, establishing, 50
Dislocation(s), of elbow, 573–574, 574t
of interphalangeal joints, distal, 592, *593*
proximal, 596–597
Distal interphalangeal (DIP) joint, fractures and dislocations of, 591–592, *592, 593*

Distal interphalangeal (DIP) joint (Continued)
joint blocking for, 605
mallet finger and, 589–591, 590t, 591
Distraction test, in low back pain evaluation, 443, 444
Disuse osteoporosis, immobilization and, 30
Dribbling, against wall, 634, 635
Duration, for exercise, 209
of electrical stimulation, 113, 114
Dynamic exercise(s), 184
Dynamic splints, 151, 152, 153
of elbow, 568, 568
Dynasplint, for knee, 152
Dysfunction syndrome, treatment for, 452–457
in extension dysfunction, 454, 454–456, 456
in flexion dysfunction, 456–457

Eccentric contractions, 183–184
Eccentric dynamic strength assessment, concentric assessment versus, 240
Eccentric elbow program, 583, 584, 585
Edema reduction, compression for, 137–139, 138
electrical stimulation for, 123
management of, 177–178
with distal interphalangeal fractures, 591, 592
Elbow(s), 554–585
adolescent injury(ies) of, 574–577
Little Leaguer's elbow as, 576, 576–577
osteochondritis dissecans and, 574–576, 575
contusions of, 573
dislocations of, 573–574, 574t
eccentric elbow program for, 583, 584, 585
epicondylitis of, 561–564, 562t, 563, 564
extension of, 668, 668
flexion of, 666, 668
isometric, 537, 538
goniometric measurements of, 63, 65, 65
implement-forearm interaction and, 556
joint mobilization techniques for, 164–166, 165, 166
Little Leaguer's, 576, 576–577
progressive-resistance exercises for, 579, 579–583, 581, 583
range-of-motion techniques for, 578, 578–579
rehabilitation program for, 557–559, 558–560
soft-tissue techniques for, 578
strains of, 573
tennis, 561–564, 562t, 563, 564
throwing and, 554–556, 555, 557t
ulnar nerve lesions of, 565, 567t
range of motion of, loss of, 565, 567–569, 568, 568t, 569, 570t
ulnar collateral ligament sprains and, 569–571, 571, 572t, 573, 573
upper extremity support of body weight and, 557
valgus extension overload and, 564–565, 566t
weighted stretching of, 149, 150
Electrical muscle stimulation (EMS), 29–30
Electrical stimulation, 106–132
basic considerations with, 106–107, 108–111, 109–112
contraindications to, 116t
direct current, 130–132
application of, 121–132, 131, 133t
for denervated muscle stimulation, 130
for iontophoresis, 130–132
for anterior cruciate ligament injuries, 368

Electrical stimulation (Continued)
indications for, 115, 116t
input parameter(s) for, 112–115
duration as, 113, 114
frequency as, 113, 114
on/off cycle as, 115, 115
polarity as, 112
strength (intensity) as, 113
waveform as, 112
interferential current, 127–130, 129
neuromuscular, 117, 117–119
of muscle, 29–30
physiologic effect(s) of, 115, 117–124
edema reduction as, 123
muscle strengthening as, 117, 117–119
pain relief as, 119–120, 121t, 122–123
wound healing as, 123–124
precautions for, 116t
pulsed, high-voltage, 124, 124–125
low-voltage, 125–126
microamperage, 132
transcutaneous electrical nerve stimulation as, 126, 126–127
Electromyography (EMG), biofeedback using, 133–137, 134
application of, 134–136, 136
"Empty can" position, for supraspinatus strengthening, 538–539, 539, 540
EMS (electrical muscle stimulation), 29–30
Epicondylitis, 561–564, 562t, 563, 564
Ergometer(s), upper body, for elbow, 559
for shoulder, 490, 491
Evaluation, 38t, 38–48. See also specific tests.
objective, 41–47
functional testing in, 47, 48
inspection in, 41, 42
muscle performance assessment in, 43–44, 44, 46
neurovascular assessment in, 44
observation in, 41
palpation in, 41–42, 43
range-of-motion testing in, 42–43, 44
special testing in, 45–47, 46, 47
sport-specific testing in, 47
repeating, 50–54
subjective history in, 39, 39–41
Exercise(s), 182–191, 183. See also specific exercises.
active. See Active exercise(s).
application of, 208–211
duration for, 209
frequency for, 210, 210
intensity for, 209
progression for, 211
specificity for, 210–211
speed for, 211
passive, 182–183
static, 182, 184
Extension, gluteal, isotonic, 641, 642
hyperextension and, on Swiss ball, 474
of elbow, 668, 668
of hip. See Hip(s), extension of.
of interphalangeal joints, metacarpopha-langeal joint flexion with, 604, 604
of knee. See Knee(s), extension of.
of shoulder. See Shoulder(s), extension of.
of spine, in lying, 441, 441
in standing, 436–437, 437, 439–440
of wrist, 607, 609, 668, 669
rotation mobilization in, for lumbar derange-ments, 463, 463

Extension (Continued)
   tibial glides in, posterior, technique for, 169–170, 170
   valgus extension overload and, 564–565, 566t
Extension dysfunction, treatment for, 454, 454–456, 456
Extension mobilization, for extension dysfunction, 456, 456
Extensor digitorum communis exercise, 604–605
Extensor exercise, for elbow, 581, 582
Extracellular matrix, of fibrous connective tissue, 21

Facet joints, 427
Fasciitis, plantar, 314–315, 316
Fatigue, 5
FCS (functional classification system), for upper extremity rehabilitation, 180, 181t
Fear, of second injury, 5
Feet. See Foot.
Fiber recruitment, submaximal exercise for, 246–247, 247
Finger(s). See also Thumb(s).
   active motion exercises for, 603–605
   boutonnière injuries of, 594–596, 596
   "coach's," 596
   goniometric measurements of, 69, 70
   jersey, 592–594, 594, 594t, 595
   joint mobilization techniques for, 167–168, 168
   mallet, 589–591, 590t, 591
   passive motion exercises for, 605–606
   pseudoboutonnière deformity of, 597
   strengthening exercises for, 606, 606
   trigger, 603
Fisting, stage, 604, 605
Fitter, 200
Flat back posture, 450, 450–451
Flexion, of elbow, 666, 668
   isometric, 537, 538
   of hip, isotonic, 641, 643
      with elastic resistance, 649–650, 650
      with multi-hip machine, 657, 659
   of interphalangeal joints, metacarpophalangeal joint flexion with, 604, 604
   of knee. See Knee(s), flexion of.
   of metacarpophalangeal joint, with interphalangeal joint flexion, 604, 604
   of shoulder. See Shoulder(s), flexion of.
   of spine, in lying, 440, 440–441
      in standing, 436, 436, 439, 439
   of wrist, 607, 607, 608, 668, 669
   plantar, closed-chain strengthening of, 304
      resisted, 646, 647
Flexion dysfunction, treatment for, 456–457
Flexion exercise(s), diagonal, throwing, 663, 664
   for elbow, eccentric, 583, 584
Flexor digitorum longus tendinitis, 293, 294
Flexor digitorum profundus, rupture of, 592–594, 594, 594t, 595
Flexor exercise, for elbow, 581, 582
Flexor hallucis longus tendinitis, 292
Flouri-Methane, for passive stretching, 149
Fluidotherapy, 97–98
Follow-through phase, of throwing, 487–488
Foot, 316–323. See also Lower extremity(ies).
   bones of, 261
   cuboid syndrome of, 318–319, 319
   fifth metatarsal of, proximal diaphysis fracture of, 320, 320–321

Foot (Continued)
   forefoot, bones of, 261
      supinatus of, 275–276, 277
      valgus of, 275, 276
   interdigital neuroma of, 321, 321–322
   metatarsal stress fractures of, 319, 319–320
   midfoot, bones of, 261
   rear. See Rearfoot.
   sesamoiditis of, 322–323
   stairclimber's transient paresthesia of, 322
   tarsal tunnel syndrome of, 318, 318
   tarsometatarsal injuries of, 316–317, 317
   turf toe of, 322, 323
Forearm, goniometric measurements of, 65, 66, 67, 67
   strengthening exercises for, 607, 607–611, 611
Forefoot, bones of, 261
   supinatus of, 275–276, 277
   valgus of, 275, 276
Forward lunge, 650, 651
   with elastic resistance, 650, 652
Four-square hopping ankle rehabilitation, 308
Fracture(s), Bennett's, 598
   hamate, 600–601
   interphalangeal, distal, 591–592, 592
   metacarpal, 597–598
   of proximal diaphysis, of fifth metatarsal, 320, 320–321
   scaphoid, 599–600
   stress, of metatarsals, 319, 319–320
   tarsometatarsal, 316, 317
French curl, 542, 544, 583, 583
Frequency, for exercise, 210, 210
   of electrical stimulation, 113, 114
Friction massage, 139–141
   application of, 139–140, 140
   contraindications to, 140–141
   deep, of elbow, 578
   indications for, 140
   physiologic effects of, 139
"Full can" position, for supraspinatus muscle isolation, 490, 491
Functional classification system (FCS), for upper extremity rehabilitation, 180, 181t
Functional hop test, for isokinetic power evaluation, 226
Functional jump test, for isokinetic power evaluation, 226, 226t
Functional performance(s), isokinetic testing related to, 240–241
Functional rehabilitation, 211–213
   aquatic, 625, 626–629, 628, 630t
   for anterior cruciate ligament injuries, 375, 376t
Functional testing, 47, 48
   lower extremity, for isokinetic power evaluation, 226–227, 227, 228t
   of knee, 395–397, 396
Functional testing algorithm (FTA), for isokinetic power evaluation, 222t, 222–228, 223, 224
   basic measurements for, 223
   closed kinetic chain squat isokinetic testing for, 225–226
   closed kinetic chain supine isokinetic testing for, 224, 225t
   functional hop test for, 226
   functional jump test for, 226, 226t

Functional testing algorithm (FTA) *(Continued)*
  kinesthesia/proprioception/balance testing
    for, 224
  KT–1000 tests for, 223–224
  lower extremity functional test for, 226–227,
    227, 228t
  open kinetic chain isokinetic testing for,
    225, 225t
  sport-specific testing for, 227–228

Gaenslen's test, in low back pain evaluation,
  446, *446*
Gait(s), dynamic assessment of, 278, 280–281,
    281, 281t, 282t
  for crutch-walking, 207, *209*
  normal, functional relationships in, 278, 279t,
    280
  pathologic, 281–283
    pronatory disorders of, 281–282, *282, 283*
    supinatory disorders of, 282–283, *283*
Ganglion cyst(s), 601
Gapping test, in low back pain evaluation, 443,
    444
Gastrocnemius, rehabilitation and treatment of,
    286t–287t
Gender differences, in response to injury, 7
Genucom arthrometer, 390, *391*, 392
Girth measurements, 55–56, *56*
Glenohumeral joint, arthrology of, 480–481
  isokinetic testing of, 235
    for muscular strength assessment, 239–240
  mobilization of, 492–493
  shoulder elevation and, 483–484
Glenoid labrum, superior labrum, anterior, and
    posterior lesion of, *525*, 525–526
  tears of, anterior, 513, *515*
Gluteal extension, isotonic, 641, *642*
Glycosaminoglycans, of fibrous connective
    tissue, 21
Goal setting, 50
Golf, interval rehabilitation program for,
    677–678
Goniometric measurement(s), 43, 56–80
  anatomic zero position and, 58, 59t
  historical background of, 57, *57–58*, *58*
  of ankle, 75, *77, 78, 79*, 79–80
  of elbow, 63, 65, *65*
  of fingers, 69, *70*
  of forearm, 65, *66, 67*, 67
  of hip, 69, *71–73*, 72
  of knee, 75, *77*
  of radius and ulna, 68–69, *69, 70*
  of rearfoot, *79*, 80, *80*
  of shoulder, 60–63, *60–64*
  of straight leg raising, 72, *73–76*, 75
  of upper extremities, 60–69
  of wrist, *67*, 67–68, *68*
  reliability of, 58–59
  technical considerations in, 59–60
  validity of, 58
Gravity, quadriceps force and, 342–345,
    343, 344
Grip exercise, for elbow, 578
Groin injury(ies), rehabilitation for, 418–421,
    420
  exercises for, 421–422, *422–424*, 425
Groin stretch(es), 422, *423*
  straddle, 421, *422*

Groin stretch(es) *(Continued)*
  wall, 422, *424*, 425

H reflex, 20
Half-sit-ups, for spondylolisthesis, 468, *468*
Hamate fractures, 600–601
Hamstring(s), function of, 349–350
  rehabilitation for injuries of, 407–410, *409–412*
    exercises for, 421–422, *422–424*, 425
Hamstring curls, *412*
  prone, 646, *646*
  standing, 646, *647*
  with multi-hip machine, *661*, 662
Hamstring stretch(es), 409, *409*, *410*, 421, 654,
    655
  straddle, 421, *422*
  supine, assisted, 421
  single, 421–422, *423*
Hand(s). See *Finger(s); Thumb(s)*; specific joints.
Healing constraints, 177
Heat, therapeutic, 92–105
  considerations for use of, 105
  deep heating modality(ies) of, 98–105
    physiologic effects of, 98
    shortwave diathermy as, 98–99
    ultrasound as, *100*, 100–105, 102t, *103, 104*
  superficial heating modality(ies) of, 92–98
    contraindications to, 94
    contrast baths as, 96
    fluidotherapy as, 97–98
    hot packs as, 94–95, *95*
    indications for, 94
    paraffin baths as, 96–97, *97*
    physiologic effects of, 92–94
    whirlpools as, 95–96, *96*
Heel bruises, 313–314
Heel raise, 646, 648, *648*
Heel slide, 637, *637*
Hemarthrosis, 16
High-voltage pulsed stimulation (HVPS), *124*,
    124–125
  for edema reduction, 123
  for wound healing, 123
Hip(s), abduction of, isotonic, 641, *642*
    with elastic resistance, 648, *648*
    with multi-hip machine, 658, *659*
  adduction of, isometric, 639, *640*
    isotonic, 641, *641*
      with elastic resistance, 648–649, *649*
      with multi-hip machine, 657, *659*
  extension of, in neutral, with Swiss ball, *473*
    isotonic, 641, *642*
      with elastic resistance, 649, *649*
      with multi-hip machine, 658, *659*
  external rotation of, 646, *646*
  flexion of, isotonic, 641, *643*
    with elastic resistance, 649–650, *650*
    with multi-hip machine, 657, *659*
  goniometric measurements of, 69, *71–73*, 72
  internal rotation of, 645, *645*
  strengthening exercises for, 375
Hip flexor stretch(es), 655, *656*
  manual, *416*
  passive, *413*
Hip spica, 419, *420*
History, in low back pain evaluation, 432,
    432–435
  subjective, *39*, 39–41

Hold-relax technique, slow reversal hold-relax technique for, 154, *156*
Hook lying position, for spondylolisthesis, 469, *469*
Hop test, functional, for isokinetic power evaluation, 226
Hopping ankle rehabilitation, four-square, *308*
Horizontal abduction-adduction, of shoulder, 531–532, *533*
Hot packs, 94–95, *95*
Humeral distraction, with anterior, posterior, and inferior glides, technique for, 162–163, *163*
Humeral glide, inferior, technique for, 163, *164*
HVPS. See *High-voltage pulsed stimulation (HVPS)*.
Hydrocollator packs, 94–95, *95*
Hydrostatic pressure, 617–618
Hydrotherapy, 615. See also *Aquatic rehabilitation*.
Hyperextension, on Swiss ball, *474*

Ice buckets (baths), 91, *91*
Ice massage, 91–92, *92*
Ice packs, 88–89, *89*
Iliopsoas stretch(es), *414*
   manual, *415*
Immobilization, effects of, 18–27
      on articular cartilage, 25–26
      on bone, 27
      on ligaments, 26–27
      on muscle, 18–20, *19*
      on periarticular connective tissue, 20–25, *22, 24, 24t*
   remobilization following. See *Remobilization*.
Inertial exercises, 185–186, *188*
   for elbow, 559, *559*
Inflammation, cryotherapy effect on, 84
Inflammatory response, 13
Inspection, in evaluation, 41, *42*
Intensity, of electrical stimulation, 113
   of exercise, 209
      submaximal, determining, 245–246
Interdigital neuroma, of foot, *321*, 321–322
Interferential current (IFC), 127–130
   application of, 128, *129*, 130
Interphalangeal (IP) joint(s), arthrokinematics of, 266
   distal, fractures and dislocations of, 591–592, *592, 593*
      joint blocking for, 605
      mallet finger and, 589–591, 590t, *591*
   distraction of, with volar, dorsal, medial, and lateral glides, technique for, 167–168, *168*
   flexion and extension of, metacarpophalangeal joint flexion with, 604, *604*
   proximal, boutonnière injuries of, 594–596, *596*
      pseudoboutonnière deformity and, 597
      sprains and dislocations of, 596–597
Interval rehabilitation programs, for golf, 677–678
   for racquetball, 676–677
   for running, 678
   for tennis, 676
   for throwing, 670–676
Interval Throwing Program (ITP), 670–675
   batting in, 673

Interval Throwing Program (ITP) *(Continued)*
   for Little Leaguers, 675–676
   individual variability and, 671
   stretching in, 672
   throwing in, *672*, 672–673
   throwing mechanics and, 672
   warm-up for, 671
   weight training in, 671
Intervertebral discs (IVDs), 427, 428–429
   pressure between, *429*, 429–430, *430*
   prolapse of, 430t, 430–431
Iontophoresis, direct current for, 130–132
   for epicondylitis, 563, *563*
Isoacceleration, isokinetic exercises and, 252
Isokinetic(s), 219–253
   advantages of, 220–221
   closed kinetic chain and, 222
   definition of, 220
   functional testing algorithm and. See *Functional testing algorithm (FTA), for isokinetic power evaluation*.
   open kinetic chain and, 221
Isokinetic exercise(s), 185, *187*, 241–253
   closed kinetic chain, 251–252
   for knee, equipment for, 362
   isoacceleration and deceleration and, 252
   of hamstrings, 409–410, *411*
   outcomes research on, 252–253
   passive, 149, *152*
   patient progression criteria and, 241–242, 242t
   progression continuum for, 242–251, *243*, 244t
      force production and, gradient increase and decrease in, 243–244
      full range-of-motion exercises and, 250–251, *251*
      multiple-angle isometrics and, 242–243, *244, 245*
      pain guidelines for, 246
      rest intervals and, 249–250, *250, 251*
      short-arc exercises and, 247–249, *248–250*
      submaximal exercise fiber recruitment and, 246–247, *247*
      submaximal exercise intensity determination and, 245–246
      trial treatment and, 246
Isokinetic testing, 44, *46*, 228–240
   data and analysis in, 229–230
   for upper extremity strength assessment, 234–240
      concentric versus eccentric considerations in, 240
      of glenohumeral joint, 235, 239–240
      of shoulder rotation, 235–237, *236*, 238t, 239t
      rationale for using, 234t, 234–235
   functional performance related to, 240–241
   of knee, 393–395, *394*
   protocol for, 228–229
   purposes of, 228
   rationale for, 230–233
      for open kinetic chain assessment, 230–233, 233t
Isometric(s), multiple-angle, 242–243, *244, 245*
   painful deformation with, 242, *245*
   physiologic overflow with, 242, 244t
Isometric exercise(s), for knee and leg, *639*, 639–640, *640*
Isometric testing, resistive, 44, 45f
Isotonic exercise(s), 185, *185*, 186
   for knee and leg, 640–641, *641–650*, 643, 645–646, 648–650

ITP. See *Interval Throwing Program (ITP)*.
IVDs. See *Intervertebral discs (IVDs)*.

Jersey finger, 592–594, *594*, 594t, *595*
Johnson antishear device, 394
Joint(s). See also specific joints, e.g., *Ankle(s)*.
  structures of, response to injury and, 15–17,
    15–17
Joint angle, quadriceps shutdown and, 20
Joint capsule, response to injury, 17
Joint distention, quadriceps shutdown and, 20
Joint effusion, reduction of, '7
Joint loading, articular cartilage and, 26
Joint mobilization, 154, 158–171
  application techniques in, for ankle, 170–171,
    171, 172
    for elbow, 164–166, *165, 166*
    for knee, 168–170, *168–170*
    for shoulder, 162–164, *163–165*
    for thumb and fingers, 167–168, *168*
    for wrist, *166*, 166–167, *167*
  for knee, 168–170, *168–170*
  grading systems for, 159–160, 160t, *161*
  joint position and force application for, 160–
    161, 161t, *162*
  physiologic effects of, 159, 159t
  techniques for, 154, 158–159
    endfeels for, 158t, 158–159
    stretching versus, 158, 158t
Joint space, solution absorption from, 16–17
Joint stiffness, therapeutic heat effects on, 94
Joint-blocking exercise(s), for fingers, 604, *605*
Jump test, functional, for isokinetic power
    evaluation, 226, 226t

Kicks, contralateral, *307*
Kinematic(s). See *Arthrokinematics*.
Kinematic chain, 178–182, *179*, 180t, 181t
Kinesthesia testing, for isokinetic power
    evaluation, 224
Knee(s), 330–397. See also specific parts, e.g.,
    Patella; Patello- entries.
  arthrofibrosis of, 22
  arthrometer testing of, 390–393, *391*, 392t
  bony anatomy of, 330–333, 331t
    of patellofemoral articulation, *332*, 332–333
    of tibiofemoral articulation, 331–332
  braces for, functional, 388–390
  capsular restraints of, 337. See also *Menis-*
    cus(i).
  closed kinetic chain exercises for, 650–654,
    650–658, 657
  extension of, 90°-to-0°, 643, *644*
    90°-to-45°, 643, *644*
    passive, *638*, 639
      prone, with weight, 356, *357*
      supine, with weight, 356, *357*
    prone, terminal, 359, *359*
    terminal, closed kinetic chain, *346*, 653
      isotonic, 641, 643, *643*
    with multi-hip machine, *661*, 662
  flexion of, active-assisted, 637, *637*
    passive, *636*, 636–637
      using body weight, 357, *358*
      using Total Gym, 357, *359*
    pulley, 637–638

Knee(s) *(Continued)*
  functional testing of, 395–397, *396*
  goniometric measurements of, 75, *77*
  isokinetic testing of, 393–395, *394*
  isometric exercises for, *639*, 639–640, *640*
  isotonic exercises for, 640–641, *641–650*, 643,
    645–646, 648–650
  joint effusion of, quadriceps reflex inhibition
    and, 348
  ligaments of, 333–337
    anterior cruciate. See *Anterior cruciate liga-*
      ment (ACL).
    lateral collateral, 337
    medial collateral. See *Medial collateral liga-*
      ment (MCL).
    posterior cruciate. See *Posterior cruciate liga-*
      ment (PCL).
  muscles of, function of, 349–351
  patellofemoral joint of. See *Patellofemoral joint*.
  range of motion of, active-assisted, 149, *151*
  range-of-motion exercises for, *636–638*, 636–
    639
  rehabilitative principles for, 355–364
    closed kinetic chain exercises and, 359–360,
      360t, *361*
    dynamic splinting and, 356
    early knee motion and, 355–357, 356t, *357,*
      358
    early quadriceps recruitment and, 355
    equipment and, 362, *363, 364*
    proprioception exercises and, 360, 362, *362–*
      364
    strengthening and, 357, 359–360, 360t, *361*
    time frames and, 355
  splints for, dynamic, *152, 153*
  stationary cycling and, biomechanics of, 351–
    355, 352t, 353t, *354*
  weighted stretching of, 149, *149*
Knee Signature System (KSS), 390, 392
KT–1000 arthrometer, for isokinetic power
    evaluation, 223–224
  knee testing using, 390, *391*, 392, 393
KT–2000 arthrometer, knee testing using, 392

Lateral collateral ligament (LCL), 337
Lateral retinaculum release, 388, 389t
Lateral shifts, correction of, 464, *465*
  in low back pain evaluation, *435*, 435–436
Lateral step-ups, 360, *361*, 653, *653*
Leg(s). See also *Lower extremity(ies)*; specific
    joints.
  closed kinetic chain exercises for, 650–654,
    650–658, 657
  isometric exercises for, *639*, 639–640, *640*
  isotonic exercises for, 640–641, *641–650*, 643,
    645–646, 648–650
  lower, 283–295
    Achilles tendinitis of, 285, 288–289, 290t–
      291t
    Achilles tendon rupture of, *284*, 284–285,
      286t–287t
    anterior tibialis tendinitis of, 289
    compartmental compression syndromes of,
      293–295, 294t, 295t
    flexor digitorum longus tendinitis of, 293,
      294
    flexor hallucis longus tendinitis of, 292
    peroneal tendinitis of, 289, 292

Leg(s) (Continued)
  posterior tibialis tendinitis of, 292, 293
  tennis leg and, 285
  tibiofibular synostosis of, 283–284
  tennis, 284, 285
Leg presses, 360, 361
  with multi-hip machine, 658, 661, 662
Ligament(s). See also specific ligaments, e.g.,
    Anterior cruciate ligament (ACL).
  immobilization and, 26–27
  in proprioception, 193
  of spine, 428
  remobilization and, 30–31
Lisfranc's joint, arthrokinematics of, 266, 266
  injuries of, 316–317, 317
Little Leaguer Interval Throwing Program,
    675–676
Little Leaguer's elbow, 576, 576–577
Low back pain, 426–475
  biomechanics of, 427–431, 429, 430, 430t
  evaluation of, 431–448
    active range of motion in, 436–438, 436–438
    history taking in, 432, 432–435
    myotomes and dermatomes in, 442–443,
      443t
    philosophy of, 431
    posture in, 435, 435–436
    progression of forces in, 467, 467t
    reflexes and cutaneous distribution in, 442,
      442t
    standing neurologic screen for, 443, 444–
      447, 446–448
    test movements for, 438–442, 439–441
  treatment of, 448–469
    for derangement, 457–466, 460–463, 465
    for dysfunction syndrome, 452–457, 454–
      456
    for postural syndrome, 449t, 449–452, 450–
      453
    for spondylolisthesis, 467–469, 468–470
    philosophy of, 431
    progression of forces in, 467, 467t
    strengthening and stabilizing exercises for,
      471, 471–474
Lower extremity(ies). See also specific regions,
    e.g., Foot.
  anthropometric assessment of, 270, 270–277
    for subtalar neutral point determination,
      271, 271, 272
    for tibial torsion determination, 277, 278
    for tibial varum determination, 276–277,
      277
    of midtarsal joint position, 275–276, 276,
      277
    of plantar flexion-dorsiflexion range of mo-
      tion, 272–273, 274
    of subtalar joint position, 273–275, 274, 275
    of subtalar range of motion, 271–272, 272,
      273
  arthrokinematics of. See Arthrokinematics.
  functional relationships of, 277–283
    dynamic gait assessment and, 278, 280–281,
      281, 281t, 282t
    in normal gait, 278, 279t, 280
    in pathologic gait, 281–283, 282, 283
  muscular function of, 267–270, 268, 268t, 269
    in anterior muscle group, 269–270
    in intrinsic muscle group, 270
    in lateral muscle group, 269
    in posterior deep muscle group, 268–269

Lower extremity(ies) (Continued)
    in posterior superficial muscle group, 267–
      268
  orthotic therapy for, 323–326, 325t
    orthosis components and, 324, 324
    orthosis types for, 324–325, 325
    post of orthosis and, 325–326
    return to competition and, 326, 327, 328
Lower extremity functional test, for isokinetic
    power evaluation, 226–227, 227, 228t
Low-voltage pulsed stimulation, 125–126
Lufkin tape measure, 56, 56
Lumbar roll. See also Low back pain.
  for sitting posture, 452, 453
Lumbar spine, biomechanics of, 427–428. See
    also Spine.
Lunge(s), cross-step, diagonal, with elastic
    resistance, 651, 652
  with elastic resistance, 650–651, 652
  diagonal, with elastic resistance, 651–652, 652
  forward, 650, 651
  with elastic resistance, 650, 652
  sidestep, with elastic resistance, 650, 652

Mallet finger, 589–591, 590t, 591
Massage, friction. See Friction massage.
  ice, 91–92, 92
Mattresses, low back pain and, 451
Measurement(s), 55–80
  circumferential, 46
  goniometric. See Goniometric measurement(s).
  of girth, 55–56, 56
Mechanoreceptors, 192t, 192–193
Medial collateral ligament (MCL), 336–337
  immobilization and, 27
  rehabilitation for injuries of, 376–377, 380t–
    382t
Medi-Ball Rebounder, 362, 364
Meniscus(i), 337–339, 338t
  rehabilitation for, 380, 382–383, 383t–386t
  response to injury, 16
Metabolism, cellular, cryotherapy effect on, 83
  therapeutic heat effects on, 93–94
Metacarpal fractures, 597–598
Metacarpophalangeal (MCP) joint(s), flexion of,
    with interphalangeal joint flexion and
    extension, 604, 604
  trigger finger and, 603
Metatarsal(s), fifth, proximal diaphysis fracture
    of, 320, 320–321
  stress fractures of, 319, 319–320
Metatarsophalangeal (MTP) joint(s),
    arthrokinematics of, 266, 266–267
  plantar glide of first metatarsal at, 313
Microamperage pulsatile stimulation, 132
Midfoot, bones of, 261
Midtarsal joint, arthrokinematics of, 265,
    265–266, 266
  dorsal glide of, 312
  plantar glide of, 312
  position of, anthropometric assessment of,
    275–276, 276, 277
Minisquats, 360, 360t, 361, 650, 650–651
  with multi-hip machine, 658, 660
Moment of force, water and, 616, 617
Mood congruence, 4–5
Movement, through water, 617
Multiaxial wobble board, 305

Multi-hip machine, 657–662
Multiple-angle isometrics, 242–243, *244, 245*
Muscle(s), denervated, direct current electrical stimulation for, 130
  force production by, gradient increase and decrease in, 243–244
  function of, of lower extremity. See *Lower extremity(ies), muscular function of.*
  immobilization and, 18–20, *19*
  patellofemoral joint and, 339–340
  remobilization and, 29–30
  strength of, cryotherapy effect on, 84–86, *85, 86*
Muscle performance assessment, 43–44, *44, 46*
Muscle spasm, cryotherapy effect on, 83
  therapeutic heat effects on, 94
Muscle spindles, proprioception and, 193
Musculoskeletal system, water immersion and, effects of, 618–619, *619*
Myofascial release techniques, 151
Myotomes, in low back pain evaluation, 442–443, 453t

Neurologic screen, standing, in low back pain evaluation, 443, *444–447,* 446–448
Neuroma, interdigital, of foot, *321,* 321–322
Neuromuscular control exercises, for elbow, 559, *560*
Neuromuscular electrical stimulation (NMES), *117,* 117–119
Neuromuscular training, before exercise, 406
Neurovascular assessment, 44
Nucleus pulposus, 428–429

Observation, in evaluation, 41
On/off cycle, of electrical stimulation, 115, *115*
Open kinetic chain (OKC), 175
Open kinetic chain exercise(s) (OKCE), 178–182, 180t
Open kinetic chain (OKC) pattern, 221
Open kinetic chain (OKC) testing, closed kinetic chain functional performance correlated with, 233
  for isokinetic power evaluation, 225, 225t
  isokinetic, rationale for, 230–233, 233t
Orthotic therapy, for lower extremity, 323–326, 325t
  orthosis components and, 324, *324*
  orthosis types for, 324–325, *325*
  post of orthosis and, 325–326
Os trigonum, injury of, 314
Osteochondritis dissecans, 574–576, *575*
Osteoporosis, disuse, immobilization and, 30
Overhead soccer throw, two-hand, 632, *633*

Pain, control of, 177
  electrical stimulation for, 119–120, 121t, 122–123
  cryotherapy effect on, 83
  during exercise, guidelines for, 246
  in low back. See *Low back pain.*
  in shoulder, beyond 90° of rotation, 497
    painful arc and, 496–497
  middle deltoid and elbow, referred from shoulder, 497

Pain *(Continued)*
  patellofemoral, rehabilitation for, 384–388, *387,* 389t
  therapeutic heat effects on, 94
  with isometrics, 242, *245*
Palpation, in evaluation, 41–42, *43*
Paraffin baths, 96–97, *97*
Paresthesia, transient, stairclimber's, 322
Passing. See *Throwing.*
Passive exercise(s), 182–183
Passive-assisted stretching techniques, 148–151
Patella, mobilization of, 636
  tracking pattern of, 340–341, *341*
Patellar glides, inferior and superior, technique for, 168, *168, 169*
  medial and lateral, technique for, 168–169, *169, 170*
Patellar tendon allografts, for anterior cruciate ligament injuries, 367–368
Patellofemoral braces, 388
Patellofemoral joint, *332,* 332–333
  biomechanics of, 339–349, 346t
    muscles and, 339–340
    patellar tracking pattern and, 340–341, *341*
    quadriceps force and, 318–319, 342–345, *343–346*
    sagittal plane mechanics and, 341–342, *342*
    static stabilizers and, 340, *340*
    valgus vector and, *347,* 347–348
  rehabilitation for injuries of, 384–388, *387,* 389t
Patellofemoral joint reaction force (PFJR), 342–346, *343, 344,* 346t
PCL. See *Posterior cruciate ligament (PCL).*
Pelvic tilt, anterior, on Swiss ball, *472*
  posterior, on Swiss ball, *472*
Pelvic torsion test, in low back pain evaluation, 446, *446*
Pendulum swings, circumduction, 528–529, *529*
Periarticular connective tissue, immobilization and, 20–25, *22, 24,* 24t
Peripheral nervous system, water immersion and, effects of, 619
Peritendinitis, lower leg, rehabilitation and treatment of, 290t–291t
Peroneal tendinitis, 289, 292
Peroneal tendons, J-pad stabilization of, *313*
Physiologic overflow, with isometrics, 242, 244t
Pitching. See *Throwing.*
Plantar fasciitis, 314–315, *316*
Plantar flexion, resisted, 646, *647*
  strengthening of, closed-chain, *304*
Plantar flexion-dorsiflexion range of motion, anthropometric assessment of, 272–273, *274*
Plyometric exercises, 186–191, *188–191*
  upper extremity, 632, *632–635,* 635
    for elbow, 559, *560*
    for shoulder, 495–496
PNF. See *Proprioceptive neuromuscular facilitation (PNF).*
Polarity, of electrical stimulation, 112
Popliteus muscle, function of, 350
Posterior cruciate ligament (PCL), 335–336, 336t
  rehabilitation for injuries of, 376
Posterior shear test, in low back pain evaluation, 443, *445*
Posterior tibialis tendinitis, 292, *293*
Posteromedial capsule, of knee, 337
Postural education, for flexion dysfunction, 457
Postural syndrome, treatment for, 449t, 449–452, *450–453*

Posture, flat back, *450*, 450–451
  in low back pain evaluation, *435*, 435–436
  sitting, low back pain and, 451, *451*, *452*
  swayback, 450, 450f
Power, isokinetic, functional testing algorithm for evaluating. See *Functional testing algorithm (FTA), for isokinetic power evaluation.*
Prehab, 205–206
PREs. See *Progressive-resistance exercises (PREs).*
Press-Grip, 558, *558*
Press-ups, 665, *667*
  for extension dysfunction, 454, *454*, *455*
Primary injury, 13
Problem identification, 48–49
ProFitter, ankle rehabilitation on, *304*
Progression, for exercise, 211
Progressive-resistance exercises (PREs), 202–205
  daily adjustable technique for, 203–204, 204t
  DeLorme program for, 202–203
  for elbow, 579, *579–583*, 581, 583
  for shoulder, 494
  high-repetition, low-weight method for, 204–205, 205t
Pronation, disorders of, pathologic gait due to, 281–282, *282*, *283*
Pronation exercise, for elbow, 581, *582*
  eccentric, 583, *584*
Proprioception, 191–202
  assessment of, 193–195, *194*
  cold effects on, 198–199
  cryotherapy effect on, 84
  physiology of, 191–193, 192t
  taping or bracing effects on, 199, 201
  testing and training, 195, *196–201*, 197–199, 201–202
Proprioception testing, for isokinetic power evaluation, 224
Proprioceptive exercises, for knee, 360, 362, *362–364*
  on inclined surface, *307*
Proprioceptive neuromuscular facilitation (PNF), 154, 406
  contract-relax technique for, 154, *155*
  for shoulder, 492, *492–495*
  hold-relax technique for, 154, *156*
  slow reversal hold-relax technique for, 154, *157*
Proximal diaphysis fracture, of fifth metatarsal, *320*, 320–321
Proximal interphalangeal (PIP) joint(s), boutonnière injuries of, 594–596, *596*
  pseudoboutonnière deformity and, 597
  sprains and dislocations of, 596–597
Pseudoboutonnière deformity, 597
Psychological factors, 1–11
  in compliance with rehabilitation program, 7–8
  injury proneness and, 1–5, *2–4*
  recovery problems and, 8–9
  responses to injury and, 5–7
  slumps and, 9–10
Punches, isotonic, 544, *545*
Push-ups, 666, *667*
  progressive, isotonic, 544, *545*

Quad set, 639
Quadriceps, function of, 350–351
  rehabilitation for injuries of, 411–417
    contusions and, 411–415, *413–416*, 417
    exercises for, *424*, *425*
    strains and, 417, *418*, *419*
  strength of, 342–345, *343–346*
Quadriceps force, strength of, 318–319
Quadriceps shutdown, 19–20
Quadriceps stretch(es), 654, *656*
  single-leg, *414*
    standing, *416*
  standing, *424*, *425*
Quadruped exercise, for spondylolisthesis, 469, *470*
Quebec Task Force on Spinal Disorders (QTFSD), 448–449

Racquetball, interval rehabilitation program for, 676–677
Radial deviation, 607, *609*
Radial deviation exercise, 579, *580*
Radiocarpal distraction, technique for, *166*, 166–167
Radiocarpal glides, dorsal and volar, technique for, 167, *167*
Radioulnar distraction, technique for, 164, *165*
Radioulnar glides, anterior and posterior, technique for, 165–166, *166*
Radius, goniometric measurements of, 68–69, *69*, *70*
Range of motion (ROM), active, in low back pain evaluation, 436–438, *436–438*
  aquatic rehabilitation to increase, 621
  goniometric measurement of. See *Goniometric measurement(s).*
  of elbow, loss of, 565, 567–569, *568*, 568t, *569*, 570t
  of shoulder, active-assisted, 149, *150*
  of subtalar joint, anthropometric assessment of, 271–272, *272*, *273*
  plantar flexion-dorsiflexion, anthropometric assessment of, 272–273, *274*
Range-of-motion exercise(s), for elbow, *578*, 578–579
  for knee, *636–638*, 636–639
  for shoulder, 528–532, *529–535*, 534
  in progression continuum, for isokinetic exercises, 250–251, *251*
Range-of-motion testing, 42–43, *44*
Reactor, *196*
Rearfoot, bones of, 261
  goniometric measurements of, *79*, 80, *80*
  valgus of, 274, *274*
  varus of, *274*, 274–275, *275*
Rectus femoris stretch(es), manual, 415
  passive, *413*
Re-evaluation, 50–54
Reflex(es), deep tendon, testing of, 442, 442t
  inhibition of, 19–20
    cause of, 19–20
    muscle atrophy and, 19, *19*
Rehabilitation, definition of, 175
Release and deceleration phase, of throwing, elbow in, 555–556
  shoulder in, 487
Reliability, of goniometric measurements, 58–59
Remobilization, effects of, 29–31

Remobilization *(Continued)*
  on articular cartilage, 30
  on bone, 30
  on connective tissue, 31
  on ligaments, 30–31
  on muscle, 29–30
Resistance, accommodating, definition of, 220
Resistive isometric tests, 44, *45*
Response to injury, 175, *176*
Rest intervals, for isokinetic exercises, 249–250, *250, 251*
Retrocalcaneal bursitis, 314, *315*
Reverse wrist curls, 579, *579*
ROM. See *Range of motion (ROM).*
Rope-and-pulley exercises, *529,* 529–530
Rotation mobilization, in extension, for lumbar derangements, 463, *463*
Rotator cuff(s), activation of, 488–490, *489, 490,* 491t
  arthrology of, *482,* 482–483
  "empty can" position for strengthening, 539, *540*
  impingement syndrome and, 499–506, *500–504,* 505t–507t, 508, *508*
  injury of, 499, 499t
  tears of, 508–511, *509, 511,* 512t–517t
  tendinitis of, 510
Rowing, prone, 666, *667*
Rowing exercise, seated, 544, 546
Running, interval rehabilitation program for, 678

Sacral thrust test, in low back pain evaluation, 447, *447*
Scaphoid fracture(s), 599–600
Scapula, mobilization, 498, *498*
  stabilizers of, weakness of, 513
Scapulothoracic joint, arthrology of, 481
  injury of, 497–499, *498*
  rehabilitation for, 493–494
Scapulothoracic testing, isokinetic, 240
Seated rowing exercise, 544, 546
Secondary injury, 13
Sesamoiditis, of foot, 322–323
Short-arc exercises, 247–249, *248–250*
Shortwave diathermy, 98–99
Shoulder(s), 478–550
  abduction of, active-assisted, *529,* 530
    horizontal, 531–532, *533*
      prone, 665, *666*
    isometric, 536, *536*
    isotonic, 538, *539*
    strength of, isokinetic testing of, 239–240
    supine, 530, *530*
    to 90°, 665, *665*
  adduction of, strength of, isokinetic testing of, 239–240
  anterior instability of, 511–519
    anterior glenoid labrum tear associated with, 513, *515*
    scapula stabilizer weakness and, 513
    surgical treatment for, 514, 516–517, 518t–524t
  arthrology of, 478–483, *479*
    acromioclavicular joint and, 479–480
    coracoacromial arch and, 481–482
    glenohumeral joint and, 480–481
    rotator cuff and, *482,* 482–483

Shoulder(s) *(Continued)*
  scapulothoracic joint and, 481
  sternoclavicular joint and, 478–479
crepitus and, 497
elevation of, 483–484, *484*
extension of, diagonal pattern of, 550, *550*
  isometric, 536, *536*
  isotonic, 541, *541*
  strength of, isokinetic testing of, 239–240
flexion of, active-assisted, 529, *529*
  diagonal pattern of, *548, 549,* 549–550
  isometric, 534, *535*
  isotonic, 538, *538*
  strength of, isokinetic testing of, 239–240
  supine, 530, *530*
glenoid labrum lesions of, *525,* 525–526
  acromioclavicular separation of, 526, *527,* 528
goniometric measurements of, 60–63, *60–64*
impingement syndrome of, 499–506, *500–504,* 505t–507t, 508
  lidocaine injections for, 504
  posterior, 506, 508, *508*
  surgical treatment for, 504–506
joint mobilization techniques for, 162–164, *163–165*
middle deltoid and elbow pain and, 497
multidirectional instability of, 522, 525
pain beyond 90° of elevation and, 497
painful arc and, 496–497
posterior instability of, 519, 522
range of motion of, active-assisted, 149, *150*
range-of-motion exercises for, 528–532, *529–535,* 534
rehabilitation program for, 488–496, 496t
  glenohumeral mobilization techniques for, 492–493
  plyometrics for, 495–496
  progressive-resistance exercise for, 494
  proprioceptive neuromuscular facilitation for, 492, *492–495*
  rotator cuff activation and, 488–490, *489, 490,* 491t
  scapulothoracic joint in, 493–494
  strengthening exercises in, 488, *489*
  Throwers' Ten Exercise Program for, 494–495
  upper body ergometer for, 490, *491*
rotation of, external, at 0° of abduction, 544, 546, 664, *664*
  at 90° of abduction, 547, 664, *664*
  isometric, 536–537, *537*
  side-lying, 541, *542*
  standing, 531, *532*
  supine, 530–531, *531*
internal, at 0° abduction, 544, 547, *547,* 664, *664*
  at 90° abduction, 547, *548, 549,* 664, *664*
  isometric, 537, *537*
  side-lying, 541–542, *542*
  standing, 531, *533*
  supine, 531, *532*
isokinetic testing of, for internal rotation and external rotation strength assessment, 235–237, *236,* 238t, 239t
strength of, bilateral differences in, 237
  isokinetic testing of, 235–237, *236,* 238t, 239t
  normative data and, 237, 238t
  unilateral strength ratios and, 237, 239t

Shoulder(s) (*Continued*)
rotator cuff of. See *Rotator cuff(s)*.
scaption internal rotation of, 665, *665*
scapulothoracic joint lesions of, 497–499, *498*
strengthening exercises for, 534–544
advanced, 544, *546–550*, 547, *549–550*
isometric, 534, *535–538*, 536–537
isotonic, 538–541, *538–546*, 544
throwing mechanism of, 484–488, *485*, *486*
acceleration and, 486–487
cocking and, 485–486
follow-through and, 487–488
release and deceleration and, 487
wind-up and, 485
Shoulder shrug, 542, *543*
Side steps, tubing-resisted, *303*
Sideglide(s), for low back pain evaluation, 437, *438*
for lumbar derangements, *462*, 462–463
Sidestep lunge, with elastic resistance, 650, *652*
Side-to-side throw, two-hand, 632, *633*
Sitting posture, in low back pain evaluation, 435
low back pain and, 451, *451*, *452*
Sitting root test, in low back pain evaluation, 443, *444*
Sit-ups, for spondylolisthesis, 468, *468*
Slide Board, 362, *363*
Slow reversal hold-relax technique, 154, *157*
Slumps, 9–10
Soccer throw, overhead, two-hand, 632, *633*
Social support system, 7
Soleus muscle, rehabilitation and treatment of, 286t–287t
Soleus pumps, *299*
Special testing, 45–47, *46*, *47*
Specific gravity, of water, 616
Specificity, for exercise, 210–211
Speed, for exercise, 211
Spica, hip, 419, *420*
thumb, *599*, *599*, *600*, 611
Spine. See also *Low back pain*.
biomechanics of, 427–431, *429*, *430*, 430t
extension of, in lying, 441, *441*
in standing, 436–437, *437*, 439–440
Splinting, dynamic, 151, *152*, *153*
of elbow, 568, *568*
for boutonnière injuries, 596, *596*
for mallet finger, 589–591, 590t, *591*
for ulnar collateral ligament injuries of thumb, 599, *600*
protective, for hand and wrist, *611*, 611–612
Spondylolisthesis, 467–469, *468–470*
Sport-specific testing, 47
for isokinetic power evaluation, 227–228
Sprain(s), of ankle, inversion, 295, 297–305, 298t
syndesmotic, 305–306, 309, *309*
of proximal interphalangeal joint, 596–597
of ulnar collateral ligament, 569–571, *571*, 572t, 573, *573*
of wrist, 601
Spray and stretch technique, 149
Stability testing, 45–46, *46*
Stabilization exercise(s), for low back, 471, *471–474*
Stage fisting, 604, *605*
Stair(s), climbing with crutches, 207–208
Stairclimber's transient paresthesia, 322
Standing neurologic screen, in low back pain evaluation, 443, *444–447*, 446–448

Standing posture, in low back pain evaluation, 435, *435–436*
Static exercise(s), 182, *184*
Stationary cycling, 654, *654*
biomechanics of, 351–355, 352t, 353t, *354*
for ankle rehabilitation, *303*
Step-ups, lateral, 360, *361*, 653, *653*
Sternoclavicular joint, arthrology of, 478–479
shoulder elevation and, 483
Stiffness, of joints, therapeutic heat effects on, 94
of soft tissues, cryotherapy effect on, 83
Stork stands, *197*, *302*
on trampoline, *198*
Straight leg raising, 640–641, *641*
goniometric measurements of, 72, *73–76*, 75
Strain(s), 405, 406t
of elbow, 573
of quadriceps, 417, *418*, *419*
Strength, immobilization and, 18
Strengthening exercise(s), for anterior cruciate ligament injuries, 375, *375*, 376t
for fingers, 606, *606*
for hip, 375
for knee, 357, 359–360, 360t, *361*
for low back, 471, *471–474*
for shoulder, 488, *489*, 534–544
advanced, 544, *546–550*, 547, *549–550*
isometric, 534, *535–538*, 537
isotonic, 538–541, *538–546*, 544
for wrist and forearm, 607, *607–611*, 611
in water, 621, *621–624*, 625
Stress fracture(s), of metatarsals, *319*, 319–320
Stretching, 146–154
biophysical considerations related to, 146–148
connective tissue properties and, 146
duration as, 147
neurophysiological, 146–147
temperature as, 147–148
of elbow extensors, *578*, 578–579
of elbow flexors, 578, *578*
of quadriceps, 412, *413–416*
techniques for, 148t, 148–154
myofascial release, 151
passive and active-assisted, 148–151
proprioceptive neuromuscular facilitation as, 154, *155–157*
Stryker knee laxity tester, 390, 392
Subjective history, *39*, 39–41
Subluxation(s), of peroneal tendon, 309, 313, *313*
of shoulder. See *Shoulder(s)*.
Subtalar joint, arthrokinematics of, 262–265, *263*, 263t, *264*
neutral point determination for, anthropometric assessment for, 271, *271*, *272*
position of, anthropometric assessment of, 273–275, *274*, *275*
range of motion of, anthropometric assessment of, 271–272, *272*, *273*
traction of, *310*
Superficial heating modalities. See *Heat, therapeutic*.
Superior labrum, anterior, and posterior (SLAP) lesion, 525, *525–526*
Superman exercises, 471
Supination, disorders of, pathologic gait due to, 282–283, *283*
Supination exercise, for elbow, 581, *582*
eccentric, *584*, 585

Supinatus, forefoot, 275–276, *277*
Supraspinatus muscle, "empty can" position for strengthening, 538–539, *539, 540*
   exercise of, 488–489, *489*
   "full can" position for isolating, 490, *491*
Surgery, for anterior cruciate ligament injuries. See *Anterior cruciate ligament (ACL).*
   for impingement syndrome, 504–506
   for lateral ankle reconstructions, postsurgical management for, 306, 306t, 309
   for meniscal injuries, 380
      rehabilitation following, 380, 382–383, 383t–386t
   for patellofemoral dysfunction, 388, 389t
   for rotator cuff tears, 510–511
   prehab before, 205–206
Swayback posture, 450, 450f
Swelling reduction. See *Edema reduction.*
Swing-through gait, 207, *209*
Synovial membrane, response to injury, *15,* 15–16, *16*
Synovitis, 16

Talar distraction, with posterior, medial, and lateral glides, technique for, 171, *171*
Talar glide, anterior, *311*
   technique for, 171, *172*
   posterior, *310*
Tall kneeling, active, on Swiss ball, *474*
Talocrural joint, arthrokinematics of, 261–262, *262,* 262t
   distraction of, technique for, 170
   talar glide and, anterior, *311*
      posterior, *310*
   traction of, *310*
Tape correction, for patellofemoral dysfunction, *387,* 387–388
Taping, effect on proprioception, 199, 201
Tarsal tunnel syndrome, 318, *318*
Tarsometatarsal joint, arthrokinematics of, 266, *266*
   injuries of, 316–317, *317*
TENS (transcutaneous electrical nerve stimulation), 120, *126,* 126–127
Tendinitis, of lower leg, Achilles, 285, 288–289
   anterior tibialis, 289
   flexor digitorum longus, 293, *294*
   flexor hallucis longus, 292
   peroneal, 289, 292
   posterior tibialis, 292, *293*
   rehabilitation and treatment of, 290t–291t
   of rotator cuff, 510
   of wrist, 601
Tendon excursions, for fingers, 604, *605*
Tendon gliding exercises, for fingers, 604, *605*
Tennis, interval rehabilitation program for, 676
   isokinetic torque-to-body weight ratios and, 238t
   isokinetic work-to-body weight ratios and, 238t
   shoulder rotation and, 238t
Tennis elbow, 561–564, 562t, *563, 564*
Tennis leg, *284,* 285
Thera-Band, 362, *362*
Therapeutic cold. See *Cryotherapy.*
Therapeutic electricity. See *Electrical stimulation.*
Therapeutic heat. See *Heat, therapeutic.*
Thigh thrust test, in low back pain evaluation, 443, *445*

Three-point crutch gait, 207, *209*
Threshold to detection of passive movement (TTDPM), 193–195, *194*
Throwers' Ten Exercise Program, 494–495, *663–666, 663–669,* 668
Throwing, backhand external rotation at 0° and, *634,* 635
   backhand internal rotation at 0° and, *634, 635*
   baseball pitching versus football passing and, 556, 557t
   baseball toss, 632, *633,* 635
   elbow biomechanics in, 554–556, *555,* 557t
   Interval Throwing Program for. See *Interval Throwing Program (ITP).*
   isokinetic torque-to-body weight ratios and, 238t
   isokinetic work-to-body weight ratios and, 238t
   shoulder mechanism of, 484–488, *485, 486*
      acceleration and, 486–487
      cocking and, 485–486
      follow-through and, 487–488
      release and deceleration and, 487
      wind-up and, 485
   two-hand overhead soccer, 632, *633*
   two-hand side-to-side, 632, *633*
Thumb(s), Bennett's fracture of, 598
   joint mobilization techniques for, 167–168, *168*
   scaphoid fracture and, 599–600
   ulnar collateral ligament injury of, 599, *599, 600*
Thumb spica, 599, *599, 600,* 611
Tibial collateral ligament, 336–337
   immobilization and, 27
   rehabilitation for injuries of, 376–377, 380t–382t
Tibial glide(s), anterior, *312*
   technique for, 169
   posterior, in extension, technique for, 169–170, *170*
   technique for, 169
Tibial plateau, inclination of, during stationary cycling, 353, 353t
Tibial torsion, anthropometric assessment of, 277, *278*
Tibial varum, anthropometric assessment of, 276–277, *277*
Tibiofemoral joint, 331–332
Tibiofibular joint, anterior tibial glide and, *312*
   arthrokinematics of, 261
Tibiofibular synostosis, 283–284
Tissue stiffness, cryotherapy effect on, 83
Tissue temperature, therapeutic heat effects on, 93
Toe, turf, 322, *323*
Torque-to-body weight relationship, in isokinetic testing, 230, 238t
Total Gym, 357, *359, 360*
Total leg strength, in isokinetic testing, 230, 231–232
Tourniquet ischemia, quadriceps shutdown and, 20
Towel roll, for sitting posture, 452, *453*
Traction, stages of, 160, 160t
   subtalar, *310*
   talocrural, *310*
Transcutaneous electrical nerve stimulation (TENS), 120, *126,* 126–127
Triceps curl, 542, *544,* 583, *583*
Trigger finger, 603

TTDPM (threshold to detection of passive movement), 193–195, *194*
Turf toe, 322, *323*
Two-hand overhead soccer throw, 632, *633*
Two-hand side-to-side throw, 632, *633*

Ulna, goniometric measurements of, 68–69, *69, 70*
Ulnar collateral ligament (UCL), injury of, of thumb, 599, *599, 600*
    sprain of, 569–571, *571,* 572t, 573
Ulnar deviation, 607, *610*
Ulnar deviation exercise, 579, 581, *581*
Ulnar nerve lesions, 565, 567t
Ultrasound, *100,* 100–105
    advantages and disadvantages of, 105
    application of, *103,* 103–105, *104*
    contraindications to, 103
    indications for, 103
    phonophoresis and, 101–103, 102t
    therapeutic actions of, 100–101
Unilateral ratios, in isokinetic testing, 230
Upper Body Ergometer, for elbow rehabilitation, 559
    for shoulder, 490, *491*
Upper extremity(ies). See also specific regions, e.g., *Forearm.*
    plyometric exercises for, 632, *632–635,* 635
        for elbow, 559, *560*
        for shoulder, 495–496

Valgus, forefoot, 275, *276*
    rearfoot, 274, *274*
Valgus extension overload, 564–565, 566t
Valgus vector, *347,* 347–348
Validity, of goniometric measurements, 58
Varus, rearfoot, *274,* 274–275, *275*
Vastus lateralis, 339–340
Vastus medialis longus, 339, 340
Vastus medialis obliquus, 339, 340

Versa-Climber, *304*
Vertebrae, motion between, 427
Viscosity, of water, 616–617

Wall dribbling, *634,* 635
Wall slide(s), 638, *638*
    supine, 357, *358*
Water. See *Aquatic rehabilitation.*
Waveform, of electrical stimulation, 112
Weight loading, static, 643, *645*
Weight machine exercises, 657–662
Weighted rods, for elbow rehabilitation, 558, *558*
Whirlpools, 95–96, *96*
Wind-up phase, of throwing, 485
Wobble board, *201*
    multiaxial, *305*
Work-to-body weight relationship, in isokinetic testing, 238t
Worry, about second injury, 5
Wound healing, electrical stimulation for, 123–124
Wrist(s), carpal tunnel syndrome and, 602–603
    de Quervain's tenosynovitis of, 601–602
    extension of, 607, *609,* 668, *669*
    flexion of, 607, *607, 608,* 668, *669*
    goniometric measurements of, *67,* 67–68, *68*
    hamate fracture and, 600–601
    joint mobilization techniques for, *166,* 166–167, *167*
    pronation of, *610,* 611, *611,* 668, *669*
    scaphoid fracture and, 599–600
    sprains of, 601
    strengthening exercises for, 607, *607–611,* 611
    supination of, *610,* 611, *611,* 668, *669*
    tendinitis of, 601
Wrist curls, 579, *579*
    reverse, 579, *579*

Zygapophyseal joint(s), 427

ISBN 0-7216-6549-7

90038

WITHDRAWN